D0939073

CRC HANDBOOK SERIES IN ZOONOSES

James H. Steele, D.V.M., M.P.H.
Editor-in Chief

SECTIONS AND SECTION EDITORS

SECTION A: BACTERIAL, RICKETTSIAL, AND MYCOTIC DISEASES

Section Editors

Herbert Stoenner, D.V.M.
Director, Rocky Mountain
Laboratory
U.S. Public Health Service
Hamilton, Montana

Michael Torten, D.V.M., Ph.D.
Israel Institute for Biological
Research
Ness-Ziona
Faculty of Medical Sciences
Tel Aviv University School of
Medicine
Israel

William Kaplan, D.V.M., M.P.H.
Mycology Division
Center for Disease Control
Atlanta, Georgia

SECTION C: PARASITIC ZOONOSES

Section Editors

Primo Arambulo, III, D.V.M.,
M.P.H., Dr.P.H.
Public Health Veterinary
Consultant
PAHO/WHO
Washington, D.C.

Leon Jacobs
National Institutes of Health
Bethesda, Maryland

George Hillyer
University of Puerto Rico
Rio Piedras, Puerto Rico

Myron Schultz
Center for Disease Control
Atlanta, Georgia

Cluff Hopla
University of Oklahoma
Norman, Oklahoma

SECTION B: VIRAL ZOONOSES

Section Editor

George W. Beran, D.V.M., Ph.D.,
L.H.D.
Professor, Veterinary
Microbiology and Preventive
Medicine
Iowa State University
Ames, Iowa

SECTION D: ANTIBIOTICS, SULFONAMIDES, AND PUBLIC HEALTH

Section Editor

George W. Beran, D.V.M., Ph.D.,
L.H.D.
Professor, Veterinary
Microbiology and Preventive
Medicine
Iowa State University
Ames, Iowa

Associate Editors:

Lowell Young
University of California

Thomas H. Jukes
University of California

Herbert Dupont, M.D.
University of Texas

Lester Crawford
University of Georgia

CRC Handbook Series in Zoonoses

James H. Steele, Editor-in-Chief

Assistant Surgeon General (Retired)
U.S. Public Health Service
Professor of Environmental Health
School of Public Health
University of Texas at Houston

Section B: Viral Zoonoses

Volume I

Section Editor

George W. Beran

Professor, Veterinary Microbiology and Preventive Medicine
Iowa State University
Ames, Iowa

CRC Press, Inc.
Boca Raton, Florida

Library of Congress Cataloging in Publication Data
Main entry under title:

Viral zoonoses.

  (CRC handbook series in zoonoses ; section B)
  Bibliography: p.
  1. Virus diseases. 2. Zoonoses. I. Beran,
George W. II. Steele, James H. III. Series.
RC113.5.C72   sect. B   [RC114.5]   616.9'59s   81-4868
ISBN 0-8493-2911-6 (v. 1)
ISBN 0-8493-2912-4 (v. 2)

This book represents information obtained from authentic and highly regarded sources. Reprinted material is quoted with permission, and sources are indicated. A wide variety of references are listed. Every reasonable effort has been made to give reliable data and information, but the author and the publisher cannot assume responsibility for the validity of all materials or for the consequences of their use.

Direct all inquiries to CRC Press, Inc., 2000 N.W. 24th Street, Boca Raton, Florida 33431.

International Standard Book Number 0-8493-2900-0 (Complete Set)
International Standard Book Number 0-8493-2910-8 (Section B)
International Standard Book Number 0-8493-2911-6 (Volume I)
International Standard Book Number 0-8493-2912-4 (Volume II)

Library of Congress Card Number 81-4868
Printed in the United States

PREFACE
CRC HANDBOOK SERIES IN ZOONOSES

The biological adventurousness of animal diseases is exceeded only by the insatiable adventuresomeness of man. The struggle of the infectious diseases of lower forms of life to adapt themselves to more highly developed hosts is unending. As these disease agents insure their continued existance by adapting themselves to a broader host spectrum, they become a greater threat to man's well-being. Man, in his most tenuous position on this earth, has been able to protect himself from this biological onslaught by his skill in developing the preventive medical practices that are the foundation of our present public health practices.

In this century, man has made greater progress in holding back or eliminating infectious diseases than since he appeared on earth. Progress in the control of host-specific human diseases, such as smallpox, diphtheria, cholera, poliomyelitis, and syphilis, has brought to the fore animal disease problems which in many areas of the world are major challenges to human health. The eradication of smallpox is one of the major health achievements of our times. One reason this was possible was that there is no animal reservoir of smallpox. The control of diphtheria, cholera, poliomyelitis, and other childhood diseases was possible because none of these diseases have an animal reservoir.

Animal diseases threaten man's health and well-being in many ways. To examine the importance of animal health to human health, it is well for us to consider the World Health Organization (WHO) definition of health as a guide. "Health is not the mere absence of disease or injury . . . it is a state of complete physical, mental, and social well-being." The contributions that veterinary medicine can make to reach the WHO objective are succinctly presented in the definition of veterinary public health: . . . "comprises all the community efforts influencing and influenced by the veterinary medical arts and science applied to the prevention of disease, protection of life, and promotion of the well-being and efficiency of man." The present epidemic of Rift Valley Fever in the Nile Valley is an example of how serious some zoonoses can be. The 1978 epidemic has effected thousands of persons and tens of thousands of cattle, sheep, and goats. Why Rift Valley Fever became so wide spread and virulent is unknown.

The definition of health, as established by WHO, provides a very broad framework upon which to develop our theme. How veterinary medicine will participate in protecting the public health and welfare is well expressed in the broad definition of veterinary public health, and the inter-relationship of disease and health in man and animals provides a challenge that tests the imagination, ingenuity, and knowledge of man.

James H. Steele
Editor-in-Chief

JAMES H. STEELE, EDITOR-IN-CHIEF
CRC HANDBOOK SERIES IN ZOONOSES

Dr. James H. Steele has held a broad and rewarding experience in veterinary medicine and public health. He entered the Michigan State Veterinary College in 1938 and completed his veterinary training in 1941 when he was awarded the D.V.M. degree. After an internship in veterinary medicine and the Michigan Public Health Laboratory, he was sent to Harvard School of Public Health on a U.S. Public Health Service Fellowship. On the completion of the M.P.H. degree in 1942, he was assigned to the Ohio Health Department as a sanitarian. In 1943, he was commissioned in the U.S. Public Health Service and assigned to Puerto Rico where he had his first opportunity to become acquainted with animal diseases in the tropics and received encouragement to develop a national and international program.

After world War II, he was called to the U.S. Public Health Service, Washington, D.C. to plan a program to deal with the zoonoses and veterinary public health. This was to be a part of the Communicable Disease Center in Atlanta, Georgia where it grew into a national program with an international influence. In addition to directing the CDC veterinary public health program, Dr. Steele was a consultant to U.S. government agencies and international organizations relating to the health of man and animals.

After the inauguration of the veterinary public health program in 1947, a category for veterinary officers was approved by the Surgeon General in 1948. In 1950 Dr. Steele was made Veterinary consultant to the Surgeon General and liaison to professional health organization. Later in 1967 he was to become the Assistant Surgeon General for Veterinary Affairs in the Public Health Service and Department of Health Education and Welfare. The first veterinary officer to be named to this post. He remained in this position until his retirement in 1971. During 1969 he was designated advisor to the White House office on Consumer Affairs.

Dr. Steele was a technical advisor to Surgeon General Thomas Parran when the United Nations organized the World Health Organization in 1946. Later he was appointed to the WHO Expert Committee on Zoonoses and served in varying roles. In 1966 he was elected Chairman. During 1946 the Food Agriculture Organization was having technical meetings at which he represented the United States. He has served as a consultant to the FAO on many occasions since. The Pan American Sanitary Bureau was the first to request his services in disease outbreaks in the Carribean and Panama during and after World War II. He has been a consultant to the Pan American Health Organization since 1945 and served as chairman of their Scientific Advisory Committee in 1970. In addition to serving as a consultant to international agencies, he has been an advisor to a number of countries and universities in developing veterinary public health programs.

He has received national and international recognition from numerous governments, agencies, and societies. The U.S. Public Health Service awarded him the Medal of Merit in 1963 and the Distinguished Service plaque on his retirement in 1971. The American Public Health Service presented Dr. Steele the prestigous Bronfman Award in 1971 and the Centennial medal in 1972. In 1966 the Conference of Public Health Veterinarians honored him the recipient of the K.F. Meyer Gold Headed Cane Award. These Handbooks of the Zoonoses are dedicated to K.F. Meyer. Dr. Steele has been made an honorary member of various scientific organizations in the Americas, Europe and Asia. In 1965 he was named president of the American Veterinary Epidemiology Society. He was instrumental in the estabblishment of the World Veterinary Epidemiology Society in 1972 which is affiliated with the World Veterinary Association. An award was established in his name by the WVES in 1976 which is presented to a young leader in international veterinary public health. He has been described by many of his colleagues as *Mister Veterinary Public Health.*

His publications span a period of almost 40 years and cover various subjects, especially the zoonoses of which there are more than 100 titles. He is a man of many interests.

INTRODUCTION

G. W. Beran

Zoonoses, diseases which are intertransmissible between animals and human beings under natural conditions,[4] encompass the largest group of unconquered infectious and parasitic diseases in human medicine, and a major unconquered group in animal medicine. Prominent among these zoonoses in human beings and animals are those caused by viruses. While many viral zoonoses, as rabies and yellow fever, have been recognized since ancient times, some of the most deadly have been recognized only very recently, as Marburg virus disease in 1967 and Ebola virus disease, which as yet is only hypothesized to be zoonotic, in 1976. Additional viral zoonoses must be anticipated to emerge. While control efforts have been fruitful in a few endemic zoonoses, as in canine but not wildlife rabies and in urban but not jungle yellow fever, most are brought under control only by massive efforts during epidemics and many still spread out of medical control as Rift Valley fever is now doing in northeast Africa, as Ebola virus disease did in eastern Africa in 1976 to 1977, and as rabies is now doing in foxes across Europe. Knowledge of the etiological agents of most zoonoses outstrips knowledge of their epidemiology. After decades of investigations, the mechanisms of overwintering of most arthropod-borne encephalitis viruses in temperature areas of the Northern Hemisphere remain incompletely elucidated; reasons for cyclical spread and retraction of several arboviral diseases in the tropics are unknown; and the appearance of "new" clinical manifestations caused by "old" viruses such as dengue hemorrhagic fever in tropical Asia remain unpredictable and only partially understandable.

Etiologically, the viral zoonoses appear to be fitting into logical groupings.[2,3] Application of virological tools presently available in many parts of the world is making it possible to recognize and classify the etiological agents of emerging viral diseases in animals and people, giving medical scientists predictive leads of clinical and epidemiological value before these aspects are recorded through field observations. For the viral diagnosticians and viral taxonomists, this seems to be a good era in which to be working; success is largely supplanting frustration. Clinicians in human and veterinary medicine, epidemiologists, and public health workers have made some strides but still find the viral zoonoses a source of frustration. Newly emerging problems have added complexities to the previously unresolved problems.

The arboviral zoonoses are considered as an epidemiological group in this volume.[1] They include 430 recognized viruses and a number of candidate strains comprising by far the largest grouping of viral zoonoses. Viruses within the arbovirus group are now classified in the Arenaviridae, Bunyaveridae, Reoviridae and Rhabdoviridae families with many viruses still not classified. The finding of previously unrecognized arboviruses continues world-wide and there are probably still more to be identified. The big problems in the arboviral zoonoses are in epidemiology and control.

The arboviral zoonoses causing encephalitis in human beings and in horses in temperate North America have been studied extensively since the 1930s. Birds are major reservoir hosts through the warm months for these viruses but mechanisms of survival through winters or of reintroduction in spring remain unelucidated. The ranges of infection by the different viruses are determined more by the ranges of the vector mosquitoes than of the reservoir hosts. The role of transovarial transmission in overwintering is in the early stages of delineation. Control is still directed toward protecting the alternate hosts and eliminating the vectors with no practicable prevention of infection in the reservoir hosts. Yellow fever stood alone in temperate North America with an entirely human-*Aedes aegypti* cycle. Colorado tick fever also fills an apparently unique ecological niche as a tick-borne zoonosis. Ticks carry the virus through the winter and possibly hibernating rodents do too. The epidemiology of vesicular stomatitis viruses has defied delineation. Overwintering mechanisms have not been identified in the temperate zone, though farther south transovarial transmission has been demonstrated in sandflies. It has been repeatedly suggested that this virus may have a plant-mammalian cycle. Arboviruses in North American which cause undifferentiated illness or inapparent infections, or which have been recognized only in limited foci in human beings or animals, have not been extensively studied. Among these, transovarial transmission has been identified in the overwintering of viruses of the California group.

In tropical and subtropical areas of the Americas, a large number of arthropod-borne viruses have been identified but their epidemiology and clinical manifestations in human and reservoir animal infections are still being identified. Rodents, and in some cases marsupials, play a role in transmission cycles that is often comparable to that of birds in temperate areas. Yellow fever persists in a jungle cycle involving forest primates, still posing a threat of extension to the human population as occurred in Trinidad in November 1978. Venezuelan equine encephalitis which moved rapidly northward through Central America and Mexico in 1969 to 1971 has been quiet since.

The major arboviral zoonoses of Europe and temperate western Asia are tick borne, with transovarial and transstadial transmission in the vector ticks important in survival of the viruses through the winter. Rodents appear to be the principal reservoir hosts and to play an essential role in the maintenance of transmission cycles. Milk-borne transmission is important in the central European tick-borne encephalitis but not in the Congo-Crimean fever viruses. Tahyna virus is the first recognized mosquito-borne arbovirus in Europe; it too has rodents and small mammals as reservoir hosts. Yellow fever and dengue never became established north of the range of the *Ae. aegypti* mosquitoes in Europe.

A very wide variety of arboviral zoonoses abound in Africa; only those which have caused widespread epidemics in people or animals have been studied extensively. Mosquitoes, and in a few cases midges, are the principal vectors, except for the tick-borne Congo-Crimean fever and the Nairobi sheep disease viruses. Rodents, primates, bats, and birds all appear to be reservoir hosts, but their role in maintaining viruses like Dengue and Chikungunya which are transmitted in human-mosquito-human cycles remains undetermined. Africa is considered to have been the source of yellow fever which spread northward and westward but for unknown reasons not eastward with the world-wide transport of the adaptable highly domesticated *Ae. aegypti* mosquito. Rift Valley fever has been extending northward in east Africa as both a human and animal epidemic of markedly increased clinical severity since 1977. Arboviral zoonoses must be expected to play an increasing public health role in the dynamics of African society.

In east and south Asia, a wide variety of arboviral diseases, most of them mosquito borne, are identified as human problems, but except for abortions in gestating swine and possible sporadic encephalitis in horses caused by Japanese encephalitis virus, domestic and wild animals and birds appear to function entirely as inapparent reservoir hosts. A jungle primate cycle of dengue appears to operate quite separate from the human-mosquito-human cycle; the infection in human beings has emerged since the early 1950s as a hemorrhagic shock syndrome with an immunopathological basis. The closely related Japanese and Murray Valley encephalitis viruses appear to be endemic north and south, respectively, of Wallace's Line which separates the Asian and Australian fauna; their distribution is associated with the mosquito vector ranges. The overwintering mechanism of arboviruses in temperate east Asia have not been identified; the possible role of hibernating snakes and other hibernating animals in maintaining

Japanese encephalitis virus is being investigated. Several tick-borne arboviruses have been recognized in southeast Asia but have been very inadequately studied.

The major arobviral zoonoses recognized for their clinical importance on a worldwide basis are discussed in individual chapters in this volume. In addition, arboviral zoonoses about which less is known are discussed on a regional basis by areas of principal occurrence in the world. There is some overlap and specific zoonoses may be considered in more than one chapter each. There is, however, remarkable regional distribution of the arboviral zoonoses. Viruses in the Arenaviridae and Rhabdoviridae families which have not been shown to be transmitted by arthropod vectors are considered seprately from arthropod-transmitted viruses of these families in this volume.

Argentine hemorrhagic fever, Bolivian hemorrhagic fever, Lassa fever of Africa, and lymphocytic choriomeningitis are caused by zoonotic viruses of the Arenaviridae family. Korean hemorrhagic fever, which has defied etiological diagnosis since its original description in 1934, has been more and more definitely associated with a specific replicating transmissible antigen called the "Korea Antigen" which may be an arenavirus. The zoonotic arenaviral infections, all of which are capable of causing severe disease in human patients, have been quite extensively studied clinically in human infections. Rodents are the principal proven or suspected reservoir hosts, but little is known of clinical disease caused in rodents by any of these viruses except the lymphocytic choriomeningitis virus. Junin virus of Argentine hemorrhagic fever is shed in the saliva and urine of persistently inapparently infected rodents. Machupo virus of Bolivian hemorrhagic fever causes persistent immunotolerant infections or transient infections with clearing of viremia and immunity depending on the age and status of maternally derived immunity in the rodents. The African multimammate rat is considered to be an inapparent persistent reservoir host of Lassa virus but the mechanisms of transmission to people have not been determined. Human-to-human transmission occurs with devastating ease from primary human cases but secondary cases seem to be less hazardous as a source of Lassa virus, and tertiary human cases have not been reported. Lymphocytic choriomeningitis virus, which has the house mouse as its natural hosts, variably produces acute disease or persistent tolerant infection depending on the virus strain and on the age and portal of exposure of the susceptible host.

Marburg, Ebola, rabies, and at least five rabies-related viruses are important possibly nonarboviral rhabdoviruses which cause zoonotic diseases. Marburg and Ebola viruses have been inadequately studied. They cause acute hemorrhagic human diseases with extreme hazard of contact transmission from patients, necropsy tissues or in vitro cultures. The reservoir hosts of these two viruses are unknown but are believed to be some wild African mammals; monkeys have served as a source of Marburg virus but have not been shown to be reservoir hosts, and animal reservoirs of Ebola virus have yet to be postulated on epidemiological bases. Much more investigation needs to be done and it will be hazardous to do it.

Rabies has been recognized through the period of recorded history and studied scientifically since early in the 19th century, but progress in elucidating its basic aspects has come slowly. The morphology of rabies virus as having bullet-shaped virions has been recognized only since the early 1960s. The cycle of transmission in wild animals is still being elucidated. Subclinical or abortive infections with immunological responses appear to play a role in the intraspecific transmission cycles of rabies virus in Mustelidae, Viverridae, Procyonidae, possibly wild Canidae and both hematophagus and nonhematophagus bats, but not in transmission from these to animals of other species. Although susceptible to rabies virus infection, birds and rodents do not appear to be important in the epidemiology of rabies; it has been suggested that scavenger birds may be infected by ingestion of carcasses of rabid animals, and inapparent infection with vertical transmission of rabies virus has been demonstrated in central Europe.

The role of inhalation and ingestion in intraspecific transmission cycles in wild animals has not been delineated; transmission from wild animals to domesticated animals and people occurs almost exclusively by bites or, rarely, under unique circumstances of severe exposure by inhalation.

Dogs and, to some extent, cats play a uniquely important role in the epidemiology of rabies. Except perhaps in certain areas of the world, the relationship between the rabies virus and its canine and feline hosts is epidemiologically primitive. Transmission in nature appears to be entirely by bites, the clinical disease appears to be uniformly fatal, and transmission to susceptible hosts is essentially limited to the period of clinical illness. The close proximity into which the ubiquitous dogs and cats come with other animals — wild, domestic, and their own kind — and with people make them historically, and to this day, the major source of human exposure to rabies world-wide. The eradication of rabies from countries where dogs are the maintaining hosts has been achieved in a few countries and could be accomplished in more by use of presently available vaccines and dog control techniques. Even in areas with endemic wildlife rabies, the control of the disease in dogs provides extensive protection to the human population. In such areas, vigilant maintenance of herd immunity in the dog population is essential; as underscored by the current epidemics of rabies in dogs, with exposures of people, which are occurring in Malaga, Spain and along the Mexico-U. S. border. Control of rabies in wild animals and in unrestricted dogs has not been achieved on any widespread bases; experimental studies on oral vaccines for such animals holds great promise for the future. In the meantime, the application of more highly effective passive and active immunizing agents for pre- and postexposure prophylactic use offers greater protection for persons at risk of exposure, or following exposure, than has been historically possible before.

Five rabies-related viruses have been recognized in Africa. Some evidence of animal infections in nature has been obtained for four; human disease has been recorded for one, and two have been recovered from insects, though arthropod transmission has not been shown. Three of these viruses are serologically related to rabies, one shows distant serological relationship, and one is related only indirectly through two of the other viruses. An additional, serologically related virus has been recovered from a horse in Nigeria. Much more investigation is needed on the epidemiology of these viruses.

The Picornaviridae comprise a very large group of viruses in terrestrial and sea mammals, birds, and people, with most transmission being intraspecific, but with some demonstrated occasions of interspecific transmission, including interspecific transmission involving people. Encephalomyocarditis virus causes widespread but uncommon disease in swine, captive primates, and people, with evidence, principally serological, that rodents may serve as inapparent reservoir hosts. Scores of enterovirus types have been recognized in a wide variety of domesticated animals and birds but only one, the swine vesicular disease virus, which is closely related to coxsackievirus B5, has been shown to be naturally pathogenic for human beings. In situations of high environmental exposure, human enteroviruses have been shown to cause inapparent infections in animals. Foot-and-mouth disease, a major infectious disease of cattle, swine, sheep, goats, and other cloven hoofed animals on every continent except North America and Australasia, has been only rarely documented as a cause of human vesicular disease. The rare human oropharyngeal carrier or clinically infected patient could presumably transmit the virus to susceptible animals but evidence that this has occurred has been entirely circumstantial. Vesicular exanthema of swine appears to have been caused by the San Miguel sea lion virus which was transmitted from these marine animals to terrestrial swine. There has been no evidence, however, of transmission of this marine calicivirus, or of any other virus of marine mammals, to human beings.

In the family Reoviridae, at least eight serotypes of human, mammalian, and avian orthoreoviruses, 43 types of orbiviruses, and many strains of rotaviruses have been identified. Reoviral infections extend from inapparent to acute upper respiratory disease in animals, a variety of acute and chronic syndromes in domestic poultry, and four clinical syndromes in human patients, limited largely to children. Transmission between mammals and people appears to take place readily, but the avian types appear to infect fowl only, either by horizontal or vertical transmission. Rotavirus infections in animals and people are associated with neonatal diarrhea. So far, no evidence has been obtained of natural cross infections among animal species or between animals and human beings, although such infections have been reported experimentally.

The influenza viruses, the family Orthomyxoviridae, are the subject of extensive interhost species investigations at this time. Animals and birds infected with influenza viruses have appeared to pose little individual hazard to persons in contact with them; a small number of infections in persons exposed directly to infected swine or in the laboratory to A equi$_2$ virus have been recorded without secondary spread. It has been postulated, but not demonstrated, that new waves of influenza in people may be initiated by establishment of strains transmitted from mammals or birds to human beings. Numerous isolations of influenza strains currently epidemic in the human population have been reported from mammals and birds surveyed in countries in various parts of the world. It has been proposed that these infections represented human-to-animal transmission. Most such reported isolations have been from clinically healthy animals but some have been from wild migratory birds showing lesions. Much further investigation and verification of the numerous extant reports are needed on this very important prospect.

The parainfluenza viruses, Newcastle disease virus, the morbilliviruses, the respiratory syncytial viruses, and the foamy virus group are placed in the Paramyxoviridae family. The five recognized types of parainfluenza viruses, except for Sendai virus infections in mice and SF-4 infections in calves appear to cause little clinical concern in people or animals. Intraspecific transmission appears to be ubiquitous on the basis of serological surveys, but interspecific transmission among animals of different species and between animals and people appears to be limited to those in very close contact. Interspecific transmission appears to lead to no more clinical disease than does intraspecific. "Simian virus" SV$_5$ appears more likely to be a human parainfluenza virus transmitted to primates than a true simian virus.

Newcastle disease, while varying from a mild respiratory disease to a peracute highly fatal respiratory-encephalitic disease in domestic and wild birds, is only occasionally transmitted to mammals or people. Human infection is usually a transient, unilateral conjunctivitis, but may include systemic involvement.

Measles, canine distemper, rinderpest, and rinderpest of small ruminants viruses share common morphological, clinical, pathological, and immunological properties in their respective hosts. Aside from the susceptibility of captive monkeys to measles virus, there is little evidence of human-animal intertransmission of these morbilliviruses. A number of studies reported in the literature have suggested that canine distemper virus may be etiologically associated with human multiple sclerosis, but the data have not been sufficiently definitive to warrant any conclusion at this time. Measles and parainfluenza type 1 viruses have also been suggested as associated with human multiple sclerosis.

Foamy virus infections have been demonstrated in clinically normal monkeys, cattle, cats, and hamsters and, in a few instances, in human beings and in normal human cell cultures. They have not been etiologically associated with disease in any species, and the only evidence of cross infections among species has been between rhesus and grivet monkeys.

Respiratory syncytial viruses cause acute respiratory infections in people, especially infants and young children, in cattle, and in chimpanzees, with additional serological evidence of infection in swine and lambs. Animal and human outbreaks have not been shown to coincide, and there is no evidence that intertransmission occurs.

The oncogenic RNA viruses are placed in the family Retroviridae. A large number of these viruses have been associated with leukemia, sarcoma, and mammary cancer in a very wide variety of poikilothermic and homeothermic vertebrate animals, but not definitively in human patients. These oncogenic animal infections provide models for studies on human malignant diseases, but none of these viruses have been definitely demonstrated to be transmissible to people. Several DNA viruses cause malignant diseases under natural or experimental conditions in animals, including Simian papovaviruses SV_{40} in experimentally inoculated hamsters, and Yabapox in naturally infected monkeys. *Herpesvirus saimiri* is oncogenic to many species of monkeys and to rabbits by experimental infection. Of these, only yabapox virus has caused transient human tumorigenesis by laboratory exposure. DNA viral oncogenic infections in animals, as well as malignant diseases of unidentified etiology in animals, are important models for studies on human malignancies.

The slow viral diseases of human beings and animals are discussed as a separate group in this volume. Most of the etiological viruses have not been classified on the basis of their nucleic acid genomes; Aleutian mink disease virus has been reported by one investigator to be a DNA virus. No evidence has been obtained of intertransmission of these viruses between animals and people, but the animal infections serve as very important models for human infections caused by viruses of this group. Scrapie and mink encephalopathy, which are considered to be caused by the same virus, elicit no demonstrated host responses and are classified with human kuru and Creutzfeldt-Jakob disease as subacute spongiform viral encephalopathies. Aleutian disease of mink and progressive interstitial pneumonia of sheep are slow viral diseases in which the host response plays a major role in the pathogenesis of the disease. These are important models for human diseases in which host responses to unknown antigens appear to be causing the conditions.

Among the DNA viruses, certain herpesviruses and the pox and parapox viruses are important as zoonoses. The poxviruses which are related to vaccinia all appear to be intertransmissible between their primary hosts and human beings, usually causing self-limiting infections without further intraspecific spread. Vaccinia virus is experimentally transmissible to animals of many species, but natural transmission has been reported principally from vaccinated people to cattle. Cowpox, monkeypox, buffalopox, horsepox, and swinepox viruses which are related to vaccinia virus are also transmissible to susceptible people. Whitepox virus and, to a lesser extent, camelpox virus, both very closely related to variola virus, are cause for concern that they or other such viruses could be established in human beings again as smallpox. Other animal poxviruses transmissible to people are contagious ecthyma virus of sheep, pseudocowpox virus of cattle, tanapox virus of monkeys, and, experimentally, Yabapox virus of monkeys.

Several additional groups of viruses causing animal infections are important in their transmissibility to human beings, their actual or potential impact on human well-being, or their use as models for study of human diseases. These are discussed together in this volume.

The cross-infection potential for viruses infectious to human beings and to nonhuman primates appears to be total, and the increasingly close contact between people and nonhuman primates in research laboratories, zoos, and other settings only promotes intertransmission. A very wide variety of viruses considered to have Simian reservoir hosts are naturally infectious to people. Several arboviruses have Simian reservoir hosts or, as yellow fever and dengue viruses, have separate Simian-mosquito and human-mosquito cycles. Naturally occurring Simian infections with rhabdoviruses, poxviruses, herpesviruses, and papovaviruses have all been transmitted to human beings. Among the herpesviruses, all of which appear to have a high degree of host specialization, *Herpesvirus simiae* is of greatest public health concern as a cause of acute encephalitis disease in human beings handling infected monkeys or their tissues. There is evidence that the Epstein-Barr virus of human lymphoma, carcinoma, and infectious mononucleosis may have been of simian origin. Simian virus SV_{40}, a papovavirus, has been of considerable public health concern as a contaminant surviving the inactivation process in poliomyelitis vaccines or in attenuated live poliomyelitis or respiratory-syncytial vaccines, but evidences of human disease associated with such exposure have not been forthcoming at this time. A wide variety of human viral infections have been naturally transmitted to nonhuman primates, some with transmission back to susceptible people, including poliomyelitis and other human enteroviruses, measles and other paramyxoviruses, hepatitis A and B viruses, and possibly the SV_5 parainfluenza virus.

A very large number of viral diseases have been recognized in fish, essentially all in fresh water fish, which are caused by viruses in the same families as those infecting human beings and animals, but no evidences of intertransmission have yet been observed. The chief impact of viral diseases of fish on public health has been the effect on the human food supply.

The adeno-associated parvoviruses are defective in that they cannot replicate except in the presence of a helper adenovirus or a partially helper herpesvirus. The SV_{40} papovavirus and adenoviruses form naturally occurring hybrids when replication takes place in the same cell. During viral replication of DNA viruses, occasionally host DNA instead of viral DNA is enclosed in the viral capsids, forming pseudovirions. The occurrence of these phenomena lies at the forefront of research in viral infections and the implications of these naturally occurring events, as well as of recombinant DNA laboratory-manipulated changes, for zoonotic viral infections remain to be discerned. Viroids, a newly recognized class of infectious agents smaller than viruses, have been associated with diseases in plants but so far are only suspected in human and animal diseases. It is hoped that this volume on viral zoonoses not only elaborates the present state of knowledge on these diseases, but that it also highlights the incompleteness of this knowledge and the need for much further study of the diseases included here and of those still emerging as zoonoses.

REFERENCES

1. Berge, T. O., Ed., *International Catalogue of Arboviruses*, 2nd ed., Publ. No. (CDC) 75-8301, U. S. Public Health Service, U. S. Department of Health, Education and Welfare, Atlanta, 1975.
2. Fenner, F., The classification and nomenclature of viruses. Summary of results of meetings of the International Committee on Taxonomy of Viruses in Madrid, September 1975, *Intervirology*, 6, 1, 1975/76.
3. Fenner, F., Classification and nomenclature of viruses: second report of the International Committee on Taxonomy of Viruses, *Intervirology*, 7, 1, 1976.
4. World Health Organization, Second Report of a Joint WHO/FAO Expert Committee on Zoonoses, *WHO Tech. Rep. Ser.*, 169, 1959.

SECTION EDITOR

George W. Beran is currently professor of Veterinary Microbiology and Preventive Medicine, College of Veterinary Medicine, Iowa State University, Ames, Iowa. He received the D.V.M. degree from Iowa State University, and the Ph.D. degree in Medical Microbiology with emphasis on epidemiology, from the University of Kansas College of Medicine. He was awarded the Doctor of Humane Letters, *honoris causa* by Silliman University, Dumaguete City, Philippines in 1973. He is a diplomate of the American College of Veterinary Preventive Medicine.

Following a short period in food animal veterinary practice, Dr. Beran joined the U.S. Public Health Service, in which he served as an epidemic intelligence officer stationed at the Communicable Disease Center field station at the University of Kansas Medical Center. From 1960 to 1973, he was a professor at Silliman University, Dumaguete City, Philippines, where he directed development of two public health laboratories, the Van Houweling Laboratory for Microbiological Research at Silliman University and the Provincial Central Laboratory of Negros Oriental Province. Through his research and community efforts, rabies control on community- and island-wide bases was successfully undertaken in the central Philippines. Since 1973, as a World Health Organization (WHO) consultant, he has been assisting the Philippine government in national rabies control. Dr. Beran has also served as a WHO consultant in India, Malaysia, Laos, and Jamaica, as well as a member of a WHO panel on Veterinary Public Health in Moscow, U.S.S.R.

Since 1973, he has been professor at Iowa State University studying epidemiology of herpesvirus infection, rabies, and enteric pathogenic bacteria of swine, in addition to teaching veterinary public health, epidemiology of disease, and world food issues. He is an honorary diplomate of the American Society of Veterinary Epidemiology and a member of Phi Kappa Phi, Phi Zeta, Gamma Sigma Delta, Alpha Zeta, Sigma Xi, and Cardinal Key Honor Societies. He is listed in *Men of Achievement, Who's Who in the Midwest,* and *American Men and Women of Science.* He is recipient of the International Award of the World Veterinary Epidemiology Society, the Wilton Park International Service Award, and the Outstanding Teacher Awards of the American Association of Food Hygiene Veterinarians, of the Iowa State University College of Veterinary Medicine, and of Iowa State University. He is author or co-author of over 75 scientific publications in the public health field, three chapters in scientific books, and two monographs on zoonoses in the Philippines.

FOREWORD

H. N. Johnson

"It is not the things I don't know that bother me, it is the things I know that aren't so" (Anonymous).

It is natural for people to want absolute answers to problems encountered in the natural environment, but the theories proposed to explain problems are difficult to prove and there is apt to be increasing uncertainty as more information is collected. In the biological sciences the data may seem to be very accurate but there are questions about objectivity and ability to observe and record all the pertinent details of studies. In biology variability exists in all living organisms, even viruses. When viruses are cloned, considerable variation appears in the virus population, requiring repeated cloning in order to obtain a high percentage of virus particles with the same characteristics; for example, pathogenicity for cells or animals, plaque size, and rate of growth at various temperatures. Variability of experimental animals makes it necessary to use large numbers in experiments to compare the effect of drug treatments or vaccinations with like numbers of control animals. Factors such as age, sex, and exposure to stress must be controlled. Male mice caged together tend to fight and kill each other when they become sexually mature. Stress of this type will alter the morbidity and mortality of male animals as compared to female animals.

The methods used in isolating viruses have much to do with the character of the virus populations. Intracerebral (i.c.) inoculation selects for neurotropism. Serial i.c. passages result in adaption to neuroglial cells as well as neurons. The ability of viruses to invade and multiply in other organ systems will be altered. The high neurotropism observed in studies of brain adapted viruses such as rabies virus, poliomyelitis viruses, and other encephalitis viruses has led to the ill-formed conclusion that these viruses were strictly neurotropic and would not multiply in other organs. Viruses adapted to experimental hosts by brain passage differ from natural viruses in tropism for non-nervous tissue. This can be confirmed by isolation of viruses from natural sources by inoculation into skin, muscle, nose, or mouth of animals and recovering them from blood, intestinal contents, or organ systems, maintaining them by the same method of inoculation. Such strains are called non-neuroadapted; for example, the viscerotropic versus neurotropic variants of yellow fever virus, and poliomyelitis viruses isolated and maintained in cell cultures inoculated with viruses obtained from fecal specimens as compared to virus strains obtained from brain tissue and maintained by i.c. passage in monkeys.

The classical varieties of viruses that produce encephalitis are brain adapted. For example, the Pasteur strain of rabies virus was isolated and studied by a method that depended on the uniform production of a fatal infection in the rabbit hosts used during the isolation and adaption of the virus by i.c. passage. Most of the stock strains of animal viruses have been prepared from infected mouse-brain tissue. Tests for tropism have shown that the various animal viruses exhibit preference for certain organ systems such as salivary glands, lungs, kidneys, pancreas, liver, mammary glands, and intestinal tract. Diseases related to involvement of the brain seem to be an unlikely event in the long-term, natural reservoir system of a virus.

Many problems in virology are unresolved, as exemplified by books with titles such as "Problems in Virology". Many of these unresolved problems are major. What are the hosts in which many dangerous viruses persist in nature between outbreaks of zoonotic diseases? What factors contribute to the variations in pathogenicity observed in the study of different strains of viruses derived from natural sources? What is the significance of the serological relationships observed between virus strains by complement fixation (CF), hemagglutination inhibition (HI), and neutralization(N) tests versus cross-protection tests? From studies of parasitism in general, minimal morbidity and mortality are expected for parasitic infections in the long-term natural host. Therefore, outbreaks of disease with high morbidity and mortality indicate involvement of alternate, or even aberrant, hosts. Changes in portals of entry of viruses play important roles in the production of disease, leading to confusion in classifying viruses by mode of transmission; for example, arthropod-borne versus direct contact transmission.

The descriptive term "arbovirus" or arthropod-borne virus" implies that a virus depends on an arthropod host for survival in nature. Birds are known to be important hosts for Western encephalitis virus, Eastern encephalitis virus, and St. Louis encephalitis virus during epidemics caused by these viruses. However, the viremia phase that serves to infect mosquitoes from birds will last only a few days. Mosquitoes, once infected, are able to transmit the virus by bites as long as they live, but the mean survival time for mosquitoes is only a few days. If these viruses must be maintained by either birds or mosquitoes, how do the viruses persist or survive during the winter in northern latitudes? One of the first theories postulated was that the viruses may be maintained in bird mites. Other theories have been postulated, but field studies have not confirmed them, for example; overwintering of the virus in birds and reactivation during the spring breeding season; overwintering in hibernating female mosquitoes; or overwintering in hibernating cold-blooded animals such as frogs, lizards, turtles, and snakes. Current studies are concerned with the role of transovarial infections in mosquitoes in the perpetuation of these viruses. Are there other possibilities? Not long ago it was believed that the encephalitis viruses were strictly neurotropic. Subsequent to the discovery that these viruses could multiply in mosquitoes and ticks, and be transmitted by these blood feeding arthropods, research on these viruses has become concentrated on the study of suspected and proven arthropod hosts. Survey studies of wild birds have rarely resulted in the isolation of these viruses from blood specimens. Only at times when paradomestic mosquitoes have been found to contain these viruses has it been easy to demonstrate the viruses in the blood of paradomestic nestling wild birds. This has shown that nestling birds serve to amplify the virus that was introduced into this environment. Studies of migratory birds have revealed that only rarely have they been found to be infected during spring migration, but that a variety of viruses could be isolated from immature birds collected during the fall migration. Tropism studies of these viruses, as well as many other viruses not suspected of being transmitted by insects, have revealed that there are certain target organs which viruses may select and that these may contain active or latent viruses for weeks or months after the viremic phase of the infection. There is little evidence to indicate that recurrent viremias play any part in the maintenance of viruses in bird hosts. Viremias in infected hosts seem to be related to the pathogenicity of these viruses for these hosts. The greater the pathogenicity of a virus, the more likely the presence of high titers of virus in the blood, suggesting that viremias, though necessary for transmission by arthropods during epidemics, may not be necessary for survival in reservoir hosts. In bacterial infections, similar differences have been observed in pathogenicity between infections of surface epithelium and of the intestinal tract, as compared to bacteremias with systemic invasion of other organs. Some flaviviruses which are closely related to mosquito and tick-borne viruses by serological tests, appear to be transmitted by inhalation or ingestion, because the virus is excreted in the saliva or urine or both over long periods of time and there is no evidence of insect transmission in nature. The abundance of shrews and bats in some endemic foci of mosquito-borne viruses underscores the need for studies of these animals as potential reservoir hosts of viruses that can produce encephalitis. Yellow fever and dengue viruses were, for a time, considered to be maintained only in human beings and mosquitoes. With the discovery of jungle yellow fever the prospect arose that monkeys may be the mammalian reservoir hosts and that the virus may be maintained in monkey-mosquito-monkey infection cycles. The most abundant small mammals in endemic foci of yellow fever and dengue are bats, and studies should be done on the various species to determine whether they can serve for the maintenance or amplification of these viruses. Survey studies of bat blood and salivary gland specimens have resulted in the isolation of many different flaviviruses which show serological relationships to yellow fever and dengue viruses. A major significance of this relationship may be whether infection by one flavivirus may prevent infections by others. Flaviviruses which have been isolated from rodents should be investigated in the same way. Modoc virus, isolated from *Peromyscus* spp. mice is an example of a flavivirus which can survive in a small mammal without transmission by arthropods.

How then should animal viruses be classified? Originally they were classified by the clinical syndromes they elicited. Electron microscopic studies have now made it possible to classify viruses on morphological bases. The relationships of viruses producing human disease to those causing diseases in domesticated animals need further study. What are the significances of the relationship of herpangina and vesicular stomatitis with exanthem in human patients caused by coxsackieviruses group A, to foot-and-mouth disease in cattle caused by a rhinovirus and of coxsackieviruses group B infections in children, to swine vesicular disease? Do they have a similar epidemiology with transmission by fecal contamination of water or food? Are they possibly derived from enteroviruses present in rodents? The Rotaviruses produce an intestinal infection with the symptom of severe diarrhea in both children and calves. Are such viruses found in wildlife? Are wild ducks the major wildlife source of influenza A viruses? Are these viruses maintained in sea birds? Are there wildlife sources of smallpox viruses? Is the lymphocytic choriomeningitis virus host system in house mice the same reservoir host system which may be operating in the hemorrhagic fever viruses encountered in South America and Africa? If so, phenotypic selection and hybridization with other viruses must occur or have occurred in order to produce the variants observed. The recent outbreaks of lymphocytic choriomeningitis in children in the U.S. and Germany were derived from pet hamsters that harbored the virus as inapparent infections. This is an example of the ease with which this virus may set up alternate or aberrant cycles of infection in laboratory animals. Human rubeola virus is related to canine distemper and bovine rinderpest viruses. Are there wildlife sources of these viruses? The parainfluenza viruses have been found to be present in mice and other laboratory animals without evidence of disease, suggesting that these viruses may be maintained in rodents. Parainfluenza 3 virus produces disease in cattle; it may be suspected that widespread use of bovine serum in cell culture media has led to the infection of cell culture lines with this virus.

All wildlife species seem to have their own viral fauna, such as the pox viruses, adenoviruses, myxoviruses, and enteroviruses. The percentage of animals suffering from disease by these viruses appears to be extremely low. How then should wildlife be studied to determine possible reservoir host systems for animal viruses? In searching for latent viruses, primary cell cultures of kidneys of the host animals have yielded the greatest number of viruses. When studying small mammals such as mice and bats, the kidneys of several animals of the same species may be pooled for the preparation of single bottle cultures. Enteroviruses can be isolated by inoculation of tube cultures of kidney cells with specimens obtained from liver or intestines.

What are some of the problems encountered in the production of viral vaccines? There are many instances where viruses other than the seed viruses have been present in live-virus vaccines. Tests developed for the identification of active seed virus in such vaccines may not reveal the presence of other viruses. Primary cell cultures from kidneys of monkeys, swine, cattle, dogs, hamsters, and embryonic cells from chicken and duck embryos all may contain latent viruses. The ease with which many different viruses may hybridize when infecting the same cell systems has been demonstrated in studies of Simian virus 40 derived from monkey kidney cells. The production of hybrids in cell cultures of the well-known animal viruses may occur if they are passed repeatedly in primary cell cultures of different animals, and some of these hybrids may be more infectious or dangerous than the natural viruses. It should be noted also that viruses attenuated by passage or clonal selection in one host system such as embryonating hens' eggs will have selected virus populations which grow best in this system, but the transfer of such viruses to other host systems, such as kidney cells of mammals, cannot be expected to produce the same populations of virions. Allergic encephalitis may occur in human patients following injection of killed-virus rabies vaccine prepared from infected rabbit brains. Sensitization to kidney tissue may similarly follow injection of a similar vaccine prepared from infected kidney cell cultures. This is related to heterologous host systems. What about human immunization with vaccines prepared in human cell cultures? With the rapid development of knowledge of human autoimmune diseases related to infections with viruses, the possibility of production of antinuclear antibodies in persons receiving such viral vaccines must be investigated.

Tools for making rapid advances in the study of animal viruses are now available. Cooperation among the specialties of microbiology, biochemistry, electron microscopy, medical zoology, medical entomology, and human and veterinary medicine is essential to the application of these tools. The veterinary profession must play a major role in the investigation of wildlife viruses. The veterinary profession must maintain closer supervision of animal colonies and monitor them for animal viruses. The development and testing of live virus and killed virus vaccines require large scale testing in animals. As effective sanitary procedures become developed for controlling the classical diseases of people and domesticated animals, these deeper problems can, and must, be brought out. Epidemics of disease tend to recur at intervals, and cyclical patterns have frequently and falsely been credited as due to control measures which were applied. Epidemics have a tendency to depopulate the highly susceptible hosts or to produce immunity in populations so that diseases die out spontaneously. The development of epidemics caused by hitherto unknown viruses such as happened with Marburg and Ebola viruses must be expected to happen again in the future. All viruses should be handled as if they were highly contagious and pathogenic. Primary cell cultures of wildlife origin should be handled as if they were known to contain pathogenic viruses, a lesson that follows from the outbreak of Marburg virus disease in which the virus was derived from supposedly normal monkey kidney cell cultures. *Herpesvirus simiae,* the monkey B virus, has caused death or severe disease in laboratory workers. Some of the original descriptions of fatal lymphocytic choriomeningitis in human patients were related to laboratory exposures, and the clinical syndromes were very similar to those observed during the recent outbreaks of Lassa fever in Africa. Scientists, physicians, and veterinarians must be open to new ideas about animal-human disease interrelationships, but must be skeptical of all theories regarding the ways viruses survive and spread in the natural environment.

ADVISORY BOARD MEMBERS
SECTION B: VIRAL ZOONOSES

CONTRIBUTORS
SECTION B: VIRAL ZOONOSES
VOLUME I

Harvey Artsob
Research Scientist
National Arbovirus Reference
  Service
Laboratory Center for Disease
  Control
Department of National Health and
  Welfare
Toronto, Ontario

V. Bardos
Institute of Parasitology
Prague, Czechoslovakia

George W. Beran
College of Veterinary Medicine
Iowa State University
Ames, Iowa

R. L. Doherty
Dean, Faculty of Medicine
University of Queensland
Brisbane, Australia

Richard W. Emmons
Chief, Viral and Rickettsial Disease
  Laboratory
California Department of Health
  Services
Berkeley, California

Akinyele Fabiyi
Director, Virus Research Laboratory
University of Ibadan
Ibadan, Nigeria

J. H. S. Gear
Consultant in Tropical Medicine
South African Institute for Medical
  Research
Johannesburg, South Africa

Milota Gresikova
Institute of Virology
Slovak Academy of Sciences
Bratislava, Czechoslovakia

Scott B. Halstead
Chairman, Department of Tropical
  Medicine and Medical Microbiology
John A. Burns School of Medicine
University of Hawaii at Manoa
Honolulu, Hawaii

Richard O. Hayes
Senior Research Associate
Department of Microbiology
Colorado State University
Fort Collins, Colorado

Harry Hoogstraal
Head, Medical Zoology Department
Naval Medical Research
Cairo, Egypt

Harald Norlin Johnson
Viral and Rickettsial Disease
  Laboratory
Berkeley, California

Graham E. Kemp
Research Veterinarian
Vector-Borne Disease Center
Center for Disease Control
Atlanta, Georgia

Lim Teong Wah
Institute for Medical Research
Jalan Pahong
Kuala Lumpur, Malaysia

Oscar de Souza Lopes
Head, Secão de Virus Transmitidos
  por Artrópodos
Instituto Adolfo-Lutz
São Paulo, Brazil

Nyven J. Marchette
Professor, Department of Tropical
  Medicine
University of Hawaii School of
  Medicine
Honolulu, Hawaii

Stuart McConnell
Professor, Department of Veterinary
Microbiology
College of Veterinary Medicine
Texas A&M University
College Station, Texas

B. M. McIntosh
Senior Virologist
National Institute for Virology
Johannesburg, South Africa

Donald M. McLean
Professor, Division of Medical
Microbiology
University of British Columbia
Vancouver, British Columbia

J. M. Meegan
Yale Arbovirus Research Unit
Yale University
New Haven, Connecticut

Joseph L. Melnick
Professor and Chairman
Department of Virology and
Epidemiology
Baylor College of Medicine
Houston, Texas

J. C. Peters
Research Scientist
U. S. Army Medical Research
Institute of Infectious Diseases
Fort Detrick Frederick, Maryland

F. P. Pinheiro
Chief, Virus Section
Instituto Evandro Chagas
Ministério da Saude
Belém, Brazil

Yves Robin
Directeur de l'Institut Pasteur
Cayenne, French Guiana

C. E. Gordon Smith
Dean, London School of Hygiene
and Tropical Medicine
London, United Kingdom

R. O. Spertzel
College of Veterinary Medicine
Texas A&M University
College Station, Texas

Wayne H. Thompson
Professor, Preventative Medicine
Department
Center for Health Sciences
University of Wisconsin
Madison, Wisconsin

M. G. Varma
London School of Hygiene
London, United Kingdom

Thomas M. Yuill
Professor and Chairman
Department of Veterinary Science
University of Wisconsin
Madison, Wisconsin

ACKNOWLEDGMENTS

Many persons to whom I owe an unending debt of gratitude have assisted me throughout my career in public health. Dr. James H. Steele has been my mentor ever since he first accepted me as a new graduate veterinarian, a recruit into the U. S. Public Health Service. Through his program in cooperation with Dr. Herbert A. Wenner of the University of Kansas College of Medicine, and later as a graduate student with Dr. Wenner, I received my first training and experience in the public health team.

Most of my career has been spent in Asia as a missionary and with the World Health Organization (WHO), and many Asians have been instrumental in guiding and assisting me. Under Dr. Federico N. Florendo and later Dr. Jose S. Garcia, medical directors of Silliman University Medical Center, and with the sponsorship and continual assistance of Dr. C. D. Van Houweling, we were able to develop the Van Houweling Laboratory for Microbiological Research in the Medical Center. The late Mariano F. Perdices, governor of Negros Oriental Province in the Philippines and a close friend, had a keen concern for the health and well-being of the people of this province where my family and I lived, and of which I am an adopted son. At his invitation, and working in close cooperation with him and the capable Provincial Health Officer Dr. Felipe S. Rustia, we were able to develop the pioneer provincial public health laboratory. I am grateful to those with whom I was privileged to work in the development of rabies control in the Philippines, Dr. Francisco J. Dy, Director of the WHO Regional Office for the Western Pacific, Dr. Clemente S. Gatmaitan, Minister of Health, and Dr. Joaquin S. Sumpaico, Director of the Bureau of Research and Laboratories of the Republic of the Philippines.

In the past several years at Iowa State University, I owe much to Dr. R. Allen Packer, Head of the Department of Veterinary Microbiology and Preventive Medicine and Dr. Phillip T. Pearson, Dean of the College of Vetcrinary Medicine for their guidance and support in teaching, research, and consultative service in public health. It has been with their continuing encouragement and forbearance that this section on viral zoonoses in this Handbook Series in Zoonoses has been achieved. In the preparation of this manuscript, my special gratitude is extended to Mrs. Marjorie Davis who handled the bulk of the typing of the correspondence and manuscripts, often through several editings, with no thought of reward. With equal capability and dedication, Mrs. Jeanne Gehm joined in the typing during the last months of preparation. Without their help I would have been in serious difficulty.

To all who contributed to writing the chapters of this section covering the diverse field of the viral zoonoses I am sincerely grateful. They have all been recognized specialists and the accumulated hours of their cfforts are beyond my estimating.

I cannot express the warmth of my gratitude to my wife, Dr. Janice A. Beran and our children, Bruce, Anne, and George with any adequacy in cold print. Somehow, while keeping dinners warm, arriving at social events late if at all, and providing a cheerful, understanding atmosphere, Jan built, and the family tolerated, the environment in which this task was completed.

TABLE OF CONTENTS
SECTION B: VIRAL ZOONOSES
VOLUME I

Introduction to Viral Zoonoses

THE CLASSIFICATION OF VERTEBRATE VIRUSES

J. L. Melnick

Until about 1950, little was known about viruses other than their pathogenic effects in causing diseases, and thus any efforts at classification tended to focus on host responses rather than on properties of the virus particles. At present, the end of an important phase of discovery and characterization of animal viruses is being approached. It is becoming apparent that most of the major groups of viruses of vertebrates, at least those of human beings and the animals important to people, have been recognized and described. The knowledge thus gained has made it possible to establish and broadly define groupings for these agents. Many of these virus groupings, initially established on tentative and provisional bases, now appear to form "real" families and genera, in which the members are indeed related in fundamental ways. For example, the validity of the original grouping of the enteroviruses based on an enteric habitat and small size is being borne out by current studies that utilize sophisticated techniques of modern molecular virology to compare the genetic makeup of different members of the group and their modes of replication.

The shift in emphasis, from sketching the broad outlines of the virus kingdom based on disease causation to filling in essential details about the viruses themselves, has been recognized by a change in the name of the International Committee on Nomenclature of Viruses (ICNV) to the International Committee on Taxonomy of Viruses (ICTV). The first report of the ICNV was published in 1971,[51] and the second report of this Committee in 1976.[12] Work of the study groups and subcommittees of the ICTV is proceeding, and they are reporting an increasing number of taxonomic articles in their special areas of virology. Reports of these groups appear regularly in *Intervirology*, the journal of the Virology Section of the International Association of Microbiological Societies. Official decisions of the ICTV made at its meetings held during the Third International Congress for Virology have recently been summarized,[27] and a full report of the results of the last five years of work by the ICTV and its committees has been published as a special triple issue of *Intervirology*.[28]

Tables 1 through 5 are schematic diagrams showing separation of viruses of vertebrates into 16 families.[32] RNA-containing viruses are presented in three tables: Table 1, those with cubic capsid symmetry; Table 2, those with helical symmetry; and Table 3, those with capsid architecture either asymmetric or unknown. Table 4 describes viruses that have a DNA genome, cubic symmetry, and a naked nucleocapsid; and Table 5, DNA-containing viruses with envelopes or complex coats. Commentaries follow on the viruses that have been definitely assigned to these groups. Also included are hepatitis viruses A and B, and some other agents whose classification is still tentative.

RNA VIRUSES

Family Picornaviridae[8,34]

These viruses are shown at the top of Table 1. Members of this family, the smallest of the viruses with RNA genomes, exist in at least four genera and in several hundred species. At least 70 members of the *Enterovirus* genus are known to infect human beings; these include polioviruses, coxsackieviruses, echoviruses, and, in recent years, new enterovirus serotypes that are assigned sequential numbers, enterovirus-68, etc., rather than being placed in ill-defined subgroups. Well over 100 viruses infecting human beings belong to the genus *Rhinovirus*. Large numbers of agents from both of these genera are indigenous to other host species. The other two genera are *Cardiovirus*, a rodent agent that may also infect human beings and *Aphthovirus*, which includes the economically important, foot-and-mouth disease viruses of cattle.

The picornavirus genome is one piece of linear, single-stranded RNA of low molecular weight (about 2.5×10^6). The RNA is infectious and serves as its own messenger for protein translation. The enteroviruses and cardioviruses are acid-stable and have a buoyant density in CsCl of about 1.34 g/cm³; the rhinoviruses and aphthoviruses, in contrast, are acid-labile, and have a higher buoyant density of about 1.4 g/cm³.

Several other groups of viruses had previously been considered for possible membership in the picornavirus family, including the ribophages, which are RNA-containing bacteriophages resembling picornaviruses in some properties, and the caliciviruses, which are several viruses that infect sea lions, swine (in which they cause vesicular exanthema) and cats (in which they cause respiratory disease). Neither ribophages nor caliciviruses have as yet been firmly placed in families, although family status has been proposed for caliciviruses. Both of these groups differ from picornaviruses in several important ways, and have been excluded from Picornaviridae.[28]

The diseases caused by picornaviruses range from severe paralysis (paralytic poliomyelitis) to aseptic meningitis, pleurodynia, myocarditis, skin rashes, and common colds; inapparent infection is very common. Different viruses may produce the same syndrome; on the other hand, the same picornavirus may cause more than a single syndrome.

After decades of investigation it now seems that hepatitis A virus is an enterovirus. Data previously unavailable and needed to settle the issue now have been obtained.[44] The nucleic acid of hepatitis A virus has been shown to be RNA, and this virus also resembles enteroviruses in many other properties (see Table 6). Similarities include the 27-nm size and spherical shape of the hepatitis A virus, its density in cesium chloride (1.34 g/cm³), its location in the cell cytoplasm, and its stability to ether and to acid pH. Both hepatitis A virus and enteroviruses are labile at 100°C temperatures, but hepatitis A virus is more consistently stable at 60°C heat, whereas enteroviruses vary in this regard. The agent is clearly distinguished from the rhinoviruses by its acid stability, from the hepatitis B virus (i.e., the Dane particle) by size, nucleic acid type, and location within the cell, and from HBsAg, not only by particle size but also by the absence of any demonstrable nucleic acid in the HBsAg. Distinction from the parvoviruses also can be made on the basis of size, nucleic acid type, and location of parvoviruses in the cell nucleus.

Family Reoviridae[21,28]

Members of this virus family share a property unique among the RNA-containing viruses of vertebrates: the possession of a double-stranded, rather than single-stranded, RNA genome. The genome consists of several segments. The capsid has a double shell, and the structure of the outer capsid layer is indistinct. However, icosahedral symmetry has been demonstrated in the inner capsid layers of all three recognized groups of reoviruses that infect vertebrates, the genera *Reovirus*, *Orbivirus*, and *Rotavirus*. Members of the genus *Reovirus* have been thought to have 92 capsomeres (this number is at present being restudied), while the other two groups have 32 capsomeres. The capsomeres of the orbiviruses are unusually large, 10 to 15 nm wide, and appear ring-shaped. The human reoviruses are found in the enteric tract, but their association with disease is not clear. Members of this genus recovered from lower animals are similar to those of humans. The *Orbivirus* genus includes viruses that infect vertebrates but also infect invertebrates; some have been considered to be arboviruses. Several have

Table 1

RNA-CONTAINING VIRUSES WITH CUBIC CAPSID SYMMETRY

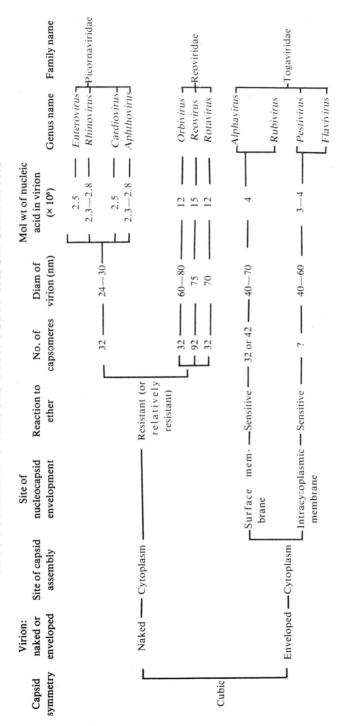

Capsid symmetry	Virion: naked or enveloped	Site of capsid assembly	Site of nucleocapsid envelopment	Reaction to ether	No. of capsomeres	Diam of virion (nm)	Mol wt of nucleic acid in virion ($\times 10^6$)	Genus name	Family name
Cubic	Naked	Cytoplasm		Resistant (or relatively resistant)	32	24—30	2.5	*Enterovirus*	*Picornaviridae*
							2.3—2.8	*Rhinovirus*	
							2.5	*Cardiovirus*	
							2.3—2.8	*Aphthovirus*	
					32	60—80	12	*Orbivirus*	*Reoviridae*
					92	75	15	*Reovirus*	
					32	70	12	*Rotavirus*	
	Enveloped	Cytoplasm	Surface membrane	Sensitive	32 or 42	40—70	4	*Alphavirus*	*Togaviridae*
								Rubivirus	
			Intracytoplasmic membrane	Sensitive	?	40—60	3—4	*Pestivirus*	
								Flavivirus	

Table 2
RNA-CONTAINING VIRUSES WITH HELICAL SYMMETRY

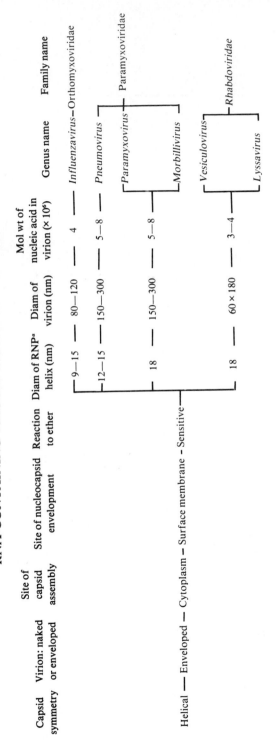

Capsid symmetry	Virion: naked or enveloped	Site of capsid assembly	Site of nucleocapsid envelopment	Reaction to ether	Diam of RNP[a] helix (nm)	Diam of virion (nm)	Mol wt of nucleic acid in virion (×10⁶)	Genus name	Family name
Helical	Enveloped	Cytoplasm	Surface membrane	Sensitive	9—15	80—120	4	*Influenzavirus*	*Orthomyxoviridae*
					12—15	150—300	5—8	*Pneumovirus*	*Paramyxoviridae*
					18	150—300	5—8	*Paramyxovirus* / *Morbillivirus*	
					18	60×180	3—4	*Vesiculovirus* / *Lyssavirus*	*Rhabdoviridae*

ᵃ   ribonucleoprotein

Table 3

RNA-CONTAINING VIRUSES WITH ARCHITECTURE UNSYMMETRIC OR UNKNOWN

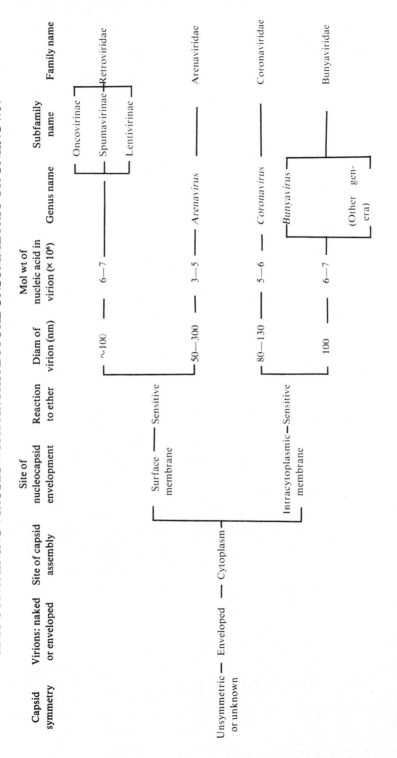

Table 4

DNA-CONTAINING VIRUSES WITH CUBIC SYMMETRY AND NAKED NUCLEOCAPSID

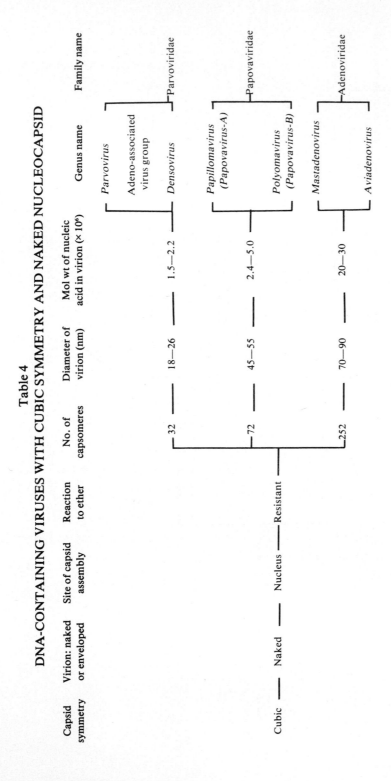

Table 5

DNA-CONTAINING VIRUSES WITH ENVELOPES OR COMPLEX COATS

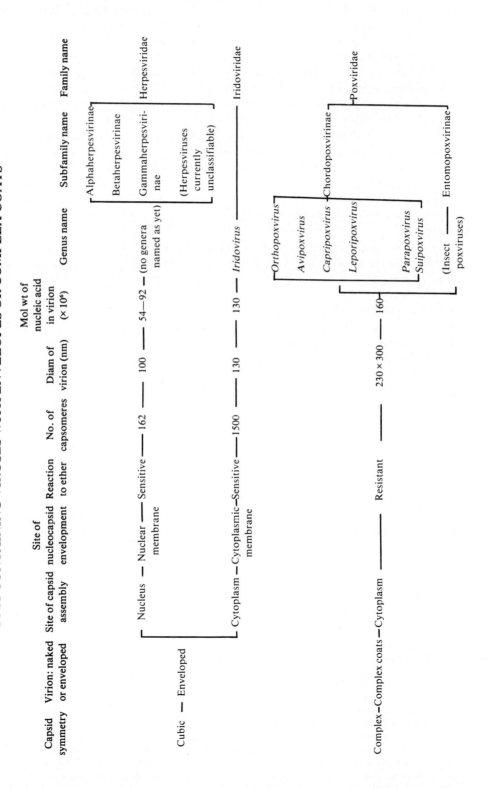

been recovered only from insects. The known diseases caused by orbiviruses include blue-tongue of sheep, African horse sickness, Colorado tick fever of human beings, and epizootic hemorrhagic disease of deer. The members of the genus *Rotavirus* that infect human beings are increasingly recognized as major pathogens of nonbacterial infantile diarrhea. The gastroenteritis syndrome is clinically more severe and of longer duration than the illness caused by the 27-nm "Norwalk agent," and occurs in sporadic rather than epidemic form. Gastroenteritis caused by these agents is one of the commonest childhood illnesses throughout the world, and in underdeveloped countries it is a leading cause of death. Other members of this antigenically interrelated rotavirus group include calf diarrhea virus, the virus of epizootic diarrhea of infant mice, SA11 rotavirus of monkeys, and similar viruses from swine and other species. Much of the initial study of the rotaviruses was accomplished by use of electron microscopy and immune microscopy, and thus far, isolation of the human members of the group has not been achieved in cell cultures. The virus does replicate in fetal intestinal organ cultures, and antibodies to the virus can be assayed by indirect fluorescent antibody techniques.[19]

In addition to the members of Reoviridae that infect vertebrates, there are other groups within the family: the cytoplasmic polyhedrosis viruses of insects and the reoviruses of plants.

Family Togaviridae[36,43]

Members of this family include most arboviruses* of antigenic groups A and B, now classed in the genus Alphavirus (group A) and the genus *Flavivirus* (group B), and in addition, include the newly designated genera *Rubivirus* and *Pestivirus*, in which non-arbo togaviruses have been placed. The virions are spherical, 40 to 70 nm in diameter, and have a lipoprotein envelope with lipid and virus-specified glycopeptide tightly applied to an icosahedral nucleocapsid. The genome is a single molecule of single-stranded RNA. The alphaviruses and flaviviruses include many of the major human arboviral pathogens.

The viruses of Venezuelan, eastern, and western encephalitis are alphaviruses, and the viruses of yellow fever, dengue, Japanese encephalitis, St. Louis encephalitis, Omsk hemorrhagic fever, and Russian spring-summer encephalitis are flaviviruses. Rubella virus thus far is the only member of the genus *Rubivirus*. Members of the *Pestivirus* genus include bovine virus diarrhea (mucosal disease complex) virus, hog cholera (European swine fever) virus, and border disease virus. Lactic dehydrogenase virus of mice, equine arteritis virus, and simian hemorrhagic fever virus may also be members of the family Togaviridae.

Family Orthomyxoviridae[6,10] (See Table 2)

The orthomyxoviruses recognized to date are influenza viruses, which may be spher-

---

*   One important and well-known virus group name that does not appear in the diagrams is a category based on ecologic properties, the arbovirus group.[4] The 359 or more arthropod-borne viruses survive through complex cycles involving vertebrate hosts and arthropods which serve as vectors, transmitting the viruses by their bites. This grouping, based on transmission, remains a useful one despite the wide diversity of its members in regard to properties of the virions. The vast majority of arboviruses now have been sufficiently well-characterized to permit their taxonomic placement. Many of the classical serologic interrelationships previously delineated by arbovirologists have been found to be paralleled by morphologic similarities, and these serologic relationships have tremendously speeded the taxonomic placement process by providing clues on where to look. Once some of the members of a serological group have been characterized in terms of biophysical and biochemical properties, attention of taxonomists can be focused on their antigenic relatives. Arboviruses now are included in a number of families, chiefly Togaviridae, Bunyaviridae, Rhabdoviridae, Arenaviridae, and Reoviridae.

Table 6
COMPARATIVE BIOPHYSICAL PROPERTIES OF
HEPATITIS TYPE A VIRUS AND POLIOVIRUS
TYPE 1

Physicochemical characteristics of major virus particle population	Hepatitis type A virus	Poliovirus type 1
Morphology		
Diameter	28 nm	28 nm
Envelope	None	None
Sedimentation rate	160S	160S
Density (CsCl)	1.34 g/ml	1.34 g/ml
Nucleic acid		
Type	Single-stranded	Single-stranded
	RNA	RNA
Length (EM)[a]	1.7 μm	2.3 μm
Mol wt	1.9×10^6	2.6×10^6
Polypeptides (major);	22,000[b]	24,000
(mol wt)	24,000	25,000
	29,000	34,000

[a] EM = as measured by electron microscopy.
[b] Values of 23,000, 25,500, and 34,000 have also been reported.

ical, elongated, or filamentous. For most members of the family, there are "spikes" projecting from the surface of the envelope; these are glycosylated protein peplomers 10 to 14 nm long and 4 nm in diameter, consisting of two types, the hemagglutinin and the neuraminidase. The helically symmetric ribonucleoprotein capsid has RNA strands 9 to 15 nm in diameter. The RNA is single-stranded, in 6 or 7 segments. An RNA-dependent RNA polymerase is associated with purified virions. During replication, the helical nucleocapsid is first detected in the nuclei, whereas the hemagglutinin and neuraminidase are formed in the cytoplasm. The virus matures by budding at the cell surface membrane.

The genus, *Influenzavirus,* has been established to include viruses of type A and type B; type C is considered a "probable genus." Antigenic variations are common, particularly among members of type A. Recombination occurs with high frequency within species, but not among types or genera. Type A influenza viruses include agents of human, equine, swine, and avian influenza and of fowl plague. For types B and C, only human strains are known.

Family Paramyxoviridae[12,24]

Usually spherical, these virions may also be pleomorphic. They are 150 nm or more in diameter and filamentous forms may be several μm long. On the lipid bilayer envelope are surface projections. The RNA is single-stranded and is in unsegmented, linear form; the helical nucleocapsid is 12 to 18 nm in diameter. Virions are formed in the cytoplasm by budding from the plasma membrane. Infectivity is sensitive to ether, acid, and heat, but paramyxoviruses are resistant to actinomycin D. The genera include *Paramyxovirus* (parainfluenza viruses 1—4, mumps virus, Newcastle disease virus, Yucaipa, and other avian paramyxoviruses), *Morbillivirus* (the viruses of measles, canine distemper, rinderpest, and peste de petiti ruminants), and *Pneumovirus* (respiratory syncytial viruses of humans and of cattle, and pneumonia virus of mice). Members of the genus *Paramyxovirus* have both hemagglutinin and neuraminidase in the virions.

Morbillivirus members have hemagglutinin in the viral envelopes but not neuraminidase, while for members of the genus *Pneumovirus,* the virions contain neither hemagglutinin nor neuraminidase. Members of Paramyxoviridae are genetically stable and genetic recombination does not occur.

Family Rhabdoviridae[5]

Members of this family have enveloped virions that are rod-shaped, resembling bullets (with one end rounded and the other flattened), or bacilliform. Enclosed within the lipoprotein envelope and membrane protein is the long tubular nucleocapsid with helical symmetry. The genome of single-stranded RNA is unsegmented, linear form. Members of some genera multiply in arthropods as well as in vertebrates or higher plants, others multiply only in insects. Infectivity is sensitive to ether, acid, and heat. The genera which have members that infect vertebrates are *Lyssavirus* and *Vesiculovirus*; these two genera also include several viruses that thus far have been isolated only from insects. Members of *Lyssavirus* include rabies, Duvenhage, and Mokola viruses that infect human beings; Lagos bat virus; and several isolates from insects. Members of *Vesiculovirus* include vesicular stomatitis virus and a number of antigenically interrelated viruses; among the vesiculoviruses are Chandipura virus (from human beings), Flanders-Hart Park virus (of mosquitoes and birds), Kern Canyon bat virus, Piry opossum virus; and probably also bovine ephemeral fever virus, Mt. Elgon bat virus, Egtved virus (viral hemorrhagic septicemia virus) of trout, and several other fish viruses. In addition, there are numerous rhabdoviruses of plants.

Marburg and Ebola viruses, serious human pathogens not yet classified, resemble rhabdoviruses in over-all bullet-like shape, but have very elongated forms. Their internal structure also apparently differs from that of the rhabdoviruses. These viruses are of extraordinary concern because, when transmitted to people from their natural animal hosts (which are as yet unknown, but are presumably one or more African jungle animals), they cause severe and often fatal hemorrhagic disease. These agents are being studied under limited conditions in maximum-containment laboratories, but are not yet understood sufficiently to permit their classification.

Family Retroviridae[9,28,49] (See Table 3)

Much remains to be settled concerning this family, but a good deal of progress has been made. The members include not only the RNA tumor viruses ("oncornaviruses," and "leukoviruses"), which are now assigned to a subfamily, Oncovirinae, but also the slow viruses of the maedi/visna group, now assigned to a subfamily Lentivirinae, and the foamy virus group (agents which form syncytia in cell cultures), now assigned to the subfamily Spumavirinae.

Members of the family characteristically have a reverse transcriptase (RNA-dependent DNA polymerase) within the virion. For the most thoroughly studied members, the lipoprotein envelope encloses an inner shell with icosahedral symmetry, and a central core, or nucleocapsid, with helical symmetry. The genome is a single molecule of single-stranded RNA which dissociates readily into two or three pieces. Infectivity is ether-, acid-, and heat-sensitive. Replication of the viral RNA involves a DNA provirus which is integrated into host-cellular DNA.

In the case of Oncovirinae, all normal cells of several animal species contain integrated copies of genes of the endogenous species of oncovirus. The oncovirus genes may not be expressed, but can be activated by physical and chemical agents, by superinfection with other oncoviruses, and even by herpesviruses. According to their host range in cell cultures, oncoviruses fall into three classes: (1) ecotropic—capable of growth in cells of the natural host; (2) xenotropic — capable of growth only in cells of a different species; and (3) amphotropic — capable of growth in both autologous and heterologous cells. According to certain morphological, antigenic and enzymatic differences, oncoviruses also have been divided into A, B, and C (and possibly D) types of viruses. Most current schemes for classifying oncoviruses utilize Bernhard's classification of A, B, and C particles. A particles, or A-type particles, are double-shelled and have an electron-lucent center. B-type particles have eccentric cores, and C-type particles have central cores. With some exceptions, oncoviruses fall into host-species-specific groups of agents inducing either leukemias or sarcomas, i.e., leukemia-sarcoma complexes of avian, murine, feline, and hamster oncoviruses. Other groups are murine mammary tumor virus and primate oncoviruses. One of the primate oncoviruses is the monkey mammary tumor virus (MoMTV — previously termed Mason-Pfizer virus) from a rhesus monkey tumor. This may be a D-type agent, with particles generally resembling B or C particles, but having a distinct configuration, with an outer unit membrane and an inner tubular or cylindrical nucleoid. Recent evidence has indicated that all strains of mice studied to date contain C-type viruses which are xenotropic (i.e., replicate in cells of other species but not in the homologous murine cells).

The ICTV[12,28] has designated two genus-level groups within this subfamily, although genus names have not been assigned. These are (i) the type C oncovirus group (including mammalian, avian, and reptilian subgenus groupings of type C oncovirus and probably also a number of ungrouped species); and (ii) the type B oncovirus group, in which the virus core is located eccentrically within the extracellular virion. These include the mouse mammary tumor virus and probably also include the similar viruses from guinea pigs and perhaps from other species. MoMTV, the monkey mammary tumor virus, now has been listed as a "proposed genus," type D oncovirus.

The members of the subfamily Spumavirinae, "foamy viruses," do not induce tumors or cellular transformation, but cause persistent asymptomatic infections in natural and experimental host animals. They have perhaps been best known for their induction of syncytia in cell cultures being prepared for cultivation of other viruses. Foamy viruses or syncytial viruses are known for a number of mammalian species, including human beings.

The slow viruses of the maedi/visna group, which have been placed in the subfamily Lentivirinae of the Retroviridae family, are morphologically and chemically like other members of the family, but do not induce tumors. A nucleoid or core forms immediately beneath the viral envelope during budding from the cellular plasma membranes, and particles lack second internal viral membranes. Natural infections are known only in sheep. Visna virus causes panleukoencephalitis. The virus infects all of the organs of the infected sheep, but pathological changes are confined chiefly to the brain, lungs, and reticuloendothelial system. There is a long incubation period, and virus can be recovered from infected animals as long as 4 years after inoculation. Several serologically related viruses, variously designated in different countries as maedi, progressive pneumonia, or Zwoegerziekte viruses, cause interstitial pneumonitis.

Family Arenaviridae[41]

Members of this family have spherical or pleomorphic virions with a dense lipid bilayer membrane bearing surface projections. Within the virion core are electron-dense RNA-containing granules about 20 to 30 nm in diameter which are ribosome-like in size, shape, and density. The RNA is single-stranded, and consists of 4 large and 1 to 3 small segments. Virions are formed by budding from the surface membranes. Viral RNA is probably transcribed by virion polymerase into complementary RNA which probably acts as mRNA. Infectivity is sensitive to ether, acid, and heat. Most member viruses have a single restricted rodent host in which persistent infections occur accompanied by viremia, viruria, or both. Spread to other mammals and to humans occurs, but it is unusual. Members include lymphocytic choriomeningitis virus which infects mice but may spread to humans: Lassa virus; and members of the Tacaribe complex: Junin and Machupo viruses of South American hemorrhagic fevers, Pichinde virus, and several other viral agents which have been isolated from arthropods, but for which natural transmission cycles involving arthropod vectors have not been demonstrated.

Family Coronaviridae[47,48]

The family is named for unique petal-shaped or club-shaped peplomers which project from the envelope. In negatively stained electron micrographs these projections form a fringe resembling the solar corona. The interior structure of the virion is not fully understood. It is probably a loosely wound helically symmetric nucleocapsid. The genome consists of one large molecule of single-stranded RNA. Infectivity is sensitive to ether, acid, and heat. Nucleocapsids develop in the cytoplasm and mature by budding through intracytoplasmic membranes. Several serotypes of human coronaviruses have been isolated from patients with acute upper respiratory tract illnesses, primarily through the use of human embryonic tracheal and nasal organ cultures. Coronaviruses are known in many lower animals, including avian infectious bronchitis virus, mouse hepatitis virus, porcine transmissible gastroenteritis virus, and hemagglutinating encephalitis virus. Probable members include turkey bluecomb disease virus, canine coronavirus, calf neonatal diarrhea coronavirus, and at least two rat coronaviruses; feline infectious peritonitis virus is a possible member.

Family Bunyaviridae[28,42]

This family is the largest and most recently recognized taxonomic grouping assigned to an antigenically interrelated set of arboviruses. There are at least 150 members, more than 114 belonging to the Bunyamwera supergroup of arboviruses, which consists of 13 serologically crossrelated groups and several ungrouped arboviruses. The virions are spherical, and on their unit-membrane envelope have surface projections which may be randomly placed or clustered in arrays with icosahedral symmetry. The envelope contains at least one virus-specified glycopeptide. The internal ribonucleoprotein is helically wound and symmetric, with long strands 2- to 2.5-nm broad. The single-stranded RNA is probably in three circular segments. The virion develop in the cytoplasm and mature by budding through intracytoplasmic membranes into smooth-surfaced vesicles in the Golgi region or nearby. Infectivity is sensitive to ether, acid, and heat. Virus particles hemagglutinate. Members of the family produce a number of important diseases of humans and of domestic animals, e.g., California encephalitis, Crimean hemorrhagic fever, sandfly fever, Rift Valley fever, and Nairobi sheep disease. Most Bunyaviridae members are mosquito-transmitted, but some are tickborne. In addition to the viruses already assigned to the genus *Bunyavirus*, confined at present to members of the serologic Bunyamwera supergroup, at least 95 other arboviruses are known which are generally very similar to bunyaviruses in most properties, but are not serologically related. These agents are considered members, or probable members, of the family, perhaps in two different genera yet to be designated. The largest antigenic grouping among these is the Uukuniemi group, antigenically unrelated to *Bunyavirus* and transmitted by ticks.

DNA VIRUSES

Family Parvoviridae[1,2]

Originally named picodnaviruses to reflect their small size and DNA-containing genome,[29] the family Parvoviridae now includes two genera with Latinized names, *Parvovirus* and *Densovirus,* and a third genus called the *Adeno-associated virus group.* These are DNA-containing viruses that have cubic symmetry and a naked (unenveloped) nucleocapsid. During replication, capsid assembly takes place in the nucleus of the host cell (see Table 4). Infectivity of these viruses is resistant to ether and other lipid solvents, and also to heating ($56°C$ for 1 hr). The capsid has 32 capsomeres. The diameter of the virus particle is 18 to 26 nm, and the molecular weight of the nucleic acid is 1.5 to 2×10^6. The capsomeres which form the outer layer of the nucleocapsid are each 3 to 4 nm in diameter.

The genus *Parvovirus* includes autonomously replicating members of the group that infect vertebrates. These are hamster osteolytic H viruses, latent rat viruses (Kilham rat virus, X14 virus), minute virus of mice (MVM), and parvoviruses of swine, cattle, cats, and other species. The members of the *Densovirus* genus are viruses of insects, but are also capable of producing cytopathic effects in L cells of vertebrates. They replicate autonomously. In contrast to the two genera that replicate autonomously, members of the *Adeno-associated virus* genus (adenosatellite viruses) are defective in that they cannot multiply except in the presence of a replicating adenovirus which serves as a helper virus. Herpesviruses can act as partial helpers. In cells coinfected with herpesviruses, infectious satellite DNA and capsid proteins are made, but they are not assembled into satellite virions. The type species of this genus is human adeno-associated virus type 1; other species include types 2, 3, and 4, and also simian, bovine, avian, and canine adeno-associated viruses. A possible member is equine adeno-associated virus.

Members of the Parvoviridae are the only DNA-containing viruses of vertebates whose DNA genome is single-stranded within the virion. All the others shown in Tables 4 and 5 have double-stranded DNA. In the case of adeno-satellite viruses and densoviruses, separate virions contain single strands of positive or negative DNA. These strands are complementary, and when isolated from the virion shells, they come together to form a double strand. However, in the members of the genus *Parvovirus* (of which Kilham rat virus is the type species), the DNA in the virion is a positive strand only. This single-stranded DNA molecule has a hairpin-like structure at both the 5' and the 3' ends. In members of this genus, about 1% of the virions form double strands similar to the self-complementary strands of the other two genera. Members of this genus show marked preference for actively dividing cells, have been shown to be transmissible transplacentally, and are receiving attention for their special disease potential in fetuses and neonatal animals.[23,25] Other members of the *Parvovirus* genus include minute virus of mice and viruses of pigs, cattle, cats, geese, and other species. In addition, probable members include the virus of Aleutian mink disease, as well as canine and lapine parvoviruses. Among possible members of the genus are certain important gastroenteritis viruses of human beings (Norwalk agent and related isolates), and also the virus of hepatitis type B.

In the light of accumulating data, it is becoming clear that hepatitis virus type B has a number of important properties similar to those of representative members of the parvovirus family. The 42-nm "Dane" particle found in the serum of hepatitis B virus-infected individuals is now recognized as the virus of this disease. The morphology, nucleic acid type, and nucleic acid strandedness of the Dane particle place it in a class by itself, unrelated to any other known viruses. However, the 25 nm central core (HBcAg, hepatitis B core antigen), which can be released from Dane particles, shares many biochemical and biophysical properties with several members of the parvovirus family. In addition to similarities in site of maturation, morphology, and size, core particles and members of the parvovirus family contain three polypeptides with similar molecular weights.[15] Moreover, they share a similar sedimentation coefficient and DNA molecular weight. The buoyant density of core particles resembles that of the defective adenosatellite viruses. However, these core particles and parvoviruses seem to differ in two major characteristics. First, the DNA of the core particles has been reported to be double-stranded,[17,39,45] whereas parvovirus virions contain single-stranded DNA.[46] It should be noted, however, that the DNA of one group of parvoviruses, the adeno-satellite (adeno-associated) viruses had been variously reported as double-stranded or single-stranded, and that this seeming contradiction was only resolved when it was found that positive and negative single strands of DNA were present within different adeno-satellite virions, and that these strands, upon extraction from the virions, united to form double-stranded DNA.[18,30] As yet, there are no reports of the isolation of the DNA of hepatitis core particles under conditions that would prevent reannealment of positive and negative single DNA strands, as has been done with the adeno-satellite viruses. Another problem to be reconciled is the fact that hepatitis core particles exist as units within the nuclei of infected hepatocytes in which they are manufactured, but when they circulate in the blood, they are present within a shell, with the entire unit being now considered a Dane particle or the virion. Hepatitis core particles (devoid of outer shells) appear to be more like members of the parvovirus family than of any other known virus group. However, other observations have suggested that there are differences which may eventually place hepatitis B virus into a new virus group that has not previously been recognized.

Family Papovaviridae[28,31,33]

These relatively small, ether-resistant viruses contain double-stranded DNA in circular form. Many are unusually heat-stable surviving temperatures that inactivate most other viruses. The representatives that infect human beings are the papilloma or wart virus and SV40-like viruses such as JC virus, which has been isolated from the brain tissues of patients with progressive multifocal leukoencephalopathy (PML), or BK virus, which has been isolated from the urine of immunosuppressed recipients of renal transplants.[40] Other members include papilloma viruses of several vertebrate species, polyoma and K viruses of mice, and vacuolating viruses of monkeys (SV40), and of rabbits. These viruses have relatively slow growth cycles characterized by replication within the nuclei of the host cells. Papovaviruses produce latent and chronic infections in their natural hosts. All are tumorigenic in at least some animal host species. The genome, a single cyclic molecule of double-stranded DNA, integrates into cellular chromosomes of transformed cells. The capsid antigens of JC and BK viruses are unique, but the tumor antigen induced by each crossreacts antigenically with that induced by SV40. Two genera have been named by the ICTV as *Papillomavirus* and *Polyomavirus*. The Study Group for Papovaviruses designated these genera as Papovavirus-A and Papovavirus-B, respectively. Genus A includes rabbit (Shope) papilloma virus, and papilloma viruses of cattle, deer, dogs, goats, hamsters, horses, human beings (several types), and sheep. For genus B the type species is polyoma virus of mice (which, as indicated by its name, induces multiple neoplasms in its host). Other members are K virus of mice, RK virus of rabbits, SA12 of baboons, and SV40 of monkeys. In addition, the human viruses, BK and JC, have been included in this genus. It is important to note that there is no evidence that these viruses are associated with human neoplasms.

When SV40 and adenoviruses replicate together within the same cell, they may interact to form various kinds of SV40/adenovirus "hybrid" virus particles, in which a portion of the SV40 genome is covalently linked to incomplete or complete adenovirus DNA and is carried within an adenovirus capsid.

Family Adenoviridae[37]

Among these medium-sized viruses, at least 33 serotypes infect human beings, and there are distinct serotypes for a number of other species. The virions are nonenveloped isometric particles with 252 capsomeres, each 7 to 9 nm in diameter. Vertex capsomeres are antigenically distinct from the other capsomeres and carry one or two filamentous projections. The adenovirus genome is a single linear molecule of double-stranded DNA.

Adenoviruses have a predilection for mucous membranes and may persist for years in lymphoid tissue. Some of the adenoviruses cause acute respiratory diseases, febrile catarrhs, pharyngitis, and conjunctivitis. Latent infections are often produced. Human adenoviruses rarely cause disease in laboratory animals, but certain serotypes produce tumors in newborn hamsters. Common antigens are shared by all mammalian adenoviruses, which now have been classed as members of the *Mastadenovirus* genus.

Family Herpesviridae[28,38]

Herpesviruses are a heterogeneous group of viruses identified by their structure. As shown in Table 5, the virus particles consist of a DNA-containing core enclosed by an icosahedral capsid with 162 partially hollow cylindrical capsomeres. The nucleocapsid is surrounded by a bilayer envelope which contains lipid, carbohydrate, and protein. The enveloped virions are 150 to 200 nm in diameter. Between the capsid and the envelope is a layer called the tegument, the size of which varies among the herpesviruses. Within the nucleocapsid, the DNA genome is spooled around a cylindrical mass (probably protein), forming the viral core. The double-stranded linear DNA of various herpesviruses differs considerably in size (80 to 150×10^6 mol wt), cytosine and guanine content (32 to 72%), and structural complexity. Herpes simplex virus has a complex structural organization, including in the genome a terminally redundant section and internal inverted repetitions of sequences present at both ends of the DNA molecule, with a long and short unique sequence region. The DNA of Herpes simplex virus is sufficiently large to code for 80 to 100 proteins, of which about 50 have been observed. As many as 30 of these may be structural proteins of the virus particle, while others may be virus-induced enzymes, including thymidine kinase, DNA polymerase, and DNase. Other members of the herpesvirus family may have simpler structural organization of the genome.

The DNA of herpesviruses replicates within the nuclei of the infected cells. Maturation of the progeny virus particles occurs by budding of nucleocapsids through the altered inner nuclear membranes of the infected cells. Thus the cell nuclear membranes contribute to the envelopes of the mature virus particles.

Most herpesviruses are exceedingly thermolabile, but some (Herpes simplex) can be stabilized by 1 M Na$_2$SO$_4$ so as to withstand heating at 50°C. They are destroyed by ether and other lipid solvents, and by photodynamically active dyes (proflavine and neutral red) in the presence of light.

Herpesviruses are noteworthy for their ability to establish latent and/or persistent infections. Latent infections may last for the lifetime of the hosts, even in the presence of circulating antibodies. Special interest has been generated by the association of Epstein-Barr (EB) herpesvirus with human Burkitt lymphomas and nasopharyngeal carcinomas, and by the possible role of the genital herpesvirus, Herpes simplex type 2 in cancers of the uterine cervix. Several simian herpesviruses have been shown to be oncogenic in experimentally infected animals. Infections of heterologous species are in many cases very serious; examples are the fatal infections of humans caused by one of the simian herpesviruses, herpesvirus simiae or B virus, and the infection of cattle by swine pseudorabies virus. Human diseases include oral and genital herpes, chickenpox, and shingles due to varicella/zoster virus, cytomegalic inclusion disease, and infectious mononucleosis.

Three subfamily groups have been established within the family Herpesviridae on the basis of differences in host range, cytopathogenic patterns, replicative cycle, latency, and properties of the viral DNA. A number of members of the family are left unclassified for the present. The subfamily Alphaherpesvirinae has human (alpha) herpesvirus 1 (the cause of the common "fever blister" or "cold sore") as the prototype. This subfamily also includes human (alpha) herpesvirus 2 (genital herpes), as well as human (alpha) herpesvirus 3 (varicella/zoster virus), suid (alpha) herpesvirus 1 (pseudorabies, bovid herpesvirus 2 (bovine mammillitis), and equid herpesvirus 1 (equine abortion). Other viruses considered probable or possible members include equid herpesviruses 3 (coital exanthema) and 2, cercopithecid herpesvirus 1 (herpes B), and herpesviruses of cats, dogs, and fowl. The subfamily Betaherpesvirinae has as its prototype human (beta) herpesvirus 5 (human cytomegalovirus, the cause of cytomegalic inclusion disease). Other members are murid herpesvirus 1, suid herpesvirus 2, and probably murid herpesvirus 2. Gammaherpesvirinae (the lymphoproliferative group) has as its prototype human (gamma) herpesvirus 4 (Epstein-Barr virus, the cause of infectious mononucleosis and associated with Burkitt lymphomas and nasopharyngeal carcinomas). Other probable members are Herpesvirus saimiri and Herpesvirus ateles of primates, and possibly also gallid herpesvirus 1 (Marek's disease herpesvirus), gallid herpesvirus 2 (turkey herpesvirus), and leporid herpesvirus 1.

Family Iridoviridae[16,22,28]

The best-known members of this family are members of the insect iridescent virus group (e.g., *Tipula* iridescent virus), now placed in the genus, *Iridovirus*. However, other important viruses that are now considered members of this family include African swine fever virus and a large number of viruses of frogs and of fish. No human iridoviruses are known. The vertebrate iridoviruses are enveloped. The iridoviruses that infect insects have a lipid fraction present in the virion shell but do not have envelopes as such. The genome is a single, very large molecule of double-stranded DNA.

Family Poxviridae[13,14,28]

These large viruses are brick-shaped or ovoid with a complex virion structure. An external coat contains lipid and tubular or globular protein structures. This coat encloses one or two lateral bodies and an internal body (core) which contains the genome. The virions contain more than 30 structural proteins and several viral enzymes including a DNA-dependent RNA polymerase. The genome consists of a single molecule of double-stranded DNA. Genetic recombination occurs within genera; nongenetic reactivation occurs both within and among genera of the poxviruses that infect vertebrates. Most poxviruses of vertebrates share at least one antigen. Members of each genus of vertebrate poxviruses have additional antigens in common. This is the major DNA-containing virus family whose members replicate entirely within the cytoplasm; a number of them produce intracytoplasmic inclusion bodies. The family has been divided into two subfamilies (see Table 5): Entomopoxvirinae, poxviruses of insects (probably with at least three genera, as yet unnamed) and Chordopoxvirinae, poxviruses of vertebrates, in which six genera have been designated. The genus *Orthopoxvirus* includes the poxviruses of human beings. This genus produces a hemagglutinin separate from the virion; this hemagglutinin is serologically specific, and is a lipid-rich pleomorphic particle 50 to 65 nm in diameter.

Table 7
USE OF POLYMERASES FOR CLASSIFICATION OF ANIMAL VIRUSES

Virus family	Example	Approximate number of genes	Polymerase
RNA Viruses			
Picornaviridae	Poliovirus	12	
Togaviridae	Japanese B encephalitis	15	Induce RNA-dependent RNA polymerase
Reoviridae	Reovirus	40	
Orthomyxoviridae	Influenza virus	15	
Paramyxoviridae	Measles virus	30	
Rhabdoviridae	Vesicular stomatitis virus	20	Carry RNA-dependent RNA polymerase
Arenaviridae	Lymphocytic choriomeningitis virus	15	
Bunyaviridae	Bunyamwera virus	15	
Coronaviridae	Human upper respiratory illness virus	30	
Retroviridae	C-type oncovirus	50	Carry RNA-dependent DNA polymerase
DNA viruses			
Parvoviridae	Adenosatellite virus	7	
Papovaviridae			
Polyomavirus	Polyoma virus	7	
Papillomavirus	Human wart virus	13	Induce DNA-dependent DNA polymerase
Adenoviridae	Human adenovirus	50	
Herpesviridae	Herpes simplex virus	180	
Poxviridae	Vaccinia virus	400	Induce DNA-dependent DNA polymerase and carry DNA-dependent RNA polymerase

OTHER CLASSIFICATION SCHEMES

While vertebrate virus families can be diagrammed and discussed conveniently in an organizational arrangement with the primary separation based upon the type of nucleic acid genome, there are other ways in which known data about groups of viruses can be organized. One interesting approach to virus classification has related to the induction or carriage of polymerases, the enzymes essential for replication of the viral genes. As shown in Table 7, among viruses with an RNA genome the viruses with fewer genes, picornaviruses and togaviruses, induce, but do not carry, RNA-dependent RNA polymerase, whereas the medium-sized RNA viruses carry this enzyme. The retroviruses are distinctive in that the enzyme which they carry is an RNA-dependent DNA polymerase (reverse transcriptase). Among the DNA-containing viruses, the small- and medium-sized viruses induce DNA-dependent DNA polymerase; only the very large poxviruses both induce this enzyme and carry DNA-dependent RNA polymerase.

Another major difference among viruses is the presence or absence of a lipid-containing envelope. Matthews[26] developed an interesting and potentially useful classification which was based in part upon the viral membrane. The system that he described was based on the relationship between the size of the viral genome and the size of the entire virion (dry mass or particle volume). Under this scheme, viruses fell into two classes: those with, and those without envelopes. The enveloped viruses have a ratio of nucleic acid molecular weight to whole virus anhydrous weight of 1 to 40, and to whole-virus volume of 1 to 0.2 (Table 8). These ratios of genome to weight and volume

Table 8
COMPARISON OF ENVELOPED
AND NONENVELOPED VIRUSES:
VIRUS AND GENOME SIZE

	Ratio of molecular weight of nucleic acid to	
Class of virus	Whole virion (dry weight)	Whole virion (vol)
Enveloped	1:40	1:0.2
Nonenveloped	1:4	1:0.01

are similar to those of prokaryotic cells. In contrast, nonenveloped viruses have a ratio of nucleic acid to whole virus dry weight of 1 to 4 and to whole virus volume of 1 to 0.01, markedly different both from the enveloped viruses and from the prokaryotic cells.

These two classes of viruses further differ in the reaction of enveloped viruses to freezing. Wallis and Melnick[50] found that enveloped viruses required the presence of the very same additives to preserve their infectivity that are required to preserve the membranes and viability of animal cells, whereas such additives were not required to stabilize nonenveloped viruses.

Further subdivisions have been made based on size of the nucleic acid genome and its mode of replication. For the enveloped viruses (Table 9), those with large genomes have double-stranded DNA and those with smaller genomes have single-stranded RNA. For the nonenveloped viruses (Table 10), those with genomes above a certain size have double-stranded nucleic acid (DNA or RNA), while those below that size have single-stranded nucleic acid (DNA or RNA).

The striking difference between the two virus classes can be brought into focus by comparing influenza virus and poliovirus. Influenza virus is only 1/1000 the size of *E. coli,* but it has a similar dry mass and particle volume per unit of nucleic acid. When influenza virus is compared with poliovirus, both have about the same amount of RNA, but the influenza virus particle has ten times the anhydrous mass, and 20 to 30 times the volume of the whole virus (Table 11). Matthews[26] has suggested that a primary division of viruses into these two classes may have more predictive value than the current schemes, and might correspond more nearly to evolution of viruses.

Cooper[7] has suggested that genome strategy may be a factor of substantial weight in indicating relatedness, and perhaps a more fundamental one than, for example, capsid structure, which might be more readily altered by mutational or environmental manipulations. While a common strategy of replication naturally includes a common particle structure, the criterion of strategy may be useful to differentiate certain viruses which have a somewhat similar structure, but which reached that structure by different evolutionary pathways. This cannot be the only criterion for degrees of relatedness, as viruses with similar genome strategies but no other properties in common could have arrived at this similarity by converging in the course of evolution. Viruses with distinct strategies would clearly be expected to have arisen through distinct phylogeny, and thus would not be placed in the same family.

EMERGING PROBLEMS IN VIRUS CLASSIFICATION

Some of the present and developing problems that viral taxonomists will have to

Table 9
MATTHEWS' CLASSIFICATION SYSTEM: ENVELOPED VIRUSES

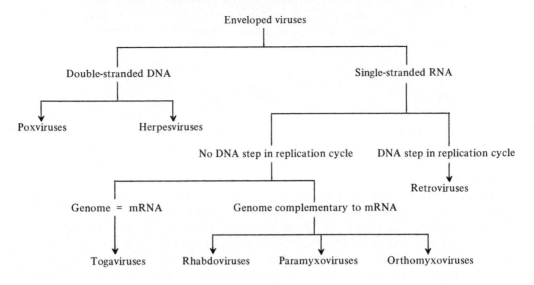

Table 10
MATTHEWS' CLASSIFICATION SYSTEM: NONENVELOPED, GEOMETRIC VIRUSES

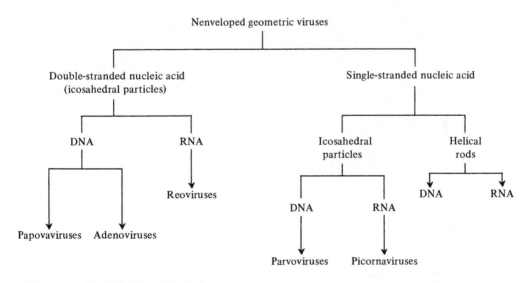

meet are those posed by the recently discovered forms of life called viroids, viral hybrids (between unrelated viruses), pseudovirions, and recombinant DNA.

Viroids

Viroids constitute a recently discovered class of infectious agents smaller than viruses. They are known to cause several diseases of plants (e.g., potato spindle tuber disease), and may ultimately be found to cause disease in humans and higher animals. For example, the agent of scrapie disease of sheep may, according to recent findings, prove to be a viroid. Viroids exhibit the characteristics of nucleic acids in crude extracts, that is, they are insensitive to heat and to organic solvents, but are sensitive to

Table 11

COMPARISON OF INFLUENZA VIRUS AND POLIOVIRUS

Virus	Mol wt (nucleic acid) (A)	Whole virion (dry mass) (B)	Whole virion (vol) (C)	Ratios	
				A/B	A/C
Influenza virus	$\sim 4 \times 10^6$	$\sim 2 \times 10^8$	$\sim 8 \times 10^5$	1:50	1:0.2
Poliovirus	2.6×10^6	8.5×10^6	1.2×10^4	1:3	1:0.005

nucleases. They do not appear to possess protein coats. Viroids known at present consist solely of short strands of RNA with a molecular weight of 75,000 to 100,000.

Virus Hybrids

The fact that virus hybrids can exist in nature should be more widely recognized. If SV40 had not already been known as a virus prior to the discovery of SV40-adenovirus "hybrid" particles, these particles would have presented viral taxonomists with a very confusing puzzle. The hybrid particles, in which portions of SV40 genome material are covalently linked to adenovirus genetic material and encased within an adenovirus coat, would have seemed to be new and very strange viruses which reacted antigenically like adenoviruses of the serotype from which its coat was derived, but which had many properties altogether unlike adenoviruses when grown in cultures.

Two types of adenovirus-SV40 hybrids have been detected. PARA-adenovirus populations consist of two kinds of particles: the first, a nonhybrid typical adenovirion, and the second, a defective adenovirus-SV40 genome encased in an adenovirus capsid (PARA). PARA can be transcapsidated from one adenovirus serotype to another. The second type of hybrid, the Ad2+ND viruses, consists of a series of nondefective adenovirus type 2 isolates carrying different amounts (5 to 44%) of the SV40 genome.

A similar problem of identification and classification does in fact exist in another type of particle found in some human adenovirus populations. This particle, termed MAC (monkey-adapting component), behaves somewhat like the PARA particle, permitting the true human adenovirus to replicate in monkey cell cultures. This particle with a MAC genome and an adenovirus coat does not contain any SV40 nucleic acid fragments, and its origin remains unknown.

Pseudovirions

The pseudovirion is another viral form that is difficult to classify. During viral replication, the capsid sometimes encloses host nucleic acid rather than viral nucleic acid. Such particles look like ordinary virus particles when observed by electron microscopy, but they do not replicate. Pseudovirions contain the "wrong" nucleic acid. For example, fragments of host-cell DNA may be incorporated into papovavirus capsids instead of viral DNA, forming pseudovirion particles. This situation resembles the phenomenon of generalized transduction by bacteriophages, i.e., transfer of random portions of nucleic acid from the donor bacterial cell to the recipient bacterium. Hybridization studies have also indicated the occurrence of covalent linkage of cell DNA segments into the circular DNA of papovaviruses during replication in cells infected at high multiplicity, similar to the situation with specialized transducing bacteriophages, i.e., transfer of a specific segment of donor bacterial cell DNA. Furthermore, under specialized experimental conditions, a DNA segment containing functional genes of lambda bacteriophage may have been incorporated into the circular DNA of papovavirus SV40. These findings may open avenues for study of possible transducing events in eukaryotic cells, whereby functionally defined segments of genetic information can be transmitted from cell to cell. Pseudovirions present the taxonomist with problems based on natural events, but future laboratory manipulations will probably add to these problems of classification.

Recombinant DNA

Recently developed techniques allow DNA to be cleaved into specific pieces, using enzymes from bacteria called restriction endonucleases. These distinct fragments have importance in two areas, (1) the physical mapping of genes in large, complicated DNA genomes, and (2) genetic engineering. In addition to the overriding concerns for safety precautions to ensure that new genetic combinations thus produced do not result in new organisms with dangerous properties, virologists must also give attention to how the new recombinant organisms should be classified. Classification of these new forms of life needs to be developed in ways that will reflect their origins and relatedness to each other and to other living things.

REFERENCES

1. **Bachmann, P. A., Hoggan, M. D., Melnick, J. L., Pereira, H. G., and Vago, C.,** Parvoviridae, *Intervirology,* 5, 83, 1975.
2. **Bachmann, P. A., Hoggan, M. D., Kurstak, E., Melnick, J. L., Pereira, H. G., Tattersall, P., and Vago, C.,** Parvoviridae: second report, *Intervirology,* 11, 248, 1979.
3. **Bellett, A. J. D.,** The iridescent virus group, *Adv. Virus Res.,* 13, 225, 1968.
4. **Berge, T. O.,** International Catalogue of Arboviruses including Certain Other Viruses of Vertebrates, 2nd ed., Publ. No. (CDC) 75-8301, Public Health Service, U.S. Department of Health, Education and Welfare, Atlanta, 1975.
5. **Brown, F., Bishop, D. H. L., Crick, J., Francki, R. I. B., Holland, J. J., Hull, R., Johnson, K., Martelli, G., Murphy, F. A., Obijeski, J. F., Peters, D., Pringle, C. R., Reichmann, M. E., Schneider, L. G., Shope, R. E., Simpson, D. I. H., Summers, D. F., and Wagner, R. R.,** Rhabdoviridae, *Intervirology,* 12, 1, 1979.
6. **Burnet, F. M.,** Portraits of viruses: influenza virus A, *Intervirology,* 11, 201, 1979.
7. **Cooper, P. D.,** Towards a more profound basis for the classification of viruses, *Intervirology,* 4, 317, 1974.
8. **Cooper, P. D., Agol, V. I., Bachrach, H. L., Brown, F., Ghendon, Y., Gibbs, A. J., Gillespie, J. H., Lonberg-Holm, K., Mandel, B., Melnick, J. L., Mohanty, S. B., Povey, R. C., Rueckert, R. R., Schaffer, F. L., and Tyrrell, D. A. J.,** Picornaviridae: second report, *Intervirology,* 10, 165, 1978.
9. **Dalton, A. J., Melnick, J. L., Bauer, H., Beaudreau, G., Bentvelzen, P., Bolognesi, D., Gallo, R., Graffi, A., Haguenau, F., Heston, W., Huebner, R., Todaro, G., and Heine, U. I.,** The case for a family of reverse transcriptase viruses: Retraviridae, *Intervirology,* 4, 201, 1974.
10. **Dowdle, W. R., Davenport, F. M., Fukumi, H., Schild, G. C., Tumova, B., Webster, R. G., and Zakstelskaja, L. Ya.,** Orthomyxoviridae, *Intervirology,* 5, 245, 1975.
11. **Fenner, F.,** The classification and nomenclature of viruses. Summary of results of meetings of the International Committee on Taxonomy of Viruses in Madrid, September 1975, *Intervirology,* 6, 1, 1975/76.
12. **Fenner, F.,** Classification and nomenclature of viruses: second report of the International Committee on Taxonomy of Viruses, *Intervirology,* 7, 1, 1976.
13. **Fenner, F.,** Portraits of viruses: the poxviruses, *Intervirology,* 11, 137, 1979.
14. **Fenner, F., Pereira, H. G., Porterfield, J. S., Joklik, W. K., and Downie, A. W.,** Family and generic names for viruses approved by the International Committee on Taxonomy of Viruses, June 1974, *Intervirology,* 3, 193, 1974.
15. **Fields, H. A., Hollinger, F. B., Desmyter, J., Melnick, J. L., and Dreesman, G. R.,** Biochemical and biophysical properties of hepatitis B core particles derived from Dane particles and infected hepatocytes, *Intervirology,* 8, 336, 1977.

16. **Goorha, R. and Granoff, A.**, Icosahedral cytoplasmic deoxyriboviruses, in *Comprehensive Virology*, Vol. 14, Fraenkel-Conrat, H., and Wagner, R. R., Eds., Plenum Press, New York, 1979, 347.

17. **Hirschman, S. Z., Gerber, M., and Garfinkel, E.**, DNA purified from naked intranuclear particles of human liver infected with hepatitis B virus, *Nature (London)*, 251, 540, 1974.

18. **Hoggan, M. D.**, Adenovirus associated viruses, *Science*, 11, 408, 1970.

19. **Holmes, I. H.**, Viral gastroenteritis, *Prog. Med. Virol.*, 25, 1, 1979.

20. **Jawetz, E., Melnick, J. L., and Adelberg, E. A.**, *Review of Medical Microbiology*, 13th ed., Lange Medical Publ., Los Altos, California, 1978.

21. **Joklik, W. K. et al.**, Reoviridae, *Intervirology*, to be published.

22. **Kelley, D. C. and Robertson, J. S.**, Icosahedral cytoplasmic deoxyvirus, *J. Gen. Virol.*, Suppl. 20, 17, 1973.

23. **Kilham, L. and Margolis, G.**, Problems of human concern arising from animal models of intrauterine and neonatal infections due to viruses: a review. I. Introduction and virologic studies, *Prog. Med. Virol.*, 20, 113, 1975.

24. **Kingsbury, D. W., Bratt, M. A., Choppin, P. W., Hanson, R. P., Hosaka, Y., ter Meulen, V., Norrby, E., Plowright, W., Rott, R., and Wunner, W. H.**, Paramyxoviridae, *Intervirology*, 10, 137, 1978.

25. **Margolis, G. and Kilham, L.**, Problems of human concern arising from animal models of intrauterine and neonatal infections due to viruses: a review. II. Pathologic studies, *Prog. Med. Virol.*, 20, 144, 1975.

26. **Matthews, R. E. F.**, A classification of virus groups based on the size of the particle in relation to genome size, *J. Gen. Virol.*, 27, 135, 1975.

27. **Matthews, R. E. F.**, The classification and nomenclature of viruses: summary of results of meetings of the International Committee on Taxonomy of Viruses in The Hague, September, 1978, *Intervirology*, 11, 133, 1979.

28. **Matthews, R. E. F.**, Classification and nomenclature of viruses: third report of the International Committee on Taxonomy of Viruses, *Intervirology*, 12, 129, 1979.

29. **Mayor, H. D. and Melnick, J. L.**, Small deoxyribonucleic acid-containing viruses (picodnavirus group), *Nature (London)*, 210, 331, 1966.

30. **Mayor, H. D., Torikai, K., Melnick, J. L., and Mandel, M.**, Plus and minus single-stranded DNA separately encapsidated in adeno-associated satellite virions, *Science*, 166, 1280, 1969.

31. **Melnick, J. L.**, Papovavirus group, *Science*, 135, 1128, 1962.

32. **Melnick, J. L.**, Taxonomy of viruses, 1979, *Prog. Med. Virol.*, 25, 160, 1979.

33. **Melnick, J. L., Allison, A. C., Butel, J. S., Eckhart, W., Eddy, B. E., Kit, S., Levine, A. J., Miles, J. A. R., Pagano, J. S., Sachs, L., and Vonka, V.**, Papovaviridae, *Intervirology*, 3, 106, 1974.

34. **Melnick, J. L., Agol, V. I., Bachrach, H. L., Brown, F., Cooper, P. D., Fiers, W., Gard, S., Gear, J. H. S., Ghendon, Y., Kasza, L., LaPlaca, M., Mandel, B., McGregor, S., Mohanty, S. B., Plummer, G., Rueckert, R. R., Schaffer, F. L., Tagaya, I., Tyrrell, D. A. J., Voroshilova, M., and Wenner, H. A.**, Picornaviridae, *Intervirology*, 4, 303, 1974.

35. **Melnick, J. L., Midulla, M., Wimberly, I., Barrera-Oro, J. G., and Levy, B. M.**, A new member of the herpesvirus group isolated from South American marmosets, *J. Immunol.*, 92, 596, 1964.

36. **Murphy, F. A.**, Taxonomy of vertebrate viruses, in *CRC Handbook of Microbiology*, Vol. 2, Lechevalier, H. A., Ed., 1978, 623.

37. **Norrby, E., Bartha, A., Boulanger, P., Dreizin, R. S., Ginsberg, H. S., Kalter, S. S., Kawamura, H., Rowe, W. P., Russell, W. C., Schlesinger, R. W., and Wigand, R.**, Adenoviridae, *Intervirology*, 7, 117, 1976.

38. **O'Callaghan, D. J. and Randall, C. C.**, Molecular anatomy of herpesviruses: recent studies, *Prog. Med. Virol.*, 22, 152, 1976.

39. **Overby, L.R., Hung, P. O., Mao, J. C. H., Ling, C. M., and Kakefuda, T.**, Rolling circular DNA associated with Dane particles in hepatitis B virus, *Nature (London)*, 225, 84, 1975.

40. **Padgett, B. L. and Walker, D. L.**, New human papovaviruses, *Prog. Med. Virol.*, 22, 1, 1976.

41. **Pfau, C. J., Bergold, G. H., Casals, J., Johnson, K. M., Murphy, F. A., Pedersen, I. R., Rawls, W. E., Rowe, W. P., Webb, P. A., and Weissenbacher, M. C.**, Arenaviruses, *Intervirology*, 4, 207, 1974.

42. **Porterfield, J. S., Casals, J., Chumakov, M. P., Gaidamovich, S. Ya., Hannoun, C., Holmes, I. H., Horzinek, M. C., Mussgay, M., Oker-Blom, N., and Russell, P. K.**, Bunyaviruses and Bunyaviridae, *Intervirology*, 6, 13, 1975/76.

43. **Porterfield, J. S., Casals, J., Chumakov, M. P., Gaidamovich, S. Ya., Hannoun, C., Holmes, I. H., Horzinek, M. C., Mussgay, M., Oker-Blom, N., Russell, P. K., and Trent, D. W.**, Togaviridae, *Intervirology*, 9, 129, 1978.

EASTERN AND WESTERN ENCEPHALITIS

EASTERN ENCEPHALITIS

R. O. Hayes

NAMES AND SYNONYMS

Eastern encephalitis (EE) and eastern equine encephalomyelitis (EEE) are the two names that have been used most frequently for this arthropod-borne viral disease of animals and people. Other references to this disease have been eastern viral encephalitis, encephalomyelitis, encephalitis, horse sleeping sickness, and sleeping sickness. The latter four terms were generally used in the U.S. prior to the recognition that several different etiologic agents existed which caused central nervous system (CNS) disease syndromes in horses and human beings in rather specific geographic regions. In 1968, the American Committee on Arthropod-Borne Viruses listed and discussed the names and abbreviations of 204 arboviral infections, including eastern equine encephalomyelitis, and recommended that the full name and the EEE abbrevaition be used; the Committee also recognized the shortened term, eastern encephalitis (EE)[1] Since the virus causes a zoonosis that is not restricted to equine hosts, the shortened term is used in this description of the infection.

HISTORY

Retrospective evidence has been reported which indicated that EE was the cause of equine epidemics in the U.S. in 1831, 1845, and 1933, and that the etiological agent had been present along the Atlantic seaboard for centuries — "even before there were horses or men in America.[92]

The initial isolation of EE virus was made from equine brain tissue during an epidemic of encephalitis in horses which occurred along the coastal areas of Delaware, Maryland, New Jersey, and Virginia during 1933.[72,230] Virus isolations, the finding of specific neutralizing antibodies in sera of horses from the 1933 outbreak area,[231] the recovery of virus from the blood of febrile horses, and successful experimental infections confirmed the virus as the causative agent for the EE epidemics.[230] The 1933 outbreak of EE in horses was followed by additional cases in Virginia in 1934 and in North Carolina in 1935, and it was noted that the outbreaks tended to be cyclic with respect to time.[73]

Although horses were the only vertebrate hosts initially demonstrated to be naturally infected, Tenbroeck, Hurst, and Traub suggested on the basis of epidemiological findings in 1935 that birds should be considered as possible reservoir hosts.[230] Their studies indicated that pigeons were susceptible to intracerebral inoculations.

In Massachusetts during 1938, the first human cases of EE were confirmed by virus isolations from brain tissue.[66,245] From 1938 through 1961, a total of 112 human cases were recorded in intermittent outbreaks in Massachusetts, New Jersey, Delaware, Florida, Louisiana, Mississippi, and Texas.[107] From 1962 through 1971, 40 additional human cases were reported from New York, Pennsylvania, and South Carolina.[161,172] Equine cases have been reported from all of these states, plus Alabama, Arkansas, Michigan, New Hampshire, North Carolina, Virginia, and Wisconsin. Equine cases of EE were reported in Ontario in 1972.[11]

During the period from 1935 through 1970, the Animal Health Division of the U.S. Department of Agriculture reported a total of 533,269 cases of arthropod-borne encephalitides in equidae in the U.S., with 41,968 associated deaths from 1939 through 1970.[21] The equine mortality rate was 28.5% for the period in which both cases (147,277) and deaths (41,968) were reported. These reports are not categorized by types of encephalitis, and include cases caused by both EE and WE (western encephalitis) virus, as well as some nonarboviral encephalitides. Furthermore, laboratory diagnoses often have been reported on the basis of high antibody titer in a single convalescent serum specimen, without supplementary information upon vaccination history.

EE case fatality rates among both human beings and horses are characteristically high, usually 80% or greater.[196,210] EE infections acquired by laboratory workers have been rare.[81,94]

The occurrence of outbreaks among flocks of pheasants was first documented by virus isolations from brains of naturally infected birds in Connecticut.[237] EE virus also was shown to cause disease in pheasants in New Jersey in 1938, 1939, 1940, and sporadically in subsequent years.[7,8] The outbreaks usually have been in commercially-reared, ring-necked pheasant flocks, and they have occurred in most of the Atlantic and Gulf Coast states, from New Hampshire through Texas. An unusual epidemic of EE in a South Dakota pheasant flock has been reported.[175] Other imported domestic birds, including Peking ducks in New York[50] and Chukar partridges in Maryland,[173] also have been shown to display symptoms and suffer mortality from EE infections.

Wild birds (pigeons and sparrows) were shown to be susceptible to infection by EE virus in the 1930s,[65,238] but the first isolation of the virus from a bird with an inapparent infection (a purple grackle from a Louisiana swamp habitat) was not obtained until 1950.[147] Subsequent studies have shown that many species of birds are infected in nature throughout regions of EE enzootic activity.[102,113,144,215]

Arthropod studies for transmission of EE virus in the laboratory incriminated mosquitoes as potential vectors of EE during the mid-1930s.[165,166] In 1940, Davis reported laboratory confirmation of these previous studies and identified six species of *Aedes* mosquitoes which were experimentally infected by feeding on viremic birds or mammals, and which successfully transmitted virus to susceptible birds or mammals. He demonstrated that the period of viremia in experimentally infected birds was less than 4 days.[46] Many species of mosquitoes have since been identified as vectors of EE virus,[32,34,35] and their importance as disease vectors has been associated with their host preferences and behavior patterns.[33,53,227] Species of arthropods other than mosquitoes also have been found naturally infected with EE virus, but laboratory studies and field epidemiological findings have not incriminated them as potentially important vectors in disease outbreaks, or in the natural cycle of transmission of the virus.[3,127,139] An excellent review covering the literature through 1952, which stresses the entomological phases and the history of EE, is available.[63]

Vertebrates other than human beings, horses, and birds have been found naturally infected with EE virus, but they have not been identified as of public health importance, or essential to maintenance of the virus in nature.[32,104,137]

The geographic distribution of EE virus extends from Canada through the U.S., Mexico,[205] Panama[219], Trinidad, the Dominican Republic, Guyana, Argentina, Brazil, Colombia,[32] and Peru.[206]

ETIOLGY

Classification

EE, as well as other arthropod-borne viruses (arboviruses), is characterized by its capability to multiply in infected arthropods without producing disease or apparent tissue damage. The history of classification of arboviruses has been reviewed meticulously by Theiler and Downs,[232] with detailed description of the application of immunological methods for determining the relationships between arboviruses. Using hemagglutination-inhibition techniques (HI), Casals and Brown were able to separate several arboviruses into two groups, A and B; the three immunologically-related equine encephalitis viruses (EE, WE, and Venezuelan encephalomyelitis) were assigned to group A.[29] EE virus strains have been isolated from the Neoarctic (North American) to the Neotropical (Central and South American) geographic regions. Antigenic variants can be separated by HI techniques into North American and South American types with distinct geographical distributions.[28]

The International Committee on Taxonomy of Viruses has classified EE in the genus *Alphavirus* of the family Togaviridae, based primarily upon its physical and chemical characteristics.[60,61] The "International Catalog of Arboviruses" has classified EE as an arbovirus on the basis of isolation from an arthropod, transmission to a vertebrate by means of the bite of an infected arthropod, and demonstration of a specific viremia in the vertebrate host:[2]

Characteristics

EE has a single-stranded RNA virion with spherical symmetry enclosed in a lipoprotein envelope. It is about 50 nm in size. It is unstable at room temperatures, but it can be preserved by freezing at $-70°C$, and it can be inactivated by sodium deoxycholate, ether, or chloroform.[62,130] The viral envelope has projections which correspond to the hemagglutinin. Viral multiplication is by budding in the host cytoplasm. EE virus may be readily cultured in the laboratory in a variety of cell lines; primary cultures of chick or duck fibroblasts and continuous cell lines of monkey kidney (e.g., Vero) have been used most frequently.

EE virus is related to Ndumu and Middleburg viruses in a complex based on antigenic relationships demonstrated by plaque reduction neutralization tests.[135] Two other complexes within the alphaviruses are the WE and the Venezuelan encephalitis (VE) complexes.

DEFINITION

Eastern encephalitis is a mosquito-borne zoonosis, primarily of wild birds, that produces acute CNS (central nervous system) infections in horses and human beings. Vertebrates which develop viremias of sufficiently high titers to infect arthropods are termed reservoir hosts, and the infected mosquitoes capable of transmitting the virus from one vertebrate host animal to another are termed vectors. EE is categorized as a vector-borne disease.

ANIMAL INFECTION

Horses

Infection of horses with EE virus often results in a fatal illness. For example, in the large 1947 outbreak in Louisiana, 11,927 deaths were reported among 14,334 equine cases with a 83% case-fatality rate.[195] The early clinical symptoms include staggering, imbalance, and a tendency to walk in circles. Stupor develops, and may be followed by convulsive seizures preceding death.[21] Four different types of clinical response to EE infections varying from subclinical to acute fatal disease have been categorized in horses.[143]

The lesions of EE were first described by Kissling and Rubin.[146] Two general types of lesions were described in the brains of horses succumbing to EE. In animals surviving 1 day or less after onset of neurologic signs, diffuse infiltrations of the gray matter with polymorphonuclear leucocytes, severe endothelial damage, perivascular hemorrhage and moderate perivascular edema were observed; the reticulum appeared swollen and fragemented, and there was some swelling of the neurofibrils, but most of the neurons were anatomically normal. In animals surviving 2 days or longer, the polymorphonuclear leucocyte response was no longer evident, and the perivascular exudate was almost entirely lymphocytic. Cellular nodular formation containing large mononuclear cells and diffuse infiltrations of microglia were prominent. In the intermediate stages observed, there was a thinning of the polymorphonuclear leucocytic infiltrate and a mobilization of the microglia. The lesions were limited almost exclusively to the gray matter of the brains. All areas of the cerebral cortex showed severe damage; the corpus striatum showed mild involvement, the lateral thalamic nuclei usually showed more damage than the anterior or the dorso-medial nuclei, the midbrain showed a random distribution of damage, and the cerebellum showed the least involvement of any portion of the brain. The lesions in the brain stem were also generally located in the gray matter, and the cervical cord showed much less damage than was observed at any level of the medulla oblongata. The severity of pathological changes observed in necropsy among horses infected with EE also has been described by Miller, Pearson, and Muhm.[168]

Definitive diagnosis of EE depends upon laboratory tests,[91] with virus isolation or specific immunologic criteria serving as the basis for diagnostic confirmation.[161] Confirmed cases fulfill one or more of the following criteria: (1) isolation and identification of EE virus; (2) a fourfold or greater change in hemagglutination inhibition (HI) or complement-fixation (CF) antibody levels between acute and convalescent serum specimens; or (3) a rise in the neutralization index (NI) of 1.7 logs or greater in unvaccinated horses. Significant levels of antibody (HI $\geq$ 1:320, CF $\geq$ 1:8 or NI $\geq$ 2.0 logs) in a single serum specimen from an unvaccinated horse may be considered to be presumptive evidence of an etiological relationship between infection and disease. Accurate vaccination history data is a prerequisite for meaningful interpretation of serological laboratory tests.

Pheasants

Clinical EE infections have been described in Chinese ring-necked, Impeyan, Mongolian, and Tragopan pheasants.[56] Fever was an early manifestation of disease, with ensuing ataxia, trembling, weakness, leg paralysis, drooping of the extremities, generalized paralysis, and death. At necropsy, vasculitis, patchy necrosis, microgliosis, and meningitis were the lesions most frequently observed. The rostellum, and secondly the cerebellum, were the most severely affected.[134] Isolation and identification of the virus from blood or brain specimens from stricken birds are needed for diagnostic confirmation.

Other Birds and Mammals

Infections in chickens more than 1 day old, in fledged birds, and in mammals other than horses are usually inapparent. They may, however, be readily infected by mosquitoes, may develop viremic levels adequate to infect mosquitoes, and thus serve as reservoirs of infection in the natural cycle of EE. They are of considerable epidemiological importance. Their roles are discussed in detail in the section on epidemiology.

HUMAN INFECTIONS

The clinical manifestations of EE in human beings are indistinguishable from those of WE, but the overall case-fatality rate following symptomatic infection with EE approaches 80%; whereas, with WE it ranges between 5 and 15%[196] Onset is characteristically abrupt, with high fever (40 to 41°C), severe headache, nuchal rigidity, nausea, stupor, coma, and convulsions.[73,98,125,244] The cerebrospinal fluid (CSF) shows pleocytosis with predominance of lymphocytes, and cell counts may range from 100 to 1000/mm[3]. The protein count is elevated, but the CSF glucose level is unchanged. The peripheral leucocyte count may be elevated. The severity of sequelae shows a marked association with age; of 16 survivors of EE studied in Massachusetts, 4 had profound residual mental retardation, 2 had marked retardation, 3 had moderate retardation, 2 slight retardation, and 5 appeared to have had no permanent cerebral damage.[57]

Clinical encephalitis is characteristically associated with severe EE virus infections. At necropsy, three principal histopathologic features in the CNS tissue have been described:[21] (1) perivascular cuffing with large numbers of mononuclear cells filling the Virchow-Robin spaces around intracerebral blood vessels, (2) neuronophagia, where some necrotic neurons become surrounded by macrophages, and (3) foci containing 20 to 100 microgleal cells scattered throughout the parenchyma of the brain and the spinal cord. The lesions observed in patients have been described in studies of outbreaks in several geographic regions.[12,133,150]

Although severe, fatal infections occur in the majority of clinically recognized cases, mild and subclinical syndromes have been described.[39] Inapparent infection rates reported from New Jersey ranged from 3.1 to 3.6% among residents in a coastal outbreak area, and up to 7.3% among 55 household contacts of overt cases.[76] Evidence of a high inapparent infection rate has been reported from the Dominican Republic,[54] but not within endemic areas if Louisiana,[204] or Massachusetts, where a serologic survey of 537 individuals residing in a known endemic area had an EE antibody prevalence rate of only 0.7%.[59]

Laboratory confirmation of clinical cases is based on virus isolation and identification (usually from post-mortem CNS tissue), or on significant changes in antibody titers between paired serum specimens.[91,161] Case records on patients with laboratory or occupational exposure should include history of use of EE or WE vaccine.

EPIDEMIOLOGY

The occurrence of an epidemic of EE depends upon the interaction of the factors determining the rate of virus transmission, including virus amplification, reservoir host populations, host susceptibility, host population immunity status, reservoir host breeding success, season, climatologic conditions, and vector population composition and abundance. Although the epidemiology of EE has been greatly elucidated since 1938, the year of the first recognized epidemic, there are still many unknown constituents which preclude a complete understanding of the natural history of the infection. Reviews of the epidemiology of EE have been published which provide detailed insights into the relationships of virus, vectors, and hosts, plus ecologic variables associated with outbreaks of EE.[33,93,117,141,142,243]

The coastal region of the eastern U.S. is the primary zone of EE virus activity. The numerous fresh-water swamp habitats in the area are an important fundamental ecologic feature; studies on EE virus within the vicinity of swamps in Alabama,[217,221] Connecticut,[242] Florida,[13,252] Louisiana,[203] Massachusetts,[109] Maryland,[202] New Jersey,[74,101] and elsewhere have provided much of the available data on the ecology and natural history of EE virus.

Most outbreaks of EE have occurred between late August and the time of the first killing frosts of the autumn, with pheasant and equine cases occurring before human cases.

Although more than 1000 isolations of EE virus from mosquitoes have been reported from the U.S. since the initial isolation in 1948 by Howitt, et al.,[126] only a few mosquito species have been shown to be important vectors of EE. The pioneering work of Chamberlain, et al.[33-35] established that a principal factor associated with transmission of EE virus to susceptible horses or human beings is the host relationship between the mosquito species and the vertebrate hosts involved. The principal endemic vector, *Culiseta melanura,* prefers to feed on birds, and only rarely feeds on horses or human beings.[53,99,153,241] Mosquitoes which frequently feed on people and horses, and which also feed on birds, are of species which are less readily infected with virus.[227] Among these, *Aedes sollicitans* and *Ae. vexans* are considered the most likely to serve as vectors during animal and human epidemics of EE.[42,58,101]

Birds were suggested as reservoir hosts for EE virus in 1935,[230] and many studies since then have provided evidence to support that hypothesis. By 1966, at least 52 species of birds were known to be naturally susceptible to EE virus.[215] Passerine birds have a generally greater potential than domestic birds or larger wild birds for serving as effective reservoir hosts.[102,113,144,147,148,214-216] The infection of these birds with EE virus has been repeatedly observed. The association of viremic immature sparrows with an outbreak of EE in pheasants was initially reported from New Jersey in 1955.[121] Studies on the natural history of EE virus in the endemic Pocomoke Cypress Swamp in Maryland showed that recently hatched birds-of-the-year soon became infected and developed EE antibody.[43]

The spread of EE among pheasants being reared in confinement has been demonstrated by contact.[121] Such transmission without vector involvement is believed to represent direct or mechanical transmission associated with picking among birds. Infection may be by ingestion of blood from a viremic bird, or by transfer and injection from one bird to another of infective blood on a bird's beak. Explosive outbreaks of EE have occurred among captive pheasants.

Several species of warm-blooded vertebrates other than horses and birds, and some cold-blooded vertebrates, have been shown to be susceptible to laboratory infections with EE virus,[104,137] and a variety of different species have been found with EE viremia or antibody titers in nature.[43,75,138] Natural and laboratory infections with EE virus have been demonstrated in swine in Georgia;[178] and naturally-occurring antibodies in swine have been reported from Massachusetts.[59] EE viremias in nonavian vertebrate hosts have been detected so infrequently, and at such low levels, that they have been considered aberrant or dead-end, rather than alternate hosts in the chain of transmission of the virus. Though an occasional horse may develop sufficient viremia to serve as an EE virus source for mosquitoes, it is thought that horses rarely play an epidemiologically important role other than as indicators of spillover of EE virus from birds.[224]

Environmental conditions such as temperature, rainfall, and unusual wind patterns are frequently mentioned in reports of EE epidemiological investigations, and attempts have been made to relate these conditions to vector population density and the outbreaks. The analysis of weather data in relation to EE epidemics occurring in the U.S. in 1963 to 1964 remains a valid hypothesis.[107] The areas of excessive rainfall in the summer months of outbreaks and also in the preceeding autumn months were strongly associated with high populations of vector mosquitoes, and consistently associated with epidemics. Weather conditions which have enhanced overwintering and subsequent summer build-ups of populations of the enzootic vector (*Cu. melanura*), and also of other mosquitoes that may serve as epidemic vectors, have been strongly associated with Massachusetts and New Jersey epidemics.

Studies on the epidemiology of EE have been reported from two areas in Brazil, but it is not known whether the virus was endemic or introduced.[155] In a tropical rain forest area near Belem, it was found that both forest-dwelling mosquitoes and birds were involved in natural cycles of EE virus; very little evidence was obtained for any involvement of forest rodents.[209] *Culex taeniopus* was the presumed vector. In the state of Sao Paulo, EE virus has caused equine epidemics, and studies have shown mosquitoes, wild birds, and wild mammals were involved.

There are still many unknown aspects of the epidemiology of EE. The principal vector species that is/are responsible for transmission to horses and human beings has/ have not been documented, although there is strong circumstantial evidence to incriminate *Ae. vexans* and *Ae. sollictans* in eastern U.S. The role of nestling birds in the summer virus amplification cycle needs clarification. The mechanisms of overwintering of the virus have not been elucidated. Evidence of birds transporting virus during migration has been reported for both southward[43,218] and northward movement,[27] but EE virus probably is not solely reintroduced into the U.S. by migratory birds. Small or large mammals (e.g., rodents or deer), bats, amphibians, and reptiles have been considered as overwintering reservoir hosts, but their importance in overwintering of EE virus remains undocumented. Similarly, larval and adult mosquitos have been tested as overwintering vectors and as transovarian transmitters of EE virus, without definitive findings as yet. Thus there are major gaps in our knowledge regarding the natural history of EE virus. There also are concurrent voids in our knowledge regarding methods for the prevention and control of EE outbreaks.

CONTROL

Prevention and Therapy In Animals and Birds

EE vaccines for immunization of horses are available from several pharmaceutical companies. They are prepared from avian origin cell culture, killed virus.[152] A bivalent vaccine containing both EE and WE virus antigen is usually used. It is formulated to be intradermally injected in 2 1.0 mℓ doses at 7 to 10 day intervals,[14]* or in 2 2.0 mℓ intramuscular doses at 4 to 8 week intervals.[240]* The control of EE among horses has recently been reviewed.[25]

Vaccine trials have been conducted in New Jersey in pheasants under epidemic and pre-epidemic conditions.[225] Each bird was administered 0.2 mℓ of undiluted, formalized chick embryo, bivalent vaccine intramuscularly in the pectoral region, using a repeating dose syringe with a single needle for 50 to 75 birds. The vaccine was termed effective under conditions of these experiments. Another recommendation is for one tenth of the equine dose of either of the EE or the bivalent EE and WE vaccine given intramuscularly in the pectoral region in pheasants at 5 to 6 weeks of age, or when they are released from the breeder houses.[164] Debeaking of young pheasants to prevent the spread of EE virus by mechanical transmission between viremic and susceptible birds is recommended as an EE preventative measure.

Prevention and Control of Human Infection

There are no licensed vaccines for immunization of human beings, but such vaccines have been considered since 1938.[5,6,44,121,156] Individuals with extensive occupational exposures may request information on the use of an investigational EE vaccine from the Center for Disease Control (CDC), Atlanta, Georgia. The vaccine is a formalin-inactivated, freeze-dried product, prepared from supernatant maintenance fluid of chick embryo monolayer cell cultures infected with a specific virus strain. The lyophilized

---

* References to products of commercial companies are for identification and as examples only, and do not constitute an endorsement by the author or Colorado State University.

material is reconstituted with sterile water, and two 0.5-mℓ doses are injected subcutaneously 28 days apart. Single annual booster doses of 0.1 mℓ administered intradermally are recommended. Significant neutralizing antibody levels have been detected in over 95% of the small number of individuals who have been vaccinated.

No specific treatment for human EE illness is available. Isolation of patients, immunization of contacts, and quarantine are not pertinent. Good nursing and supportive care, including drugs to alleviate convulsions, should be given to patients.

Vector Control

Control of mosquito populations is the only available method for minimizing the risk of EE infections. Many of the areas in which EE epidemics have occurred in the U.S. now have well organized, effective mosquito control districts; New Jersey, Massachusetts, and Florida are outstanding examples of states with such programs. Two principal approaches include: (1) control of the endemic vector *(Cu. melanura)*,[100] and (2) control of mosquitoes associated with epidemic spread (*Ae. vexans* and *Ae. sollicitans*). Control of other species of mosquitoes (*Coquillettidia perturbans* and *Culex spp.*) which develop in relatively permanent water habitats are considered in EE control. Integrated mosquito control by destruction of mosquito larval habitats, use of biological control methods, water management procedures, and application of chemical larvicides approved for such use is of major importance.[45]

Epidemic control measures for interrupting transmission of EE virus are usually directed against the adult mosquitoes. Aerial spraying of insecticides approved for such usage at ultra low volumes (ULV) is usually the method of choice for wide area control measures, usually at rates of 0.5 to 3.0 oz/acre. ULV ground applicators also have been developed by several companies, and several insecticides are labeled for such use.

Health education measures are also needed to instruct the public to avoid exposure to mosquito bites, to protect infants from being bitten, to eliminate or report potential mosquito larval habitats to mosquito control agencies, and to understand the ULV fogging or misting control procedures that are being used against the adult mosquitoes. Radio, television, and newspaper descriptions of health education items are an important part of vector control during outbreaks of EE. Personal protection from exposure to mosquito bites through the use of repellents, by screening houses, sleeping and living quarters, and by placing netting over otherwise unprotected infants in cribs and baby carriages is recommended.

PUBLIC HEALTH ASPECTS

EE is a reportable, communicable disease in most of the states in the U.S. Although the total number of cases is small, the disease can have major economic impact and cause widespread alarm. It was estimated that the hotel industry in a single city experienced a loss of $2 million due to an outbreak of EE.[17] The public concern, fear, and anxiety expressed during epidemics of EE are due in part to the severity of the clinical disease, public unfamiliarity with the disease, and the lack of effective measures for human immunization or treatment. Often the panic situation has been aggravated by publicity from the news media, even though the same media also may be playing an important role in an EE health education program.

Several approaches to EE surveillance are utilized to provide information on the level of EE virus activity in an area, and serve as a basis for initiation of preventative measures. Vector population indices obtained by several types of mosquito collection methods, EE infection rates among mosquito vector species, wild bird virus infection rates (or antibody rates among birds-of-the-year), and pheasant flock and equine EE case reports are the types of data that can be sought and obtained for surveillance. Correlation of such data in epidemic years also could provide data on threshold of parameters that preceded the cases. Field and laboratory methods for collecting, processing, and testing arthropod and vertebrate specimens for arbovirus surveillance and studies have been described in detail.[220,222] Such studies are often difficult to financially support during interepidemic periods, but through such programs, Massachusetts obtained sufficient data for serving as a basis for successfully initiating preventative measures against an outbreak of EE in 1973. In Maryland, areas with characteristics similar to those at sites deep in swamps were suggested as being most suitable for obtaining data for surveillance.[248] In Trinidad, lowland areas with high rainfall were chosen as the best sites for surveillance of EE virus activity.[236] Currently, in New Jersey, a surveillance system based on the vector potential of *Ae. sollicitans* populations and epizootic potential of *Cu. melanura* populations is being evaluated using physiological aging, gonotrophic development, and adult mosquito population indices.[239]

An unusual measure was taken to "control" an epidemic of EEE which occurred in southeastern New Hampshire during 1973. Illness among pheasants at a state-operated pheasant farm at Brentwood in Rockingham County was noted about August 1, 1973, and by mid-August horse cases were reported from nearby Exeter. Adult mosquito control measures, using aerial applications of malathion applied by ULV techniques, were undertaken in a 100-square mile area. Single isolations of EE virus were obtained from *Ae. vexans, Anopheles punctipennis, An. quadrimaculatus,* and *Cx. salinarius* and there were six isolations of the virus from *Cu. melanura** Because the focus of the epidemic was within a 100-square mile area round the pheasant farm, with EE virus isolations from pheasants, horses, and mosquitoes, the governor ordered the extermination of all the pheasants at the state farm. Approximately 12,000 pheasants were exterminated on August 25, 1973, which was 4 days before the aerial spraying of the region was completed.

WESTERN ENCEPHALITIS

R. O. Hayes

NAMES AND SYNONYMS

Western encephalitis (WE) and western equine encephalomyelitis (WEE) are the names and abbreviations that have been generally used for this arboviral disease of horses and human beings. Other terms such as sleeping sickness and horse sleeping sickness have been used. The American Committee on Arthropod-Borne Viruses recommended that the full name, western equine encephalomyelitis and the abbreviation WEE be used, but it noted that the shortened term, western encephalitis and the WE abbreviation as used in this section also were acceptable.[1]

HISTORY

Meyer, Haring, and Howitt reported scattered cases of a peculiar CNS disease in

---

* Hayes, R. O., Newhouse, V. F., Mason, A. H., Lazuick, J. S., and Francy, D. B., unpublished data, 1973.

horses during early July 1930 in the San Joaquin Valley of California.[167] The peak of the epidemic was reached during September, and no case was reported after November. Nearly 6000 horses were stricken in the epidemic, and about 50% of the cases terminated fatally. A filterable virus isolated from equine brain material was shown to be the etiologic agent. Laboratory-infected *Aedes aegypti* mosquitoes experimentally transmitted the virus to guinea pigs in 1933,[140] and to a horse which developed subsequent viremia, but a subclinical infection in 1936.[230] In 1938, the virus was recovered from the brain of a child who died of encephalitis.[123] By that same year, a variety of wild and domestic birds and animals were shown to be susceptible to intracerebral inoculation of WE virus.[124] WE virus was first isolated from naturally infected mosquitoes (*Culex tarsalis*) collected in Washington during 1941.[84] By 1942, epidemiological evidence indicated that *Cx. tarsalis* was an important vector of the virus,[85] and by 1943 it was hypothesized that WE was mosquito-borne, and that birds were the principal source of mosquito infection.[89] An excellent literature review of the history of WE through 1952 has been cited previously.[62]

In the 1940s, various studies provided evidence for the presence of WE virus in much of the western, midwestern, and central portions of the U.S. Epidemic investigations, animal and bird serologic surveys, and field virus isolation studies in mosquitoes outlined a distribution of WE, covering Arizona, California, Colorado, Minnesota, Montana, Nebraska, North Dakota, Texas, and Washington.[22,80,82,87,88,176,246] The presently known geographic distribution of WE virus includes western and central Canada and U.S., eastern U.S., Mexico, Guyana, Brazil, Uruguay, and Agrentina.[186]

During 1941, a major epidemic of WE with at least 2792 cases occurred in Mainitoba and Saskatchewan and the north-central U.S.[49] The recorded attack rates ranged from 22.9 to 171.5 (mean = 55.3) per 100,000 population and the case fatality rates from 8.1 to 15.3 (mean = 12.4). It is now known that the virus is endemic in western Canada and causes epidemics in horses and human beings at irregular intervals.[47,62,68] The Central Valley of California, eastern Colorado, and the high plains of Texas have been long recognized as endemic areas of WE virus activity, and both human and equine cases have occurred there over many years.[71,79,90,190,207] WE epidemics also have been reported from Iowa, Kansas, Nebraska, Utah, Washington, and Wyoming.[115] Although the virus is endemic in birds in the eastern U.S., only sporadic cases among horses have been reported from states such as Florida,[132] Maryland, and Virginia.[26]

WE virus is seldom associated with devastating outbreaks among captive pheasants, as has been so frequent in EE. However, WE virus has been isolated during outbreaks of encephalitis among Chukar partridges being reared in Florida,[180] among pheasants in Massachusetts,[56] and from a Chukar in Rhode Island.[44]

Human laboratory infections with WE virus have been uncommon, but two of the five laboratory infections known to have occurred up to 1968 resulted in death.[81,94]

ETIOLOGY

Classification

WE virus is classified in the *Alphavirus* genus of the family Togaviridae along with EE.[60,61] As there are for EE virus, antigenic differences also exist among strains of WE virus, and strains isolated in the eastern U.S. have sufficient antigenic differences from WE strains isolated in the western U.S. that they can be readily separated.[136] These differences among strains of WE virus may be important in the selection of proper screening antigens in serologic surveys, and in determining the patterns of virulence.

Characteristics

WE is a single-stranded RNA virus with spherical symmetry enclosed in a lipoprotein envelope. It can be inactivated by sodium deoxycholate, ether, or chloroform.[60,130] It is unstable at room temperature, but can be preserved by freezing at −70°C. At −62°C, no significant loss in virus titer was recorded in positive mosquito suspensions stored 33 months in diluting fluid containing 33% normal rabbit serum in phosphate-buffered normal saline (pH 7.4) containing antibiotics.[188,208] The structure and development of WE virus in cell cultures of chick embryo fibroblasts was described in detail in 1961;[170] replication is by budding in the host cytoplasm. WE virus may be readily cultured in a variety of cell lines as well as in many types of susceptible laboratory animals.[30] Large and small size plaques often are produced in cell cultures, and the types of host cells, the inocula dilutions, and the composition of culture media have been shown to affect plaque size.[30,154,158]

DEFINITION

Western encephalitis is a zoonotic infection, primarily of wild birds, that produces acute CNS disease in infected horses and human beings. The infections may be apparent or inapparent, and they are transmitted among susceptible hosts by mosquitoes. Infected vertebrates which develop viremias with sufficiently high titers of virus in their blood to be infective for the hematophagous arthropods are termed reservoir hosts. The infected mosquitoes capable of transmitting the virus from one vertebrate host animal to another are termed vectors. Thus WE is categorized as a vector-borne disease.

ANIMAL INFECTION

Horses
WE virus is generally less virulent for horses than EE virus; the case fatality rate may be as high as 50%, but averages from 20 to 30%.[196] The incubation period in horses is 1 to 3 weeks, a febrile reaction is usually the first clinical manifestation of the infection, and CNS involvement with signs of fatique, somnolence with occasional excitability, followed by incoordinated movement of the limbs, disturbed equilibrium, grinding of teeth, and in severe cases, encephalitic signs including inability to swallow, paralysis of the lips and inability to stand or rise may or may not occur.[167]

There are no gross lesions that may be considered characteristic of WE in horses.[210] Histologically, the virus causes degenerative changes in neurons, culminating in necrosis. The gray matter of the brain around affected neurons also may become edematous and diffusely infiltrated with lymphocytes, neutrophils, and some erythrocytes. Lymphocytic perivascular cuffing may extend into the white matter, which is otherwise unaffected. Small neuronal intranuclear acidopholic inclusion bodies have been described. The lesions in the gray matter are most prominent in the olfactory bulb, thalamus, pons, medulla, and in both the dorsal and the ventral columns of the spinal cord. Diagnosis should be confirmed by virus isolation or serological laboratory tests, since neither the clinical nor the pathological signs can differentiate WE from EE with certainty.[91,161]

Other Birds and Mammals,
Domestic poultry have been shown to be highly susceptible to infection, but not to disease.[124] Swine have been shown to develop clinical illness. Experimentally infected cattle did not develop detectable viremia, but did form antibody.[250] None of the domestic animal species is currently believed to be important as a reservoir host of WE virus for arthropod vectors.

Laboratory studies have shown that a wide variety of wild birds and mammals are susceptible to WE virus, serve as hosts for virus multiplication, undergo viremia, develop immunological responses, and display different levels of clinical or pathological responses. Most of the natural isolations of WE virus obtained from vertebrate hosts have been from wild birds, and only a relatively few isolations of virus have been obtained from a wide variety of mammal species.[186] For many years, the suckling mouse (usually 1 to 3 days of age) was used as the laboratory animal for isolation of arboviruses; suckling hamsters, guinea pigs, and wet chicks (less than 1 day old) also have been successfully used for isolation of WE virus strains.[91]

HUMAN INFECTIONS

During 1952, a total of 348 human cases of WE were laboratory confirmed in an encephalitis epidemic in California. The clinical features of the disease were analyzed and considered within four age groups,[149] with the following clinical categories:

1. Less than 1 year of age: fever and convulsions
2. One through four years old: fever, headache, vomiting, drowsiness, irritability, restlessness, muscle rigidity, tremors, and sometimes convulsions
3. Five through fourteen years old: headache, fever, drowsiness, nausea, vomiting, muscular pain, photophobia, limitation of neck and back flexion, and sometimes convulsions and intention tremors
4. Fifteen or more years old: drowsiness, lethargy, malaise, fever, stiffness of back and neck, usually with severe occipital headache, disturbance of vision, nausea, photophobia, and vertigo

The attack rate during the 1952 epidemic was reported to be 36.1/100,000 among residents of the Central Valley. One third of the confirmed we cases were among infants of less than 1 year of age.[122] Generally, similar clinical findings in WE patients during sporadic outbreaks in the endemic area of Texas during 1963, 1964, and 1965 have been reported in detail.[181,207]

Subclinical infections among human beings also are known to be relatively common in regions where WE virus is endemic in nature and where recognized cases of the disease occur. WE antibody was detected among 10.9% of a population sampled in Colorado,[151] and 8.6% of a population sampled in northern Utah,[131] indicating that human infections were occurring during years in which clinical cases of WE had not been recognized or reported. More detailed studies of subclinical infections with antibody conversion from negative to positive, have been conducted in California and Texas.[67,108]

Follow-up studies on survivors of WE virus infections have revealed that neurologic, intellectual, and psychologic sequellae may occur. A strong correlation has been reported between the age of the patient at the time of illness and the incidence and severity of permanent residuum. In California, long-term studies of patients who were less than 1 month of age at onset showed residual brain damage among 55% of the survivors; of those 1 month of age at onset, 12% had severe sequellae; of those 2 to 11 months old, 6% had severe sequellae, whereas not more than 5% of the stricken adults had severe sequellae.[64,197] Similar results were obtained from a study of a small number of confirmed patients in Texas.[51]

The lesions of WE virus infection in human patients involve widespread microscopic changes throughout the central nervous system.[179] Lesions are found particularly in the gray matter in the thalamus, striated body nuclei, pontine nuclei, Purkinje cells, and molecular cells of the cerebellar cortex. Ganglion cells are involved in many different regions and layers of the cerebral cortex, and lesions also are found in the spinal cord.[64] Perivascular cuffing with leukocytes and small focal areas of necrosis and inflammatory infiltration also have been reported.[200] Specific WE diagnosis cannot be made upon the basis of pathologic examination of neuroanatomic material.

Diagnosis of clinical cases based upon virus isolation and serologic procedures has been previously described for EE,[91] and the same criteria are used for WE.[161] A refined serologic procedure for differentiating maternal antibodies and antibodies being produced in response to a WE infection in infants has been described to aid in the early diagnosis of infection.[118]

EPIDEMIOLOGY

Many studies of the natural history and the epidemiology of WE virus have provided insight into ecological details and interrelationships involved in the maintenance of this virus in nature and in the conditions associated with epidemics of the disease.[33,93,117,141,142] The geographic distribution of large WE epidemics has been essentially west of the Mississippi River,[21,93,117,141,142,196,210] but special ecologic conditions have provided for either permanent or temporary WE virus activity in many eastern states including Alabama,[217] Florida,[132,180] Georgia,[38] Maryland,[132,202] Massachusetts,[56,103] New Jersey,[75,121] Rhode Island,[44] and Virginia.[26]

The seasonal occurrence of WE outbreaks is associated with the warm summer and autumn months, during which populations of vector mosquitoes increase and become abundant. WE epidemics often begin to involve people in June or early July, whereas the occurrence of human EE cases usually does not begin until August. The onset of a killing frost usually terminates epidemics of the disease. The dynamics of WE virus activity during the overwintering period, the spring amplification cycle, the summer period of activity, and the fall subsidence have been reviewed and discussed.[116] It has been reported that most WE outbreaks have occurred at or above the area of 21.1°C (70°F) June isotherms, and indices have been suggested for use in predicting endemic activity levels of WE virus using the dates when 10 and 50 day-degrees above 21.1°C are first accumulated.[114] Excessive summer rainfall is conducive to build-up of large vector mosquito populations.[163] In California, the role of temperature in relation to virus activity, the amount of river flow correlated with *Cx. tarsalis* populations, plus rainfall and snowpack effect upon vector populations have been reported.[191]

Since the initial isolation of WE virus from mosquitoes in 1941 by Hammon, et al.,[84] there have been thousands of isolations of the virus from mosquitoes of many genera.[186] The greatest number of isolations have been from *Cx. tarsalis*, and this mosquito has been repeatedly shown to be the principal vector of the virus in the western U.S.[40,110,191] In the eastern U.S., the mosquito from which WE virus has been most frequently isolated has been *Cu. melanura*.[31,37,38,103,202] The widespread detection of virus-infected *Cx. tarsalis*,[186] along with information on the significance of vector infection and vector infectivity,[188] on the seasonal feeding pattern and host preferences of this species on vector virus infection thresholds,[227] and on the correlations between the *Cx. tarsalis* population indexes, *Cx. tarsalis* infection rates, and the vertebrate infection rates[110] have comprised epidemiologic evidence that substantiates the importance of that species of mosquito as the most important vector of WE virus. *Cx. tarsalis* has been shown in laboratory studies to have a low threshold of infection with WE virus and following exposure, to have high infection and lifelong transmission potential.[36,233] The age and history of blood feeding in a population of mosquitoes have been shown to be related to its potential for virus infection and virus transmission;[188] whereas, mosquito population densities alone may have no direct relationship to virus activity.[16] Direct relationships between *Cx. tarsalis* WE virus infection rates, WE virus infection and antibody rates among wild and domestic birds and mammals, and infections among people have been documented.[96,110] In three principal endemic areas of California, Colorado, and Texas, a higher rate of *Cx. tarsalis* feeding on mammals during the summer months when the mosquito populations are the highest[183] has been shown to enhance its role as a WE vector.[112,228,229]

Many other species of mosquitoes have been found infected with WE virus in nature, including: *Cx. quinquefasciatus, Cu. inornata, Ae. melaminon, Ae. nigromaculis, Ae. vexans, Anopheles freeborni,* and *Psorophora* species. However, one or a variety of factors have been shown to limit the importance of these species as vectors of WE virus, including natural resistance to virus infection, poor transmitting efficiency, specific host preferences which limit the likelihood of feeding on reservoir hosts and subsequently upon people or horses, single-brood (univoltine) physiologic characteristics that reduce the chance for repeatedly taking blood meals, and seasonal population patterns which exclude the mosquito species from becoming involved in epidemic transmission cycles.

Mosquitoes often have been considered as having a possible role in the overwintering of WE virus. Various studies have provided evidence that they probably are not involved as overwintering-hibernating adult hosts,[9,10,201] and the possible role of transovarial transmission in maintaining WE virus has not been delineated.[184]

A variety of other insects (also mites) have intermittently yielded WE virus in nature.[117] These infections have been thought to be of a mechanical type and not of epidemiological importance. Recently, an *Alphavirus* related to WE virus has been shown to overwinter in cliff swallow nest bugs (*Oeciacus vicarius*) in Colorado.[106] To date, the virus strains isolated appear to be antigenically distinct from WE virus.

In laboratory studies, horses, rodents, rabbits, and other mammals have been experimentally infected, and many species have been shown to develop viremias without apparent illness.[95,186,190,226] Usually these viremias are of such low level to be insufficient to infect most vector species, and generally of a duration of only for 2 to 5 days. Field studies on wild mammals in many geographic regions have shown that they are seldom found infected with WE virus, and that WE antibody prevalence rates are considerably lower than those detected among birds from the same locations.[24,53,83,129,149] The information obtained to date indicates that small mammals are not basically involved in the maintenance of WE virus in nature. However, small mammals are important indicator hosts of levels of virus activity as they become infected during periods of epidemic transmission. It should be noted that the black-tailed jack rabbit (*Lepus californicus*) appears to be one of the most frequently involved mammals.[19,96,129]

Numerous data are available from both laboratory and field studies on wild birds, indicating their importance as the principal reservoir hosts for WE virus. Although the earliest studies led to a hypothesis that domestic fowl were the principal reservoir hosts of WE virus,[89] additional data have subsequently indicated that wild birds more frequently develop effective viremias than domestic fowl.[145,160,190,212,214] Laboratory studies show that a wide range of wild bird species are susceptible to the virus, and that they circulate WE virus at high titers.[186] The period of viremia among birds is generally of 3 to 6 days duration.[113] The virus titers attained, the clinical response, and the lesions elicited vary greatly with the age and the species of birds.[124,142]

Scattered reports of WE virus infections among nestling birds in Colorado from 1950 through 1953,[40,211] in California during 1958,[187] and in Texas in 1965[110] led to greater consideration of the role of nestling birds rather than adult birds in transmission of the virus. Studies in California and Colorado showed a preference by *Cx. tarsalis* for younger birds.[15] Subsequent field and laboratory studies showed that nestling house sparrows were involved in the amplification cycles and in summer epidemic cycles in Hale County, Texas and that nestling house sparrows were excellent sentinel hosts for monitoring WE virus activity.[119,120]

Birds have been considered as possible overwintering reservoir hosts because of occasional winter isolations from resident birds, and because of evidence of chronic persistent infections.[97,194] It has also been hypothesized that migrant birds reintroduce WE virus into the U.S. each year upon returning from their southern wintering grounds in subtropical or tropical areas.[148,184]

Amphibians and reptiles also have been investigated to determine their roles as reservoir and overwintering hosts for WE virus.[124,184] There are reports of natural isolations of WE virus from snakes and frogs collected in Utah and in Saskatchewan.[23,70,213] WE virus also has been isolated from a tortoise in Texas.[223] Laboratory studies on poikilothermic vertebrates have demonstrated that they are susceptible to WE virus infections and that they undergo prolonged viremias which could carry the virus through the winter and infect mosquitoes the following year.[18,69,234,235] However, field data from highly endemic areas of California, Colorado, and Texas have not supported an epidemiological role for amphibians and reptiles in the maintenance of WE virus in nature.

Many epidemiologic factors involved in the maintenance, amplification, and epidemic cycling of WE are known because of long-term ecologic studies in California,[189] in Colorado,[211] and in Texas,[110,120] but much more remains to be delineated.

CONTROL

Prevention and Therapy

Prevention of WE in horses may be enhanced by annual immunization with commercially available vaccines. Vaccines are available for WE and each of the other specific equine arboviruses, and as bivalent (WE-EE) and trivalent combinations (WE-EE-VE). Some formulations also include tetanus toxoid.[152] The vaccines are administered intradermally at 7- to 10-day intervals,[14] or intramuscularly at 4- to 8-week intervals.[240] Annual revaccination each spring is recommended in endemic areas.[225] An attenuated live WE virus vaccine has been developed and field tested for immunization of horses, and although the results indicated a high efficacy,[128,199] it has not been licensed and is not commercially available.

No WE vaccine is licensed for immunization of people, but investigative vaccines containing WE virus grown in chick embryos have been tested for immunization of laboratory workers with satisfactory results.[4,6,159] A procedure for producing WE vaccine from avian chick embryo cell culture that is similar to the methods used for EE vaccine has been developed and demonstrated to develop good immunological responses in laboratory and field workers subject to a high risk of infection.[198] Information on the use of investigational human vaccines may be obtained from the Center for Disease Control, Atlanta, Georgia.

No specific treatment is available for WE illness. Supportive nursing care is important, especially in cases with severe neurologic illness.

Vector Control

Control of vector mosquitoes is the most effective method of reducing the risk of WE in human beings, and organized mosquito control districts have been shown to be most efficient and effective ways to obtain protection for populations at risk. Lower rates of arbovirus activity were found among indicator animals within areas of California treated for mosquito control, than were found in the untreated areas, as early as 1948.[86] WE attack rates in human beings in western Texas were 4 to 5 times lower in an area having an effective mosquito control program than in adjacent untreated areas,[117] and in 1958, successful mosquito control activities contributed towards aborting a WE epidemic in California.[187] Extensive use of insecticides for agricultural purposes in Washington was shown to reduce vector populations and decrease WE virus activity.[193] In 1968, Reeves indicated that when mosquito control procedures in California could reduce female *Cx. tarsalis* population indices to 1 or less per light-trap night, then WE virus would "probably disappear from the environment."[185] Ultra low volume applications of insecticide have been used for controlling adult mosquitoes during encephalitis epidemics, but repeated treatments at about 2-day intervals probably would be necessary to attain continuing protection against mosquito infiltration from adjacent untreated areas.[169] Integrated mosquito control programs are needed to eliminate aquatic habitats that are breeding places of mosquito vectors, to biologically or chemically control mosquito larvae and adults, to reduce exposure to mosquito bites by screening of houses and sleeping quarters, to encourage avoidance of being bitten (through the use of repellants or avoiding exposure to mosquitoes), and to educate the public about mosquito control and preventive measures.

PUBLIC HEALTH ASPECTS

In fiscal year 1975—76, nearly $70 million were spent by 533 mosquito control agencies in Canada and the U.S.,[48] aimed, in part at least, at reducing the risk of WE and other arboviral diseases. In 1969, at least $1.25 million were expended to prevent an encephalitis outbreak in California, in addition to the estimated $10 million already scheduled that year for mosquito control.[182] More recently, dire consequences for WE epidemics in California were predicted because of reduced tax support for mosquito control in areas of increasingly large populations of susceptible persons.[192] In a study of the benefits and costs of physically modifying playa lakes, which are one of the principal *Cx. tarsalis* larval habitats in western Texas, the estimated health benefits were only 2.9% of the modification costs on a 20-year projection, and were 3.5% for a 40-year projection. The average annual health benefits to the study area from the playa lake modifications were estimated at $146,000,[78] while the estimated costs for each epidemic year in one county in the same study area had been above $320,000.[51]

Social services that need to be considered in relation to WE epidemics include fears and psychological problems aggravated by uncertainties of diagnosis and prognosis, costs of medical, hospital, and convalescent care, and long-range medical and social planning for patients with severe sequellae, including instruction and assistance with special therapy and equipment, with care for patients at home, and with psychological adaptation to handicaps.[157]

Cases of primary viral encephalitis, including WE, are among those required by regulations in most states to be reported to the local health authorities. Such reporting is a necessary part of surveillance measures designed for early detection and control of communicable diseases.

WE virus surveillance involves reporting of suspected equine and human cases, and monitoring vector populations or infection indexes among arthropods and/or vertebrate reservoir hosts.[55,105] Evidence of current WE virus activity in young chickens,[114,116,171,190,253] pigeons,[174,251] quail, and in other avian species[84] has frequently been used to obtain seasonal transmission indexes and to assay recent serological conversions among sentinel animals. For example, in South Dakota during 1975, evidence of

125. **Howitt, B. F., Bishop, L. K., Gorrie, R. H., Kissling, R. E., Hauser, G.H., and Trueting, W. L.,** An outbreak of equine encephalomyelitis, eastern type, in southwestern Louisiana, *Proc. Soc. Exp. Biol. Med.,* 68, 70, 1948.

126. **Howitt, B. F. Dodge, H. R., Bishop, L. K., and Gorrie, R. H.,** Recovery of the virus of eastern equine encephalomyelitis from mosquitoes (*Mansonia perturbans*) collected in Georgia, *Science,* 110, 141, 1949.

127. **Howitt, B. F., Dodge, H. R., Bishop, L. K., and Gorrie, R. H.,** Virus of eastern equine encephalomyelitis isolated from chicken mites (*Dermanyssus gallinae*) and chicken lice (*Eomenacanthus stramineus*), *Proc. Soc. Exp. Biol. Med.,* 68, 622, 1948.

128. **Hughes, J. P. and Johnson, H. N.,** A field trial of a live-virus western encephalitis vaccine, *J. Am. Vet. Med. Assoc.,* 150, 1967.

129. **Hutson, G. A., Howitt, B. F., and Cockburn, T. A.,** Encephalitis in Midwest. VII. Neutralizing antibodies in sera of small wild mammals. Colorado, 1950, *Proc. Soc. Exp. Soc. Med.,* 78, 290, 1951.

130. **Jawetz, E., Melnick, J. L., and Adelberg, E. A.,** *Review of Medical Microbiology,* 6th ed., Lange Medical Pub., Los Altos, Calif., 1964, 325.

131. **Jenkins, A. A. and Donath, R.,** The 1958 encephalitis outbreak in northern Utah. I. Human aspects, *Mosq. News,* 19, 221, 1959.

132. **Jennings, W. L., Allen, R. H., and Lewis, A. L.,** Western equine encephalomyelitis in a Florida horse, *Am. J. Trop. Med. Hyg.,* 15, 96, 1966.

133. **Jordan, R. A., Wagner, J. A., and McCrumb, F. R.,** Eastern equine encephalitis: report of a case with autopsy, *Am. J. Trop. Med. Hyg.,* 14, 470, 1965.

134. **Jungherr, E. L., Helmboldt, C. F., Satriano, S. F., and Luginbuhl, R. E.,** Investigations of eastern equine encephalomyelitis. III. Pathology in pheasants and incidental observations in feral birds, *Am. J. Hyg.,* 67, 10, 1958.

135. **Karabatsos, N.,** Antigenic relationships of group A arboviruses by plaque reduction neutralization testing, *Am. J. Trop. Med. Hyg.,* 24, 527, 1975.

136. **Karabatos, H., Bourke, A. T. C., and Henderson, J. R.,** Antigenic variation among strains of western equine encephalomyelitis virus, *Am. J. Trop. Med. Hyg.,* 12, 408, 1963.

137. **Karstad, L.,** Reptiles as possible reservoir hosts for eastern encephalitis virus, *N. Am. Wildl. Conf. Trans.,* 26, 186, 1961.

138. **Karstad, L., Vadlamudi, S., Hanson, R. P., Trainer, D. O., and Lee, V. H.,** Eastern equine encephalitis studies in Wisconsin, *J. Infect. Dis.,* 106, 53, 1960.

139. **Karstad, L. H., Fletcher, O. K., Spalatin, J., Roberts, R., and Hanson, R. P.,** Eastern equine encephalomyelitis virus isolated from three species of Diptera from Georgia, *Science,* 125, 395, 1957.

140. **Kelser, R. A.,** Mosquitoes as vectors of the virus of equine encephalomyelitis, *J. Am. Vet. Med. Assoc.,* 82, 767, 1933.

141. **Kissling, R. E.,** The arthropod-borne viruses of man and other animals, *Ann. Rev. Microbiol.,* 14, 261, 1960.

142. **Kissling, R. E.,** Host relationships of the arthropod-borne encephalitides, *Ann. N. Y. Acad. Sci.,* 70, 320, 1958.

143. **Kissling, R. E., Chamberlain, R. W., Eidson, M. E., and Bucca, M. A.,** Studies on the North American arthropod-borne encephalitides. II. Eastern equine encephalitis in horses, *Am. J. Hyg.,* 60, 237, 1954.

144. **Kissling, R. E., Chamberlain, R. W., Sikes, R. K., and Eidson, M. E.,** Studies on the North American arthropod-borne encephalitis. III. Eastern equine encephalitis in wild birds, *Am. J. Hyg.,* 60, 251, 1954.

145. **Kissling, R. E., Chamberlain, R. W., and Sudia, W. D., and Stamm, D. D.,** Western equine encephalitis in wild birds, *Am. J. Hyg.,* 66, 48, 1957.

146. **Kissling, R. E. and Rubin, H.,** Pathology of eastern equine encephalomyelitis, *Am. J. Vet. Res.,* 12, 100, 1951.

147. **Kissling, R. E., Rubin, H., Chamberlain, R. W., and Eidson, M. E.,** Recovery of virus of eastern equine encephalomyelitis from blood of purple grackle, *Proc. Soc. Exp. Biol. Med.,* 77, 398, 1951.

148. **Kissling, R. E., Stamm, D. D., Chamberlain, R. W., and Sudia, W. D.,** Birds as winter hosts for eastern and western equine encephalomyelitis viruses, *Am. J. Hyg.,* 66, 42, 1957.

149. **Kokernot, R. H., Shinefield, H. R., and Longshore, W. A., Jr.,** The 1952 outbreak of encephalitis in California. Differential diagnosis, *Calif. Med.,* 79, 73, 1953.

150. **Konzelmann, F. W.,** Pathology of eastern encephalitis, *Public Health News (New Jersey),* 41, 128, 1960.

151. **LaVeck, G. D., Winn, J. F., and Welch, S. F.,** Inapparent infection with western equine encephalitis virus: epidemiological observations, *Am. J. Public Health,* 45, 1409, 1955.

152. **LeClaire, R. A. and Johnston, D. E.,** *A Comprehensive Desk Reference of Veterinary Pharmaceuticals and Biologicals 76/77,* F. A. Davis, Philadelphia, 1976, 6—2.

153. **LeDuc, J. W., Suyemoto, W., Eldridge, B. F., and Saugstad, E. S.,** Ecology of arboviruses in a Maryland freshwater swamp. II. Blood feeding patterns of potential mosquito vectors, *Am. J. Epidemiol.,* 96, 123, 1972.

154. **Lee, Y. T. and Park, Y. S.,** The enhancement of plaque formation in tissue culture (Vero-cell) by arboviruses, *N. Med. J.,* 12, 51, 1969.

155. **Lopes, O. and Sacchetta, L.,** Epidemiological studies on eastern equine encephalitis virus in Sao Paulo, Brazil, *Rev. Inst. Med. Trop., Sao Paulo,* 16, 253, 1974.

156. **Maire, L. F., III, McKinney, R. W., and Cole, F. E., Jr.,** An inactivated eastern equine encephalomyelitis vaccine propagated in chick-embryo cell culture. I. Production and testing, *Am. J. Trop. Med. Hyg.,* 19, 119, 1970.

157. A Manual for the Control of Communicable Diseases in California, California State Department of Public Health, Sacramento, Calif., 1971, 145.

158. **Marshall, I. D., Scrivani, R. P., and Reeves, W. C.,** Variations in the size of plaques produced in tissue culture by strains of western equine encephalitis virus, *Am. J. Hyg.,* 76, 216, 1962.

159. **Maurer, F. D., Kuttler, K. L., Yager, R. H., and Warner, A.,** Immunization of laboratory workers with purified trivalent equine encephalomyelitis vaccine, *J. Immunol.,* 68, 109, 1952.

160. **McClure, H. E., Reeves, W. C., and Hammon, W. McD.,** Ornithological Investigations, in *Epidemiology of the Arthropod-Borne Viral Encephalitides in Kern County, California, 1943—1952,* Reeves, W. C. and Hammon, W. McD., Eds., University of California Press, Berkeley, 1962, 109.

161. **McGowan, F. E., Jr., Bryan, J. A., and Gregg, M. B.,** Surveillance of arboviral encephalitis in the United States, 1955—1971, *Am. J. Epidemiol.,* 97, 199, 1973.

162. **McLintock, J.,** The arbovirus problem in Canada, *Can. J. Public Health,* 67, 8, 1976.

163. **McLintock, J., Burton, A. N., Dellenberg, H., and Rempel, J. G.,** Ecological factors in the 1963 outbreaks of western encephalitis in Saskatchewan, *Can. J. Public Health,* 57, 561, 1966.

164. The Merck Veterinary Manual, Siegmund, O. H., Ed., 4th ed., Merck and Co., Rahway, N. J., 1973, 251, 1032.

165. **Merrill, M. H., Lacaillade, D. W., Jr., and Ten Broeck, C.,** Mosquito transmission of equine encephalomyelitis, *Science,* 80, 251, 1934.

166. **Merrill, M. H. and Ten Broeck, C.,** The transmission of equine encephalomyelitis virus by *Aedes aegypti, J. Exp. Med.,* 62, 687, 1935.

167. **Meyer, K. F., Harring, C. M., and Howitt, B.,** The etiology of epizootic encephalomyelitis of horses in the San Joaquin Valley, 1930, *Science,* 74, 227, 1931.

168. **Miller, L. D., Pearson, J. E., and Muhm, R. L.,** A comparison of clinical manifestations and pathology of the equine encephalitides: VEE, WEE, EEE, *U.S. Animal Health Assoc. Proc.,* 77, 629, 1973.

169. **Mitchell, C. J., Hayes, R. O., Holden, P., Hill, H. R., and Hughes, T. B., Jr.,** Effects of ultra-low volume applications of malathion in Hale County, Texas. I. Western encephalitis virus activity in treated and untreated towns, *J. Med. Entomol.,* 6, 155, 1969.

170. **Morgan, C., Howe, C., and Rose, H. M.,** Structure and development of viruses as observed in the electron microscope. V. Western equine encephalomyelitis virus, *J. Exp. Med.,* 113, 219, 1961.

171. **Morgante, O., Shemanchuk, J. A., and Windsor, R.,** Western encephalomyelitis virus infection in "indicator" chickens in southern Alberta, *Can. J. Comp. Med.,* 33, 227, 1969.

172. **Morris, C. D., Whitney, E., Bast, T. F., and Deible, R.,** An outbreak of eastern equine encephalomyelitis in upstate New York during 1971, *Am. J. Trop. Med. Hyg.,* 22, 561, 1973.

173. **Moulthrop, I. M. and Gordy, B. A.,** Eastern viral encephalomyelitis in chukar (*Alectoris graeca*), *Avian Dis.,* 4, 4, 1960.

174. **Olson, T. A., Kennedy, R. C., Rueger, M. E., Price, R. D., and Schlottman, L. L.,** Evaluation activity of viral encephalitides in Minnesota through measurement of pigeon antibody response, *Am. J. Trop. Med. Hyg.,* 10, 266, 1961.

175. **Parikh, G. C., Colburn, Z. D., and Larson, D. R.,** 1967 eastern equine encephalitis outbreak on a South Dakota pheasant farm, *Bacteriol. Proc.,* 69, 159, 1969.

176. **Philip, C. B., Cox, H. R., and Fountain, J. H.,** Protective antibodies against St. Louis encephalitis virus in the serum of horses and man, *Public Health Rep.,* 56, 1388, 1941.

177. **Pigford, C. A.,** Infectious encephalitis in West Texas — report of an epidemic, *Tex. Med.,* Sept. 1957, 708.

178. **Pursell, A. R., Packham, J. C., Cole, J. R., Stewart, W. C., and Mitchell, F. E.,** Naturally occurring and artificially induced eastern encephalomyelitis in pigs, *J. Am. Vet. Med. Assoc.,* 161, 1143, 1972.

179. **Quong, T. L.,** The pathology of western equine encephalomyelitis, *Can. J. Public Health,* 33, 300, 1942.

180. **Ranck, F. J., Jr., Gainer, J. H., Hanley, J. E., and Nelson, S. L.,** Natural outbreak of eastern and western encephalitis in pen-raised chukars in Florida, *Avian Dis.,* 9, 8, 1965.

181. Ray, C. G., Sciple, G. W., Holden, P., and Chin, T. D. Y., Acute febrile CNS illness in an endemic area of Texas, *Public Health Rep.*, 82, 785, 1967.
182. Reeves, W. C., The impact of mosquito-borne diseases on organized mosquito control districts, *Mosq. News*, 31, 319, 1971.
183. Reeves, W. C., Mosquito vector and vertebrate host interaction: the key to maintenance of certain arboviruses, in *Ecology and Physiology of Parasites, A Symposium*, Fallis, A. M., Ed., University of Toronto Press, 1971, 223.
184. Reeves, W. C., Overwintering of arboviruses, *Prog. Med. Virol.*, 17, 193, 1974.
185. Reeves, W. C., A review of developments associated with the control of western equine and St. Louis encephalitis in California during 1967, *Proc. Calif. Mosquito Control Assoc.*, 36, 65, 1968.
186. Reeves, W. C., Western equine encephalomyelitis, in *International Catalogue of Arboviruses*, 2nd ed., Publ. No. (CDC) 75-8301, Berge, T. O., Ed., Public Health Service, U. S., Department of Health Education, and Welfare, Atlanta, 1975, 759.
187. Reeves, W. C., Bellamy, R. E., Geib, A. F., and Scrivani, R. P., Analysis of the circumstances leading to abortion of a western equine encephalitis epidemic, *Am. J. Hyg.*, 80, 205, 1964.
188. Reeves, W. C., Bellamy, R. E., and Scrivani, R. P., Differentiation of encephalitis virus infection rates from transmission rates in mosquito vector populations, *Am. J. Hyg.*, 73, 303, 1961.
189. Reeves, W. C. and Hammon, W. McD., *Epidemiology of the Arthropod-Borne Viral Encephalitides in Kern County, California, 1943—1952*, University of California Press, Berkeley, 1962, 257.
190. Reeves, W. C. and Hammon, W. McD., Infection in other vertebrate hosts, in *Epidemiology of the Arthropod-Borne Viral Encephalitides in Kern County, California, 1943—1952*, Reeves, W. C. and Hammon, W. McD., Eds., University of California Press, Berkeley, 1962, 46.
191. Reeves, W. C. and Hammon, W. McD., The role of arthropod vectors, in *Epidemiology of the Arthropod-Borne Viral Encephalitides in Kern County, California, 1943—1952*, Reeves, W. C. and Hammon, W. McD., Eds., University of California Press, Berkeley, 1962, 75.
192. Reeves, W. C. and Milby, M. M., Encephalitis viral activity and vector populations in California — presented future concerns, *Proc. Calif. Mosq. and Vector Control Assoc.*, 47, 1, 1979.
193. Reeves, W. C., Hammon, W. McD., Lazarus, A. S., Brookman, B., McClure, H. E., and Doetschman, W. H., The changing picture of encephalitis in the Yakima Valley, Washington, *J. Infect. Dis.*, 90, 291, 1952.
194. Reeves, W. C., Hutson, G. A., Bellamy, R. E., and Scrivani, R. P., Chronic latent infections of birds with western equine encephalomyelitis virus, *Proc. Soc. Exp. Biol. Med.*, 97, 733, 1958.
195. Report on Infectious Equine Encephalitis in the United States in 1947, Bureau of Animal Industry, U.S. Department of Agriculture, abstracted in *J. Am. Vet. Med. Assoc.*, 113, 123, 1948.
196. Rhodes, A. J. and von Rooyen, C. E., *Textbook of Virology*, 4th ed., Williams & Wilkins, Baltimore, 1962, 300.
197. Riggs, N. and Finley, K. H., Sequelae of western encephalitis and St. Louis encephalitis, *Calif. Vector Views*, 7, 35, 1960.
198. Robinson, D. M., Berman, S., Lowenthal, J. P., and Hetrick, F. M., Western equine encephalomyelitis vaccine produced in chick embryo cell cultures, *Appl. Microbiol.*, 14, 1011, 1966.
199. Roca-Garcia, M., Jungherr, E. L., Johnson, H. N., and Cox, H., An attenuated strain of western equine encephalitis virus as a possible live immunizing agent, *U.S. Livestock Sanit. Assoc. Proc.*, 68, 24, 1964.
200. Rozdilsky, B., Robertson, H. E., and Chorney, J., Western encephalitis. Report of eight fatal cases: Saskatchewan epidemic, 1965, *Can. Med. Assoc. J.*, 98, 79, 1968.
201. Rush, W. A., Kennedy, R. C., and Eklund, C. M,. Evidence against winter carry-over of western equine encephalomyelitis virus by *Culex tarsalis*, *Mosq. News*, 23, 285, 1963.
202. Saugstad, E. S., Dalrymple, J. M., and Eldridge, B. F., Ecology of arboviruses in a Maryland freshwater swamp. I. Population dynamics and habitat distribution of potential mosquito vectors, *Am. J. Epidemiol.*, 96, 114, 1972.
203. Schaeffer, M. and Arnold, E. H., Studies on the North American arthropod-borne encephalitides. I. Introduction. Contributions of newer field-laboratory approaches, *Am. J. Hyg.*, 60, 231, 1954.
204. Schaeffer, M., Kissling, R. E., Chamberlain, R. W., and Vanella, J. M., Studies on the North American arthropod-borne encephalitides. IV. Antibody in human beings to the North American arthropod-borne encephalitides, *Am. J. Hyg.*, 60, 266, 1954.
205. Scherer, W. F., Campillo Sainz, C., de Mucha Macias, J., Rubio-Brito, R., Miura, T., Dickerman, R. W., Warner, D. W., and Dyer, M., Serological survey for neutralizing antibodies to eastern equine and western equine encephalitis viruses in man, wild birds and swine in southern Mexico during 1961, *Am. J. Trop. Med. Hyg.*, 15, 211, 1966.
206. Scherer, W. F., Madalengoitia, J., Flores, W., and Acosta, M., The first isolations of eastern encephalitis, group C, and Guana group arboviruses from the Peruvian Amazon region of western South America, *Pan. Am. Health. Organ. Bull.*, 9, 19, 1975.

207. **Sciple, G. W., Ray, C. G., Holden, P., La Motte, L. C., Jr., Irons, J. V., and Chin, T. D. Y.,** Encephalitis in the high plains of Texas, *Am. J. Epidemiol.,* 87, 87, 1968.

208. **Scrivani, R. P. and Reeves, W. C.,** Comparison of hamster kidney and chick embryo tissue cultures with mice for primary isolation of western equine and St. Louis encephalitis viruses, *Am. J. Trop. Med. Hyg.,* 11, 539, 1962.

209. **Shope, R. E., Homobono Paes de Andrade, A., Bensabath, G., Causey, O. R., and Humphrey, P. S.,** The epidemiology of EEE, WEE, SLE, and Turlock viruses, with special reference to birds, in a tropical rain forest near Belem, Brazil, *Am. J. Epidemiol.,* 84, 467, 1966.

210. **Smith, H. A., Jones, T. C., and Hunt, R. D.,** *Veterinary Pathology,* 4th ed., Lea & Febiger, Philadelphia, 1974, 356.

211. **Sooter, C. A., Howitt, B. F., Gorrie, R., and Cockburn, T. A.,** Encephalitis in midwest. IV. Western equine encephalomyelitis virus recovered from nestling wild birds in nature, *Proc. Soc. Exp. Biol. Med.,* 77, 393, 1951.

212. **Sooter, C. A., Howitt, B. F., and Gorrie, R.,** Encephalitis in Midwest. IX. Neutralizing antibodies in wild birds of midwestern states, *Proc. Soc. Exp. Biol. Med.,* 79, 507, 1952.

213. **Spalatin, J., Connell, B., Burton, A. N., and Gollop, B. J.,** Western equine encephalitis in Saskatchewan reptiles and amphibians, 1961—1963. *Can. J. Comp. Med. Vet. Sci.,* 28, 131, 1964.

214. **Stamm, D. D.,** Arbovirus studies in birds in South Alabama, 1959—1960, *Am. J. Epidemiol.,* 87, 127, 1968.

215. **Stamm, D. D.,** Relationships of birds and arboviruses, *Auk,* 83, 84, 1966.

216. **Stamm, D. D.,** Susceptibility of bird populations to eastern, western and St. Louis encephalitis viruses, 13th Int. Ornithol. Cong. Proc., 1963, 591.

217. **Stamm, D. D., Chamberlain, R. W., and Sudia, W. D.,** Arbovirus studies in South Alabama 1957—1958, *Am. J. Hyg.,* 76, 61, 1962.

218. **Stamm, D. D. and Newman, R. J.,** Evidence of southward transport of arboviruses from the U.S. by migratory birds, *Am. Microbiol.,* 11, 123, 1963.

219. **Steele, J. H. and Habel, K.,** Observations on an outbreak of encephalomyelitis in Panama, *J. Am. Vet. Med. Assoc.,* 61, 263, 1947.

220. **Sudia, W. D. and Chamberlain, R.W.,** Collection and Processing of Medically Important Arthropods for Arbovirus Isolation, Center for Disease Control, U.S. Department of Health, Education, and Welfare, Atlanta, 1967, 29.

221. **Sudia, W. D., Chamberlain, R. W., and Coleman, P. H.,** Arbovirus isolations from mosquitoes collected in South Alabama 1959—1963, and serologic evidence of human infection, *Am. J. Epidemiol.,* 87, 112, 1968.

222. **Sudia, W. D., Lord, R. D., and Hayes, R. O.,** Collection and Processing of Vertebrate Specimens for Arbovirus Studies, Center for Disease Control, U.S. Department of Health, Education, and Welfare, Atlanta, 1970, 65.

223. **Sudia, W. D., McLean, R. G., Newhouse, V. F., Johnston, J. G., Jr., Miller, D. L., Trevino, H., Bowen, G. S., and Sather, G.,** Epidemic Venezuelan equine encephalitis in North America in 1971. Vertebrate field studies, *Am. J. Epidemiol.,* 10, 36, 1975.

224. **Sudia, W. D., Stamm, D. D., Chamberlain, R. W., and Kissling, R. E.,** Transmission of eastern equine encephalitis to horses by *Aedes sollicitans* mosquitoes, *Am. J. Trop. Med. Hyg.,* 5, 802, 1956.

225. **Sussman, O., Cohen, D., Grende, J. E., and Kissling, R. E.,** Equine encephalitis vaccine studies in pheasants under epizootic and pre-epizootic conditions, *Ann. N. Y. Acad. Sci.,* 70, 328, 1958.

226. **Syverton, J. T. and Berry, G. P.,** Host range of equine encephalomyelitis susceptibility of the North American cottontail rabbit, jack rabbit, field vole, woodchuck, and opossum to experimental infection, *Am. J. Hyg.,* 32(B), 19, 1940.

227. **Tempelis, C. H.,** Host-feeding patterns of mosquitoes with a review of advances in analysis of blood meals by serology, *J. Med. Entomol.,* 11, 635, 1975.

228. **Tempelis, C. H., Francy, D. B., Hayes, R. O., and Lofy, M.,** Variations in feeding patterns of seven Culicine mosquitoes on vertebrate hosts in Weld and Larimer Counties, Colorado, *Am. J. Trop. Med. Hyg.,* 16, 111, 1967.

229. **Tempelis, C. H., Reeves, W. C., Bellamy, R. E., and Lofy, M.,** A three year study of the feeding habits of *Culex tarsalis* in Kern County, California, *Am. J. Trop. Med. Hyg.,* 14, 170, 1965.

230. **Ten Broeck, C., Hurst, E. W., and Traub, E.,** Epidemiology of equine encephalitis in the eastern United States, *J. Exp. Med.,* 62, 677, 1935.

231. **Ten Broeck, C. and Merrill, M. H.,** A serological difference between eastern and western equine encephalomyelitis viruses, *Proc. Soc. Exp. Biol. Med.,* 31, 217, 1933.

232. **Theiler, M. and Downs, W. G.,** *The Arthropod-Borne Viruses of Vertebrates,* Yale University Press, New Haven, 1973, 95.

233. **Thomas, L. A.,** Distribution of the virus of western equine encephalomyelitis in the mosquito vector, *Culex tarsalis, Am. J. Hyg.,* 78, 150, 1963.

234. Thomas, L. A. and Eklund, C. M., Overwintering of western equine encephalomyelitis virus in experimentally infected garter snakes and transmission to mosquitoes, *Proc. Soc. Exp. Biol. Med.,* 105, 52, 1960.

235. Thomas, L. A., Eklund, C. M., and Rush, W. A., Susceptibility of garter snakes (*Thamnophis* Spp.) to western equine encephalomyelitis virus, *Proc. Soc. Exp. Biol. Med.,* 99, 698, 1958.

236. Tikasingh, E. S., Worth, C. B., Jonkers, A. H., Aiken, T. H. G., and Spence, L., A three year surveillance of eastern equine encephalitis virus activity in Trinidad, *West Indian Med. J.,* 22, 24, 1973.

237. Tyzzer, E. E., Sellards, A. W., and Bennett, B. L., Occurrence in nature of "equine encephalomyelitis" in the ring-necked pheasant, *Science,* 88, 505, 1938.

238. Van Roekel, H. and Clarke, M. K., Equine encephalomyelitis from ring-necked pheasant, *J. Am. Vet. Med. Assoc.,* 94, 466, 1939.

239. New Jersey State Mosquito Control Commission, Vector Surveillance Report, Period Spring Survey June-July, Intensive Survey Aug 1—2, 1977, 2, 1, 1977.

240. Veterinary Biologicals and Pharmaceuticals Catalog, Fort Dodge Laboratories, Fort Dodge, Iowa, 1975, 11.

241. Wallis, R. C., Howard, J. J., Main, A. J., Jr., Frazier, C., and Hayes, C., An increase of *Culisita melanura* coinciding with an epizootic of eastern equine encephalitis in Connecticut, *Mosq. News,* 34, 63, 1974.

242. Wallis, R. C., Jungherr, E. L., Luginbuhl, R. E., Helmboldt, C. F., Satriano, S. F., Williamson, L. A., and Lamson, A. L., Investigations of eastern equine encephalomyelitis. V. Entomologic and ecologic field studies, *Am. J. Hyg.,* 67, 35, 1958.

243. Wallis, R. E. and Main, A. J., Jr., Eastern equine encephalitis in Connecticut, progress and problems, *Mem. Connecticut Entomol. Soc.,* 1974, 117.

244. Webster, H. D. F., Eastern equine encephalomyelitis in Massachusetts. Report of two cases, diagnosed serologically, with complete clinical recovery, *N. Engl. J. Med.,* 255, 267, 1956.

245. Webster, L. T. and Wright, F. H., Recovery of eastern equine encephalomyelitis virus from brain tissue of human cases of encephalitis in Massachusetts, *Science,* 88, 305, 1938.

246. Wenner, H. A., Kamitsuka, P., Kramer, M. C., Cockburn, T. A., and Price, E. R., Encephalitis in the Missouri River basin. II. Studies on a focal outbreak of encephalitis in North Dakota, *Public Health Rep.,* 66, 1075, 1951.

247. White, A., Berman, S., and Lowenthal, J. P., Inactivated eastern equine encephalomyelitis vaccines prepared in monolayer and concentrated suspension chick embryo cultures, *Appl. Microbiol.,* 22, 909, 1971.

248. Williams, J. E., Young, O. P., and Watts, D. M., Relationships of density of *Culiseta melanura* mosquitoes to infection of wild birds with eastern and western encephalitis viruses, *J. Med. Entomol.,* 11, 352, 1974.

249. Williams, J. E., Young, O. P., Watts, D. M., and Reed, T. J., Wild birds as eastern (EEE) and western (WEE) equine encephalitis sentinels, *J. Wildl. Dis.,* 7, 188, 1971.

250. Winn, J. F., Kaplan, W., Palmer, D. F., and Solomon, G., Sensitivity of swine and cattle to artificial infection with western equine encephalitis virus, *J. Am. Vet. Med. Assoc.,* 133, 464, 1958.

251. Winn, J. F., Palmer, D. F., and Kaplan, W., Development and persistence of western equine encephalitis virus antibodies in experimentally infected pigeons, *Cornell Vet.,* 47, 337, 1957.

252. Winn, J. F. and Scatterday, J. E., Equine encephalomyelitis in Florida, *J. Am. Vet. Med. Assoc.,* 125, 115, 1954.

253. Wong, F. C., Lillie, L. E., and Drysdale, R. A., Sentinel flock monitoring procedures for western encephalomyelitis in Manitoba — 1975, *Can. J. Public Health,* 67 (Suppl. 1), 15, 1976.

VENEZUELAN EQUINE ENCEPHALOMYELITIS (VEE)

S. McConnell and R. O. Spertzel

NAME AND SYNONYMS

The English-language name of the disease is Venezuelan equine encephalomyelitis, in both human and animal patients. In Central and South America, it is called *peste loca* or *derrengadera*.[40]

HISTORY

The early history of VEE virus infection is highlighted by a few scattered outbreaks of disease, confirmed in only a few instances by actual virus isolations. The records[22] show that the first publication on VEE was based on clinical diagnosis only.[1] The etiology was established in 1938 when the virus was first isolated by Kubes and Rios,[33] and characterized by Beck and Wyckoff.[5]

A number of outbreaks have been recorded since this early period. During the years 1935 and 1959, VEE was reported from Colombia, Venezuela, Trinidad, and Peru, reflecting a limited geographic distribution. The major movement of the virus occurred during the decade from 1961 to 1971, with extension of its geographic range northward. Epidemics or outbreaks have now been recorded in 11 countries extending from Peru to the central part of Texas.

VEE exists in two general forms, a severe epidemic form, in which horses are the principal hosts, and an endemic form, in which rodents appear to be the main hosts. Epidemic strains are believed to have been involved in the horse epidemics reported between 1939 and 1959 in Venezuela, Ecuador, Peru, Colombia, Argentina, Trinidad, and probably in Guyana and Mexico. A rapidly spreading variant epidemic strain (IB) was recognized in Ecuador and Peru in 1969; the origin of this variant remains undetermined but is postulated to have existed, perhaps in endemic form in the highlands of Ecuador. In May and June 1969, the same strain was identified in Guatemala and spread from there to Honduras, El Salvador and Nicaragua (1969), Costa Rica and Mexico (June-July, 1970), and southern U.S. (April 1971).[33,42,44,48]

Endemic or sylvatic foci of VEE have been recognized in eight countries extending from Colombia in the south to the Everglades of Florida in North America.[58] In addition to the original isolate from Venezuela and the isolate from Florida, two additional subtypes of VEE have also been isolated and identified from Brazil, Trinidad, and Surinam.[58] The accuracy of the early information on episodes of VEE is complicated by current knowledge of the existence of a number of strains of VEE with recorded differences in pathogenicities. The known geographic distribution of the sylvatic types of VEE virus is shown in Figure 1. For a more complete history of the origin and distribution of VEE, the reader is referred to the articles by Groot[22] and Kubes.[4]

ETIOLOGY

Venezuelan equine encephalomyelitis is caused by an arthropod-borne virus maintained in the ecosystem through biological transfer between vectors and susceptible hosts. The virus replicates in both its vertebrate hosts and in haemophagous arthropods and is transmitted to new hosts following an extrinsic incubation period.

Classification

The VEE virus is classified as a species in the VEE complex,[9,57] of the Alphavirus

(Group A) genus of the family Togaviridae. Four subtypes are recognized: (I) VEE, original, (II) Florida, (III) Mucambo, and (IV) Pixuna. Within subtype I are three epidemic variants: (IA) Trinidad, (IB) Ica, IC, and two sylvatic variants, ID and IE. Of the five subtype I variants, only three (IA, IB, and IC) are considered to be of epidemiologic importance.[17] Infection with one of these variants generally results in immunity to the others. Subtypes 1A through 1E have always been recognized as VEE virus. Subtype II is sometimes referred to as the Florida strain.[12] Subtype III is better known as Mucambo virus, and subtype IV is commonly identified as Pixuna virus.[46]

Characteristics

VEE virus subtypes have single-stranded RNA genomes with a molecular weight of 4 million daltons. The virions are replicated in the cytoplasm, and mature by budding from cytoplasmic membranes. The virions have icosahedral symmetry with 32 capsomeres; intact virions are between 60 and 70 nm in diameter, and consist of 30 to 35 nm nucleocapsids contained within membranous envelopes.[38] The virions of VEE, like other alphaviruses, contain two polypeptides with molecular weights of 30,000 and 53,000.[13] VEE virus shows serological cross reaction in the hemagglutination-inhibition (HI) test with alphaviruses, especially EEE and WEE. VEE virus multiplies in cell cultures of the arthropod vectors.

The virus is lethal for weanling and suckling mice, guinea pigs, hamsters, and wet chicks, and is excreted in their nasal secretions, urine, and feces. It produces a cytopathogenic effect in many types of cell cultures: duck and chicken embryo fibroblasts, Vero, HeLa, and baby hamster kidney cell cultures. VEE virus is sensitive to heat, acid, and to lipid solvents such as chloroform and ether.[2]

DEFINITION

VEE is a mosquito-borne viral disease of variable severity in susceptible hosts. The disease affects primarily horses and human beings.[29] A wide variety of other hosts and vectors may be infected.[35,52] In horses, the infection may be manifested as an acute, fulminating disease without encephalitis signs, terminating in death or recovery, or the more classical disease with a progressing encephalitis. In human patients, an influenza-like syndrome predominates with an accompanying high fever and frontal headache.

ANIMAL INFECTION

Clinical

The viruses of the VEE complex are pathogenic for a variety of animal species under natural and experimental conditions. The host-virus interactions vary from inapparent or subclinical to severe, ending in paralysis and death. This variation in response is a function of both the virus strains and susceptibility or resistance of the host species.

Clinically inapparent to mild disease is seen in a number of domestic animal species. The disease in cattle, sheep, and goats[24,55] exposed to the Texas 1B isolate is subclinical and is characterized by a transient temperature rise and leucopenia. Such a response suggests that these species of animals serve, as suggested by Johnson,[26] as "guests" rather than as "hosts" for the virus.

Dogs[24,53] and swine[55] experimentally infected with VEE virus have responded in a more positive manner. The disease was mild, and clinical signs usually included anorexia, depression, huddling, reluctance to move, aggressive behavior, and death. In experimentally infected dogs, the incubation period was short, 12 to 24 hr, followed

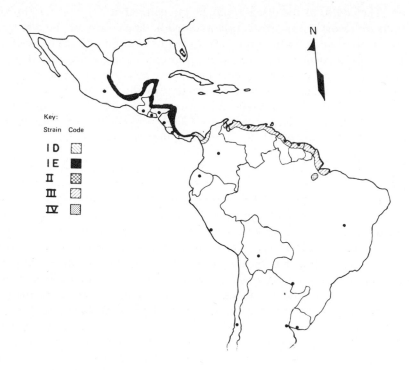

FIGURE 1.   Geographical distribution of VEE subtypes and variant strains.

by a marked elevation in temperature to 40.5 to 41°C, returning to base values in 4 to 5 days. Viremia preceeded pyrexia by 12 to 24 hr and terminated abruptly in 48 to 72 hr. Recovery was rapid and uneventful. Dogs challenged with the Texas 1B isolate did not show the aggressive behavior and death pattern elicited by exposure to the Trinidad 1A isolate.[53] Swine exposed to the Texas 1B isolate showed a mild febrile response, anorexia, depression, and leucopenia. Recovery was rapid and no untoward sequelae were observed. The severity of disease in dogs and swine is virus strain dependent. Cattle are not as severely affected by VEE virus as are the other two species.

In horses, two general forms of the disease exist, a fulminating form, in which signs of acute febrile systemic disease predominate, and an encephalitic form, in which encephalitic signs dominate. The severity may vary from (a) subclinical with no overt manifestations, to (b) moderate with anorexia, high fever, and depression, to (c) severe nonfatal disease characterized by anorexia, high fever, stupor, weakness, staggering, blindness, and occasionally with permanent sequelae, to (d) severe fatal disease with the same sequence of symptoms but terminating in death.[28,29,30,35] Not all fatal cases of VEE in horses are accompanied by definite neurologic signs. An incubation period of 1 to 5 days precedes the rise in body temperature to 103 to 105°F, accompanied by hard, rapid pulse, loss of appetite, and depression. Although fever is the earliest sign of VEE infection, the onset is insidious with inappetence and mild excitability as the earliest outward signs of disease. Frequently, a rapid progression ensues with depression, weakness, and ataxia occurring, followed by overt signs of encephalitis such as muscle spasms, chewing movements, uncoordination, and convulsions. Early encephalitic signs include loss of both cutaneous neck reflexes and visual response; diarrhea and colic may also develop. Some animals stand in an extremely depressed or somnolent position and show no responsiveness to their surroundings, others may wander aimlessly or press against solid objects. A braced stance or circling may occur late in the disease. The course of the disease may be interrupted at any point in this sequence of symptoms by recovery, or prostration and death. The course of the disease may be rapid, with death ensuing within hours after the observation of first signs (during epidemics reports of sudden death are not uncommon), or more protracted, with dehydration and extreme loss of weight occurring prior to an encephalitic death or recovery.

The length of the incubation period is related to the size of the virus inoculum. Typically, detectable viremia precedes the onset of fever by 12 to 24 hr, and persists for 2 to 4 days. Onset of encephalitic signs follows the peak of the viremia by 2 to 4 days, and occurs at a time when the circulating virus is disappearing, and body temperature is falling.

Pathology

Gross pathological lesions of VEE in sheep, goats, cattle, swine, and dogs are minimal to nonexistent. The macroscopic appearance of CNS tissues in horses which have succumbed to experimental VEE have varied from no visible lesions to extensive necrosis and hemorrhages. Lesions reported in other tissues have been too variable to be of diagnostic significance. Early in the course of the disease, leukopenia of varying degree and duration occurs and, on necropsy, severe depletion of the myeloid elements of the bone marrow, spleen, and lymph nodes can be seen. Necrotic foci involving the acinar cells of the pancreas are a variable finding. Necrotic lesions may involve the adrenal cortex, liver, myocardium, and the walls or small- and medium-sized blood vessels.[20] In the CNS, a diffuse necrotizing meningoencephalitis may be seen, ranging from a slight perivascular mixed-cellular reaction to marked vascular necrosis with hemorrhages, gliosis, and frank neuronal necrosis.[37,39] Endothelial cells may be swollen, accompanied by perivascular edema and extravasation of blood. Lesions are usually most severe in the cerebral cortex, becoming progressively less severe toward the cauda equina. The degree and severity of the CNS lesions vary with the progression and duration of the clinical signs. Microlesions in experimentally infected domestic animals other than horses are nonexistent.

Diagnosis

Field diagnosis of VEE can rarely be made. In domestic animal species other than horses, signs observed are minimal and not suggestive of VEE. In horses, the initial signs may go undetected, and index cases are often missed. Reports of sudden deaths of apparently healthy animals are not uncommon. When encephalitic signs predominate, the disease in horses is indistinguishable from Eastern equine encephalomyelitis (EEE) and Western equine encephalomyelitis (WEE).[29] In contrast to EEE or WEE, herd morbidity with VEE is higher, and diarrhea and colic are more common.[8,17]

Specific diagnoses can be made by laboratory procedures, i.e., virus isolation or demonstration of specific rises in hemagglutination-inhibiting or neutralizing antibodies with paired (acute and convalescent) sera. Frequently, animals die before convalescent sera can be obtained. Virus may be isolated from brain, pancreas, or whole blood of dead or dying animals, but the frequency of success is low. A herd diagnosis by viral isolation and identification from the blood of horses which are in contact with suspect animals, and which show marked elevations in temperature, is often possible.

A variety of diseases may produce signs which resemble one or more of the clinical signs of VEE infection, but since none of the clinical signs of VEE (including encephalitis) are pathognomonic for VEE, an all-encompassing list of differential diagnoses is virtually impossible. The more obvious diseases which may be confused with VEE include toxic encephalitis, mineral poisoning, botulism, African horse sickness, EEE, and WEE. During the Texas epidemic of 1971, VEE was initially diagnosed presumptively as equine infectious anemia, colic, and shock. Any conditions which produce fever and depression, with or without signs of CNS involvement, must be considered in differential diagnosis.

HUMAN INFECTION

Clinical

In human beings, the disease occurs most commonly as a mild to severe respiratory illness, associated with severe frontal headache, muscle pains, and high fevers. Overt encephalitis is rare, and occurs primarily in children. The incubation period ranges from 1 to 4 days. Earliest signs are fever, headache followed shortly by, or associated with myalgia (especially in the lower back and legs), and chills. Vomiting occurs as an early sign in some patients. During the course of the illness, sore throat, diarrhea, and drowsiness may also develop.[7] Most patients recover in 3 to 5 days without sequelae. Encephalitis occurs in approximately 0.4/100 infections in adults and 4.0/100 infections in children.[41] Mortality is usually very low, but rates as high as 36/1000 have been reported in epidemics in the absence of adequate medical care.[4]

Pathology

Histopathologic lesions in patients who died following neurologic signs consisted of leptomeningitis, interstitial pneumonia, bronchopneumonia, hemorrhagic infarction and passive congestion of lungs, inflammatory infiltration of the liver with fatty metamorphosis, and centrolobular necrosis.[22]

Diagnosis

Diagnosis is usually made by virus isolation from whole blood drawn during the first 2 to 3 days after onset of clinical signs, or by recognition of seroconversion using paired acute and convalescent sera.[7]

EPIDEMIOLOGY

Occurrence

VEE virus is endemic throughout major portions of Central (ID, IE) and South America (III, IV) and parts of North America (IE, II), as shown in Figure 1.[58] While major epidemics have occurred in these regions, no evidence of the virus has been found during interepidemic periods. The maintenance in nature of the variants of VEE during interepidemic periods remains one of the unresolved mysteries of this disease.[17]

Reservoirs

The host patterns of VEE have been shown to relate to the antigenic variants involved and their relative virulence for different hosts. Over 150 different animal species have been found infected naturally in the field, or have been infected artificially in the laboratory. Horses have been of the highest importance in the explosive spread of epidemic VEE (IA, IB, and IC). Infected human beings develop high enough viremic levels to infect mosquitoes, but probably play little role in transmission of the virus. Dogs and their wild relatives, and swine, develop high levels of viremia and may serve as reservoir hosts of the virus. Cats, sheep, goats, cattle, and bats have been shown to function as propagative hosts. Birds, although developing only relatively low viremic levels, may infect mosquitoes, and have been considered as playing a possible role in long distance transport of the virus. During epidemics, many other domestic and wild species have been shown to seroconvert to VEE, but have not been considered to play a role in its transmission.[7,14,16,17,28,35]

Small rodents appear to be the reservoir hosts of endemic VEE (ID, IE, II, III, IV), the virus smoldering in subclinical infections and rarely producing clinical disease in these animals. In endemic VEE foci, where in depth studies have been conducted, ground dwelling rodents of several species have been regularly implicated.[27] Cotton mice (*Peromyscus gossypinus*), which are found only in the southern U.S., and cotton rats (*Sigmodon hispidus*) are two of the principal hosts for VEE virus subtype II (Florida) in the Everglades ecosystem.[34] Rodent hosts for subtype III (Mucumbo) include spring rats (*Proechimys spp.*), and rice rats (*Oryzomys capito*).[45,56] Similar spectra of VEE infections in rodents have been reported from Panama, Mexico, and Colombia.[21,35,43] The exact role of rodents in the ecology of VEE infections remains to be determined. They do serve as a large potential population of susceptible hosts with a short lifespan and rapid turnover rate.[27] Horses may be infected, but no clinical disease has been recognized in them. Human infections are occasionally characterized by mild disease. A number of other species of vertebrates, opossums, bats, birds, and monkeys (in the Amazon basin) have shown serological evidence of infection.[17,28]

Transmission

Epidemic VEE — During epidemics involving horses and people, many species of mosquitoes, *Culex, Anopheles, Mansonia, Deinocereites, Psorophora,* and *Aedes spp.* have been shown to be infected. Black flies (*Simuliidae*) have been suspected.[10] During the epidemics of 1969, the virus (variant IB) is believed to have been transported from Ecuador over 2000 km to Guatemala, possibly through infected adult *Cx. nikini* mosquitoes carried on floating water lettuce, or through infected birds, particularly herons.[3]

Endemic VEE — Variants, ID, IE, and subtypes II, III, and IV have been invariably associated with endemic VEE in a rodent-mosquito-rodent cycle, with people and horses only incidental victims of the virus. The vectors appear to be limited to *Culex,* Subgenus *Melanoconion spp.,* and *Deinocereites spp.* mosquitoes, which act as highly efficient vectors in rodent to rodent transmission.[10,17] Generally the virus appears to cycle in rodents where the highly efficient *Culex (Melanoconion) spp.* vector mosquitoes are present.[10,17,19]

Direct contact transmission among horses has been demonstrated on occasions, but is not postulated as playing an important role in the maintenance of epidemics or in spread to new foci.[31] Recent studies have demonstrated transplacental transmission of the virus in horses, but the epidemiological significance of this finding has not been elucidated.[6] Human exposures by inhalation have occurred in numerous laboratory accidents, but no evidence exists to suggest that direct human to human transmission occurs in nature.[4,25,41,47]

Environment

The relative abundance of vectors and susceptible hosts provides VEE virus with some degree of protection to environmental pressures. Mechanisms for survival include a relatively long extrinsic incubation period in the vector, averaging 3 weeks at 26.5°C; possibly transovarian transmission in mosquitoes or overwintering in hibernating animals; and long range transport in infected birds. For the endemic virus, environmental conditions play a major role in regulating vector mosquito populations, as feral rodent populations are relatively ubiquitous. In subtropical and tropical America where the efficient transmitters *Culex (Melanconium) spp.* are present, endemic foci of VEE are likely to be found. The habitats of these mosquitoes are located in regions of moderate to high rainfall throughout the year,[15,54] are generally near sea level, and are extremely focal in nature.[18,54] Epidemic VEE has caused disease in horses from at, or near, sea level (Venezuela, Mexico, U.S.) to high altitudes (Colombia and Guatemala), and in regions with low to moderate rainfall.[15] Recent evidence has suggested a unique beach environment in which an epidemic strain of VEE virus may have been transmitted by the crab hole mosquito *Deinocereites pseudes*.[17]

Human Host

Small human epidemics in which no horses were involved have been reported in human-mosquito-human cycles with variant ID in Panama and the Canal Zone. At least 118 laboratory-acquired human infections with one death have been recorded, with 24 cases following inhalation of dust contaminated with lyophilized virus following accidental breakage of nine ampules in a single accident, placing the VEE virus into a category as a definite laboratory biohazardous agent.[25,47]

CONTROL

Prevention and Treatment

There is no specific treatment other than good supportive care for human or equine patients. Effective control must be based on restricting the movement of viremic animals from infected to noninfected areas, mosquito-control measures during periods of epidemics, and immunization of susceptible horses. Immunization with an attenuated virus vaccine can provide long term protection to horses.[50,51] Inactivated VEE vaccines for animal use also have been developed and are in widespread use in the U.S. No specific, preventive measures for human beings exist, except for high risk laboratory personnel for whom the attenuated virus vaccine is recommended.[17,25,36,51] No preventive measures for horses or people have been indicated for endemic VEE areas.

Regulatory Measures

During nonepidemic periods, no regulatory measures exist. Continual surveillance of vector mosquitoes is recommended for countries with risk of epidemic VEE.

Epidemic Measures

During epidemics, restriction of movement of horses between epidemic zones and noninfected areas is of prime importance in controlling the spread of VEE. Because of the high levels of VEE viremia in horses ($\geqslant 10^6$/mℓ blood), introduction of infected animals into noninfected areas may readily establish new foci of infection.[50] Mosquito control measures are an essential adjunct to the regulation of horse movement during epidemics. Experience has been that vector control in the absence of other control measures has only slowed the spread of VEE to horses and man, but has not halted it.[11]

Large-scale equine immunization programs have been highly effective in protecting horses, and in conjunction with vector control and horse movement control, in controlling epidemics.[46] Currently, an attenuated VEE vaccine is widely used and strongly recommended in many areas of the Americas where the virus is active, and used to protect nonepidemic areas where a high risk of infection is present.[50,51] During the 1971 epidemics, the U.S. government emergency program coordinated the vaccination of 2,854,191 horses across the southern half of the U.S.; vector control programs in 22 counties of Texas and 2 parishes of Louisiana; and a 22-state surveillance program. In a cooperative effort to halt the spread of VEE, 200,000 doses of horse vaccine were supplied by the U.S. government to the Mexican government. During 1972, no cases in horses were documented in the U.S.; two human cases which occurred in California resulted from exposures in Mexico. No human or animal cases were reported in the U.S. from 1973 to 1976. From 1972 to 1975, approximately 2/3 to 3/4 of the horses in Mexico were vaccinated against VEE.[3]

Eradication

Eradication measures for endemic strains have not been attempted, and probably would not be successful. In epidemic areas, when successful control measures, vaccination, vector control, and horse movement regulation have been achieved, the epidemics have been halted and no evidence for persistence of the epidemic virus has been found.

Health Education

No specific measures have been indicated. During epidemics, or threat of epidemics, personal measures to avoid mosquito bites, including local mosquito control and use of repellents, may be indicated.

PUBLIC HEALTH ASPECTS

Economic and Social Impact

VEE virus infections are of importance in human medicine, veterinary medicine, public health, and economies of countries in general. As cited by Groot,[22] an estimated 60,000 human cases of VEE were recorded in Colombia, Venezuela, and Ecuador between 1962 and 1970, with over 1,200 neurologic cases and approximately 500 deaths occurring in these populations. During the 1969 to 1970 outbreak in Mexico, 16,922 human cases were reported, with 42 deaths. In the Texas outbreak in 1971, 84 confirmed cases of VEE were recorded. The figures on equine losses reflect the economic effect of this disease in veterinary medicine. The estimated number of equine deaths for all outbreaks 1967 to 1971 ranges from a low of 113,000 to a high of 164,000. This loss is staggering for replacement of animals which die, for losses in income derived from work and transportation uses of these animals, and for burdensome costs of treatment, care, management, medicine, and other expenditures in efforts to save affected animals. Preventive measures are costly, but where adequately applied, the benefits have far outweighed the costs.

Reporting

VEE is now a reportable disease in the U.S.; however, the difficulty encountered in distinguishing this disease from EEE and WEE, which are both widely distributed, makes a complete task difficult. An extensive surveillance system is in operation to monitor movement of the virus in both domestic and feral animals, and to identify, as accurately as possible, all vector species involved in the extension of disease. The necessity for surveillance cannot be underestimated. The role of silent vertebrate host(s) involved in epidemics still needs to be defined, as does the possible role of such unusual hosts as the vampire bats, *Desmodus rotundus,* virus types involved in outbreaks and their specific host interactions, and the role of birds and of people in the movement of VEE virus from area to area.

The primary means of controlling VEE continues to be the use of effective vaccines. The attenuated TC-83 strain of VEE virus, which has been used in over 10 million horses, has served to contain VEE virus transmission in the U.S., Mexico, Central America, and in a number of other countries. The complete cessation of VEE activity in Texas, and the maintenance of this status, speaks well for presently implemented programs for control and prevention of this disease. Immunization of horses serves two purposes, to protect individual horses (and as a consequence reduce economic losses from this disease), and secondly to remove horses as reservoir hosts for mosquito vectors, and thus to halt the extension of this infection to such other hosts as people, dogs, and other mammals.

REFERENCES

1. **Albornoz, J. E.,** La pest loca de las bestiae, (enfermedad de Borna), *Bol. Agr. Suppl.,* 26, 1, 1935.
2. **Andrewes, C. H. and Pereira, H. G.,** in *Viruses of Vertebrates,* 3rd. ed. Balliere Tindall, London, 1972, 82.
3. The origin and spread of Venezuelan equine encephalomyelitis, Animal and Plant Health Inspection Service, U.S. Department of Agriculture, Hyattsville, Md., 1973, 1.
4. **Avilan Rovira, J. (Discussant),** in *Venezuelan Encephalitis,* Pan American Health Organization, Washington, D.C., 1972, 189.
5. **Beck, E. C. and Wyckoff, R. W. G.,** Venezuelan equine encephalomyelitis, *Science,* 88, 530, 1938.
6. **Benenson, A. S.,** 56th Annual Meeting, Gorgas Memorial Institute of Tropical and Preventive Medicine, Washington, D.C., 1979.
7. **Bowen, G. S.,** Human disease: USA, in *Venezuelan Encephalitis,* Pan American Health Organization, Washington, D.C., 1972, 231.
8. **Bryne, R. J.,** The control of Eastern and Western arboviral encephalomyelitis of horses, in *Equine Infectious Diseases III — Proc. 3rd Int. Conf. Equine Infectious Disease, Paris, 1972,* Bryans, J. T. and Allen, G. P., Eds., S. Karger, Basel, 1973, 115.
9. **Casals, J.,** Antigenic characteristics of Venezuelan equine encephalitis (VEE) virus: relation to other viruses, in *Venezuelan Encephalitis,* Pan American Health Organization, Washington, D.C., 1972, 77.
10. **Chamberlain, R. W.,** Venezuelan equine encephalitis: infection of mosquitoes and transmission, in *Venezuelan Encephalitis,* Pan American Health Organization, Washington, D.C., 1972, 144.
11. **Chamberlain, R. W.,** Venezuelan encephalitis prevention and vector control, in *Venezuelan Encephalitis,* Pan American Health Organization, Washington, D.C., 1972, 390.
12. **Chamberlain R. W., Sudia, W. D., Coleman, P. H., and Work, T. H.,** Venezuelan equine encephalitis virus from South Florida, *Science,* 145, 272, 1964.
13. **Dalrymple, J. M.,** Biochemical and biophysical characteristics of Venezuelan equine encephalitis virus, in *Venezuelan Encephalitis,* Pan American Health Organization, Washington, D.C., 1972, 56.
14. **Davis, M. H., Hogge, A. L., Corristan, E. C., and Ferrell, J. F.,** Mosquito transmission of Venezuelan equine encephalomyelitis virus from experimentally infected dogs, *Amer. J. Trop. Med.,* 15(2), 227, 1966.
15. **Dickerman, R. W., (Discussant),** in *Venezuelan Encephalitis,* Pan American Health Organization, Washington, D.C., 1972, 313.
16. **Dickerman, R. W., Baker, G. J., Ordonez, J. F., and Scherer, W. F.,** Venezuelan equine encephalomyelitis viremia and antibody responses of pigs and cattle, *Am. J. Vet. Res.,* 34, 357, 1973.
17. **Eddy, G. A., Martin, D. H., and Johnson, K. M.,** Epidemiology of the Venezuelan equine encephalomyelitis virus complex, in *Proc. 3rd. Int. Conf. Equine Infectious Disease, Paris, 1972,* S. Karger, Basel, 1973, 126.
18. **Frack, P. T. and Johnson, K. M.,** An outbreak of Venezuelan equine encephalitis in man in the Panama Canal Zone, *Amer. J. Trop. Med.,* 19(5), 860, 1970.
19. **Galindo, P.,** Endemic vectors of Venezuelan encephalitis, in *Venezuelan Encephalitis,* Pan American Health Organization, Washington, D.C., 1972, 249.
20. **Gochenour, W. S., Jr.,** The comparative pathology of Venezuelan encephalitis virus infection in selected animal hosts, in *Venezuelan Encephalitis,* Pan American Health Organization, Washington, D.C., 1972, 113.
21. **Grayson, M. A. and Galindo, P.,** Epidemiologic studies of Venezuelan Equine encephalitis virus in Almirante, Panama, *Am. J. Epidemiol.,* 88, 80, 1968.
22. **Groot, H. L.,** The health and impact of Venezuelan equine encephalitis (VEE), in *Venezuelan Encephalitis,* Pan American Health Organization, Washington, D.C., 1972, 7.
23. **Gutierrez, E., (Discussant),** in *Venezuelan Encephalitis,* Pan American Health Organization, Washington, D.C., 1972, 195.

24. **Harris, S. K.,** The Role of Domestic Animals in the Epidemiology of Venezuelan Equine Encephalomyelitis, master's thesis, Texas A & M University, College Station, 1972.
25. **Hanson, R. P., Sulkin, S. E., Buescher, E. L., Hammon, W. McD., McKinney, R. W., and Work, T. H.,** Arbovirus infections of laboratory workers, *Science,* 158, 1283, 1967.
26. **Johnson, K. M., (Discussant),** in *Venezuelan Encephalitis,* Pan American Health Organization, Washington D.C., 1972, 244.
27. **Jonkers, A. H.,** Silent hosts of Venezuelan equine encephalitis (VEE) virus in endemic situations: mammals, in *Venezuelan Encephalitis,* Pan American Health Organization, Washington, D.C., 1972, 263.
28. **Kissling, R. E.,** Epidemic behavior of Venezuelan encephalitis infection. Disease hosts: equines, in *Venezuelan Encephalitis,* Pan American Health Organization, Washington, D.C., 1972, 170.
29. **Kissling, R. E. and Chamberlain, R. W.,** Venezuelan equine encephalitis, *Adv. Vet. Sci.,* 11, 65, 1967.
30. **Kissling, R. E., Chamberlain, R. W., Nelson, D. B., and Stamm, D. D.,** Venezuelan equine encephalomyelitis in horses, *Amer. J. Hyg.,* 63, 274, 1956.
31. **Kissling, R. E. and Chamberlain, R. W.,** Venezuelan equine encephalitis, in *Advances in Veterinary Science,* Vol. II, Brandly, C. A. and Cornelius, C., Eds., Lea & Febiger, Philadelphia, 1967, 11, 65.
32. **Kubes V.,** Origins of Venezuelan equine encephalomyelitis. Isolations of its etiological agent, VEE complex, and preventive vaccines, in *Venezuelan Encephalitis,* Pan American Health Organization, Washington, D.C., 1972, 18.
33. **Kubes, V. and Rios, F. A.,** The causative agent of infectious equine encephalomyelitis in Venezuela, *Science,* 90, 20, 1939.
34. **Lord, R. D., (Discussant),** in *Venezuelan Encephalitis,* Pan American Health Organization, Washington, D.C., 245, 1972.
35. **Mackenzie, R. B.,** The role of silent vertebrate hosts in epidemics of Venezuelan encephalitis, in *Venezuelan Encephalitis,* Pan American Health Organization, Washington, D. C., 1972, 239.
36. **McKinney, R. W., Berge, T. O., Sawyer, W. D., Tigertt, W. D., and Crozier, D.,** Use of an attenuated strain of Venezuelan equine encephalomyelitis virus for immunization in man, *Amer. J. Trop. Med.,* 12(4), 597, 1963.
37. **Monlux, W. S., Luedke, A. J., and Bowne, J.,** Central nervous systems response of horses to Venezuelan equine encephalomyelitis vaccine (TC-83), *J. Am. Vet. Med. Assoc.,* 161 (2), 265, 1972.
38. **Murphy, F. A. and Harrison, A. K.,** The virus: morphology and morphogenesis, in *Venezuelan Encephalitis,* Pan American Health Association, Washington, D.C., 1972, 28.
39. **Roberts, E. D., Sanmartin, C., Payan, J., and Mackenzie, R. B.,** Neuropathologic changes in 15 horses with naturally occurring Venezuelan equine encephalomyelitis, *Amer. J. Vet. Res.,* 21(7), 1223, 1970.
40. **Sanmartin, C., (Discussant),** in *Venezuelan Encephalitis,* Pan American Health Organization, Washington, D.C., 1972, 26.
41. **Sanmartin, C.,** Diseases hosts: man, in *Venezuelan Encephalitis,* Pan American Health Organization, Washington, D.C., 1972, 231.
42. **Sanmartin, C., Groot, H., and Osorno-Mesa, E.,** Human epidemic in Colombia by the Venezuelan equine encephalomyelitis virus, *Amer. J. Trop. Med.,* 3, 283, 1954.
43. **Scherer, W. F., Dickerman, R. W., LaFiandra, R. P., Wong Chia, C., and Terrian, J.,** Ecologic studies of Venezuelan encephalitis virus in Southeastern Mexico. IV. Infections of wild mammals, *Amer. J. Trop. Med.,* 20, 980, 1971.
44. **Sellers, R. F., Bergold, G. H., Suarez, O. M., and Morales, A.,** Investigations during Venezuelan equine encephalitis outbreaks in Venezuela — 1962—1964, *Amer. J. Trop. Med.,* 14(3), 460, 1965.
45. **Shope, R. E., (discussant),** in *Venezuelan Encephalitis,* Pan American Health Organization, Washington, D.C., 1972, 271.
46. **Shope, R. E., Causey, O. R., deAndrade, A. H. P., and Theiler, M.,** The Venezuelan equine encephalomyelitis complex of group A arthropod-borne viruses, including Muco and Pixuna from the Amazon region of Brazil, *Am. J. Trop. Med.,* 13, 723, 1964.
47. **Slepushkin, A. N.,** An epidemiological study of laboratory infections with Venezuelan equine encephalomyelitis, *Probl. Virol. (USSR),* 4, 54, 1959.
48. **Sotomayor, C. G.,** A study of the virus of equine encephalomyelitis in Ecuador, *J. Am. Vet. Med. Assoc.,* 109, 478, 1946.
49. **Spertzel, R. O.,** Overview of the 1971 Texas Venezuelan equine encephalitis epizootic, in Proc. 75th Annual Meeting, U.S. Animal Health Assoc., Oklahoma City, October, 1971, 162.
50. **Spertzel, R. O.,** Venezuelan equine encephalomyelitis (sic), vaccination and control, in *Proc. 3rd Int. Conf. Equine Infectious Diseases, Paris, 1972,* S. Karger, Basel, 1973, 146.
51. **Spertzel, R. O. and Kahn, D. E.,** Safety and efficacy of an attenuated Venezuelan equine encephalomyelitis vaccine for use in equidae, *J. Am. Vet. Med. Assoc.,* 159(4), 731, 1971.

52. **Sudia, W. D.**, Arthropod vectors of epidemic Venezuelan equine encephalitis in *Venezuelan Encephalitis,* Pan American Health Organization, Washington, D.C., 1972, 157.

53. **Tabor, L. E., Hogge, A. L., Jr., and McKinney, R. W.**, Experimental infection of dogs with two strains of Venezuelan equine encephalomyelitis virus, *Am. J. Trop. Med. Hyg.,* 14, 647, 1975.

54. **Trapido, H.**, Geographic distribution and ecologic setting, in *Venezuelan Encephalitis,* Pan American Health Organization, Washington, D.C., 1972, 302.

55. **Whitford, H. W.**, The evaluation of jet injection for use in veterinary medicine, Dissertation, Texas A & M University, College Station, 1976, 1.

56. **Woodall, J. P.**, (discussant), in *Venezuelan Encephalitis,* Pan American Health Organization, Washington, D.C., 273, 1972.

57. **Young, N. A.**, Serologic differentiation of viruses of the Venezuelan encephalitis (VEE) complex, in *Venezuelan Encephalitis,* Pan American Health Organization, Washington, D.C., 1972, 77.

58. **Young, N. A. and Johnson, K. M.**, Antigenic variants of Venezuelan equine encephalitis virus: their geographic distribution and epidemiological significance, *Am. J. Epidemiol.,* 89, 286, 1962.

SAINT LOUIS ENCEPHALITIS (SLE)

G. E. Kemp

NAME AND SYNONYMS

St. Louis encephalitis is named for the initial recognition of the etiological virus during a large human encephalitis epidemic in and around St. Louis, Mo. The name is applied world-wide.

HISTORY

During 1932, an epidemic of encephalitis (38 cases) occurred in Paris, Ill. During the following summer more than 1000 clinically similar cases appeared in and around St. Louis, Mo. adjacent to the Mississippi River. During this latter outbreak, virus was isolated from brain material from a human being who had died of the disease.[28] Although arthropod transmission was postulated, no vector was incriminated.

Investigations conducted during the early 1940s in rural Yakima Valley, Washington, resulted in the isolation of the St. Louis encephalitis (SLE) virus from *Culex tarsalis* (flood plain and irrigation water) mosquitoes.[14,15,16] In the late 1950s, SLE virus isolations were obtained from *Cx. pipiens* and *Cx. quinequefaciatus* mosquitoes, later recognized as "dirty water" mosquitoes so important in urban epidemics. Since 1933, human cases have been reported from every state in continental U.S. except Maine, New Hampshire, Massachusetts, Connecticut, Rhode Island, and South Carolina.[27] Outside the U.S., epidemics have occurred in such widely separated locations as Hermosillo, Mexico, and Ontario, Canada.[13,38] One human case has been reported in Manitoba, Canada.[37]

In 1958, human cases in the Caribbean area were recorded from Miami, Jamaica, Panama, and Trinidad.[5] In Florida, the tropical mosquito *Cx. nigripalpus* has been incriminated as the principal urban vector. Through the years, SLE outbreaks have been principally in the Mississippi and Ohio River valleys, and the warmer states of California, Texas, and Florida. However, an epidemic occurred in New Jersey in 1964, and in 1975, sizable epidemics occurred as far north as Chicago, Ill., and Ontario, Canada, as well as in Tennessee, Alabama, Kentucky, Texas, Mississippi, Ohio, and Michigan.[27]

ETIOLOGY

SLE is an RNA virus recently placed in the family Togaviridae, in the genus *Flavivirus*, along with yellow fever (YF) and dengue (DEN).[9,12,40] The virions are uniformly 40 to 50 nm, spherical, have a dense core, and an envelope with surface projections.[29] SLE virus is sensitive to lipid solvents. It readily agglutinates chick and goose erythrocytes in a pH range of 6.0 to 7.9, with an optimal pH of 7.0. Agglutination occurs at a temperature of 4°C to 37°C, with the optimal temperature being 22°C.

The morphogenetic events of SLE virus replication in mammalian cells are not yet clear. The nucleus is almost certainly involved in replication, but cytoplasmic structures are severely altered before structures in the nucleus.[30,41] A conventional budding process similar to that seen with alphaviruses has been difficult to document with certainty.[29]

In ultrastructural studies on intracerebrally inoculated newborn mice, Murphy et al. have shown a severe progressive encephalitis with virus titers of 10^9 to 10^{11} LD$_{50}$/g of brain tissue.[29,30] The first change in neurons was hypertrophy of cytoplasmic membranes to such an extent, that in moribund animals, cells were filled with convoluted membranous inclusion bodies and rapidly increasing numbers of virus particles in cisternae.

Murphy, et al. also studied SLE virus in *Cx. pipiens pipiens* mosquitoes.[29] They detected virus in the mid-gut epithelium at 6 days, first at the basal ends of cells and subsequently secreted directly from intact cells into hemolymph. Salivary glands were infected within 8 days, and numbers of viral particles increased spectacularly in the salivary gland cells and the saliva for as long as 32 days. Crystalline arrays of virus particles were noted at 25 days, with some crystals containing greater than 50,000 virions.

DEFINITION

SLE is the most important mosquito-borne human encephalitis in the U.S. Sporadic cases occur each summer, and periodic urban and rural epidemics result in as many as 1000 cases per year. Since SLE virus is an arbovirus transmitted by infected invertebrates (mosquitoes) to vertebrates (usually birds), all the ecologic factors affecting these vectors and their hosts must be considered in any meaningful discussion of the disease. Successful parasitism depends on the virus being introduced into an appropriate, susceptible vertebrate-host, such as a bird, after which for a brief period of time it is latent and difficult to detect. The virus is then replicated within host cells and ultimately escapes into the general circulatory system. Duration and titer levels of viremia must be sufficient to ensure infection of blood-sucking arthropods. The replicative cycle in vertebrate hosts is referred to as the intrinsic incubation period. A similar sequence of events takes place in mosquitoes, except that the virus must exit from the mosquitoes' mouth part with saliva. The development in mosquitoes (extrinsic incubation phase) is dependent on relatively high environmental temperatures. Neither the invertebrate mosquito vectors nor any of the economically important animals are harmed by this infection. Therefore, all efforts to elucidate the factors involved in surveillance and control of SLE are directed toward recognizing viral activity in a community early, and preventing or minimizing human infections.

ANIMAL INFECTION

Susceptibility

Most animals, including birds, are probably susceptible to natural infection with SLE virus. Whether they become exposed depends to a great extent on the host preferences of the particular vector mosquitoes, the amount of virus inoculated by the vectors, and the immune status of the hosts. Infection is not synonymous with illness, and a number of individuals and species will incur only inapparent infections, which can only be detected if specific antibodies subsequently develop. Many hosts, including human beings and the economically important animals, are not epidemiologically important, in that they develop viremias of such low magnitude as to render them noninfectious to biting mosquitoes. Wild birds and fowl are the principal reservoir hosts for SLE virus, and in urban situations pigeons and house sparrows play an important role in amplifying virus.

Laboratory Diagnosis

White mice are the laboratory animals of choice. They can be consistently infected intracerebrally i.c. and can also be infected intranasally and less regularly orally. After a 3- to 4-day incubation period, mice inoculated i.c. show an acute illness characterized by ataxia, ruffled fur, convulsions, and paralysis. Total prostration and death follow in 1 to 4 or 5 days, depending on the strain of virus and the dosage. Suckling mice are more susceptible than older mice and can be readily infected peripherally as well as i.c. Young rats, hamsters, horses, and rhesus monkeys can be infected i.c., but pathogenicity varies considerably depending on the strain of SLE virus. Adult rats, adult sheep, and kittens are not susceptible. Although guinea pigs and rabbits develop inapparent infections following exposure by any route, they do produce antibodies. Small doses of virus given to chickens, ducks, and some wild birds result in inapparent infection, viremia, and specific antibody production.[10]

Chicken embryos 10 to 12 days of age may be infected by inoculation of the yolk-sacs or the chorioallantois. Virus can be recovered at increased titers following 3 to 4 days incubation at 37°C.

At our laboratory, Pekin duck embryo and Vero cell cultures are routinely used for SLE detection and research studies but numerous other cell culture systems can support SLE virus replication.

HUMAN INFECTION

CLINICAL

Most persons have a relatively mild illness characterized by fever and headache lasting for several days, followed by a complete and uneventful recovery. A few persons may have life-threatening central nervous system (CNS) involvement. The clinical features of SLE meningitis and encephalitis are not specific, and "no pathognomonic profile based on symptoms, physical findings, clinical laboratory abnormalities, radiographic or electroencephalographic features can be derived to formulate a specific clinical diagnosis of SLE in an individual case."[7] The clinician can, however, combine the above findings with epidemiologic information regarding location, patient's age, season of year, presence of virus in the area as determined by isolations from mosquitoes, seropositive birds, or the presence of other diagnosed local human infections to increase the index of suspicion toward SLE. Since no specific therapy is available for SLE infections, a differential diagnosis is essential, principally to allow therapeutic intervention in non-SLE cases in which it could be life-saving. The reader is directed to the comprehensive review of "The Human Disease: Acute Central Nervous System Infection."[7]

Differential Diagnosis

The following diseases, infections, and conditions should be considered:

- Viral infections — California encephalitis, Eastern encephalitis, Western encephalitis, Powassan infection, Venezuelan encephalitis, Colorado tick fever, echovirus infections, coxsackievirus infections, poliomyelitis, adenovirus infections, mumps, influenza, respiratory syncitial virus infections, lymphocytic choriomeningitis, rabies, herpes virus infections including *Herpes simplex* infections, Epstein-Barr infections, mononucleosis, cytomegalovirus infections, hepatitis, spongiform encephalopathies, post-infectious vaccination encephalitis, and serum sickness
- Bacterial — tuberculosis, leptospirosis, pyogenic infections including brain abscesses, meningitis, cerebral thrombophlebitis, brain emboli, syphilis, typhoid, salmonellosis

- Fungal infections
- Trichinosis, malaria, toxoplasmosis, amebic dysentery
- Rickettsial infections, Rocky Mountain spotted fever, Q fever
- Chlamydia infections, psitticosis, ornithosis, lymphogranuloma venereum
- Neoplastic diseases
- Metabolic conditions

Pathology

Visual examinations reveal vascular congestion, small hemorrhages and edema of the brain and spinal cord. Microscopic findings are characterized by cellular infiltration, principally of lymphocytes; engorgement of meningeal blood vessels and small hemorrhages in brain tissue. Degeneration and necrosis of neurons and neuronophagia, very small sterile abscesses and necrosis of grey and white matter, are the most outstanding features. Perivascular demyelination is not seen.

Laboratory Diagnosis

Human SLE infections range from inapparent infection, through mild febrile reactions with headache, to frank encephalitis followed by death. Since the clinical disease may easily be confused with a number of other infections, laboratory assistance is essential in establishing its etiology. Virus is almost never isolated from cerebrospinal fluid (CSF) in human patients and only occasionally from blood. Thus to a great extent the confirmation of SLE infections in human beings depends on the demonstration of specific antibody formation in patients' serum. Although it may be possible on some occasions to make "presumptive" diagnoses from low antibody levels in single serum specimens, more accurate determinations can be made from paired specimens from the same patients taken 2 to 3 weeks apart — the first (acute) as early in the course of the disease as possible, and the second (convalescent) about 3 weeks later. A fourfold rise (or fall, if the first specimen is taken late in the course of the illness) in antibody levels is considered diagnostic. In certain areas of the U.S. where other related flaviviruses (chiefly dengue) may be present, laboratory diagnoses may be more difficult because of wide sharing of antigenic components among members of this genus. The two most common laboratory tests used to detect antibodies are the complement fixation (CF) and the hemagglutination inhibition (HI) tests, both of which can be performed rapidly and accurately by competent laboratory personnel, and which may be used in testing large numbers of specimens during epidemics. When questions arise concerning specificity of results, a greater number of specific antigens can be included in the tests. When doubt still exists or in specific research projects, neutralization (N) tests may be used. N tests can be conducted in vivo using suckling mice inoculated with appropriate dilutions of serum-virus combinations, or in vitro in appropriate cell cultures. Numerous other tests are applicable to special circumstances.

In fatal infections, virus can usually be recovered by homogenizing small portions of brain material in suitable diluent and inoculating animals or cell cultures with the brain suspensions. Animals will sicken, or cell cultures will show plaques. Viral isolates may then be identified using tests mentioned above.

Antibodies contained in serum are relatively stable. Once blood clots have been aseptically removed from serum samples, appropriately labeled specimens can be shipped to a laboratory by mail on wet ice or, if shipment time is brief, simply by first class mail. Specimens intended for virus isolation must be handled more carefully to protect the virus. Brain samples should be removed aseptically, placed in suitable airtight containers, placed at 50°C or lower, and shipped to a laboratory with an adequate supply of dry ice. Persons who handle tissues, including blood, should exercise adequate precautions to protect themselves and others from acquiring infectious hepatitis or other infections, but there are no recorded human SLE infections from handling clinical specimens.

Persons taking histories from possible SLE-infected patients should be aware of locations to which patients have previously been exposed. These which might include parts of the world having such related viruses as yellow fever, Illeus, Japanese B encephalitis, West Nile, Uganda S, Rocio, and dengue.

EPIDEMIOLOGY

SLE virus most often produces inapparent human infection, a fact which was recognized in the 1940s during investigations conducted in Yakima, Washington, and which has been supported in numerous subsequent studies.[15,16] Antibody studies in Canada, Mexico, and Louisiana showed that SLE virus was present before the first clinical human infections were diagnosed in those areas.

During 1962, 1964, and 1966, SLE caused 20% of all encephalitides in the U.S. with known etiology, and in 1975 it was the most important cause of human encephalitis.[27] In interepidemic years, SLE infections cause less than 5% of all cases of encephalitis and less than 10% of encephalitis cases with known etiology as officially reported to the Center for Disease Control (CDC), Atlanta, Ga.

Inapparent-apparent infection rates have varied widely in different reports, from a low of 19 to 1 to a high of 425 to 1. Most serologic surveys have been conducted during or after urban epidemics and have been based on single serum samples taken from sample populations. In such surveys, HI or neutralizing antibody tests have most frequently been used, and the results have provided prevalence rather than incidence figures since these antibodies are of very long-lasting, if not lifelong, duration. Because CF antibodies are estimated to last only 2 to 5 years, CF tests have been used to assay incidence from single serum samples. In areas having no previous SLE or other flavivirus activity, the results of tests are probably valid, but more accurate information can be obtained only by testing repeated samples from the same individuals. It must be remembered that dengue virus has circulated in the southern U.S. in the past (and may again); it is broadly reactive in both CF and HI tests, and may falsely inflate SLE incidence estimates if not taken into consideration.

Age Relationship

In Houston (1964), a study conducted during the epidemic showed a seroconversion rate of 6.6% further supported by a postepidemic random survey using N tests,[18,23] with comparable seroconversion rates for all age groups. In this study, age-specific rates of inapparent to apparent infections varied inversely with age, decreasing from over 800:1 in children 0 to 9 years old, to 85:1 in persons 60 years old or older, indicating that older persons had a greater likelihood of clinical illness. Other studies have yielded conflicting findings, varying from inapparent infection rates in all ages[1,8,21] to some indicating increasing infection rates and clinical disease with age.[22,33,39] In the western U.S., where SLE virus is endemic and active in rural areas, antibody levels increase with age and are logically accompanied by a decrease in clinical infections. Children appear to be highly resistant to clinically apparent SLE infection, in contrast to their reaction to western encephalitis (WEE), in which a high proportion of infected children develop clinical infections.[27]

Sex Effects

The effects of sex difference are difficult to analyze in SLE infections. In some urban outbreaks, the incidence has been higher in females than males. In Louisville

(1956) and New Jersey (1964), the differences were statistically significant, but in other outbreaks, differences have not been significant. In Kern County, California, sex-specific antibodies were higher in males than females under 10 years, showed no difference in children 10 to 19 years, and were significantly higher in males than females over 20 years of age.[35]

Race Effects

The effects of racial difference in SLE outbreaks were investigated in Florida in 1959 and 1962.[5] Blacks showed lower incidence of clinical disease than whites in Tampa in 1959, and similarly showed lower prevalence of specific SLE N antibodies. Subsequent studies conducted after 1962 were confounded by the widespread prevalence of neutralizing antibodies identifiable as resulting from dengue infections. It was postulated that among both blacks and whites the presence of pre-existing antibodies against dengue afforded some protection against SLE infection.[3,4]

Following the Houston SLE epidemic of 1964, serological HI survey results indicated a high percentage of flavivirus antibodies which increased with age. N-test results showed about 20% of the HI-positive sera represented dengue infections presumably acquired during or before 1922. Dengue antibody prevalence was highest in central Houston, which was also the center of the SLE outbreak. No racial differences in attack rates were noted, and it was concluded that pre-existing dengue antibodies probably did not provide protection from SLE infection.[18]

Socioeconomic Effects

These have been examined in a number of outbreaks. Air conditioning, adequate screening, and closed foundations on houses were shown to have had a protective effect in Houston, as measured by inapparent infection rates.[18] Residents in towns bordering the Trinity River between Houston and Dallas had higher infection rates if their homes had open foundations, inadequate screens, no air conditioners, and fowl in their yards.[24] Following the 1964 Houston outbreak, it was shown that none of 249 persons who lived in a suburban area with effective mosquito control had antibodies, whereas matched suburban control persons in an area without mosquito control had a 9% antibody prevalence.[32]

Human Case Definition

This needs to be standardized for SLE investigations.[27] The Center for Disease Control (CDC) has recently proposed guidelines to this effect.[11] In the past, varying clinical criteria have been used, making comparisons among outbreaks difficult. Reports of clinical cases without laboratory confirmation have probably inflated some outbreaks, since enteroviral and other infections may clinically simulate SLE and occur during the same time-periods. During epidemics, cases should be first screened clinically and classified according to sites and extent of CNS involvement, e.g., as aseptic meningitis, encephalitis, or other clinical syndromes. Appropriate specimens should be taken for laboratory examination. As results accumulate, additional specimens should be taken, and gradually cases be classified as confirmed or presumptive SLE or other infections. When SLE, WEE, and enteroviral infections occur simultaneously in some areas (particularly southern), existing dengue antibody prevalence must be considered, particularly when only single-serum samples are available from patients.

Urban and Rural SLE

The vectors of SLE provide a ready way to divide human infections into urban and rural. Since the 1940s, urban outbreaks transmitted by *Culex pipiens* complex mosquitoes have increased both in intensity and expanse. *Cx. pipiens* is a "dirty water" breeding mosquito which proliferates in urban waste waters high in organic matter. The urbanization of America and its attendant concentration of human populations and increase in waste water management problems have contributed to the production of vast populations of this peridomestic mosquito. Rural outbreaks of SLE have diminished in relative importance. The principal vector in much of rural America is *Cx. tarsalis,* the flood plain or irrigation water mosquito. In Florida, *Cx. nigripalpus,* a tropical mosquito, is the epidemic vector. SLE virus is also transmitted by other *Culex* species (*Cx. salinarius* and *restuans*), but their exact role is less understood than that of the principal vectors.

Wild birds maintain and amplify virus in urban transmission cycles to levels sufficient to infect mosquitoes. Sparrows and pigeons are the principal avian hosts, but a number of other birds participate in the cycles. When conditions are met for the successful amplification of virus in birds and mosquitoes, aberrant hosts, such as people and other animals, become involved. These are not epidemiologically important in the basic cycle, as they produce viremia levels insufficient to infect mosquitoes.

Morbidity in Urban Epidemics

Between 1932 and 1976, a total of 5292 SLE infections were reported in Canada and the U.S. in urban outbreaks.[27] Laboratory examinations were conducted on 1851 specimens. Of 4230 SLE infections officially reported to CDC between 1955 and 1975, about 3150 were likely to have been transmitted by urban vectors. Epidemics have involved from 5 (Memphis, 1964) to 1095 (St. Louis, 1933) clinically diagnosed infections, with the largest number occurring in large urban areas. However the highest attack rates were in small communities where there was a concentrated source of urban vectors. In cities of over 500,000, attack rates have ranged from 5 to 20/100,000 population, whereas in small communities, rates of 100 to 800/100,000 have been recorded. In urban SLE, occupational associations have not been striking, although elderly urban housewives have had greater morbidity in some outbreaks. Unemployed and nonlaborer persons appeared to have been at higher risk in the Danville, Kentucky epidemic (1964).[25]

Morbidity in Rural Epidemics

SLE occurred in various rural areas of the western and midwestern U. S. from 1932 to 1942. Laboratory diagnoses were less sophisticated during those years and were frequently retrospective. Many outbreaks were definitely mixed SLE and WEE by laboratory studies, i.e., the Yakima Valley outbreaks from 1932 to 1942 were both WEE and SLE, and the Weld County, Colorado epidemic in 1940 showed evidence that 7 of 35 encephalitis infections were SLE.[31] In rural outbreaks since 1950, when techniques became available to separate SLE from WEE and other viral agents, 538, or 16%, of 3416 have been SLE infections. Generally, *Cx. tarsalis* transmitted outbreaks have been mixed WEE and SLE; morbidity in western U.S. has been highest in areas associated with irrigated farm lands. In Kern County, California (1954 to 1962), the encephalitis incidence was 340/100,000 in the rural part of the county compared to 61/100,000 for the urban part. In the rural cycle of SLE in Kern County, agricultural workers were at considerably higher risk. Similarly, in Pinal County, Arizona (1941), migrant workers and their families were at high risk of acquiring SLE infection.[26] Long-term residents in these areas had high antibody prevalence rates, and clinical infections most often occurred among newcomers.

Mortality and Case Fatality Rates

Very high morbidity and mortality rates were recorded in early outbreaks of SLE in urban areas. Considering clinically diagnosed infections only, these rates may be explained by inclusion of non-SLE infections because of inadequate diagnosis, less sophisticated patient care, greater virulence of the virus, or other reasons. In recent years, mortality rates in large urban-suburban outbreaks have varied between 0 and 5/ 100,000.[27] Case fatality rates in urban outbreaks having 30 or more laboratory-diagnosed infections have varied from 2.6 to 19.4%. Old age is definitely a factor in increased case fatality rates in urban outbreaks. In the Tampa Bay epidemic (1962), the mortality rate increased 2.5 times for each 10-year age group beyond 44.[2] The fatality rate for SLE in western U.S. has been lower than that for outbreaks in southern and eastern U.S., leading to speculation that the western SLE strains might be less virulent. Serologic diagnoses in fatal infections has been difficult, as death has commonly occurred before the appearance of specific antibodies.

Surveillance
Weather

Hess et al. showed that SLE outbreaks have mainly occurred south of the 21°C June isotherm, and that rural SLE outbreaks cycle with spring temperatures.[19] Reeves and Hammon associated SLE virus activity with very hot summers.[36] An analysis by Monath of 15 localities during epidemic and nonepidemic years provided the following information: Excessive rainfall in January and February and relative drought in July preceded outbreaks.[27] Warm temperatures in January and February, cool temperatures in April, and warm temperatures from May through August often preceded outbreaks. Such associations were most clearly seen in northern areas where natural temperature differences were greater.

Vectors

Interpretation of vector indices depends on baseline values collected systematically over a period of years, including vector populations, age and parity of females, and biting preferences. Vector competence has received increased attention in recent years. Vector data in conjunction with information regarding vertebrate availability and composition of susceptible populations, provide insight into epidemic potential in an area. In California, Reeves and Hammon concluded that vector population indices alone correlated poorly with occurrence of human infections.[36] In subsequent studies, Reeves postulated that a *Cx. tarsalis* population level of 12 per trap night was the threshold to sustain SLE virus transmission in Kern County, California.[34] Direct counts of infected mosquitoes assayed by isolation of virus from them are potentially useful, but require careful collection, accurate identification of mosquitoes, biocontainment facilities, and identification of isolates, all of which are costly and time-consuming. Bowen and Francy have summarized data on mosquito minimum infection rates (MIR) in major outbreaks of SLE.[6] MIR have ranged from 0.3 to 20.3 virus positive per 1000 mosquitoes, but most have been between 2.2 and 6.9. MIR of *Cx. tarsalis* during high transmission years in rural cycles were 1.8 to 2.9 in Kern County, California, and 0.8 to 1.7 in Hale County, Texas. In urban cycles in Memphis in 1975 and 1976, the MIR rose from an initial 1 to 2 at the time of the first viral isolation, to 3 to 21 during the epidemics. Mosquito MIR correlated with host preferences, vector populations, and percentage of immune people in the community at risk of being bitten must be considered in transmission predictions. Clearly, a vector population composed of older, parous, and engorged females has a greater transmission potential than a mosquito population composed of juvenile, nulliparous, nonengorged female mosquitoes.

Wild Vertebrates

The principal wildlife cycle of SLE virus occurs between mosquitoes and small vertebrates, principally birds. Since clinical illness and death rarely occur in any naturally infected vertebrates, this cycle is essentially inapparent. A number of techniques have been devised to detect this cycle and use it as a predictive mechanism to alert public health authorities before epidemics occur: 1. Free-flying birds can be caught for sampling in nylon mist nets. Age and species are determined, blood samples taken, and birds released. Blood samples can be assayed for SLE virus by laboratory inoculation of infant mice or cell cultures, though these procedures are costly and time consuming. Serological evidence of virus activity has usually been based on HI serological tests using SLE antigen. Results must be interpreted with caution, as older birds may have pre-existing antibody from the prior year, but if age data are recorded on the birds sampled, it becomes possible to show the incidence rate of infections for the year in question. Repeated samplings over a summer period, combined with a knowledge of local and migratory birds in the area, will give information about serologic conversions and virus activity in localized areas. It is advisable to capture sizable numbers of birds in several different locations in order to increase the sensitivity and reliability of the procedure. Since birds vary in their daily flight ranges and roosting locations, only general locations of acquired infections can be determined. 2. Resident nesting birds such as house sparrows and pigeons, which may be present in sizable numbers and may also have several clutches of young per year, can be sampled on a regular basis from spring through late summer. In Texas, nestling house sparrows were shown to be involved in SLE virus amplification and mosquito infection.[20] In intensive studies carried out over a number of years in Hale County, Texas, it was shown that in 1965 and 1966, when 3 to 5% of nestling sparrows were viremic, human infections were recorded. In 1967, when only 0.3% of birds were viremic, no human cases occurred despite a very high *Cx. tarsalis* infection rate. The demonstration of specific virus or antibodies in nestling birds indicates that transmission is occurring in a specific location at a specific time. The rapidity of serologic conversion in a population of nestlings from one bleeding to the next gives an indication of intensity of activity. 3. Small mammals may be assayed for viral infection or antibody conversion, but much less information is available relating to the susceptibility of small mammals to SLE infection than has been ascertained for birds. The nonavailability of persons skilled in trapping, handling, identifying, and bleeding small mammals might be a deterrent to its general use.

Sentinel Animals and Birds

Sentinel chickens may be placed in strategic locations early in the spring, and bled periodically, usually weekly or every other week, to show HI seroconversion to SLE virus. Large numbers of serum samples may be rapidly screened by this technique at relatively low cost. Seroconversions in sentinel chickens have a high correlation with the presence or absence of human disease, and a high rate of antibody titers in sentinel flocks has been correlated with epidemics in a number of instances.

Bird surveillance of this type is generally more efficient than mosquito sampling surveillance which, as in the case of *Cx. pipiens*, must be captured at rest, identified, and then assayed by relatively complex virological procedures. Even if virus is recovered from mosquitoes, this does not mean that they are transmitting the virus to susceptible hosts.

In its most primitive passive form, surveillance may consist simply of recognizing clinically suspect human encephalitis infection, followed by confirmatory diagnoses by competent laboratory personnel. Even such surveillance requires an index of suspicion that SLE may be occurring in a community in order to request the appropriate laboratory tests. By the time human cases are recognized, a high threshold of infection has usually already developed in vertebrate hosts and invertebrate vectors. Control efforts may be too late to prevent a sizable human epidemic from occurring if total reliance is placed on human surveillance. The more reliance which can be placed on detection of SLE virus activity in reservoir hosts and vectors, the greater is the possibility of predicting events in advance of the occurrence of clinical illness in human beings.[6]

CONTROL

In rural agricultural areas where *Cx. tarsalis* breeds in flood waters and irrigation water runoff areas, much can be accomplished by good water management practices. Knowledge of the biology of mosquitoes can aid greatly in directing control measures against the principal vectors' habitats, rather than against noninvolved species which may only have nuisance value. Improved agricultural practices designed to prevent the occurrence of free-standing water will reduce breeding sites for mosquitoes.

Irrigation projects should be built with no low areas or catchments which will retain water following irrigation, and naturally occurring low areas may be drained. Reservoir construction techniques which involve the use of concrete-lined banks and ditches, proper attention to steepness of banks, and avoidance of shallow water, all contribute to lowering mosquito populations. Controlling vegetation on the banks of reservoirs helps to destroy mosquito habitats. Controlling vegetation in feeder canals and ditches allows the free flow of water and prevents mosquito oviposition. In urban areas where *Cx. pipiens* complex mosquitoes are the principal vectors, the breeding sites are frequently man-made, and are caused by poorly designed or inadequate sewage and waste water disposal. Often very small breeding areas, even such sites as rain barrels, tanks, tin cans, and other artificial containers may be responsible for tremendous numbers of mosquitoes. Minimal efforts may be required to remedy the situation in some instances, while major engineering projects may be required in others. When habitat reduction by physical alteration cannot be carried out, the relatively more costly larval and adult destruction programs may be most practical. These vary, from the use of fish which eat larvae, to the use of oily films such as fuel oil (which prevents larvae from breathing), to application of larvicides which destroy the larvae directly. If environmental measures and larvicides fail to control developing immature forms, efforts must be directed toward control of adult mosquitoes, usually with appropriate insecticides of various types.

Emergency Measures

An early assessment of the problem is essential. This usually involves a multidisciplinary effort in order to evaluate the various factors including virus, vectors, wildlife hosts, geographical factors, and host populations. In order to formulate a control strategy, information on the following parameters is usually required as quickly as possible: size and species of adult mosquito population, infection rates in mosquitoes and birds, extent of mosquito breeding, extent and area of human disease, and changes in mosquito activity that can be anticipated as a result of climate and season. The success of control measures may be diminished by delays in decision making.[6]

Because human SLE infection may be confused clinically with several other illnesses, institution of most appropriate control measures must be based on correct diagnoses. Alert surveillance is essential, with prompt collection of serum samples from the earliest occurring cases, and second samples taken from those persons 2 to 3 weeks later. A communications center should be set up as a matter of high priority, and all accumulated data should be controlled and analyzed from this point. Much of this can be done by telephone, between local clinics and hospitals and the communications center.

Local physicians and health services must be informed of the surveillance program and their full assistance enlisted.

During an epidemic situation, the principal efforts must be directed toward the immediate destruction of adult mosquitoes carrying the virus. This can usually be accomplished by the application of ultra low volume (ULV) insecticides. If the area is small, this can be done from the ground; if not, aerial applications may be required to accomplish this task in the shortest possible time period. This is usually done in the late evening, as still air is essential for effective application, and the evening cool air inversion helps to keep the insecticides from dispersing too rapidly.

Health Education

The timely and appropriate release of information to the public is essential to the success of the program in mosquito spraying operations, disease intelligence gathering, and personal protection of individuals. These efforts should be centrally coordinated so that confusion does not result from changing plans of operation. Public information should include the nature of the disease and its transmission, mosquito involvement, timing and nature of mosquito control measures, the safety of mosquito control operations, and information on what individuals can do to protect themselves and their families. Community participation in destroying breeding sites of peridomestic mosquitoes in the vicinity of their own homes may greatly affect mosquito populations, and public information on biting habits of vector mosquitoes may enable people to avoid sites where and times when they are most likely to be exposed.

REFERENCES

1. **Altman, R. A., Goldfield, M., and Sussman, O.,** The impact of vector-borne viral diseases in the Middle Atlantic states, *Med. Cl. North Am.,* 51, 661, 1967.
2. **Azar, G. J., Bond, J. O., and Lawton, A. H.,** St. Louis encephalitis: age aspects of 1962 epidemic in Pinellas County, Florida, *J. Am. Geriatr. Soc.,* 14, 326, 1966.
3. **Bond, J. O.,** St. Louis encephalitis virus infection in man, *Fl. State Board Health, Monogr. Ser.* 12, 1, 1969.
4. **Bond, J. O.,** St. Louis encephalitis and dengue fever in the Caribbean area: evidence of possible cross-protection, *Bull. WHO,* 40, 160, 1969.
5. **Bond, J. O., Ballard, W. C., Markush, R. E., and Alexander, E. R.,** The 1959 outbreak of St. Louis encephalitis in Florida, *Fl. State Board Health. Monogr. Ser.* 5, 2, 1963.
6. **Bowen, G. S. and Francy, D. B.,** Surveillance, in *St. Louis Encephalitis,* Monath, T. P., Ed., American Public Health Association, Washington, D.C., 1980, 473.
7. **Brinker, K. R. and Monath, T. P.,** The human disease: acute central nervous system infection, in *St. Louis Encephalitis,* Monath, T. P., Ed., American Public Health Association, Washington, D.C., 1980, 503.
8. **Brody, J. A., Burns, K. F., Browning, G., and Schattner, J. D.,** Apparent and inapparent attack rates for St. Louis encephalitis in a selected population, *N. Engl. J. Med.,* 261, 644, 1959.
9. **Casals, J.,** Arboviruses: incorporation in a general scheme of virus classification, in *Comparative Virology,* Maramorosch, K. and Kurstak, E., Eds., Academic Press, New York, 307, 1971.
10. **Chamberlain, R. W., Kissling, R. E., Stamm, D. D., and Sudia, W. D.,** Virus of St. Louis encephalitis in three species of wild birds, *Am. J. Hyg.,* 65, 110, 1957.
11. Center for Disease Control, Control of St. Louis Encephalitis, Vector Topics, No. 1., Center for Disease Control, Atlanta, Georgia, 1976.
12. **Fenner, F.,** Classification and nomenclature of viruses, *Intervirology,* 7, 115, 1976.
13. **Gonzalez Cortes, A., Zarat Aquino, M. L., Guzman Bahena, J., Miro Abella, J., Cano Avila, G., and Aquilera Arrayo, M.,** St. Louis encephalomyelitis in Hermosillo, Sonora, Mexico, *Bull. PAHO.,* 9, 306, 1975.

14. **Hammon, W. McD.,** Encephalitis in the Yakima Valley. Mixed St. Louis and western equine types, *JAMA,* 117, 161, 1941.

15. **Hammon, W. McD. and Howitt, B. F.,** Epidemiological aspects of encephalitis in the Yakima Valley, Washington: mixed St. Louis and western equine types, *Am. J. Hyg.,* 35, 163, 1942.

16. **Hammon, W. McD., Reeves, W. C., Benner, S. R., and Brookman, B.,** Human encephalitis in the Yakima Valley, Washington, 1942, *JAMA,* 128, 1133, 1945.

17. **Harford, C. G. and Bronjenbrenner, J.,** Infection of mice by feeding with tissues containing the virus of St. Louis encephalitis, *J. Infect. Dis.,* 70, 62, 1942.

18. **Henderson, B. E., Pigford, C. A., Work, T., and Wende, R. D.,** Serologic survey for St. Louis encephalitis and other group B arbovirus antibodies in residents of Houston, Texas, *Am. J. Epidemiol.,* 91, 87, 1970.

19. **Hess, A. D., Cherubin, C. E., and LaMotte, L.,** Relation of temperature to activity of western and St. Louis encephalitis viruses, *Am. J. Trop. Med. Hyg.,* 12, 657, 1963.

20. **Holden, P., Hayes, R. O., Mitchell, C. J., Francy, D. B., Lazuick, J. S., and Hughes, T. B.,** House sparrows, *Passer domesticus* (L.) as hosts of arbovirus in Hale County, Texas, I. Field studies, 1965—1969, *Am. J. Trop. Med. Hyg.,* 22, 244, 1971.

21. **Kokernot, R. H., Hayes, J., Rose, N. J., and Work, T. H.,** St. Louis encephalitis in McLeansboro, Illinois, 1964, *J. Med. Entomol.,* 4, 255, 1967.

22. **Kriel, R. L., Poland, J. D., Johnson, V., and Chin, T. D. Y.,** St. Louis encephalitis in St. Louis County, Missouri during 1966, *Am. J. Trop. Med. Hyg.,* 18, 460, 1969.

23. **Luby, J. P., Miller, G., Garner, P., Pigford, G. A., Henderson, B. E., and Eddins, D.,** The epidemiology of St. Louis encephalitis in Houston, Texas, 1964, *Am. J. Epidemiol.,* 86, 584, 1967.

24. **Luby, J. P., Sanders, C. V., Johanson, W. G., Jr., McCubbin, J. H., Barnett, J. A., Sanford, J. P., and Sulkin, S. E.,** Trinity River serologic survey. A survey of residents of communities along the course of the Trinity River between Houston and Dallas, Texas, for antibodies to the viruses of St. Louis encephalitis, western equine encephalitis, and California encephalitis, *Am. J. Epidemiol.,* 94, 479, 1971.

25. **Mack, T. M., Brown, B. F., Sudia, W. D., Todd, J. C., Macfield, H., and Coleman, P. H.,** Investigation of an epidemic of St. Louis encephalitis in Danville, Kentucky, 1964, *J. Med. Entomol.,* 4, 70, 1967.

26. **Meiklejohn, G. and Hammon, W. McD.,** Epidemic of encephalitis, predominantly St. Louis type, in Pinal County, Arizona, *JAMA,* 118, 961, 1942.

27. **Monath, T. P.,** Epidemiology, *St. Louis Encephalitis,* Monath, T. P., Ed., American Public Health Association, Washington, D. C., 1980, 239.

28. **Muckenfuss, R. S., Smadel, J. E., and Moore, E.,** The neutralization of encephalitis virus (St. Louis, 1933) by serum, *J. Clin. Invest.,* 17, 53, 1938.

29. **Murphy, F. A.,** Morphology, *St. Louis Encephalitis,* Monath, T. P., Ed., American Public Health Association, Washington, D.C., 1980, 65.

30. **Murphy, F. A., Harrison A. K., Gary, G. W., Jr., Whitfield, S. G., and Forrester, F. T.,** St. Louis encephalitis virus infection of mice. Electron microscopic studies of central nervous system, *Lab. Invest.,* 19, 652, 1968.

31. **Philip, C. B., Cox, J. R., and Fountain, J. H.,** A preliminary report of human and equine encephalitis in Weld County, Colorado in the late summer and fall of 1940, *J. Parasitol.,* Suppl. 26, 24, 1940.

32. **Phillips, C. A., and Melnick, J. L.,** Community infection with St. Louis encephalitis virus, *JAMA,* 193, 207, 1965.

33. **Razenhofer, E. R., Alexander, E. R., Beadle, L. D., Bernstein, A., and Pickard, R. C.,** St. Louis encephalitis in Calvert City, Kentucky, 1955. An epidemiologic study, *Am. J. Hyg.,* 65, 147, 1957.

34. **Reeves, W. C.,** A review of developments associated with the control of western equine and St. Louis encephalitis in California during 1967, *Proc. Pap. Ann. Conf. Calif. Mosq. Control Assoc.,* 36, 1968.

35. **Reeves, W. C. and Hammon, W. McD.,** *Epidemiology of the Arthropod-borne Viral Encephalitides in Kern County, California, 1943—1952.* Vol. 4, University of California Public Health, University of California Press, Berkeley, 1962.

36. **Reeves, W. C. and Hammon, W. McD.,** *Epidemiology of the Arthropod-Borne Viral Encephalitides in Kern County, California, 1954—1962,* Vol. 4, University of California Publ. Public Health, University of California Press, Berkeley, 1962.

37. **Sekla, L. H. and Stackiw, W.,** Laboratory diagnosis of western encephalomyelitis, *Can. J. Public Health,* 67 (Suppl. 1), 33, 1976.

38. **Spence, L., Artsob, J., Grant, L., and Th'ng, C.,** St. Louis encephalitis in southern Ontario: Laboratory studies for arboviruses, *Can. Med. Assoc. J.,* 116, 35, 1977.

39. **Steigman, A. J.,** Influence of age of infection with St. Louis encephalitis virus, *J. Infect. Dis.,* 123, 1971.
40. **Wildy, P.,** Classification and nomenclature of viruses, *Monogr. Virol.,* 5, 1, 1971.
41. **Yazuzumi, G., Tsubo, T., Sugihara, R., and Nakai, Y.,** Analysis of the development of Japanese B encephalitis (JBE) virus. I. Electron microscope studies of microglia infected with JBE virus, *J. Ultrastruct. Res.,* 11, 213, 1964.

YELLOW FEVER

Y. Robin and G. W. Beran

NAME AND SYNONYMS

Many synonyms have been used for yellow fever (YF) world-wide, including fievre jaune, typhus amaril, typhus icteroide, yellow jack, black vomit, febris flava, typhus amarillo, vomito prieto, vomito negro, Gelbfieber, and *Flavivirus hominis* fever. The virus exists in two cycles; an urban cycle involving human beings and *Aedes aegypti* mosquitoes, and a sylvatic or jungle yellow fever cycle involving forest primates, principally monkeys, and forest canopy mosquitoes, with human infections tangential to the transmission cycle.[33,73]

HISTORY

The origin of yellow fever is considered to have been West Africa, although it was first clinically described in the "peste" encounterd by Spanish explorers in the Yucatan peninsula in 1648.[19] It was probably transported with the transplanting of *Ae. aegypti* mosquitoes from Africa to the Western Hemisphere. In Africa, yellow fever was first described in the epidemic which ravaged St. Louis du Senegal in 1778.[61] During the eighteenth and nineteenth centuries, it was one of the great plagues of the world,[73] occurring along eastern U.S. from Maryland to Florida, in Central America, in South America from Brazil to Argentina, and in Africa throughout the tropical area and as far south as Zimbabwa. Although transported northward, it never became established in Europe above the range of the *Ae. aegypti* mosquitoes. Yellow fever has never been reported from Asia and Australia, despite the endemic presence of *Ae. aegypti* in tropical Asia.[73] In 1900, a U.S. Army Yellow Fever Commission under Major Walter Reed was assigned to Cuba, where its studies demonstrated that a filterable agent present in the blood of acute phase patients could be transmitted by *Ae. aegypti* mosquitoes.[55,56,57] Eradication efforts directed toward *Ae. aegypti* mosquitoes were successfully achieved under the direction of Dr. William Gorgas by 1901 in Havana, and by 1905 in the Panama Canal Zone. At that very period of dramatic conquest of yellow fever and of optimistic prediction of its world-wide eradication, Franco et al.,[28] in Colombia, South America, described a forest-centered epidemic transmitted by daylight-biting mosquitoes other than *Ae. aegypti*.[28,69] In 1914, Balfour reported that people of Trinidad predicted outbreaks of human yellow fever whenever sick or dead red howler (*Alouatta spp.*) monkeys were found in the forests.[3] YF virus was first isolated from blood samples from human patients by inoculation into monkeys and transmitted among monkeys by *Ae. aegypti* mosquitoes in a series of studies in the late 1920s in South America and Africa.[2,4,26,72] Theiler's demonstration in 1930 of the susceptibility of laboratory mice to YF virus by intracerebral (IC) inoculation opened a new era in laboratory studies.[77] The elucidation of the epidemiology of jungle yellow fever was principally achieved in Africa and South America under the auspices of the U.S. Rockefeller Foundation.[70,73] The earliest human vaccine, an infected mouse brain tissue suspension administered simultaneously with human immune serum, was put into use in 1931.[60] Theiler's attenuated live virus vaccines introduced in 1937 form the basis for the present day products.[11,78]

Great epidemics occurred in New Orleans in 1905, in Brazil in 1928 and 1932, in the southern Sudan in 1940, in Nigeria in 1951 to 1954, in Trinidad in 1954, in Central

America from 1948 to 1957, in Zaire, in 1958, in southwest Ethiopia in 1960—1962, and in Senegal in 1965 to 1966.[10,47,73] A jungle yellow fever epidemic decimated the monkey population from Panama to Guatemala in 1955.[9] A single, human, fatal case of yellow fever along with reports of deaths in monkeys in southeastern Trinidad in 1978 was considered to constitute an epidemic, with attendant international reporting and prompt institution of epidemic control measures.[81]

ETIOLOGY

Classification

Yellow fever virus is the prototype strain of the genus *Flavivirus* (group B arboviruses) of the family Togaviridae.[27] Yellow fever virus shows antigenic relatonships by hemagglutination inhibition (HAI) tests to other flaviviruses.[16,17] Antibody absorption tests have shown that African YF strains have an antigenic component which is not shared by New World strains.[21] The type strain of YF virus is the Asibi strain,[73] a viscerotropic strain which has been maintained by serial passage in rhesus monkeys, in which it produces fatal illness.[80]

Characteristics

Yellow fever virions are spherical, and show a limiting membrane, possibly an envelope. Electron microscopic studies have established a size of 38 ± 5 nm diameter.[8] The genome is single stranded RNA with a molecular weight of 3×10^6 daltons. The virus is extremely fragile in the absence of a protein milieu, and is sensitive to the action of lipid solvents, chemical disinfectants, acid, and heat.

DEFINITION

Yellow fever is an infection of human beings and primates, characterized by icteric disease in human patients. It is transmitted by a variety of mosquitoes breeding in human inhabited areas and in jungle forest canopies.

ANIMAL INFECTION

All primate species are considered susceptible to YF virus infection. African species are considered to be most resistant, showing inapparent to very mild, nonfatal illness. South American and Indian monkeys are considered much more susceptible. Baboons and some marsupials develop viremias but show no clinical signs.[5,37,68,73] Wild rodents and birds are resistant to experimental infections. At necropsy, most infected African monkeys show no lesions. The lesions in experimentally infected rhesus monkeys involve principally liver and kidneys. The marked, distinctive, midzonal, hyaline necrotic areas in the liver are called Councilman bodies, and are very similar to those seen in naturally occurring human infections.[6,36,73] Yellow fever diagnosis is based on virus isolation and identification or development of specific antibodies.[35,85]

HUMAN INFECTION

Most YF patients have a characteristic but nondiagnostic febrile disease with fever, headache, backache, nausea, variable epistaxis, and a lack of correlation between pulse and body temperature. The clinical course is 2 to 3 days, followed by uneventful recovery. Many tropical diseases, including a variety of arboviral infections, malaria, and relapsing tick fever may present similar clinical syndromes, making a clinical diagnosis of suspected yellow fever appropriate only if seen during a recognized epidemic. The development of icterus occurs following a remission of the general manifestations in a serious form of the disease. It develops as a yellowish tinge of the sclera, a very important diagnostic sign in black people, and only rarely becomes marked. Hemorrhagic signs and vomiting of blood characterize the most serious form of disease, and are common preceding death within 9 days of onset. Icteric yellow fever must be differentiated from infectious and serum hepatitis, leptospirosis, and poisoning.[40,58,78] Because of these uncertain clinical criteria, use must be made of laboratory diagnostic tests.[86]

Pathology

At necropsy of patients who succumb to yellow fever, icterus and hemorrhage are common in various organs, and the stomach and intestines may contain partially digested blood. Histologically, hepatic lesions are characterized by midzonal necrosis, trabecular disorganization with absence of stromal damage, acidophilic degeneration, and fatty metamorphosis, forming masses called Councilman bodies which are scattered through the lobules. Histologic lesions of hemoglobinuric lower nephron nephrosis are seen in kidneys, small perivascular hemorrhages in brain, and degenerative changes may be present in myocardium.[13,14,59] In many areas, these lesions must be differentiated from those of malaria, measles, or kwashiorkor.[14,59]

Diagnosis

Isolation and identification of YF virus in blood samples or necropsy specimens, or demonstration of specific antibody titer rises are definitive.[35,86] Demonstration of pathognomonic hepatic lesions in necropsy specimens is used when applicable, but needle biopsies of the liver have proven so hazardous that the procedure is contraindicated.

EPIDEMIOLOGY

Occurrence

Eastern Hemisphere

Numerous extensive epidemics of yellow fever have been recorded in Africa in the past 30 years. Control had been achieved since 1939 in the francophone nations of West Africa through widespread vaccination. After 1960, with the relaxation of immunization efforts, epidemics occurred in six countries between 1965 and 1969.[12,15,19] Recent data have shown that the virus is circulating in nature in Central African Republic,[29] Ivory Coast,[20] and Senegal.[23]

Year around endemic activity of yellow fever occurs in rain forests where the virus is transmitted in the forest canopies in monkey-*Ae. africanus* mosquito-monkey cycles. Both monkeys and vector mosquitoes are relatively scarce, and endemic areas are limited but continuous. In the savannahs of southern Sudan, virus circulates only in the rainy and early part of the dry seasons. Populations of *Ae. africanus* become large and the virus is readily transmitted to people, with resultant high prevalence of antibody titers in people. In these areas, called emergence areas, susceptible populations of people or monkeys do not build up, and epidemics are rare.[29]

In the northern part of the Sudanese savannah and cape of Sahel, rainy seasons are short, and virus circulates only for a brief period each year. The virus does not persist endemically and must be periodically reintroduced from emergence areas into these areas, which are called relay areas.[23] The introduction may be by infected people, wild vertebrates, or vector mosquitoes, which in these areas are *Ae. luteocephalus*, *Diceromyia* spp., and *Ae aegypti*. Where populations of susceptible people and vector mosquitoes reach sufficient levels, introduction of the virus may lead to epidemics with human-*Ae. aegypti*-human transmissions. Such an epidemic took place in Diourbel, Senegal in 1965.[11,19] Similar introductions of YF virus led to epidemics in Ghana and Upper Volta in 1969 transmitted by *Ae. aegypti*, in the Nuba Mountains of Sudan in 1940 transmitted by *Ae. vittatus* and *Ae. furcifer-taylori*,[41,46] on the Jos plateau of Nigeria in 1969 transmitted by *Ae. luteocephalus*,[15,45] and in the Omo valley of Ethiopia in 1960 to 1962 transmitted by *Ae. simpsoni*.[65,66]

Western Hemisphere

Yellow fever has occurred in extensive epidemics throughout the islands of the Caribbean, Mexico (especially southeastern Mexico), Central America, and the most populated areas of both Atlantic and Pacific coastal South America, with inland epidemics in Colombia, Brazil, Bolivia, and Paraguay.[7] The introduction of *Ae. aegypti* mosquitoes from Africa to the Western Hemisphere during the period of slave trading made possible the great urban outbreaks with human-mosquito-human transmission cycles.[73] The speed with which *Ae. aegypti* adapted to the habitats of the Western Hemisphere and became endemic over vast areas is one of the marks of the domestication of this species to living in immediate proximity to people. Whether jungle yellow fever was historically present in the Western Hemisphere in monkey-mosquito-monkey cycles, or whether it developed as an extension from urban yellow fever, cannot be assessed with certainty; the latter premise appears to have the greater weight. The rather voluminous records of the pre-Colombian Native American civilizations, as well as of the earliest Spanish and Portugese invaders, give no hint of clinical yellow fever in people or animals.[73] Considerable emphasis is placed on the observation that African monkeys and people native to West Africa have a relatively greater tolerance to yellow fever than do monkeys and human populations of South America. Findings have provided evidence that yellow fever is a more ancient infection in Africa than in South America. Resistance patterns there have developed through an older process of association and selection. The mildness of YF virus infections in South American marsupials must be considered. Until evidence to the contrary may be obtained, it is postulated that this is more related to a lack of adaptation of the virus to these hosts than to genetically acquired tolerance of the hosts to the virus.[19]

In the Western Hemisphere, urban yellow fever was solely transmitted by *Ae. aegypti* mosquitoes. It was seasonally epidemic in temperate climatic areas where these mosquitoes failed to overwinter but were reintroduced by extension or transport, and was epidemic in tropical communities too small to maintain a continuouly susceptible population which would support an endemic state. It was endemic where *Ae. aegypti* survived year around and the concentration of people was sufficient to maintain a continual human-mosquito-human cycle. The chain of *Ae. aegypti* transmission cycle began to be broken with the *Ae. aegypti* eradication program in Cuba in 1901 and ended with the elimination of the last endemic focus of *Ae. aegypti* transmitted yellow fever in northeastern Brazil in 1934.[73]

Jungle yellow fever in the Western Hemisphere is transmitted chiefly among monkeys, marmosets, and possibly other forest dwelling animals, commonly causing fatal infections. The vectors are mosquitoes of the forest canopy, chiefly of *Haemagogus* spp. and to lesser extent, *Ae. leucocelaenus, Sabethes chloropterus* and possibly *Ae. fulvus* in Brazil. The endemic zone appears to be a continuous dynamic area with wandering epidemics in susceptible populations of monkeys where the virus persists in epidemic foci not longer than 1 to 2 seasons. This zone extends along the Amazon-Orinoco basin, down the forested coast of Brazil, in forested watersheds of the Amazon-Orinoco system in Guyana and Venezuela, in the Magdalena Basin, and in eastern

Panama. From this endemic area, periodic epidemics radiate outward up to 1500 km, characterized by seasonally rapid spread. In 1955, such spread took place from Panama northward to Guatemala at a rate of about 13 miles/month, essentially exterminating the forest primate population along its path. Wind drift is believed to play an important role in transporting infected mosquitoes beyond the periphery of infected monkey populations.[9]

Reservoir

Human beings of all races, sexes, and ages are susceptible to infection and may infect biting mosquitoes during the first 3 to 4 days after onset of symptoms. Human patients are the important hosts of urban yellow fever. Infected people may transport the virus following sylvatic exposure back to communities outside the forest cycle and serve as sources of exposure to *Ae. aegypti* mosquitoes initiating urban yellow fever epidemics. Theoretically at least, the reverse human transport of YF virus could also take place. The wild hosts of jungle yellow fever in Africa are nonhuman primates, principally cercopithecid monkeys (grivet, tantalus, diana, patas, and mona) of the genus *Cercopithecus,* chimpanzees (*Pan* spp.), mangabey (*Cercocebus* spp.), baboons (*Papio* spp.), bush babies (*Galago* spp.), and possibly hedgehogs (*Erinaceus* spp.) Infected forest primates have a period of viremia from 1 to 6 days during which they may transmit virus to mosquitoes, followed by disappearance of virema, and development of presumably lifelong immunity. All African nonhuman primates except bush babies appear to be reatively tolerant to YF virus infection, usually developing negligible symptoms and only rarely fatal disease. Serological evidence of infections in baboons has been obtained in the absence of any clinical disease.[34,75]

In Central and South American monkeys and marmosets, fatal infections are the rule and extermination of focal primate populations rather than development of immune animals commonly accounts for termination of epidemics. The animals chiefly involved are capuchin (*Cebus* spp.), spider (*Ateles* spp.) and howler (*Alouatta* spp.) monkeys and marmosets (*Hapale* spp.), and possibly, based largely on experimental evidence of susceptibility, in squirrel (*Saimiri* spp.) and woolly (*Lagothri* spp.) monkeys, bats, coatis, wildcats, agoutis, and more likely in armadillos and opossums resident in forest habitats. Experimental studies have shown that Asian monkeys, rhesus, bonnet, and kra (*Macaca* spp.) are very susceptible to YF virus infection, commonly developing acute and fatal disease by parenteral routes of exposure.[24]

Transmission

As early as 1881, Dr. Carlos Finley of Havana, Cuba put forth the hypothesis of mosquito transmission of yellow fever, and in 1900 he placed his colony of *Ae. aegypti* mosquitoes at the disposal of Major Walter Reed.[54] By human volunteer experiments from 1900 to 1901, Rccd and his associates demonstrated the transmission of yellow fever by these mosquitoes, leading to the prompt development of *Ae. aegypti* eradication programs.[82] After taking infective blood meals, mosquitoes are not immediately able to transmit the virus during an extrinsic incubation period of 9 to 30 days, depending upon the species, temperature, and humidity. Once they become infectious, high levels of virus persist and transmission is continuous through the life span.

Eastern Hemisphere

Seven species of *Aedes* mosquitoes are of practical importance in the transmission of YF virus. In Africa, *Ae. aegypti* in forests and savannahs breed as a wild population in impounded water and show primarily zoophylic feeding habits.[32] In human inhabited areas, this mosquito breeds as a domestic or subdomestic population dependent on stored water or water collecting in natural or waste containers during periods of rainfall. In urban habitats in Africa, and apparently exclusively in the Western Hemisphere. *Ae. aegypti* is highly anthropophilic in feeding habits. The species is largely exophilic with peak acvity in late afternoons.[4,67] *Ae. africanus* a forest canopy dwelling mosquito, breeding almost exclusively in tree holes during rainy seasons. In forest galleries, the female mosquitoes feed at ground level during daylight with a peak of activity at dusk, and more sparcely during the night. Human beings and primates are preferred to rodents or birds for blood meals.[53] *Ae. luteocephalus* has similar habitat and feeding preferences to *Ae. africanus* but can persist in areas of greater drought.[4] *Ae. metallicus* is found in dry savannah and southern Sahel areas. It is most active at dusk and continues to feed through the night. *Ae. simpsoni* commonly acts in estblishing a secondary cycle of yellow fever in banana plantation areas. This moquito breeds in vegetation around human habitations, is infected by feeding on monkeys which raid plantations, and then transmits the virus to people.[3] Once infected people and infected mosquitosdevelop, human-mosquito-human cycles may build to epidemic proportions as occurred in Ethiopia in 1960 to 1962.[65,66] On the other hand, the presence of *Ae. simpsoni* mosquitos in an are dose not always pose a human vector threat because of the nonanthropophilic populations of these mosquities as described in Uganda by Gillett.[30] *Ae. vivattatus* has very wide distribution in Africa. It breeds in rock holes and exceptionally in tree holes. The eggs are extremely resistant to drought and complete larval development takes less than 1 week. Population levels fluctuate greatly with seasons. *Aedes* of the furcifer-taylori group are forest dwelling mosquitoes. Larvae develop in tree holes but are rarely encountered in surveys. Female mosquities are highly anthropophilic and bite at ground level during the night. *Ae. opok*, which is very similar to *Ae. africanus*, has been found to be infected in nature. It prefers monkeys to human beings for blood meals.

Western Hemisphere

The vector of urban yellow fever in the Western Hemisphere was entirely the *Ae. aegypti* mosquito. Jungle yellow fever is transmitted in nature and tangentially to people by *Haemagogus capricorni, H. spegazzinii falco, H. mesodentatus, H. equinus, Ae. leucocelaenus, Sabethes chloropterus* and possibly *Ae. fulvus*[1,7,43,73] Human infection results almost exclusively from direct forest contact with exposure to infected forest canopy mosquitoes. It is suspected that occasional infections are acquired around and even in houses located near foests.[9] Human infections always pose a threat to initiation of epidemics of urban yellow fever if *Ae. aegypti* mosquitoes are present. In Central and South America, all *Haemagogus* spp. mosquitoes which have been implicated in the transmission of YF virus breed primarily in forest tree holes, ut occasionally are found to breed in bamboo stubs or in suitable sites in adjacent parks or residential premises. They have been shown to follow people several hundred meters into clear areas in pursuit of blood meals. In forest habitats, they select upper levels of the forest canopies. *Haemagogus* spp. Mosquitoes are daylight biters, being most active at midday when for occupational or recreational reasons, people are most likely to infringe upon their habitats, often in search of shady spots to eat lunch or relax. *Ae. Leucocelaewus* mosquitoes, although classified in the genus *Aedes*, have characteristics intermediate between this and the *Haemgogogus* genus. They are forest dwelling, tree hole breeders with a diurnal breeding cycle, frequently at ground level. This species is fairly common in many parts of the yellow fever endemic region of Central and South America.[43] *S. chloropterus* mosquitoes are arboreal, tree hole, or bamboo stump breeding, day-feeding mosquitoes. They are a hardy vector and considered to be responsible for maintaining transmission during prolonged dry seasons.[73]

Environment

Yellow fever occurs only in areas where climatic conditions support sufficient numbers of both vectors and hosts. Natural foci of infection are maintained in rain forest galleries where temperatures and humidity are highly stable and vertical stratification of microclimates favors specific species. Both host and vector populations are small in these foci and the cycle of endemic yellow fever is very slow. Outside the forest areas and in areas of human habitation, mosquito populations are directly dependent on natural or man-made breeding sites and on seasonal levels of rainfall.

Human Hosts

The two basic patterns of yellow fever infection are jungle or sylvatic yellow fever and urban or epidemic yellow fever. In jungle yellow fever, the infection is maintained in an endemic state through monkey-mosquito-monkey trnsmission cycles. The virus may be transmitted to people by these same mosquitoes or secondary mosquitoes as *Ae. simpsoni* which may feed on infected monkeys and then transmit the virus to people. The infected human patients may serve as aberrant hosts or as alternate hosts initiating urban yellow fever epidemics in which a human-mosquito-human transmission cycle occurs. Because this cycle depends upon the coexistence of many susceptible persons and abundant vector mosquites, urban yellow fever may not become endemic but usually disappears only to be reintroduced.

Laboratory and field study acquired infections have been many and tragic through the history of the conquest of yellow fever. Some were acquired during human volunteer studies in early years of research. Others followed inadvertent exposure by infected mosquitoes and only recently has the importance of exposure by inhalation of high virus titering aerosols been recognized. The prompt application of the earliest yellow fever vaccine, a simultaneous virulent virus-human immune serum injection regimen, for protection of research and diagnostic personnel had an immediate impact on the occurrence of lavoratory acquired infections. It is essential that all persons in occupational contact with yellow fever virus be effectively immunized against it.[50]

CONTROL

Prevention and Therapy

No specific therapeutic regimen is available for yellow fever, and treatment is chiefly supportive.[40] Prevention is based both on protection from exposure and on vaccination. The French, or Dakar, vaccine was developed at the Institute Pasteur de Dakar, Senegal from the French neurotropic virus (FNV) strain,[49,71] isolated from a human patient in 1927 and adapted to laboratory cultivation by Theiler and associates. For vaccine production, it is cultivated in mouse brain and is administered by cutaneous scarification.[62] It is used only in persons above 14 years of age, due to a risk of post-vaccinal encephalitis. FNV is commonly used in performing neutralization tests in mice. The 17D vaccine was developed by Theiler at the Rockefeller Institute in 1937. The 17D strain was attenuated in cell cultures and is cultivated for vaccine production in embryonating hens' eggs. It is administered by subcutaneous injection. Complications are extremely rare except in children under 7 months of age.[79] Following either, vaccine neutralizing antibodies appear within 10 days and persist at least 10 years.

Vaccination is the only practical preventive measure which may be effectively used by persons entering endemic or epidemic areas as forest workers, game management persons, hunters, medical personnel, migrant workers, or travellers. In endemic areas, a variable proportion of the older population has naturally acquired immunity, so priority should be given to children above 6 months of age in vaccination campaigns.

In epidemic areas, the goal should be to vaccinate 100% of the population above 6 months of age, unless serological survey data are available to identify the portions of the population at risk. With population growth at 2.5% per year by births and 1.5 to 2% by urban immigration, 20% of the population may be expected to be susceptible within 4 to 5 years after a vaccination campaign. With this large a portion of the population at risk, vaccination campaigns should be mounted to prevent recurrence of an epidemic.

Eradication of *Ae. aegypti* mosquitoes may be feasible in areas at risk of epidemics of yellow fever. Breeding site removal, larvicidal treatment of impounded water, and insecticide applications for adult mosquitoes on a community or residence basis are important with or without adjunct vaccination programs. Entomological surveys show that *Ae. aegypti* are still prevalent throughout East, Central, and West Africa and the Caribbean Islands. Vector control is not applicable in areas of jungle yellow fever.

Regulatory Measures

Yellow fever is one of four diseases under the International Health Regulations of 1969. Notification of cases to World Health Organization (WHO) and to authorities of neighboring countries is required. Travellers coming from or through "infected local areas" and proceeding to "yellow fever receptive areas" may be required to present valid international certificates of vaccination. The validity of international certificates extends for 10 years beginning 10 days after vaccination. Revaccination performed before expiration of the validity period renders the certificate valid for a further 10 years beginning on the day of revaccination.

Epidemic Measures

Both mass vaccination and *Ae. aegypti* mosquito control should be initiated as promptly as possible. Depending on the epidemiological pattern of spread, vaccination may be started at the periphery of the focus or at its center. Adult mosquito control provides the most immediate description of the transmission cycle. In nonforested rural areas, ultra low volume (ULV) application of malathion at 22 ℓ/km^2 gives good results for control of moquitoes on vegetation. In inhabited areas, double the volume gives control of mosquitoes in residences as well, and in densely vegetated areas, 58 to 147 ℓ/km^2 may be required. Application may be performed on a limited scale in urban areas with portable equipment and on a larger scale by tractor drawn equipment or by airplane.[44]

In Africa, WHO collaborating reference centers in Entebbe, Uganda and Dakar, Senegal have teams available to give prompt aid to local authorities in epidemiological investigation, institution of vaccination campaigns, and initiation of vector control. Expanded vaccination and vector control projects may obtain supplies from the West African Epidemiological Surveillance Center at Abidjan, Ivory Coast.[33]

In the Americas, the Pan American Health Organization, WHO coordinates control activities.[83] Most recently, one documented and one additional suspected human death from jungle or sylvatic yellow fever in Trinidad were reported in WHO in November, 1978. Reports of monkeys dying in forested areas of southeastern Trinidad led to the finding of the virus in both monkeys and mosquitoes. In response to this outbreak, intensified vaccination of people in both rural and urban areas, with surveillance for infections and efforts to control *Ae. aegypti* mosquitoes were promptly instituted.[81]

Eradication

Due to the sylvatic cycle of jungle yellow fever, eradication is not possible at the level of present technology.

CALIFORNIA GROUP VIRAL INFECTIONS IN THE U.S.

W. H. Thompson

NAME AND SYNONYMS

California group arbovirus infections are so named because of first isolations from mosquitoes in California and presence of antibodies in three young persons with encephalitis there. Following isolation of the antigenically related but distinct La Crosse (LAC) virus from a fatal case in Wisconsin[52] and subsequent cases serologically diagnosed in children each year[50] in midwestern and eastern states, it has become known locally as La Crosse encephalitis. In the Indiana area, the disease has been referred to as rural encephalitis. The disease is officially reported as California encephalitis.

HISTORY

Several thousand isolates of California group arboviruses have been obtained from mosquitoes (mainly *Aedes*) from many states,[46] and from other parts of the world including Canada, Trinidad, Europe, Africa, and Finland. Those studied in detail so far have been grouped into interrelated but distinct subtypes.[7]

The first California group arbovirus was isolated from *Aedes* mosquitoes in California,[16] and during 1945 was serologically related with three cases of encephalitis. Subsequent cases have not been reported from the state.

Following isolation of La Crosse (LAC) virus from the brain of a 4-year-old girl who died of encephalitis in a Wisconsin hospital during 1960,[52] over 800 cases of California encephalitis have been reported from midwestern and eastern states. Antibodies to LAC virus have been documented in convalescent sera from most California encephalitis patients in Wisconsin and neighboring states.[50] Antibodies to other California group arboviruses occasionally have been found in man, but without proven relationship to the disease.

Epidemiological studies on LAC virus infections have linked their occurrence to hardwood deciduous forest areas and rural and suburban resident areas. Small forest-dwelling mammals including chipmunks and tree squirrels have been implicated as the main vertebrate hosts. *Ae. triseriatus* mosquitoes have been shown to be the main vector,[48] with an overwintering mechanism for LAC virus in eggs and progeny through transovarial transmission.[55] Transovarial transmission in infected mosquitoes maintains infection in these vectors and leads to transmission to human and animal hosts each season in endemic areas. Other California group arboviruses have recently been isolated from mosquito larvae.

The natural maintenance cycle of LAC virus has been found to include vertical transmission through transovarial transmission in *Ae. triseriatus*, and horizontal transmission to adult female mosquitoes by blood meals on viremic vertebrate hosts.[35] Venereal transmission of LAC virus from transovarially infected male to female *Ae. triseriatus* has recently been demonstrated in this laboratory.[49] This provides a second biological mechanism of horizontal transmission.

Studies so far have indicated that different primary vectors and vertebrate hosts may be involved in the natural cycles of each of the California group arboviruses[46] relating these viruses to endemic regions, sometimes overlapping those of others.

ETIOLOGY

Classification

The California arbovirus group is an antigenically related group classified within the family Bunyaviradae on the basis of morphologic, morphogenetic, and other similarities.[40]

Within the California group of arboviruses those so far sufficiently studied have been placed in 12 major subtypes,[32,44a] 7 of which have been found in the U.S. Three antigenic complexes have been defined within the group. The California encephalitis complex includes the original California encephalitis virus[16] Keystone,[9] La Crosse (LAC),[52] San Angelo, Jamestown Canyon, Jerry Slough (and closely related South River virus), and snowshoe hare virus[10] in the U.S. The California encephalitis complex also includes several foreign strains; Tahyna in Europe and Africa and Inkoo virus in Finland.

The other two complexes within the California group each include single arboviruses; Trivittatus virus found in the U.S., and Melao virus found in Trinidad.

Characteristics

California group arboviruses replicate and produce cellular degeneration and plaques in many cell culture systems, including baby hamster kidney. Electron microscopic studies have revealed spherical, enveloped virions, 90 to 100 nm in size, with single stranded RNA genomes.[40] Viral assembly is in the cytoplasm of cells and involves budding into cysternal and vesicular lumina, the virons thereby acquiring their limiting membranes.[33] Like other arboviruses, California group virus infectivity is susceptible to lipid solvents as ether and chloroform, heat, and radiation. It is unstable below pH 6.7. As a group hemagglutinating ability is poor.

DEFINITION

California encephalitis is a febrile, central nervous system disease of children caused by La Crosse virus. It occurs each year in the midwestern and eastern U.S. Serologic evidence of infections caused by other California group arboviruses is present in animals and people in many parts of the country, but isolations of virus from infected persons, or conclusive, continuing serological evidence of disease in people has not been obtained so far, except with LAC virus.

INFECTIONS IN ANIMALS

Laboratory Animals

Most California group arbovirus strains multiply readily in young mice, usually producing encephalitis and death within 2 to 6 days following inoculation.[19] Because of their high susceptibility to infection, their short viremic state and rapid immunologic response with several California group arboviruses, laboratory rabbits have been used as sentinel hosts for detection of virus activity in nature. Chimpanzees have been used successfully in transmission studies. Hamsters, guinea pigs, and monkeys are less susceptible to the virus than rabbits or chimpanzees, but have been used for production of specific antisera for laboratory studies.

Wild Animals

A variety of small wild mammals are susceptible to experimental inoculation with California group arboviruses, including rabbits and hares with Trivittatus and snowshoe hare viruses; and ground squirrels with California encephalitis and snowshoe hare viruses. Chipmunks, woodrats, deer mice, woodchucks, and meadow voles can be infected with snowshoe hare virus, and cotton rats with California encephalitis and Keystone viruses. Mature birds, including pheasants, are refractory to infection with most California group viruses.[19]

Snowshoe hare virus was first isolated from the blood of a snowshoe hare (*Lepus americanus*) in Montana.[10] White-tailed deer are natural vertebrate hosts for Jamestown Canyon virus.

Antibodies to LAC are commonly present in sera of chipmunks and tree squirrels in endemic areas.[31] High viremic levels and antibody responses occur in chipmunks and squirrels following experimental infection wth LAC virus,[35] but associated disease has not been observed in inoculated adult animals.

Domestic Animals

Antibodies to California group viruses have been found occasionally in sera of horses, cattle, dogs, and other domestic animals, but durable high level viremias have not been reported.[19] Chickens and other mature domestic birds have been refractory to experimental infection with most California group arboviruses.

HUMAN INFECTIONS

Clinical Manifestations

California encephalitis is most commonly diagnosed as a clinical disease in children in the U.S. It is characteristically an acute central nervous system disease ranging in severity from mild transient aseptic meningitis to encephalitis and occasionally death.[50,51] Symptoms reported have included initial fever (95%) and headache (86%) with nausea or vomiting (70%), nuchal rigidity (55%), convulsions or seizures (37%), and lethargy (28%).[2] Other neurologic signs have included paresis, aphasia, and coma lasting five or more days. Hospitalization has occurred in most cases 1 or 2 days after onset of the acute febral stage and the duration has been 5 to 10 days. Encephalogram abnormalities are present during the acute phase of the disease, and residual abnormalities have occasionally persisted. In 35 children studied as late as 8 years following infection, frequency of residual neurological findings reported were meningeal signs (24); Babinsky's reflex (8); paresis (6); tremor (3); abnormal optic disc margin (3); aphasia (2), and chorea (1). Abnormalities reported have indicated persistent focal or diffuse cerebral neuronal dysfunction.[14]

More than 800 human cases of LAC virus infection have been reported from midwestern and eastern states since the initial 17 cases described in Wisconsin between 1960 and 1963.[50] California encephalitis ranked second only to St. Louis encephalitis in reported incidence of arthropod-borne viral encephalitides in the U.S. during the past decade. The disease is endemic in nature, with cases occurring each year.

In the U.S., a few cases of clinical disease characterized by fever, headache, and other symptoms with subsequent serological response to California group arboviruses other than LAC virus have been reported, but clinical patterns have not been established as yet. California group arboviruses other than LAC have not been isolated from human patients in the U.S.

In Europe, Tahyna virus has been isolated from blood and has been serologically related to disease in children. Clinically, Tahyna fever is a relatively mild respiratory disease with fever, pharangitis, and occasional acute central nervous system involvement.[4]

Diagnosis

Cases of California encephalitis usually have been serologically diagnosed by four-fold or greater rises in antibody levels between acute and convalescent serums. Hemagglutination inhibiting and virus neutralizing antibodies usually appear several days after onset of disease, followed in 2 to 3 weeks by antibodies detectable in complement-fixation, immuno-diffusion,[3] or other tests. Prompt laboratory diagnosis is needed to differentiate California encephalitis caused by LAC virus from encephalitis from other causes.

Serologic surveys have usually been based on virus neutralization or hemagglutination tests which detect antibodies for many years following infection, while complement fixing antibodies are usually detectable for only a year or so after infection.

Comparative neutralization tests[22,27] have commonly been used to differentiate between antibodies from LAC and other California group arboviruses endemic in various parts of the country. Although cross-reactions occur at low serum dilutions, convalescent sera from cases of California encephalitis have consistently shown higher titer to LAC virus antigen than other California group virus antigens.

Virus isolations from human cases have been difficult because of the short viremia and early appearance of circulating antibodies with accompanying loss of viral infectivity. Virus isolations from mosquitoes and viremic vertebrate hosts have frequently been obtained from properly collected and preserved mosquitoes and viremic vertebrate hosts.

Sequelae

Major sequelae have been uncommon following cases of California encephalitis in children. However, electroencephalogram studies of 35 former cases in Wisconsin revealed 10 with residual abnormalities when examined up to 8 years after their acute illness. Residual neurological findings included meningeal signs (24), Babinsky's reflex (8), paresis (6), tremors (3), abnormal optic disc margins (3), aphasia (2), and chorea (1).[14,29] The abnormalities reported indicated persistent focal or diffuse cerebral neuronal dysfunction.[14] In Ohio, most of 14 children studied were typically nervous, hyperactive, and restless.[11,20,23,41,43]

Pathology

The initial recognized case of California encephalitis, from which the prototype strain of LAC virus was recovered from brain tissues, has been described.[52] It occurred in a 4-year-old girl hospitalized during September of 1960 with high fever, severe headache, vomiting, convulsions, and pleocytosis. She died on the 6th day of hospitalization with respiratory distress and hypotension. Pulmonary and brain edema were observed at necropsy. Histological changes were most apparent in the cerebral cortex and basal ganglia, with neuronal degeneration and patches of inflammation and perivascular cuffing and edema. Histologic changes were similar to those of other arthropod-borne viral encephalitides.

EPIDEMIOLOGY

Occurrence

California group arboviruses are endemically maintained in nature in specific geographic regions recognized by the distribution of virus isolates from mosquitoes,[46] virus neutralizing antibodies[30] in people and animals, and occasional virus isolations from human beings and other vertebrates. There is some geographic overlap between endemic regions, with several different California group viruses being present in some regions.

The more than 800 cases of California encephalitis reported to the Center for Disease Control (CDC) between 1963 and 1976 have occurred in the midwestern and eastern part of the U.S.[46] No cases have been found in California since the three index cases recognized in 1945.[17,37] Most cases have been reported from Wisconsin,[50,51] Ohio,[8] Minnesota,[2] and other states which have eastern hardwood deciduous forest regions. Cases have occurred only during the mosquito season, June through October, in this temperate climate. The distribution of LAC virus activity as indicated by isolates reported from mosquitoes throughout the U.S.[46] shows a geographic distribution for the virus similar to that of the reported cases of California encephalitis in human patients.

Other California group arboviruses have distributions which encompass most parts of the country. Trivittatus and Jamestown Canyon viruses have been recovered from endemic foci in most states. Snowshoe hare virus has been found in northern states and Canada.[10] Keystone virus has been isolated from mosquitoes in eastern and southweastern seacoast states,[47] and California encephalitis virus in western states.[45] San Angelo and South River viruses have been isolated in Texas and New Jersey.[7]

Vertebrate Hosts

Primary vertebrate hosts as well as vectors involved have indicated different natural cycles for each California group arbovirus. Chipmunks (*Tamias striatus*) and squirrels (*Sciurus spp.*) have been shown to be principal hosts for LAC, with viremic levels during natural infection sufficient to infect female *Ae. triseriatus* mosquitoes.[35] Other vertebrate hosts occasionally infected with LAC have not been shown to develop viremic levels which would contribute significantly to the natural cycle.

Principal vertebrate hosts reported for other California group arboviruses have included snowshoe hares (*L. americanus*) and ground squirrels (*Cittelus* spp.) for snowshoe hare virus,[34] and white-tailed deer for Jamestown Canyon virus.[21] Hares, rabbits, and tree squirrels may often be infected with Trivittatus virus,[39] cotton rats with Keystone,[47] and rabbits and ground squirrels with California encephalitis viruses.[15]

Human beings and other vertebrates tangentially infected in nature have not been shown to play a significant role in the natural maintenance of LAC or other California group arboviruses in the U.S.

VECTORS

The vector status of *Ae. triseriatus* for LAC virus has been defined by: (1) repeated isolates of LAC virus from *Ae. triseriatus* collected in the field,[48] (2) field association of infected mosquitoes with infected vertebrate populations,[31] (3) experimental infection of mosquitoes by controlled blood meals on viremic vertebrates,[35] and (4) by demonstration of the transmission of LAC virus by infected mosquitoes allowed to bite susceptible vertebrate hosts after a period of extrinsic incubation. LAC virus has also been shown to be transmitted transovarially[36,55] and venereally in *Ae. triseriatus* mosquitoes.[49]

Ae. triseriatus is endemic in the California encephalitis area in midwestern and eastern states in deciduous forested areas where cases of California encephalitis are found. Well protected oviposition sites needed by *Ae. triseriatus* are found in basal tree holes and other water-holding containers on forested hillsides.

LAC virus has been obtained repeatedly from *Ae. triseriatus* larvae reared from overwintered eggs.[54,55] LAC virus is widespread throughout many tissues of *Ae. triseriatus* larvae, pupae, and emerging adults developing from eggs infected transovarially. In these transovarially infected mosquitoes, LAC virus is present in salivary glands and accessory sex organs in both females and males upon emergence as adults.[6] Venereal transmission of LAC from transovarially infected males to previously non-infected females has been demonstrated in this laboratory.[49]

Although most isolates of LAC virus have been from *Ae. triseriatus,* some isolates have occasionally been obtained from other species such a *Ae. canadensis* in Ohio.[8] Vertical transmission studies have not been reported for these species.

California group arboviruses other than LAC have been isolated from a number of different *Aedes* mosquitoes. Isolates of Keystone virus have been mainly from *Ae. atlanticus-tormentor, Ae. infirmatus,* and *Ae. taeniorhynchus* mosquitoes in southeastern states.[26,42] Trivittatus virus has been obtained mainly from *Ae. trivittatus* mosquities in midwestern states,[13,24,38,53] and from *Ae. infirmatus* in Florida.[46] Jamestown Canyon virus has been isolated from at least 12 *Aedes* species including the *Ae. communis* group, and from biting flies in Wisconsin,[12] although the vector status of the flies has not been demonstrated.

A few isolates of additional California group arboviruses have been reported from other *Aedes* spp. mosquitoes but sufficient studies have not been carried out to implicate vector relationships.

Isolates of California group arboviruses other than LAC have been obtained recently from larvae of vector mosquito species, including Keystone virus in Maryland[25] and Trivittatus virus in Iowa,[1] implicating these species in transovarial transmission of the viruses.

Environment

The survival of LAC and other California group viruses depends upon environmental factors affecting survival of primary vector and host species. The effective oviposition sites of *Ae triseriatus,* the main vector of LAC virus, are in the basal tree holes,[18] old tires, and other water holding containers on forested hillsides. These provide a protected habitat for the survival of eggs and larvae of the vector during winter seasons when adults could not otherwise survive the rigid climate, as in Wisconsin and other midwestern states. The overwintering of LAC virus in diapause phase eggs,[6] and a long emergence period continuing throughout the next season in installment hatching[5] maintains the endemic nature of LAC virus. Limited studies have indicated that similar maintenance mechanisms may also be responsible for the continuing endemic existence of other California group arboviruses in their selected geographic areas.

CONTROL

Prevention and Treatment

Endemic areas can be defined by epidemologic studies of cases in children, antibody surveys in people or other vertebrates, sentinel animal studies, or by virus isolation studies in vector mosquitoes. In LAC infection foci, the adult *Ae. triseriatus* are difficult to collect in ordinary light traps and are usually collected by aspirations from human volunteers. Collections of larvae for virus isolation studies from oviposition sites, best observed in the prefoliage period of spring, provide opportunity for preseasonal surveillance.

Prevention of California encephalitis and other infections by California group arboviruses in endemic areas focuses mainly upon a protection of the population at risk from bites by primary mosquito vectors. Since the primary vector of the LAC virus, *Ae. triseriatus* emerges from specialized oviposition in basal tree holes, old automobile tires, or other water holding containers on forested hillsides, and has a limited flight range, mosquito populations can be effectively reduced in high risk park and suburban areas by filling or removing these oviposition sites. Because of the greater severity of the infection in children than in adults, they must be considered the population at the greatest risk.

Reducing mosquito bites in children by the use of repellants, proective clothing covering arms and legs, room screening, and by avoiding contact with forested areas during highest summer season or daily (morning and late afternoon) peaks in mosquito activity are also helpful for control.

Treatment of cases of California encephalitis is mainly symptomatic. No vaccines or antisera are commercially available. Laboratory tests are necessary to differentiate causes of encephalitis. Many cases have been missed because timely samples were not submitted to diagnostic laboratories. Prompt diagnosis and treatment reduces complications and long-term damage to brain and other tissues. Medical histories of exposure are helpful not only for presumptive diagnosis but for control purposes. Although this disease does not usually affect more than one or two siblings or playmates in a neighborhood during a season, infections during subsequent years have been common in endemic foci. Health education of parents and the public is important in the control of California (La Crosse) encephalitis.

PUBLIC HEALTH ASPECTS

Economic and Social Impact

The average California (La Crosse) encephalitis case has a period of 5 to 10 days hospitalization. The endemic nature of these infections, as with other forms of encephalitis, generates community as well as family concern.

Most infections with LAC virus in children have produced disease severe enough for medical attention or hospitalization. Most children with antibodies to LAC virus in the suburbs of La Crosse, Wisconsin also have a history of hospitalization or medical attention for encephalitis. Early diagnosis is essential for prompt, proper treatment, and better early diagnostic tests are needed. The medical importance of California group arbovirus infections other than LAC commonly occurring throughout the U.S. also needs further study.

Reporting

California encephalitis is a reportable disease. The Encephalitis Surveillance Unit of the CDC in Atlanta regularly collects incidence data from state health departments, and reports national data on California encephalitis.

Surveillance

Early detection of suspected cases by physicians, prompt and early laboratory differential diagnostic assistance in arboviral and other encephalitides, and prompt reporting to city, county, state, and federal agencies are necessary to define disease levels and endemic areas. This information is needed by physicians, health officials, and others concerned wth control efforts.

REFERENCES

1. **Andrews, W. N., Rowley, W. A., Wong, Y. W., Dorsey, D. C., and Hausler, W. J., Jr.,** Isolation of trivittatus virus from larvae and adults reared from field-collected larvae of *Aedes trivittatus* (Diptera: Culicidae), *J. Med. Entomol.,* 13, 699, 1977.
2. **Balfour, H. H., Jr., Edelman, C. K., Bauer, H., and Siem, R. A.,** California arbovirus (La Crosse) infections. III. Epidemiology of California encephalitis in Minnesota, *J. Infect. Dis.,* 133, 293, 1976.
3. **Balfour, H. H., Jr., Majerle, R. J., and Edelman, C. K.,** California arbovirus (La Crosse) infections. II. Precipitin antibody tests for the diagnosis of California encephalitis, *Infect. Immun.,* 8, 947, 1973.
4. **Bardos, V., Medek, M., Kania, V., and Hubalek, Z.,** Isolation of Tahyna virus from the blood of sick children, *Acta Virol. (Engl. Ed.),* 19, 447, 1975.
5. **Beaty, B. J. and Thompson, W. H.,** Emergence of La Crosse virus from endemic foci. Fluorescent antibody studies of overwintered *Aedes triseriatus, Am. J. Trop. Med. Hyg.,* 24, 685, 1975.
6. **Beaty, B. J. and Thompson, W. H.,** Delineation of La Crosse virus in developmental stages of transovarially infected *Aedes triseriatus, Am. J. Trop. Med. Hyg.,* 25, 505, 1976.
7. **Berge, T. O., Ed.,** International Catalogue of Arboviruses Including Certain Viruses of Vertebrates, 2nd ed., Pub. No. (CDC) 75-8301, Public Health Service, U.S. Department of Health, Education and Welfare, Atlanta, 1975.
8. **Berry, R. L., Parsons, M. A., LaLonde, B. J., Stegmiller, H. W., Lebio, J., Jalil, M., and Masterson, R. A.,** Studies on the epidemiology of California encephalitis in an endemic area in Ohio in 1971, *Am. J. Trop. Med. Hyg.,* 24, 992, 1975.
9. **Bond, J. O., Hammon, W. McD., Lewis, A. L., Sather, G. E., and Taylor, D. J.,** California group arboviruses in Florida and report of a new strain, Keystone virus, *Public Health Rep.,* 81, 607, 1966.
10. **Burgdorfer, W., Newhouse, V. G., and Thomas, L. A.,** Isolation of California encephalitis virus from the blood of a snowshoe hare (*Lepus americanus*) in western Montana, *Am. J. Hyg.,* 73, 344, 1961.
11. **Cramblett, H. G.,** California encephalitis virus infections in children: clinical and laboratory studies, *JAMA,* 198, 108, 1966.
12. **DeFoliart, G. R., Anslow, R. O., Hanson, R. P., Morris, C. D., Papadopoulos, O., and Sather, G. E.,** Isolation of Jamestown Canyon serotype of California encephalitis virus from naturally infected *Aedes* mosquitoes and tabanids, *Am. J. Trop. Med. Hyg.,* 18, 440, 1969.
13. **DeFoliart, G. R., Anslow, R. O., Thompson, W. H., Hanson, R. P., Wright, R. E., and Sather, G. E.,** Isolation of trivittatus virus from Wisconsin mosquitoes, 1964—1968, *J. Med. Entomol.,* 9, 67, 1972.
14. **Grabow, J. D., Matthews, C. G., Chun, R. W. M., and Thompson, W. H.,** The electroencephalogram and clinical sequelae of California arbovirus encephalitis, *Neurology,* 19, 394, 1969.
15. **Gresikova, M., Reeves, W. C., and Scrivani, R. P.,** California encephalitis virus: an evaluation of its continued endemic status in Kern County, California, *Am. J. Hyg.,* 80, 229, 1964.
16. **Hammon, W. McD. and Reeves, W. C.,** California encephalitis virus; a newly described agent, *Calif. Med.,* 77, 303, 1952.
17. **Hammon, W. McD. and Sather, G.,** History and recent reappearance of viruses in the California encephalitis group, *Am. J. Trop. Med. Hyg.,* 15, 199, 1966.
18. **Hanson, R. P. and Hanson, M. G.,** The effect of land use practices on the vector of California encephalitis (La Crosse) in north central United States, *Mosq. News,* 30, 215, 1970.
19. **Henderson, B. E. and Coleman, P. H.,** The growing importance of California arboviruses in the etiology of human disease, in *Progress in Medical Virology,* Melnick, J. L., Ed., S. Karger, Basel, 1971, 404.
20. **Hilty, M. D., Haynes, R. E., Azimi, P. H., and Cramblett, H. G.,** California encephalitis in children, *Am. J. Dis. Child.,* 124, 530, 1972.
21. **Issel, C. J., Trainer, D. O., and Thompson, W. H.,** Serologic evidence of infections of white-tailed deer in Wisconsin with three California group arboviruses (La Crosse, Trivittatus, and Jamestown Canyon), *Am. J. Trop. Med. Hyg.,* 21, 985, 1972.
22. **Johnson, K. P.,** California encephalitis epidemiologic studies in Ohio using a quantitative metabolic inhibition test, *Am. J. Epidemiol.,* 92, 203, 1970.
23. **Johnson, K. P., Lepow, M. L., and Johnson, R. T.,** California encephalitis. I. Clinical and epidemiological studies, *Neurology,* 18, 250, 1968.
24. **Kokernot, R. H., Hayes, J., Chan, D. H. M., and Boyd, K. R.,** Arbovirus studies in the Ohio-Mississippi basin, 1964—1967, V. Trivittatus and western equine encephalomyelitis viruses, *Am. J. Trop. Med. Hyg.,* 18, 774, 1969.
25. **Le Duc, J. W., Suyemoto, W., Eldridge, B. F., Russell, P. K., and Barr, A. R.,** Ecology of California encephalitis viruses on the Del Mar Va Peninsula. II. Demonstration of transovarial transmission, *Am. J. Trop. Med. Hyg.,* 24, 124, 1975.

26. Le Duc, J. W., Suyemoto, W., Keefe, T. J., Burger, J. F., Eldridge, B. F., and Russell, P. K., Ecology of California encephalitis viruses on the Del Mar Va Peninsula, I. Virus Isolations from mosquitoes, *Am. J. Trop. Med. Hyg.*, 24, 118, 1975.

27. Lindsey, H. S., Calisher, C. H., and Mathews, J. H., Serum dilution neutralization test for California group virus identification and serology, *J. Clin. Microbiol.*, 4, 503, 1976.

28. Masterson, R. A., Stegmiller, H. W., Parsons, M. A., Croft, C. C., and Spencer, C. B., California encephalitis — an endemic puzzle in Ohio, *Health Lab. Sci.*, 8, 89, 1971.

29. Matthews, C. G., Chun, R. W. M., Grabow, J. D., and Thompson, W. H., Psychological sequelae in children following California arbovirus encephalitis, *Neurology*, 18, 1023, 1968.

30. Monath, T. P. C., Nuckolls, J. G., Berall, J., Bauer, H., Chappell, W. A., and Coleman, P. H., Studies on California encephalitis in Minnesota, *Am. J. Epidemiol.*, 92, 40, 1970.

31. Moulton, D. W. and Thompson, W. H., California group virus infections in small, forest-dwelling mammals of Wisconsin: some ecological considerations, *Am. J. Trop. Med. Hyg.*, 20, 474, 1971.

32. Murphy, F. A. and Coleman, P. H., California group arboviruses: immunodiffusion studies, *J. Immunol.*, 99, 276, 1967.

33. Murphy, F. A., Harrison, A. K., and Whitfield, S. G., Bunyaviridae: morphologic and morphogenetic similarities of Bunyamwera serologic supergroup viruses and several other arthropod-borne viruses, *Intervirology*, 1, 297, 1973.

34. Newhouse, V. F., Burgdorfer, W., and Corwin, D., Field and laboratory studies on the hosts and vectors of the snowshoe hare strain of California virus, *Mosq. News*, 31, 401, 1971.

35. Pantuwatana, S., Thompson, W. H., Watts, D. M., and Hanson, R. P., Experimental infection of chipmunks and squirrels with La Crosse and trivittatus viruses and biological transmission of La Crosse virus by *Aedes triseriatus*, *Am. J. Trop. Med. Hyg.*, 21, 476, 1972.

36. Pantuwatana, S., Thompson, W. H., Watts, D. M., Yuill, T. M., and Hanson, R. P., Isolation of La Crosse virus from field collected *Aedes triseriatus* larvae, *Am. J. Trop. Med. Hyg.*, 23, 246, 1974.

37. Parkin, W. E., Hammon, W. McD., and Sather, G. E., Review of current epidemiological literature on viruses of the California arbovirus group, *Am. J. Trop. Med. Hyg.*, 21, 964, 1972.

38. Pinger, R. R. and Rowley, W. A., Host preferences of *Aedes trivittatus* (Diptera: Culicidae) in central Iowa, *Am. J. Trop. Med. Hyg.*, 24, 889, 1975.

39. Pinger, R. R., Rowley, W. A., Wong Y. W., and Dorsey, D. C., Trivittatus virus infections in wild mammals and sentinel rabbits in central Iowa, *Am. J. Trop. Med. Hyg.*, 24, 1006, 1975.

40. Porterfield, J. S., Casals, J., Chumakov, M. P., Gaidamovich, S. Ya., Hannoun, C., Holmes, I. H., Horzinek, M. C., Mussgay, M., Oker-Blom, N., and Russell, P. K., Bunyaviruses and Bunyaviridae, *Intervirology*, 6, 13, 1975—76.

41. Rie, H. E., Hilty, M. D., and Cramblett, H. G., Intelligence and coordination following California encephalitis, *Am. J. Dis. Child.*, 125, 824, 1973.

42. Roberts, D. R. and Scanlon, J. E., The ecology and behavior of *Aedes atlanticus* D. and K. and other species with reference to Keystone virus in the Houston area, Texas, *J. Med. Entomol.*, 12, 537, 1976.

43. Sabatino, D. A. and Cramblett, H. G., Behavioral sequelae of California encephalitis virus infection in children, *Dev. Med. Child Neurol.*, 10, 331, 1968.

44. Sather, G. E. and Hammon, W. McD., Antigenic patterns within the California-encephalitis-virus group, *Am. J. Trop. Med. Hyg.*, 16, 548, 1967.

44a. Porterfield, J. S., National Institute for Medical Research, London, England, personal communication, 1977.

45. Smart, K. L., Elbel, R. E., Woo, R. F. N., Kern, E. R., Crane, G. T., Bales, G. L., and Hill, D. W., California and western encephalitis viruses from Bonneville Basin, Utah in 1965, *Mosq. News*, 32, 382, 1972.

46. Sudia, W. D., Newhouse, V. F., Calisher, C. H., and Chamberlain, R. W., California group arboviruses: isolations from mosquitoes in North America, *Mosq. News*, 31, 576, 1971.

47. Taylor, D. J., Lewis, A. L., Edman, J. D., and Jennings, W. L., California group arboviruses in Florida: host-vector relations, *Am. J. Trop. Med. Hyg.*, 20 139, 1971.

48. Thompson, W. H., Anslow, R. O., Hanson, R. P., and DeFoliart, G. R., La Crosse virus isolations from mosquitoes in Wisconsin, 1964—68, *Am. J. Trop. Med. Hyg.*, 21, 90, 1972.

49. Thompson, W. H. and Beaty, B. J., Venereal transmission of La Crosse (California Encephalitis) arbovirus in *Aedes triseriatus* mosquitoes, *Science*, 196, 530, 1977.

50. Thompson, W. H. and Evans, A. S., California encephalitis virus studies in Wisconsin, *Am. J. Trop. Med. Hyg.*, 81, 230, 1965.

51. Thompson, W. H. and Inhorn, S. L., Arthropod-borne California group viral encephalitis in Wisconsin, *Wis. Med. J.*, 66, 250, 1967.

52. Thompson, W. H., Kalfayan, B., and Anslow, R. O., Isolation of California encephalitis group virus from a fatal human illness, *Am. J. Trop. Med. Hyg.*, 81, 245, 1965.

53. **Watts, D. M., DeFoliart, G. R., and Yuill, T. M.,** Experimental transmission of trivittatus virus (California virus group) by *Aedes trivittatus, Am. J. Trop. Med. Hyg.,* 25, 173, 1976.

54. **Watts, D. M., Pantuwatana, S., DeFoliart, G. R., Yuill, T. M., and Thompson, W. H.,** Transovarial transmission of La Crosse virus (California encephalitis group) in the mosquito, *Aedes triseriatus, Science,* 182, 1140, 1973.

55. **Watts, D. M., Thompson, W. H., Yuill, T. M., DeFoliart, G. R., and Hanson, R. P.,** Overwintering of La Crosse virus in *Aedes triseriatus, Am. J. Trop. Med. Hyg.,* 23, 694, 1974.

56. **Wong, Y. W., Rowley, W. A., Rowe, J. A., Dorsey, D. C., Humphreys, M. J., and Hausler, W. J., Jr.,** California encephalitis studies in Iowa during 1969, 1970 and 1971, *Health Lab. Sci.,* 10, 88, 1973.

57. **Young, D. J.,** California encephalitis virus. Report of three cases and review of the literature, *Ann. Intern. Med.,* 65, 419, 1966.

CALIFORNIA GROUP VIRAL INFECTIONS OF CANADA

D. M. McLean

NAME AND SYNONYMS

Most strains of the California encephalitis (CE) complex of mosquito-borne arboviruses which have been isolated in Canada have shown serologic identity with the Montana snowshoe hare subtype, and are usually termed snowshoe hare (SSH) virus isolates. Occasional isolates from Alberta mosquitoes have been typed serologically as the Jamestown Canyon (JC) subtype of CE virus.

HISTORY

Initial Canadian isolates of CE virus (snowshoe hare subtype) were achieved from the blood of sentinel rabbits at Richmond, Ontario (45°N, 75°W) during summer 1963,[10] following the isolation of the prototype strain from the blood of a snowshoe hare (*Lepus americanus*) collected in the Bitter Root Valley near Hamilton, Montana (46°N, 114°N) in summer 1959.[1] Subsequent investigations of arbovirus prevalence in mosquitoes have resulted in virus isolations in northern Alberta 1964 to 68,[5] southern British Columbia 1969,[12] Saskatchewan 1972,[7] the Yukon Territory 1971 to 78,[14,17] and the Keewatin 1973[21] and Mackenzie 1976,[16] districts of the Northwest Territories, extending as far north as Inuvik (69°N, 135°W) in 1976 and 1978. Serologic evidence of infection of the central nervous system by SSH virus was first detected during 1978 among human residents of the boreal forest of the province of Quebec, Canada.[3] From 1964 through 1976, 42 to 160 cases of encephalitis per year affecting residents of U.S. have been attributed to infection with viruses of the CE complex.[2]

ETIOLOGY

Classification

The California encephalitis complex comprises 12 serotypes within the virus family Bunyaviridae.[19] This family comprises at least 93 members in 12 antigenic groups which comprise the Bunyamwera supergroup. Morphologically they exhibit spherical, helically symmetrical, envcloped virions containing single-stranded RNA, with average particle diameters 90 to 100 nm. Within the California encephalitis complex, there are three main serological species ("types") Melao, Trivittatus, and California encephalitis. The latter type includes ten serotypes ("subtypes") which share common antigenic cross-relationships in mouse neutralization tests, and to some extent complement fixation tests also. However, they are clearly separable into ten subtypes by gel diffusion (Ouchterlony) and plaque-reduction neutralization tests in tissue culture.[9] Snowshoe hare virus is a subtype of California encephalitis.

DEFINITION

California encephalitis group virus infections in Canada have induced nonfatal encephalitis in two patients only during 1978.[3] In wild mamals, CE group infections have been confined to asymptomatic viremia followed by antibody production in rodents, principally squirrels, and lagomorphs, principally snowshoe hares, of the boreal forest and adjacent vegetation zones. Encephalitis[2] which may terminate fatally, has been associated etiologically with the La Cross subtype of CE virus in the U.S.,[20], especially in the Ohio-Mississippi River Basin.

ANIMAL INFECTION

Clinical

Suckling mice aged less than 2 days at the time of intra-cerebral inoculation develop fatal encephalitis 2 to 4 days later.[13] Weaned mice aged 3 to 4 weeks develop fatal encephalitis 5 to 7 days after intracerebral inoculation.[13] Domestic rabbits and snowshoe hares develop inapparent infections which are manifested by transient viremia followed by antibody production, after exposure to SSH virus in nature or by intravenous injection.[10,13] Ground squirrels *Citellus undulatus* and *Citellus columbianus*), tree squirrels, (*Tamiasciurus hudsonicus*) and marmots (*Marmota flaviventris* and *M. monax*) develop inapparent infections accompanied by antibody production following natural infections.[12,14] Wild and domestic birds, including newly hatched chickens are not susceptible to infection with SSH virus.

Diagnosis

In serological surveys for natural infection of wild animals with SSH virus, the mouse neutralization test has been the most reliable technique, in which weaned mice are inoculated intracerebrally with mixtures of undiluted test sera and virus dilutions containing 100 mouse LD_{50}.[14]

HUMAN INFECTION

The first two cases of human infection with SSH virus in Canada were reported in 1978.[3] Both patients recovered after mild encephalitis. Antibody conversions to SSH virus have been demonstrated in paired sera from human residents of an endemic focus in east-central Alaska in the absence of identifiable clinical illness.[4] Serological surveys of human residents of boreal forest regions have shown CE antibodies in 48 of 1936 (2.5%) in British Columbia[8] and 51 of 160 (32%) in Alberta.[6]

Diagnosis in suspected cases of SSH infection in humans with acute meningitis or encephalitis is achieved by demonstration of rising SSH antibody titers in neutralization and/or complement fixation tests in paired sera collected within 2 days after onset, and again within 2 to 7 days after defervescence.

EPIDEMIOLOGY

Occurrence

Isolations of CE virus (snowshoe hare subtype) have been achieved from wild-caught unengorged female mosquitoes collected in British Columbia, the Yukon Territory, the Northwest Territories, Alberta, Saskatchewan, and Ontario[11] and serological infection of *Lepus americanus* and squirrels has been demonstrated in each of these jurisdictions except Saskatchewan. The boreal forest areas of the Yukon (60 to 66°N), northern British Columbia, Alberta, and Saskatchewan north of about 53°N comprise the prime region of prevalence of SSH virus, but its prevalence extends northwards into the open woodland zone of the Mackenzie District (60 to 69°N) in the Northwest Territories. The virus is also prevalent in the southeastern mixed forest regions of Ontario at latitudes 45 to 46°N.

Reservoir

The principal wildlife reservoir is *Lepus americanus* wherever this species is abundant, and subsidiary, but important, reservoirs are squirrels.[11] In the Yukon Territory, for example, during summers 1971 to 74, SSH antibody was detected in 430 of 1076 (40%) *Lepus americanus*.[14] Although the population of *L. americanus* declined drastically during 1974, the 5% antibody rate among arctic ground squirrels (*C. undulatus*) during that year was similar to the 4-year total of 266 of 3610 (7%). In British Columbia, 20 of 31 (64.5%) *L. americanus* had antibody during 1969 and 1970,[11], while in Alberta, between 1964 and 1968, 111 of 216 *L. americanus* had antibody,[6] and in Ontario, during 1963, 9 of 107 (8%) *L. americanus*.[11] Viremia with SSH virus was demonstrated in 1 *L. americanus* plus 3 of 36 sentinel rabbits in Alberta[22] and in 5 of 9 sentinel rabbits in Ontario.[10]

Vector

Aedes spp. mosquitoes, especially *A. communis* and *A. hexodontus*, which form major components of the mosquito population in the boreal forest, open woodland, and tundra vegetation zones of Canada, are the principal natural vectors of CE group arboviruses in Canada. Minimum field infection rates among mosquitoes[11] are 1 to 1300 *A. canadensis* in British Columbia during 1969,[12] and 1 to 8 *A. fitchii* in 1973;[11] 1 to 496 *A. canadensis*, 1 to 1179 *A. cinereus*, 1 to 1765 *A. communis* and 1 to 1778 *Culiseta inornata* in the Yukon Territory between 1971 and 1974;[14] 1 to 1189 *A. hexodontus* in the Keewatin District during 1973;[7] and 1 to 6358 *A. communis*, 1 to 1274 *A. hexodontus* and 1 to 1404 *A. punctor* in the Mackenzie District of the Northwest Territories during 1976;[16] 1 to 2000 *A. communis* and 1 to 3032 *A. stimulans* in Alberta during 1964—68; 1 to 313 *A. cataphylla*, 1 to 201 *A. excrucians*, 1 to 3072 *A. fitchii* and 1 to 238 *A. punctor* in Saskatchewan during 1972.[7]

After *A. communis* mosquitoes, which were collected wild in the Arctic, imbibed blood meals containing 1000, 100, 1, or 0.01 mouse LD_{50} of mouse passage SSH virus, transmission was demonstrated following 13 days incubation at 13°C. Virus transmission was attained 20 days after mosquitoes imbibed 100 mouse LD_{50}, following incubation at 0°C.[16] Transmission of unpassaged SSH virus recovered from arctic mosquitoes was demonstrated 13 days after *A. communis* imbibed one mouse LD_{50} following incubation at 13°C and at 23°C.[15] These laboratory results show clearly that *A. communis* may serve as a natural summer vector of SSH virus, due to: (1) the ability of this mosquito to support virus replication at frigid summertime environmental temperatures 0 to 13°C which prevail through the Canadian Arctic and (2) its susceptibility to infection and subsequent ability to transmit virus following 2 weeks of extrinsic incubation after imbibing as little as 1 mouse LD_{50} of wild SSH virus. This virus dose is usually exceeded in the blood of naturally infected snowshoe hares.[10]

Transovarial transfer may provide an important overwintering mechanism for SSH virus. In the Yukon Territory during late April 1975, and in mid-May 1974, three virus strains were recovered from 302 pools of *Aedes* sp. larvae collected in boreal forest locations at 61°N before any adult mosquitoes had emerged from water in semifrozen roadside ditches.[11,14] Since *Aedes* mosquitoes characteristically lay only one batch of eggs each summer, it seems clear that these larvae become infected through eggs deposited by infected female mosquitoes during the previous summer. However, it is also possible that SSH virus may overwinter in tissues of infected adult mosquitoes, since virus has been recovered from thoraces of *Culiseta inornata* and *A. communis* 138 days after intrathoracic injection following incubation at 0°C[14] and in the salivary gland of *Cs. inornata* mosquitoes after 329 days incubation at 4°C.[18]

CONTROL

Since infection of mosquitoes with SSH virus is distributed widely through several thousand miles of sparsely populated boreal forest, open woodland, and tundra regions of northern Canada, effective control is impossible except in small areas where humans live and work in close proximity to each other. General measures aimed at substantial reduction of numbers of *Aedes* mosquito larvae by effective drainage of swamps, possibly accompanied by application of larvicides, together with abatement of adult mosquitoes by adulticide spraying programs and universal coverage of windows of dwellings by wire screens, should result in eradication of small foci of SSH virus infection.

REFERENCES

1. **Burgdorfer, W., Newhouse, V. F., and Thomas, L. A.,** Isolation of California encephalitis virus from the blood of a snowshoe hare (*Lepus americanus*) in western Montana, *Am. J. Hyg.,* 73, 346, 1961.
2. Center for Disease Control, Encephalitis Surveillance, annual summary, 1976, Center for Disease Control, Atlanta, December 1978.
3. **Fauvel, M., Artsob, H., Davignon, L., and Chagnon, A.,** First recorded clinical cases of California encephalitis in children in Canada, *Can. J. Public Health,* 70, 48, 1979.
4. **Feltz, E. T., List-Young, B., Ritter, D. G., Holden, P., Noble, G. R., and Clark, P. S.,** California encephalitis virus: serological evidence of human infection in Alaska, *Can. J. Microbiol.,* 18, 757, 1972.
5. **Iversen, J. O., Hanson, R. P., Papadopoulos, O., Morris, C. V., and De Foliart, G. R.,** Isolation of viruses of the California encephalitis virus group from boreal *Aedes* mosquitoes, *Am. J. Trop. Med. Hyg.,* 18, 735, 1969.
6. **Iversen, J. O., Seawright G., and Hanson, R. P.,** Serologic survey for arboviruses in central Alberta, *Can. J. Public Health,* 62, 125, 1971.
7. **Iversen, J. O., Wagner, R. J., De Jong, C., and McLintock, J. R.,** California encephalitis virus in Saskatchewan: isolation from boreal *Aedes* mosquitoes, *Can. J. Public Health,* 64, 590, 1973.
8. **Kettyls, G. D., Verrall, V. M., Wilton, L. D., Clapp, J. B., Clarke, D. A., and Rublee, J. D.,** Arbovirus infections in man in British Columbia, *Can. Med. Assoc., J.,* 106, 1175, 1972.
9. **Lindsey, H. S., Calisher, C. H., and Mathews, J. H.,** Serum dilution neutralization test for California group virus identification and serology, *J. Clin. Microbiol.,* 4, 503, 1976.
10. **McKeil, J. A., Hall, R. R., and Newhouse, V. F.,** Viruses of the California encephalitis complex in indicator rabbits, *Am. J. Trop. Med. Hyg.,* 15, 98, 1966.
11. **McLean, D. M.,** Arboviruses and human health in Canada, Publ. No. 14106, National Research Council of Canada, Ottawa, 1975.
12. **McLean, D. M., Crawford, M. A., Ladyman, S. R., Peers, R. R. and Purvin-Good, K. W.,** California encephalitis and Powassan virus activity in British Columbia 1969, *Am. J. Epidemiol.,* 92, 266, 1970.
13. **McLean, D. M., Goddard, E. J., Graham, E. A., Hardy, G. J., and Purvin-Good, K. W.,** California encephalitis virus isolations from Yukon mosquitoes, 1971, *Am. J. Epidemiol.,* 95, 347, 1972.
14. **McLean, D. M., Bergman, S. K. A., Gould, A. P., Grass, P. N., Miller, M. A., and Spratt, E. E.,** California encephalitis virus prevalence throughout the Yukon Territory 1971—74, *Am. J. Trop. Med. Hyg.,* 24, 676, 1975.
15. **McLean, D. M., Grass, P. N., and Judd, B. D.,** California encephalitis virus transmission by arctic and domestic mosquitoes, *Arch. Virol.,* 55, 39, 1977.
16. **McLean, D. M., Grass, P. N., Judd, B. D., Ligate, L. V., and Peter, K. K.,** Bunyavirus isolations from mosquitoes in the western Canadian Arctic, *J. Hyg. (Camb.),* 79, 61, 1977.
17. **McLean, D. M., Grass, P. N., and Judd, B. D.,** Bunyavirus infection rates in Canadian Arctic mosquitoes, 1978, *Mosq. News,* 39, 364, 1979.
18. **McLean, D. M., Grass, P. N., Judd, B. D., and Stolz, K. J.,** Bunyavirus development in arctic and *Aedes aegypti* mosquitoes as revealed by glucose oxidase staining and immunofluorescence, *Arch. Virol.,* 62, 313, 1979.

19. **Porterfield, J. S., Casals, J., Chumakov, M. P., Gaidamovich, S. Ya., Hannoun, C., Holmes, I. H., Horzinek, M. C., Mussgay, M., Oker-Blom, N., and Russell, P. K.,** Bunyaviruses and Bunyaviridae, *Intervirology,* 6, 13, 1976.
20. **Sudia, W. D., Newhouse, V. F., Calisher, C. H. and Chamberlain, R. W.,** California group arboviruses: isolations from mosquitoes in North America, *Mosq. News,* 31, 576, 1971.
21. **Wagner, R. R., De Jong, C., Leung, M. K., McLintock, J., and Iversen, J. O.,** Isolations of California encephalitis virus from tundra mosquitoes, *Can. J. Microbiol.,* 21, 574, 1975.
22. **Yuill, T. M., Iversen, J. O., and Hanson, R. P.,** Evidence for arbovirus infections in a population of snowshoe hares: a possible mortality factor, *Bull. Wild. Dis. Assoc.,* 5, 248, 1969.

COLORADO TICK FEVER

R. W. Emmons

NAME AND SYNONYMS

Colorado tick fever (CTF) is the accepted name for this disease and there are no synonyms now used. Historically, it was referred to as "mountain fever" or "American mountain tick fever" before the viral etiology was established.

HISTORY

Priority for the recognition and description of CTF is uncertain, since many physicians from the 1850s to early 1900s mentioned "mountain fever" cases, but were unable to differentiate them with certainty from typhus, typhoid fever, malaria, and other diseases. There were many reports by Wilson and Chowning, Kieffer, Becker, Toomey, Schaffer, and others of a disease following tick bite which was not typical of Rocky Mountain spotted fever (RMSF), and which many Colorado physicians called "Colorado tick fever". There are conflicting published claims for the first recognition of the disease as a separate entity. Topping and co-workers[1] gave the first detailed clinical account of the disease in Colorado. Credit is generally given to Florio[2-4] and various collaborators (Stewart, Mugrage, Miller, and others) for the isolation and characterization of the virus from human cases and from *Dermacentor andersoni* ticks. They wrote extensively on the subject from 1944 to 1950. The virus was also adapted to the mouse and chick embryo by Koprowski, Cox, and collaborators, leading to the preparation of an experimental vaccine and study of the complement-fixation (CF) and neutralization test (NT) antibody responses in human volunteers during the period 1946 to 1950.[5,6] The reader is referred to Lloyd[7] and to Drevets[8] for more detailed accounts of the early history of CTF.

Oliphant and Tibbs[9] succeeded in isolating the virus in suckling mice, a more specific test procedure than the previous one which was based on the leucopenia produced in virus-infected hamsters. Field studies by Eklund, Kohls, Philip, Burgdorfer, Jellison, and others at the U.S. Public Health Service Rocky Mountain Laboratory in Hamilton, Montana, during the 1950 to 1960s elucidated the vector role of *D. andersoni* and other tick species, the most common vertebrate hosts, the geographic distribution, and other ecologic features of the CTF virus cycle, and the clinical and epidemiologic features of the human disease. These and other recent contributions to knowledge of CTF will be discussed and more fully referenced in the following sections. However, this is not a complete review of all published work on this disease.

ETIOLOGY

Classification

CTF virus is a member of the large and heterogenous group of arthropod-borne viruses (arboviruses), and is classified in the genus *Orbivirus,* of the family Reoviridae.[10,11] Minor serologic differences can be demonstrated among strains of CTF virus, but since the clinical disease, vectors, vertebrate hosts, and ecologic factors are essentially the same, only a single virus type is presently recognized. It was long considered to be an ungrouped virus, but a serologically-related virus (Eyach), isolated from *Ixodes ricinus* ticks in the Federal Republic of Germany, has recently been reported.[12]

Synonyms

As described in the preceding section, there are no currently used synonyms for the virus or for the disease it causes.

Characteristics

The virion consists of a double-stranded RNA genome,[13] the central core being about 50 nm in diameter, and the outer diameter about 80 nm. Viral development in cell culture results in cytoplasmic granular matrices and mature virions, and distinctive cytoplasmic and nuclear fibrillar or filamentous structures.[14,15]

The virus is relatively stable at room temperature, and is readily preserved by drying or freezing, particularly if protected by a protein-containing diluent. It is acid-labile; the optimum pH for maintenance of infectivity is from 7.5 to 7.8.[16] It is partially resistant to lipid solvents. Many cell culture types can be infected with or without the production of cytopathic effect (CPE), including primary cultures or established lines of avian, mammalian, and arthropod origin.[16-24] Interferon induction in infected cell cultures and mice has been reported.[25] In vertebrate hosts, including human beings, the virus infects hematopoietic cells and causes a prolonged viremia of weeks to months duration, due largely to the intraerythrocytic location of virions, where they are protected from antibodies or other host defense mechanisms.[26,27]

DEFINITION

The term Colorado tick fever refers to the disease in human patients, caused by the CTF virus. It consists of an acute, noncontagious, self-limited febrile illness following the bite of an infected tick (see section on Human Infection). The virus is not known to cause illness in the natural vertebrate hosts or tick vectors.

ANIMAL INFECTION

Clinical

The epizootic cycle of CTF virus consists of serial, apparently innocuous, infections of small, medium, and large mammals acquired via blood feeding by the various stages of tick species (primarily *D. andersoni*) which parasitize them (see section on Epidemiology), reflecting a long and successful adaptation to a stable ecologic niche. Large populations of both ticks and mammals are necessary to maintain these infections. It is possible that the virus is maintained in reservoir hosts by some mechanism other than tick transmission, but this has not been sufficiently investigated as yet. Experimental infections of such natural hosts as ground squirrels, chipmunks, deer mice, and porcupines result in viremias of up to a month or more, with titers of 10^3 to 10^6 (or higher) suckling mouse intracerebral (i.c.) LD_{50}/ml (SMICLD$_{50}$). A threshold viremia level of about 10^2 SMICLD$_{50}$ was estimated to be sufficient to infect larval or nymphal ticks feeding on such hosts; and the ticks retained infection after molting to the next developmental stage.[28-31] Viremia persisted over 5 months in experimentally-infected, hibernating, golden-mantled ground squirrels.[32]

When adapted to chick embryos or by i.c. passage to mice or hamsters, the virus becomes lethal for these hosts, as shown by early workers.[5,33] However, *unadapted* virus is usually lethal only for suckling mice. A standard strain (Florio) of the virus, pathogenic for adult mice, is available.[34] A transient depression of the peripheral leucocyte count is typical in infected hosts, and was used as an assay system in hamsters proir to 1950. Experimentally-infected rhesus monkeys developed prolonged viremia and depressed leucocyte count; fever developed in a few, but there were no other obvious signs of illness.[35] Baby chicks are also susceptible to infection, suggesting the possible role of ground-feeding birds in CTF ecology (H. N. Johnson, personal communication).

Pathology

Pathologic changes have not been described in naturally infected species. In laboratory animals, the virus has been found in a wide variety of tissues, perhaps because the test methods reflected the persistent viremia rather than virus production locally. However, there is apparent predilection of the virus for brain, spleen, lymphoid tissue, bone marrow , and heart muscle of laboratory mice.[36] Black, et al. found that infected hamsters had loss of lymphoid cells and appearance of large, pale inclusion-bearing mononuclear cells in the splenic follicles. The total leucocyte count was decreased, and some circulating lymphocytes had cytoplasmic inclusions.[37] Hadlow[38] described pathologic changes in mice, consisting of necrosis and mononuclear cell infiltration of cardiac muscle fibers and brain, liquefaction necrosis in the cerebellum, necrosis of fat and striated muscle, pericentral hepatic necrosis thymic involution, and pulmonary congestion. Miller, et al.[39] reported generalized cerebral vascular engorgement, petechial hemorrhages, and damage to the cerebellar Purkinje cell and granular cell layers, and formation of intracytoplasmic inclusion bodies in mice, hamsters and guinea pigs. Lesions were more severe in suckling mice than in older mice, and were more severe after i.c. than after i.p. inoculation. Infection of pregnant mice led to resorption of fetuses, stillbirths, or neonatal deaths, with replication of the virus to high titer in placental and fetal tissues.[40,41]

Most experimental infection studies have been done using virus strains passaged in animals by the i.c. route, which selects for neurotropism and reduces the ability of the virus to multiply in other tissues. Therefore, experimental findings may not reflect what occurs in natural infections. Isolation of the virus by i.m. inoculation, then subpassage of virus obtained from blood, is preferable for maintaining its natural tropism characteristics.

Diagnosis

The early developments in diagnostic methods utilized for animal hosts have been mentioned previously. Virus isolation and antibody assay methods, currently used for ecologic or pathogenetic studies, are the same as those used for the clinical disease (see section on Human Infection Diagnosis).

HUMAN INFECTION

Clinical

Mild or subclinical infections probably occur, but typically the onset of CTF is sudden, with chilly sensations, high fever, severe headache, photophobia and ocular pain, mild conjunctivitis, lethargy, myalgias, and arthralgias. The illness usually begins 3 to 6 days after tick bite, although not all patients are aware of having had a tick bite. The temperature pattern is often biphasic, with a 2 to 3 day febrile period, a remission of 1 to 2 days, then another 2 to 3 day febrile period, sometimes with worse symptoms. Rarely, there is a third febrile episode. Anorexia, nausea and vomiting, cloudy sensorium, disorientation, hallucinations, stiff neck, encephalitis, or a hemorrhagic diathesis may rarely occur, most frequently in children.[42-47] The spleen is sometimes palpable. A transient, petechial, or macular trunkal rash is sometimes observed, but is not persistent nor of the characteristic appearance and distribution of RMSF rash. Evidence of pericarditis and involvement of myocardium has been reported[48,49] of interest in view of the pathologic lesions noted in experimentally-infected mice (see section on Diagnosis).

The peripheral WBC usually falls dramatically to 2000 to 3000 or less, sometimes with a relative lymphocytosis. A "left shift" of granulocytes may occur, with meta-myelocytes and occasionally myelocytes in peripheral blood. Mild anemia may be noted. Thrombocytopenia may be marked in some cases.[50,51] The CSF may show lymphocytosis in cases with encephalitis. The persistent viremia so characteristic of the disease is due to the presence of the virus within erythrocytes, up to 120 days or more after onset of symptoms.[26,27,52,53] These infected cells can be detected by fluorescent antibody (FA) staining of peripheral blood smears (see section on Human Infection Diagnosis). One case of CTF inadvertently induced by blood transfusion has been documented.[54] and accidental transmission via needle sticks to hospital personnel or laboratory workers is a distinct hazard, but otherwise the disease is not contagious.

Recovery is usually prompt, but convalescence can be prolonged, with slow return to normal physical and mental functioning.[55] Only a few fatal cases have been described (see below), but others may have occurred and been erroneously attributed to RMSF. Infection apparently confers lasting immunity, although there are anecdotal reports of second attacks, and at least one instance in which two infections with CTF virus in the same person (1973 and 1974) were documented.[44]

Pathology

In one fatal patient, a 4-year-old boy, faint rash, purpura and petechiae, gross hemorrhage in the bowel, alveolar hyaline membrane, and capillary endothelial cell changes in lymph nodes were noted.[42] A second patient, a 10-year-old girl, showed acute renal failure, epistaxis, hematemesis, petechial rash, and disseminated intravascular coagulation syndrome; focal necrotic changes were seen in the liver, myocardium, spleen, intestine, and brain, with rare neuronal intracytoplasmic inclusion bodies in (the midbrain[56] (D. L. Dawson, personal communication). Three cases of CTF during early pregnancy have been noted.[42] (Poland, J. D., personal communication), one terminating in spontaneous abortion, and the other two resulting in healthy, full-term infants.

Diagnosis

Isolation of the virus from blood, by i.p. and/or i.c. inoculation of suspensions of blood clot or erythrocytes washed free of plasma into 1 to 3 day old mice is the preferred method for diagnosis, although the virus can also be isolated in various cell culture systems. Mice sicken or die from about the 4th to the 8th day, and specificity of the isolation is confirmed by FA staining of brain or blood smears, or by a standard neutralization test using harvested mouse brain tissue. The cross-immunity test is useful for identifying and characterizing strains of CTF virus isolated from wildlife or ticks: i.e., immunization of young adult mice by i.c. inoculation, then i.c. challenge of these mice along with control mice 3 to 4 weeks later, using the Florio strain of CTF virus (H. N. Johnson, personal communication). One "blind" passage of mouse brain harvested on about the 5th day has been suggested by some to enhance chances of isolating virus, although the increased danger of laboratory contamination and spurious "isolation" by this procedure should be recognized. The virus has also occasionally been isolated from the cerebrospinal fluid (CSF). When testing tick specimens, it is advisable to double the usual concentration of antibiotics, and to add normal rabbit serum or fetal bovine serum to a concentration of 50%. In studies of organ tropism of the virus, organs to be tested must be taken with separate sterile instruments and rinsed in sterile saline (or the animal should first be perfused with saline) to remove blood, thus avoiding cross-contamination and reflecting only the virus growth in tissue cells.

The use of the FA test on mouse tissues, first described by Burgdorfer and Lackman,[57] also has been used for detection of viral antigen in peripheral blood smears, allowing rapid and early confirmation of the disease, often within a day or two of onset of the disease.[58] Although in routine practice, some cases are missed if only the earliest blood smears are tested,[55] skill and persistence in applying the test are nearly always rewarded, and it should be a routine test available for all endemic areas of the disease. Rapid confirmation of CTF removes concern about the similar and more serious disease, RMSF, and helps reduce unnecessary antibiotic treatment.

Antibody tests may be used for serologic surveys, or as a diagnostic test if a rising titer between acute- and convalescent-phase sera can be demonstrated. The standard type of neutralization test in mice has traditionally been used for this purpose. Gerloff and Eklund[18] reported on a cell culture neutralization test (NT) method, and a standard complement-fixation (CF) test is useful also.[59,60] The CF antibody response may be slow. However, neutralizing antibody usually appears earlier than CF antibody, but may also be slow. The utility of an indirect FA antibody assay has been emphasized, since antibodies detected by this test may appear even earlier and in higher titer than neutralizing antibody.[23] Other experimental methods, such as indirect hemagglutination[61] and immunoperoxidase staining[41] have not yet been put into routine use.

EPIDEMIOLOGY

Occurrence

Colorado tick fever is known to occur in mountainous or highland regions (from about 4,000 feet to over 10,000 feet) of at least 11 western states (South Dakota, Montana, Wyoming, Colorado, New Mexico, Utah, Idaho, Nevada, Washington, Oregon, and California) and in the Canadian provinces of Alberta and British Columbia.[43,62-64] Sagebrush-juniper-pine vegetation is typical for endemic areas. The distribution has been determined primarily by virus isolations from ticks and mammalian hosts and the occurrence of human cases, and coincides generally with the range of the principal vector, *D. andersoni,* as outlined by Eklund et al.[62] Isolates from ticks[62] (C. M. Eklund, personal communication), and from a *Lepus californicus* hare (R. S. Lane and R. W. Emmons, unpublished) outside the distribution area of *D. andersoni* indicate that there are alternate cycles for the virus, and not a strict limitation to a *D. andersoni* cycle. The occurrence of virus is more widespread than the occurrence of human cases indicates, because of virus cycles involving tick species which do not readily feed on human beings and because the disease may not be suspected and diagnosed outside the presumed endemic areas. An early report by Florio, Miller, and Mugrage[63] of CTF virus in *D. variabilis* on Long Island could not be confirmed by Eklund and co-workers[62] nor by Miller,[65] so it has been considered of doubtful validity. A report by Newhouse, et al.[66] of CTF neutralizing antibody in 5 of 49 snowshoe hares (*Lepus americanus*) from the Ottawa region of Ontario reopened this question and indicated the need for further study.

Reservoir

The virus is maintained by cycles of infection in various small mammals and ticks which parasitize them, principally *D. andersoni*. The golden-mantled ground squirrel [*Spermophilus (Citellus) lateralis*] Columbian ground squirrel (*Citellus columbianus columbianus*), yellow pine chipmunk (*Eutamias amoenus*) and least chipmunk (*E. minimus*) are important amplifying hosts for the virus.[30,31,67] Other naturally infected species (determined by virus isolation and/or antibody tests) include the porcupine (*Erethizon dorsatum epixanthum*), pine squirrel (*Tamiasciurus hudsonicus richardsoni*), tassel-eared squirrel (*Sciurus aberti*), Richardson ground squirrel [*Spermophilus (Citellus) richardsoni*], Uinta chipmunk (*Eutamias umbrinus*), deer mouse (*Peromyscus maniculatus*), piñon mouse (*P. truei*), California ground squirrel (*Spermophilus (Citellus) beecheyi*), meadow vole (*Microtus pennsylvanicus*), California vole (*Microtus californicus*), boreal redback vole (*Clethrionomys gapperi*), kangaroo rat (*Dipodomys californicus*), Great Basin pocket mouse (*Perognathus parvus*), bushytail woodrat (*Neotoma cinerea*), dusky-footed woodrat (*N. fuscipes*), mountain cottontail (*Sylvilagus nuttalli*), snowshoe hare (*Lepus americanus*), black-tailed jackrabbit (hare) (*Lepus californicus*), marmot (*Marmota flaviventris*), elk (*Cervus canadensis*), coyote (*Canis latrans*), and mule deer (*Odocoileus hemionus*)[30,67-72] (Robert G. McLean, personal communication; R. S. Lane and R. W. Emmons, unpublished). Neutralizing antibody has also been found in domestic horses (H. N. Johnson, personal communication) and sheep (R. S. Lane and R. W. Emmons, unpublished). The possible role of ground-feeding birds such as quail, which are hosts for larval *D. andersoni* and other ticks, is suggested by the known susceptibility of domestic chicks to the virus, but this has not been investigated.

The indirect FA method for antibody titration is also useful for conducting serologic surveys, when specific antispecies gamma globulin conjugates are available. A number of species of possible importance as basic maintenance hosts for CTF virus have not yet been adequately studied, and knowledge of this area should not be considered complete. For example, it has been suggested that *Perognathus parvus* could be a reservoir host, since CTF virus has been isolated from this species. It is a host for larval and nymphal *D. andersoni*, and its geographic distribution fits the known endemic area for CTF.[68,72]

At least eight tick species have been found naturally infected, but *D. andersoni* is by far the most common, and as yet is the only proven vector for man. Other tick species found positive for virus include *D. parumapertus*, *D. occidentalis*, *D. albipictus*, *Otobius lagophilus*, *Haemaphysalis leporis-palustris*, *Ixodes spinipalpis*, and *Ixodes sculptus*.[62,66,70,73,74] (Carl M. Eklund and Thomas P. Monath, personal communications.) Other records of infection in vertebrate hosts or ticks probably exist, but have not reached the published literature. The involvement of *D. variabilis* is disputed, as mentioned previously,[63,65] although this species can be experimentally infected, as can *Ornithodoros savignyi*.[75] In addition to the reports to which reference has already been made which analyzed the dynamics of the tick and mammal cycles, one should also refer to the recent studies of Clark et al.[71] and Sonenshine et al.[76].

The tick is generally considered the long term reservoir for the virus, but the prolonged viremia and tissue infections in mammals also contribute to the stability of the virus in its ecologic niche. There is no evidence of transovarial transmission of CTF virus[77] but trans-stadial transmission (larva to nymph to adult stage) consistently occurs. Direct animal-to-animal transmission, by ingestion, is also postulated (H. N. Johnson, personal communication) and can be demonstrated in laboratory animals. The sequence of events and dynamics of infection in *D. andersoni* feeding on infected hamsters were studied in detail by Rozeboom and Burgdorfer.[78] The minimum infectious viremia level was estimated to be 10^2 to 10^3 mouse $ICLD_{50}/m\ell$. In both male and female ticks fed as larvae or nymphs, there was an increase in virus titer of about 10^2 to 10^3 mouse $ICLD_{50}$ following molting to the next stage. Infected adult ticks maintained the virus at titers of $10^2 f^3$ to $10^5 f^3$ mouse $ICLD_{50}/m\ell$ for periods of 10 to 13 months.

Ticks are more frequently found on grass and brush, near streams, lava rims, and on south-facing rocky slopes, since temperature moisture, shelter, and other focal climatic and geographic conditions influence the availability of the vertebrate hosts. For example, in the Bitteroot Valley in Montana, infected ticks are plentiful, whereas they are more scarce in nearby eastern Montana. Even within a single mountain canyon in the Bitteroot Valley, the infection rate in *D. andersoni* varied from 1 to 14%.[62]

The *D. andersoni* life cycle involves four stages: egg, larva, nymph, and adult; a blood meal is required by each larva and nymph in order to molt to the next stage, and by each adult female in order to lay eggs. The life cycle can be completed in 1 year, but more commonly takes 2 years. Larvae and nymphs acquire infection by feeding on viremic hosts during the spring to fall period. CTF virus survives the winter period in hibernating unfed nymphs (and adults), then is transmitted to small rodents by the nymphs in the spring. The possible role of hibernating rodents in overwintering the virus was studied by Emmons.[32] The adult tick may also contribute to virus spread by feeding jointly with nymphs on such mammals as porcupines, but its usual hosts (such as deer) or accidental hosts (human beings) are "dead-end" hosts for the virus.

Transmission

An adult *D. andersoni* male or female tick is the usual vector for infection of people, although some persons do not recall a bite or find an attached tick. The tick salivary glands are the source of virus, but hemocytes and other tissues are also infected, and the possible role of coxal fluid or fecal contamination of skin breaks or mucus membranes in transmitting the virus has not been investigated. Direct transmission from infected mammalian blood or tissues is possible (as in laboratory infections), although unlikely as a natural event. One case of blood-transfusion-induced CTF has been recorded, as mentioned earlier.[54]

Environment

The virus is quite stable in blood samples, persisting for weeks at room temperature, to over a year at 4°C, but this is probably because it is protected intracellularly in the erythrocytes (see above section). The natural cycle involves biological transmission via the tick, and the virus does not survive significantly on fomites or in the environment. Temperature, rainfall, humidity, altitude, solar rays, vegetation, and geophysical features have significant influence on the distribution of mammalian hosts and tick vectors, and thus are determining factors in the occurrence of the virus.

Human Host

The epidemiological aspects of CTF are consistent with its status as a zoonosis acquired from a focal ecologic niche. Case occurrence by residence generally coincides with the endemic area for the virus, but cases also occur in visitors after they have returned home, perhaps to far distant states or even outside the U.S. It is likely that such cases are not recognized as CTF. Rarely, acquisition of the disease has occurred outside the endemic area, apparently from a tick transferred on clothing or in some other way. The possibility of "new" endemic areas and "new" cycles for CTF virus becoming apparent should also be kept in mind, as discussed in a previous section. As with Rocky Mountain spotted fever, the virus is most prevalent in areas of reforestation where small mammals and ticks are most abundant.

Persons of all ages of both sexes are susceptible to infection, with no evidence at present of any age- or sex- specific variation; however, male cases consistently outnumber female cases two- to three-fold, and cases predominate in persons most exposed to the tick vector because of residence, occupational, or recreational pursuits. The complications of encephalitis and hemorrhagic diathesis have been observed more often in children, presumably because of less resistance to the infection. No variation in susceptibility by racial or ethnic background has been noted.

Seasonal occurrence reflects activity and host-seeking of the adult *D. andersoni* ticks. The earliest cases occur in late February or early March, and the latest in mid-October, but most occur from May through July. The length of the season varies from region to region and from year to year, depending on the climate and abundance of vector and mammalian host populations. Long term cycles of CTF incidence have not been noted, except for a gradual rise in reported cases due to increasing human population and better recognition, laboratory diagnosis, and case reporting.

CONTROL

Prevention and Treatment

Prevention consists of avoiding tick-infested areas and tick bites, via protective clothing, removing ticks before they attach and begin to feed, and possibly the use of repellants (such as diethyltoluamide or dimethylphthalate) on clothing. An experimental formalin-killed vaccine was developed for protection of laboratory workers.[79,80] Immunization is not practical for the general public. There is no specific treatment for the disease, but rest, antipyretics, analgesics, and general supportive care are helpful. The serious complications, such as encephalitis and hemorrhage, require appropriate special supportive care. The patient should not serve as a blood donor for at least 6 months after recovery, because of the persistent viremia. The patient usually does not need to be hospitalized, and need not be isolated, since the disease is not contagious, but the difficulty of differentiating CTF from RMSF in the early stages may lead to hospitalization and treatment with antibiotics.

Regulatory Measures

There are no significant regulatory measures applicable to cases of the disease. The virus has been considered a Class 3 agent,[81] but this may be changed to Class 2. One strain (VR-90, Florio, N-7180) is listed in the American Type Culture Collection Catalogue,[34] and is designated "LD" (limited distribution), meaning it may be released only with specific approval of the ATCC Advisory Committee or its designated representative.

Epidemic Measures

Large-scale epidemics have not been described, although an unusual cluster of cases, indicating a focus of high tick population and virus activity, may justify tick control measures. No quarantine or isolation of the patient is needed.

Eradication

The virus cannot be eradicated totally from its endemic foci, but it can be restricted or perhaps temporarily eliminated from small geographic areas which pose high risk (such as campgrounds) by rodent control and use of acaricides (consult appropriate state or federal officials for currently approved chemicals). However, these methods are too difficult and expensive to be of much practical value, and are rarely implemented. Clearing of brush and logs from forested areas will reduce small mammal and tick populations.

Health Education

Health education should emphasize the nature of the disease, its clinical and laboratory differentiation from RMSF, the need for better reporting of the disease occurrence, and how to prevent tick bites and properly remove attached ticks. The tick does not "screw itself into" the skin (a widely held misconception), so should not be "unscrewed'' (which will just break off the capitulum or ''head''). A lighted match should not be held to its posterior to ''make it let go'', since this is not effective and may only burn the patient. Instead, grasp the tick as close to the capitulum as possible, with forceps or tissue paper (not with the bare fingers), and exert a steady pull to remove it without breaking off the capitulum. Application of such things as alcohol, nail-polish remover, lighter fluid, or gasoline may cause the tick to relax thus aiding in its detachment. Rarely, surgical removal of an embedded tick or the detached mouthparts may be necessary to prevent secondary infection or granuloma formation. The tick should be saved alive for species identification and virus isolation attempts, should the patient develop CTF or other illness during the following week. The bite wound should be cleansed and disinfected, and the patient observed for signs of illness. Besides CTF and RMSF, *D. andersoni* ticks can also transmit tularemia and Q fever, and may secrete the toxin causing tick paralysis. Prophylactic antibiotic treatment for a tick bite is not indicated, but prompt, specific treatment should be given if signs compatible with RMSF, Q fever, or tularemia appear.

PUBLIC HEALTH ASPECTS

Economic and Social Impact

There are few significant community-wide economic effects from CTF, although the costs of medical care and impact on the individual case can be severe. The fear that a case may actually be the more serious disease, RMSF, is probably the most significant effect of CTF. High prevalence of CTF in certain areas may have an inhibiting effect on their development as recreational, residential, or occupational sites. Medical or medical-legal costs may be considered compensable for persons in occupational groups placed at risk of exposure by their jobs.

Reporting

In endemic areas, case reporting to local authorities is requested, but not required (Class 3B); in most states CTF is not considered a reportable disease, although voluntary reporting of imported cases is encouraged. The Center for Disease Control now lists CTF cases optionally reported in the annual supplements to the *Morbidity and Mortality Weekly Report.* The annual incidence of reported cases ranges from several hundred in highly endemic states such as Colorado, to dozens or only a few cases in other states. Cases are undoubtedly much more common, but no attempt is made in this review to estimate the true incidence. More complete reporting is to be encouraged.

Surveillance

In addition to reporting of human cases, active surveillance by isolation and/or antibody tests of suspected natural host species is encouraged to more accurately delineate the geographical distribution of CTF virus. Wider collaboration in sharing of serum banks and field data between various wildlife research groups would be helpful in this regard. Much yet remains to be learned about this relatively ''new'', fascinating, and unique American disease.

REFERENCES

1. **Topping, N. H., Cullyford, J. S., and Davis, G. E.,** Colorado tick fever, *Public Health Rep.,* 55, 2224, 1940.
2. **Florio, L., Steward, M. O., and Mugrage, E. R.,** The experimental transmission of Colorado tick fever, *J. Exp. Med.,* 80, 165, 1944.
3. **Florio, L. and Miller, M. S.,** Epidemiology of Colorado tick fever, *Am. J. Public Health,* 38, 211, 1948.
4. **Florio, L., Miller, M. S., and Mugrage, E. R.,** Colorado tick fever. Isolation of the virus from *Dermacentor andersoni* in nature and a laboratory study of the transmission of the virus in the tick, *J. Immunol.,* 64(4), 257, 1950.
5. **Koprowski, H. and Cox, H. R.,** Adaptation of Colorado tick fever virus to mouse and developing chick embryo, *Proc. Soc. Exp. Biol. Med.,* 62, 320, 1946.
6. **Koprowski, H., Cox, H. R., Miller, M. S., and Florio, L.,** Response of man to egg adapted CTF virus, *Proc. Soc. Exp. Biol. Med.,* 74, 126, 1950.
7. **Lloyd, L. W.,** Colorado tick fever, *Med. Clin. North Am.,* 2587, 1951.
8. **Drevets, C. C.,** Colorado tick fever. Observations on eighteen cases and review of the literature, *J. Kans. Med. Soc.,* 58, 448, 1957.
9. **Oliphant, J. W. and Tibbs, R. O.,** Colorado tick fever. Isolation of virus strains by inoculation of suckling mice, *Public Health Rep.,* 65(15), 521, 1950.
10. **Berge, T. O., Ed.,** *International Catalogue of Arboviruses Including Certain other Viruses of Vertebrates,* 2nd ed., Pub. No. (CDC) 75-8301, Public Health Service, U.S. Department of Health, Education and Welfare, Atlanta, 1975.
11. **Fenner, F.,** Classification and nomenclature of viruses. Second report of the International Committee on Taxonomy of Viruses, *Intervirology,* 7(1), 1, 1976.
12. **Rehse-Küpper, B., Casals, J., Rehse, E., and Ackerman, R.,** Eyach — an arthropod-borne virus related to Colorado tick fever virus in the Federal Republic of Germany, *Acta Virol.,* 20, 339, 1976.
13. **Green, I. J.,** Evidence for the double-stranded nature of the RNA of Colorado tick fever virus; an ungrouped arbovirus, *Virology,* 40, 1056, 1970.
14. **Murphy, F. A., Coleman, P. H., Harrison, A. K., and Gary, G. W., Jr.,** Colorado tick fever virus: an electron microscopic study, *Virology,* 35(1), 28, 1968.
15. **Oshiro, L. S. and Emmons, R. W.,** Electron microscopic observations of Colorado tick fever virus in BHK_{21} and KB cells, *J. Gen. Virol.,* 3, 279, 1968.
16. **Trent, D. W. and Scott, L. V.,** Colorado tick fever virus in cell culture. II. Physical and chemical properties, *J. Bacteriol.,* 91(3), 1282, 1966.
17. **Pickens, E. G. and Luoto, L.,** Tissue culture studies with Colorado tick fever virus. I. Isolation and propagation of virus in KB cultures. *J. Infect. Dis.,* 103(1), 102, 1958.
18. **Gerloff, R. K. and Eklund, C. M.,** A tissue culture neutralization test for Colorado tick fever antibody and use of the test for serologic surveys, *J. Infect. Dis.,* 104(2), 174, 1959.
19. **Deig, E. F. and Watkins, H. M. S.,** Plaque assay procedure for Colorado tick fever virus, *J. Bacteriol.,* 88(1), 42, 1964.
20. **Trent, D. W. and Scott, L. V.,** Colorado tick fever virus in cell culture. I. Cell-type susceptibility and interaction with L cells, *J. Bacteriol.,* 88(3), 702, 1964.
21. **Yunker, C. E. and Cory, J.,** Growth of Colorado tick fever (CTF) virus in primary tissue cultures of its vector, *Dermacentor andersoni* Stiles (Acarina: Ixodidae), with notes on tick tissue culture, *Exp. Parasitol.,* 20(3), 267, 1967.
22. **Yunker, C. E. and Cory J.,** Colorado tick fever virus: growth in a mosquito cell line, *J. Virol.,* 3(6), 631, 1969.
23. **Emmons, R. W., Dondero, D. V., Devlin, V., and Lennette, E. H.,** Serologic diagnosis of Colorado tick fever. A comparison of complement-fixation, immunofluorescence, and plaque-reduction methods, *Am. J. Trop. Med. Hyg.,* 18(5), 796, 1969.
24. **Eklund, C. M.,** Colorado tick fever (CTF), in *International Catalogue of Arboviruses,* 2nd ed., Pub. No. (CDC) 75-8301, Berge, T. O., Ed., Public Health Service, U.S. Department of Heath, Education and Welfare, Atlanta, 1975, 226.
25. **Dubovi, E. J. and Akers, T. G.,** Interferon induction by Colorado tick fever virus: a double-stranded RNA virus, *Proc. Soc. Exp. Biol. Med.,* 139(1), 123, 1972.
26. **Emmons, R. W., Oshiro, L. S., Johnson, H. N., and Lennette, E. H.,** Intraerythrocytic location of Colorado tick fever virus, *J. Gen. Virol.,* 17(2), 185, 1972.
27. **Oshiro, L. S., Dondero, D. V., Emmons, R. W., and Lennette, E. H.,** The development of Colorado tick fever virus within cells of the haemopoietic system, *J. Gen. Virol.,* 39, 73, 1978.

28. **Burgdorfer, W.,** Colorado tick fever. The behavior of CTF virus in the porcupine, *J. Infect. Dis.,* 104(1), 101, 1959.

29. **Burgdorfer, W.,** Colorado tick fever. II. The behavior of Colorado tick fever virus in rodents, *J. Infect. Dis.,* 107(3), 384, 1960.

30. **Burgdorfer, W. and Eklund, C. M.,** Studies on the ecology of Colorado tick fever virus in Western Montana, *Am. J. Hyg.,* 69(2), 127, 1959.

31. **Burgdorfer, W. and Eklund, C. M.,** Colorado tick fever. I. Further ecological studies in Western Montana, *J. Infect. Dis.,* 107(3), 379, 1960.

32. **Emmons, R. W.,** Colorado tick fever: prolonged viremia in hibernating *Citellus lateralis, Am. J. Trop. Med. Hyg.,* 15(3), 428, 1966.

33. **Koprowsi, H. and Cox, H. R,.** Colorado tick fever. I. Studies on mouse brain adapted virus, *J. Immunol.,* 57, 239, 1947.

34. **Stevens, D. Ed.,** Animal viruses and antisera, Chlamydiae and Rickettsiae, in *Catalogue of Strains II,* American Type Culture Collection, 2nd ed., Rockville, Md., 1979, 143.

35. **Gerloff, R. K. and Larson, C. L.,** Experimental infection of rhesus monkeys with Colorado tick fever virus, *Am. J. Pathol.,* 35(5), 1043, 1959.

36. **Eklund, C. M. and Kennedy, R. C.,** Preliminary studies of pathogenesis of Colorado tick fever virus infection of mice, in *Biology of Viruses of the Tick-borne Encephalitis Complex, Proc. Symp.,* Libikova, H., Ed., Academic Press, New York, 1962, 286.

37. **Black, W. C., Florio, L., and Stewart, M. O.,** A histologic study of the reaction in the hamster spleen produced by the virus of Colorado tick fever, *Am. J. Pathol.,* 23, 217, 1947.

38. **Hadlow, W. J.,** Histopathologic changes in suckling mice infected with the virus of Colorado tick fever, *J. Infect. Dis.,* 101, 158, 1957.

39. **Miller, J. K., Tompkins, V. N., and Sieracki, J. C.,** Pathology of Colorado tick fever in experimental animals, *Arch Pathol.,* 72(2), 149, 1961.

40. **Harris, R. E., Morahan, P., and Coleman, P.,** Teratogenic effects of Colorado tick fever virus in mice, *J. Infec. Dis.,* 131(4), 397, 1975.

41. **Desmond, E. P., Schmidt, N. J. and Lennette, E. H.,** Immunoperoxidase staining for detection of Colorado tick fever virus, and study of congenital infection in the mouse, *Am. J. Trop. Med. Hyg.,* 28(4), 729, 1979.

42. **Eklund, C. M., Kohls, G. M., Jellison, W. L., Burgdorfer, W., Kennedy, R. C., and Thomas, L.,** The clinical and ecological aspects of Colorado tick fever, Proc. 6th Int. Congr. Tropical Medicine and Malaria, Vol. 5, Lisbon, 1959, 197.

43. **Eklund, C. M., Kennedy, R. C. and Casey, M.,** Colorado tick fever, *Rocky Mountain Med. J.,* 58, 21, 1961.

44. **Goodpasture, H. C., Poland, J. D., Francy, D. B., Bowen, G. S. and Horn, K. A.,** Colorado tick fever: clinical, epidemiologic, and laboratory aspects of 228 cases in Colorado in 1973—1974, *Ann. Intern. Med.,* 88, 303, 1978.

45. **Fraser, C. H. and Schiff, D. W.,** Colorado tick fever encephalitis. Report of a case, *Pediatrics,* 29(2), 187, 1962.

46. **Draughn, D. E., Sieber, O. E., Jr., and Umlauf, H. J., Jr.,** Colorado tick fever encephalitis, *Clin. Pediatr. (Philadelphia),* 4(10), 626, 1965.

47. **Spruance, S. L. and Bailey, A.,** Colorado tick fever. A review of 115 laboratory confirmed cases, *Arch. Intern. Med.,* 131(2), 288, 1973.

48. **Hierholzer, W. J. and Barry, D. W.,** Colorado tick fever pericarditis, *JAMA,* 217, 825, 1971.

49. **Emmons, R. W. and Schade, H. I.,** Colorado tick fever simulating acute myocardial infarction, *JAMA,* 222(1), 87, 1972.

50. **Johnson, E. S., Napoli, V. M., and White, W. C.,** Colorado tick fever as a hematologic problem, *Am. J. Clin. Pathol.,* 34(2), 118, 1960.

51. **Markovitz, A.,** Thrombocytopenia in Colorado tick fever, *Arch. Intern. Med.,* 111(3), 307, 1963.

52. **Hughes, L. E., Casper, E. A., and Clifford, C. M,.** Persistence of Colorado tick fever virus in red blood cells, *Am. J. Trop. Med. Hyg.,* 23(3), 530, 1974.

53. **Philip, R. N., Casper, E. A., Cory, J., and Whitlock, J.,** The potential for transmission of arboviruses by blood transfusion with particular reference to Colorado tick fever, in *Transmissible Diseases and Blood Transfusion,* Greenwalt, T. J. and Jamieson, G. A., Eds., Grune & Stratton, Inc. New York, 1975, 175.

54. **Randall, W. H., Simmons, J., Casper, E. A., and Philip, R. N.,** Transmission of Colorado tick fever virus by blood transfusion, — Montana, *Morbidity and Mortality Weekly Report,* Vol. 24, No. 50, Center for Disease Control, Public Health Service, U.S. Department of Health, Education and Welfare, Atlanta, 1975, 422.

55. **Earnest, M. P., Breckinridge, J. C., Barr, R. J., Francy, D. B., and Mollohan, C. S.,** Colorado tick fever. Clinical and epidemiologic features and evaluation of diagnostic methods, *Rocky Mountain Med. J.*, 68(2), 60, 1971.

56. **Dawson, D. L., Vernon, T. M., and an EIS Officer,** Colorado tick fever. *Colorado, Morbidity and Mortality Weekly Report,* Vol. 24, No. 44, Center for Disease Control, Public Health Service, U.S. Department of Health, Education and Welfare, Atlanta, 1972, 374.

57. **Burgdorfer, W. and Lackman, D.,** Identification of the virus of Colorado tick fever in mouse tissues by means of fluorescent antibodies, *J. Bacteriol.*, 80(1), 131, 1960.

58. **Emmons, R. W. and Lennette, E. H.,** Immunofluorescent staining in the laboratory diagnosis of Colorado tick fever, *J. Lab. Clin. Med.*, 68(6), 923, 1966.

59. **DeBoer, C. J., Kunz, L. J., Koprowski, H., and Cox, H. R.,** Specific complement-fixing diagnostic antigens for Colorado tick fever, *Proc. Soc. Exp. Biol. Med.*, 64, 202, 1947.

60. **Thomas, L. A. and Eklund, C. M.,** Use of the complement fixation test as a diagnostic aid in Colorado tick fever, *J. Infect. Dis.*, 107(2), 235, 1960.

61. **Gaidamovich, S. Ya., Klisenko, G. A., and Shanoyan, N. K.,** New aspects of laboratory techniques for studies of Colorado tick fever, *Am. J. Trop. Med. Hyg.*, 23(3), 526, 1974.

62. **Eklund, C. M., Kohls, G. M., and Brennan, J. M.,** Distribution of Colorado tick fever and virus-carrying ticks, *JAMA*, 157(4), 335, 1955.

63. **Florio, L., Miller, M. S., and Mugrage, E. R.,** Colorado tick fever. Isolation of virus from *Dermacentor variabilis* obtained from Long Island, New York, with immunological comparisons between eastern and western strains , *J. Immunol.*, 64(4), 265, 1950.

64. **Hall, R. R., McKiel, J. A., and Gregson, J. D.,** Occurrence of Colorado tick fever virus in *Dermacentor andersoni* ticks in British Columbia, *Can. J. Public Health,* 59(7), 273, 1968.

65. **Miller, J. K.,** Colorado tick fever: failure to isolate the virus from *Dermacentor variabilis* on Long Island, N.Y., *Publ. Health Lab.*, 18(3), 53, 1960.

66. **Newhouse, V. F., McKiel, J. A., and Burgdorfer, W.,** California encephalitis, Colorado tick fever and Rocky Mountain spotted fever in Eastern Canada, *Can. J. Public Health,* 55(6), 257, 1964.

67. **Eklund, C. M., Kohls, G. M., and Jellison, W. L.,** Isolation of Colorado tick fever virus from rodents in Colorado, *Science,* 128, 413, 1958.

68. **Johnson, H. N.,** The ecological approach to the study of small mammals in relation to arboviruses, in *Anais de Microbiologia*, Vol. 11 Parte A, 7th Int. Congr. Tropical Medicine and Malaria, Bruno-Lobo, M. and Shope, R., Eds., Rio de Janeiro, Sept. 6, 1963.

69. **Eklund, C. M.,** Role of mammals in maintenance of arboviruses, in *Anais de Microbiologia*, Vol. 11 Parte A, Proc. 7th Int. Congr. Tropical Medicine and Malaria, Bruno-Lobo, M. and Shope, R., Eds., Rio de Janeiro, Sept. 6, 1963, 199.

70. **Eklund, C. M,.** Colorado tick fever, in *Diseases Transmitted from Animals to Man,* Hull, T. G., 5th ed., Charles C. Thomas, Springfield, Ill., 1963.

71. **Clark, G. M., Clifford, C. M., Fadness, L. V., and Jones, E. K.,** Contributions to the ecology of Colorado tick fever virus, *J. Med. Entomol.*, 7, 189, 1970.

72. **Johnson, H. N.,** Keynote address: The ecological approach to the study of zoonotic diseases, *J. Wildl. Dis.*, 6, 194, 1970.

73. **Kohls, G. M.,** Colorado tick fever discovered in California, *Calif. Vector Views,* 2(4), 17, 1955.

74. **Philip, C. B., Bell, J. F., and Larson, C. L.,** Evidence of infectious diseases and parasites in a peak population of black-tailed jack rabbits in Nevada, *J. Wildl. Manage.*, 19(2), 225, 1955.

75. **Hurlbut, H. S. and Thomas, J. I.,** The experimental host range of the arthropod-borne animal viruses in arthropods, *Virology,* 12, 391, 1960.

76. **Sonenshine, E. D., Yunker, C. E., Clifford, C. M., Clark, G. M., and Rudbach, J. A.,** Contributions to the ecology of Colorado tick fever virus. 2. Population dynamics and host utilization of immature stages of the Rocky Mountain wood tick, *Dermacentor andersoni, J. Med. Entomol.*, 12(6), 651, 1976.

77. **Eklund, C. M., Kohls, G. M., and Kennedy, R. C.,** Lack of evidence of transovarial transmission of Colorado tick fever virus in *Dermacentor andersoni*, in *Biology of Viruses of the Tick-borne Encephalitis Complex, Proc. Symp.,* Libikova, H., Ed., Academic Press, New York, 1962, 401.

78. **Rozeboom, L. E. and Burgdorfer, W.,** Development of Colorado tick fever virus in the Rocky Mountain wood tick, *Dermacentor andersoni, Am. J. Hyg.,* 69(2), 138, 1959.

79. **Thomas, L. A., Eklund, C. M., Philip, R. N., and Casey, M.,** Development of a vaccine against Colorado tick fever for use in man, *Am. J. Trop. Med. Hyg.*, 12(4), 678, 1963.

80. **Thomas, L. A., Philip, R. N., Patzer, E., and Casper, E.,** Long duration of neutralizing-antibody response after immunization of man with a formalinized Colorado tick fever vaccine, *Am. J. Trop. Med. Hyg.*, 16(1), 60, 1967.

81. **Ad Hoc Committee, U.S. Public Health Service,** *Classification of Etiologic Agents on the Basis of Hazard,* Public Health Service, U.S. Department of Health, Education and Welfare, Atlanta, November, 1969.

VESICULAR STOMATITIS

T. M. Yuill

NAME AND SYNONYMS

Vesicular stomatitis (VS) was formerly termed erosive stomatitis[110] or stomatitis contagiosa of horses[21] and aphtous stomatitis of cattle and swine.[71] North American livestockmen have termed it sore nose or sore mouth.[65] In Latin America it has been called *mal de tierra* or *seudoaftosa*[65]

HISTORY

The early history and distribution of VS New Jersey (VSNJ) and VS Indiana (VSI) have been reviewed by Hanson.[63] The clinical disease was recognized in horses and mules in South Africa in the late 19th century, but the etiology was not confirmed. A vesicular disease of horses compatible with VS was described in horses during the Civil War in the U.S., and in cattle in eastern and western central states in 1904. Shortly after that time, other outbreaks were reported in Colorado and in the Chicago stockyards. The French reported a comparable disease in horses arriving from the U.S. in 1915. In 1916 there was a massive epidemic involving cattle and horses from Utah and Montana, through the Great Plains and the Midwest, and extending as far east as Virginia. In 1925, a virus was isolated from vesicular lesions in cattle arriving in Richmond, Indiana from Kansas City; this strain became the prototype VSI virus. The next year, a serologically distinct virus was isolated from cattle in an extensive outbreak of vesicular disease in New Jersey; this strain became VSNJ virus. VSI and VSNJ have been reported from southern Mexico.[1]

VS was first recognized in South America in 1939 in horses and cattle in Argentina, later in cattle, swine and horses in Venezuela, and in swine in Colombia. Both VSNJ and VSI have been reported to be endemic in Central America and Northern South America.[65]

Cocal (COC) virus was first isolated from *Gigantolaelaps* sp. mites in Trinidad in 1961; from rodents and later from horses with vesicular disease in Argentina;[48] and later from *Gigantolaelaps* sp. mites near Belem, Brazil.[84] Alagois (ALA) virus was isolated from horses and mules with vesicular disease in Alagoas and Pernambuca States of Brazil in 1964.[48] Piry (PIR) virus was recovered from a spleen-liver pool from an opossum captured in the Utinga forest near Belem, Brazil in 1960. Chandipura (CHP) virus was first recovered from the blood of a patient with a dengue/chikungunya-like illness in Nagpur City, Maharashtra, India, in 1965,[11] and later from *Phlebotomus* sandflies captured in the same state.[42] Serological evidence suggested that CHP was widely distributed in India.[11] The virus was subsequently also isolated from the liver of two different species of hedgehogs in Nigeria. Isfahan (ISF) virus was isolated from pools of *Phlebotomus papatasi* collected in Isfahan, Iran, in 1975, and serological evidence indicated that the virus was present in several regions of that country.[153]

ETIOLOGY

Classification

The vesicular stomatitis viruses are classified as rhabdoviruses (Rhabdoviridae family).[92] VS viruses are a complex of seven agents including VSNJ, VSI, ALA (also termed Brazil), PIR, CHP, and ISF. VSI and VSNJ were the only two VS viruses recognized for many years. These two viruses were recognized as serologically distinct, but sharing a common soluable antigen demonstrable by agar gel precipitation tests.[115] Subsequent isolation and characterization of COC and ALA has show these two viruses to be closely related to VSI.[26,48] A virus designated Argentina was found to be antigenically indistinguishable from COC[48] virus, and consideration of Argentina virus as a separate type has not seemed warranted. It has been proposed that VSI, COC (including Argentina strain), and ALA be designated Indiana$_1$, $_2$, and $_3$,[48] and that a third serotype including PIR and CHP[8] which are clearly related to each other and to the most recently reported VS virus, be designated ISF.[153] The data establishing the relationship of PIR and CHP to VSNJ or the VSI viruses have been conflicting. In one laboratory, neutralization tests indicated very slight antigenic relationship between PIR and both VSNJ and VSI,[8] and ISF antiserum gave a very low-titer crossreaction with COC virus in the plaque reduction neutralization test.[153] However, studies from another laboratory did not demonstrate any heterologous neutralization with PIR and CHP viruses and their antisera versus VSI, COC, and ALA viruses and antisera.[26] Differences in methods employed make it difficult to reconcile the reported differences.

Characteristics

The morphology, structure, and chemical composition of VS viruses have been well studied and several excellent reviews have been published.[2,74,92] In summary, the structure and composition of all VS viruses studied have been very similar. All seven are enveloped and bullet-shaped, and are approximately 177 (range 160 to 188) nm long by 75 (range 68 to 78) nm wide.[9,14,40,92] ISF virus appears to be somewhat longer and thinner (211 by 64 nm).[153] The virions are cylindrical, rounded on one end and flat on the other, although one report suggested that the bacilliform particles seen with the electron microscope following critical-point drying are the true morphology.[118] The virus particles have a density in potassium tartrate gradients of 1.14 g/mℓ.[28] Much shorter, even almost spherical, noninfectious truncated or "T" particles are sometimes observed.[7,75]

The virions are covered with approximately 500[29] surface projections 9 to 10 nm long extending from a membranous envelope.[14,74] The type-specific antigenic components of the virus reside in the projections.[25,27] The capsids are comprised of beaded capsomeres arranged in helical form.[9,14] The beads are 4.5 nm in diameter with 24 beads per turn,[9,14] giving the appearance of cross striations.[74] The inner nucleoprotein core, a single helix of about 35 turns, is 15 to 19 nm in diameter and is comprised of an estimated 1000 subunits.[14,74] The core may or may not have an axial hollow.[14]

The virus is 64 to 69% protein.[92,104] Five polypeptides have been described for VS viruses and their proposed designations are L (large protein) of mol wt 190,000, G (glycoprotein) of mol wt 69,000, N (nucleoprotein) of mol wt 50,000, NS (nonstructural protein) of mol wt 45,000 and M (matrix) of mol wt 29,000.[159] The virions are 20% lipid, 13% carbohydrate,[92,104] and contain neuraminic acid but no neuraminidase.[20,30,91,105] The RNA is single-stranded with mol wt of 3.6 to 4.0 × 10^6 daltons.[29,76,134]

VS viruses are sensitive to chloroform, ether, calcium and sodium desoxycholate,[8,153,99] and trypsin.[99] These viruses hemagglutinate within a very narrow pH range, and at a low temperature (0 to 4°C), with goose erythrocytes.[3,4,8] VSI and COC were reported to replicate to higher titer in cell cultures maintained at 28°C than did VSNJ, but VSNJ multiplied and formed plaques at incubation temperatures up to

41°C, whereas COC did so only up to 39°C.[57,155] A variety of plaque types have been observed for both VSI and VSNJ, but plaque morphology has not been found to be dependent on the serotype of virus tested.[57]

The VS viruses replicate in many different types of primary and secondary cell cultures. Vero and BHK-21 cell lines appear to be quite susceptible to VS viruses.[11,21,57,81,153,154] Various of the VS viruses have been shown to replicate and produce cytopathogenic changes or plaques in mouse L-cells,[103,117] kidney cells from several species of primates,[8,11] several types of bovine cells,[49,59,160] human monocytes,[46] cell lines (HeLa,[103] bat kidney,[11] shrew tumor),[11] and cells from cold-blooded species (turtle heart, gecko lung, and viper spleen,[102] and red swordtail fish).[90] Some of the VS viruses will also replicate in insect cell cultures, without cytopathogenic effect, including those from mosquitoes (*Aedes aegypti, Ae. albopictus, Ae. w-albus,* and *Anopheles stephensi*),[5,6,135,139] from the fruit fly *Drosophila melanogaster,*[111] and from the moth *Antheraea eucalypti.*[163,164]

DEFINITION

Vesicular stomatitis is a disease of cattle, swine, horses, and variety of wild vertebrate animals caused by a group of morphologically related viruses recognized in North America, South America, and Asia. Human infections have occurred in nature and especially following laboratory exposures. The clinical disease is characterized by fever and by vesicles on mucus membranes of the mouth and epithelium of the tongue, coronary bands, and soles of the feet. Many cases are subclinical. Reservoirs of the virus and possible role, if any, of insect vectors in transmission remain incompletely identified.

ANIMAL INFECTION

Vesicular stomatitis is of economic concern both because of the losses it causes in milk and beef production and the severe lameness it produces in cattle, swine, and horses; and because its clinical signs are indistinguishable from those of the more contagious foot-and-mouth disease.[34,101]

Clinical

The incubation period of VSNJ or VSI in cattle, horses, or swine varies from 24 hr to several days.[35,110,137] Excessive salivation is frequently the first clinical manifestation in cattle and horses, though swine frequently show an initial lameness. Fever usually appears at the time of these initial signs. Raised, blanched vesicles, varying in size from ½ to several centimeters then appear.

In cattle, horses, and swine, vesicles are common in the mouth, in and on the lips and on the muzzle.[71] Vesicles have been reported in horses' ears.[71] Swine may develop lesions on the snout.[35,137] Foot lesions also occur in all these species, especially on the coronary bands.[35] Hooves may slough, and lameness, often complicated by secondary infection, may result.[107] Teat lesions commonly occur in cattle,[1,15,98-100] making the cows nearly impossible to milk.[47,71] Mastitis may result, with a total or partial loss of mammary function. Abortions have been reported in VS infected cows but have not been confirmed in laboratory studies.[97] During the febrile and vesicular stages of the disease, the animals are often anorexic and depressed. Excessive salivation often occurs during vesicle formation, rupture and early healing; cattle may make a characteristic sucking noise, and horses may grind their teeth.[34,110] Cattle may slough large areas of the muzzle integument.[15] The fever declines, but a biphasic second peak may occur later, particularly in older calves.[15] The erosions heal quickly, barring secondary bacterial or mycotic infection, and the animals return to normal within 2 weeks of vesicle rupture.[15] No viremia has been demonstrated in cattle, horses, or swine,[56,86] although viremia has been shown in experimentally infected laboratory animals.

There is some evidence for subclinical VS infection in cattle.[83] Cattle without histories of vesicular disease have been shown to have antibodies.[99] Calves in a VSI and VSNJ endemic area in Colombia, South America, were monitored for signs of vesicular disease and development of neutralizing antibodies. During a year period, none developed vesicular disease, but several acquired high titers of antibodies to VSNJ, and several others to VSI.*

Pathology

Virus replicates in the prickle cells of the Malpighian layer of the epithelium.[34,35] As viral maturation takes place, the virions bud from the cell surfaces and intracytoplasmic vacular membranes, accumulate in intercellular spaces[112,114] and infect adjoining cells. The infected keratinocytes contain numerous desmosomes and cytoplasmic vacuoles, the plasma membranes become thickened and the tonofilaments become scattered in the cytoplasm.[124] The cytoplasm of the infected cells shrinks and intercytoplasmic bridges become marked.[128] The infected animals become febrile. Epithelium becomes edematous and leads to spongiosis.[34,35] Papules become visible and erythema of the general area may occur.[15] Extreme cytoplasmic shrinkage is followed by nuclear shrinkage and degeneration.[128] Transudates form in lacunae, coalesce, and finally form vesicles. Polymorphonuclear cells infiltrate the area of the vesicles. The thin tissue overlying the vesicles quickly breaks, and raw erosions, or occasionally ulcers are exposed (Figure 1). Erosions without vesiculation followed by necrosis have been observed in experimentally infected cattle.[136] Extravasation of red blood cells may be seen microscopically in the dermal ridges near the vesicles.[34]

Development of vesicular lesions in experimentally infected laboratory animals inoculated in the tongues or foot pads with VSNJ or VSI follows essentially the field pattern,[141] but some experimental VS virus infections in laboratory animals may be fatal. Visceral organs, usually liver and kidneys, are the primary target organs,[113] or virus may invade (or be inoculated into) the brain[109] and produce acute encephalitis.[125] Central nervous system signs may develop more slowly, often with hind limb paralysis and with spongiform changes of the gray matter of the spinal cord.[125] Lethality is determined by host factors as species,[133] race (strain), age, sex, environmental factors, and stressors.[58,80] Young of several species have been shown to be more susceptible to fatal VS virus infections than older individuals.[131,152] Some strains of Colombian VSNJ virus produce generalized fatal infection in young adult male but not female ICA strain guinea pigs by foot pad inoculation. VECOL strain guinea pigs of either sex are resistant to experimental VSNJ infection. Virus factors as strains, passage histories, routes of inoculation,[113,132] and virus titers also affect virulence and lethality. None of the VSI strains tested in ICA or VECOL strain guinea pigs[57] produced generalized disease.

High-titered or long-duration viremia in experimentally-infected laboratory animals does not usually occur. Transient, low-titered viremias have occurred in some *Zygodontomys* sp. inoculated with COC. These animals subsequently developed hind limb paralysis and died.[86] Inoculation of opossums and hamsters with PIR and marmosets with VSI also produced viremia and death.[152] Karyorrhexis and distinctive destruction of cells of the ependymal canal of the spinal medula have been reported in COC virus infections.[154]

---

*   G. J. Noreña, Zuluga, F. N., and Yuill, T. M., Universidad de Anti Colombia, and University of Wisconsin, Madison. Personal communication, 1977.

Diagnosis

The signs and symptoms of VS infection are not pathognomonic. In cattle and swine, VS can not be distinguished from foot-and-mouth disease (FMD).[34,101] The differential diagnosis must be established in the laboratory by isolation of the virus or demonstration of the development of specific antibodies.

Virus isolation is best attempted from throat swabs, vesicle fluid, or epithelial tissue from ruptured vesicles.[107] Material for virus isolation can be inoculated into cell cultures or laboratory animals. Several types of cell primary cultures and lines have been employed. Vero cells have been reported more sensitive than mice for recovery of VSI from sandflies.[150] A microtiter system employing pre-formed monolayers has been described as more sensitive for virus detection than plaque formation,[130] although plaquing efficiency can be influenced by several factors including the volume of inoculum,[158] pH of absorption, and composition and charge of the overlay medium.[156,158] Passage of undiluted virus in cell cultures may result in production of defective interfering T particles with little yield of infective virus. This can be avoided by inoculation of cell cultues with diluted passage materials.[37] In circumstances where tests in cell cultures are difficult, embryonated chicken eggs[51,89] or suckling or weanling mice can be successfully employed for isolation of VSI or VSNJ from livestock.[51]

Rapid typing of virus isolates is essential, particularly in outbreaks of vesicular disease in cattle when VS must be differentiated from FMD. Vesicular fluid or suspensions of epithelial tissues from lesions as well as laboratory passaged virus have been successfully employed as typing antigens in the direct complement-fixation (CF) test.[79,107,144] For safety, this antigen can be heat inactivated (56 to 60°C for 30 min) without significant loss of antigenic reactivity.[43] Virus neutralization tests and fluorescent antibody[73,106] tests have also been used for specific VS virus typing. VS viruses have also been differentiated by autointerference tests with defective T particles.[39]

VS diagnosis can be established by serological means. Animals develop type-specific antibodies[13] following infection with VS viruses. Infected cattle,[56,78] horses,[56] and swine[72] develop CF antibodies within 1 to 2 months of infection, acquire peak antibody titers at 2 to 3 weeks, and then show declines in titer to undetectable levels within 2 to 4 months. Swine sera may have procomplementary substances that can be eliminated by acidification to pH 4.2 to 4.4 over night and the readjustment of pH to neutral.[12]

Serum neutralizing antibodies appear in the sera of infected cattle[56] and swine[72] about as rapidly as do CF antibodies, but persist at relatively high, but fluctuating values.[56,12] Serodiagnosis of VSNJ and VSI in cattle and swine and assessment of herd immunity by serum neutralization (N) tests can be difficult because immunity is not lasting.[35] Animals convalescent from VS can still have significant N titers to VS virus at the time they become susceptible to reinfection,[32,56,72,142] but their CF titers have declined below detectable levels at this time.

A variety of N tests have been developed utilizing several types of cell cultures and laboratory animal hosts. An efficient Vero cell plaque-reduction test has been developed.[45] Micro-N tests on established monolayers[130] and metabolic inhibition tests employing cell suspensions[31] have also been used for antibody assays. VS virus antibodies have also been assayed in mouse protection tests,[31] and in mouse and embryonated chicken egg neutralization tests.[157] Plaque-reduction neutralization test results can be complicated by the presence of nonspecific substances, particularly in the sera of rodents, bats, opossums, and birds, which inhibit VSNJ plaques. Because of this lack of specificity and because neutralizing antibodies to VS viruses may be present in both acute- and in convalescent-phase sera of infected animals, the CF test is usually preferred to the N test for assessing herd immunity and detecting reinfection.[72]

VS viruses have been shown to hemagglutinate[3,4] and hemagglutination inhibition

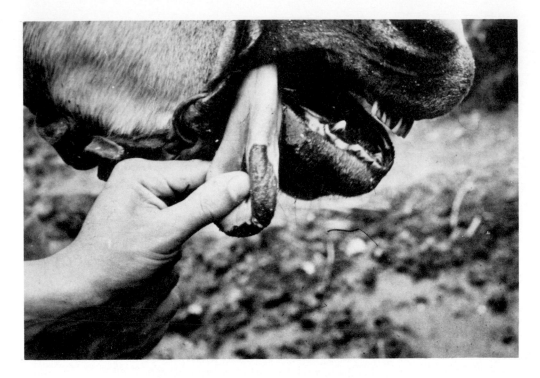

FIGURE 1.   An extensive erosion following rupture of the vesicle in a horse experimentally infected with vesicular stomatitis Indiana. (Photograph by Mr. N. E. Peterson.)

(HI) is type specific.[61] The HI test is too insensitive and subject to too many nonspecific inhibitors in sera to be a useful serological tool in diagnosis.[61,62]

HUMAN INFECTION

Clinical

VS virus infections in people appear to be common. Overt disease has occurred in individuals in contact with naturally or experimentally infected livestock, and people exposed to the virus in the laboratory.[16,50,69,121] Signs and symptoms have appeared to be the same regardless of the source of exposure VSNJ and VSI have produced an acute, febrile influenza-like illness.[81] Fever with chills has occurred 30 hr following laboratory exposure to VSI virus[82] or 30 hr following handling VSNJ virus-infected cattle.[69] The febrile response has usually been biphasic,[69] high and spiking (to 40°C), and persisting as long as 6 days.[50] General malaise, myalgia, headache, sometimes with eye and chest pains, and vomiting have been common.[47,53,69,82] There has been mild leukopenia and relative lymphocytosis.[82] In a minority of cases, vesicles have formed in the mouth (tongue and buccal and pharyngeal mucosae), lips, and nose.[33,47,54,69,71] Flat, yellow throat lesions were noted in one patient who contracted VSNJ from exposure to an infected cow.[50] Pharyngitis has occurred,[53,69] and the virus has been isolated from throat washings but not blood.[54] Pneumonitis was reported in one case.[69] Asymptomatic or very mild human cases probably have occurred frequently. One case of VSNJ contracted during an epidemic in cattle was asymptomatic except for mild coryza.[69] In human beings, both in temperate and tropical areas of endemic VSNJ and VSI, antibodies have been shown to be prevalent,[16,81,127] yet no epidemics in these areas have been reported. It is possible, however, that scattered cases of influenza-like disease have occurred regularly in these areas but that infected individuals have not sought medical attention or that diagnostic specimens were not taken to establish VS diagnosis.

Human infections with ALA, PIR, and CHP viruses also have appeared as acute, febrile diseases. Agricultural workers on farms where horses and mules have had ALA-virus infection reportedly developed fever headache, and malaise.[48] Six individuals who were infected with PIR in the laboratory had fever, headache, anorexia, and right upper quadrant tenderness.[8] CHP has produced epidemic dengue/chikungunya-like syndromes.[11] No human infections with COC virus have yet been reported.

Diagnosis

The human disease must be differentiated from acute febrile diseases as influenza or dengue/chikungunya syndromes. Virus isolation techniques, principally using throat swabs or throat washings, have been applied in diagnosis, but most identification of human infections has been by serological tests. Both CF and N tests have been used to show antibody rises in patients but the CF test has been more widely used.[82]

EPIDEMIOLOGY

The VS viruses have a truly remarkable host range. In nature and experimentally, this group of viruses has been shown to infect a variety of mammals, some birds, and insects.

Reservoirs and Vectors

The principal natural hosts of VSNJ among the domesticated animals are horses, cattle, and swine.[65,107] Sheep appear to be insusceptible.[15] Vesicular disease has been observed in dogs on farms during outbreaks of VSNJ in livestock, but the VS etiology of this canine disease was never confirmed.[15] In the southeastern U.S., deer[87,88] and raccoons[66,87] appear to be the wild mammals having highest VSNJ antibody prevalence rates. In wildlife in Panama, VSNJ antibody prevalence rates were highest among bats, carnivores, and certain rodents.[151] Experimental inoculation of VSNJ into animals of several wildlife species in Panama resulted in the rapid development of antibodies in 13 rodent species, 1 rabbit species, 2 species of marsupials, 1 of 2 species of edentates, 2 bat species, 1 carnivore species, 2 species of primates, but of no species of bird.[152] Several common laboratory small mammals have been shown to be susceptible to VSNJ,[93,116,140,141] as have ferrets,[94] chicken embryos,[140] baby chicks,[140] and adult chickens.[51] The route, dose, virus strain, and perhaps passage history have appeared to influence the outcome of experimental infection attempts. VSNJ virus persisted for up to 6 weeks in inoculated leopard frogs (*Rana pipiens*) held at 4°C, but virus replication was not demonstrated.[67] Insects have been experimentally infected, including *Ae. aegypti*, which transmitted VSNJ by bites to suckling mice,[10] and *Dr. melanogaster*.[22]

VSI has caused extensive epidemics of vesicular disease in cattle and horses,[107] but not swine. The principal wildlife hosts in North America have not been determined. In tropical America, antibody prevalence rates[151] were highest in arboreal and semiarboreal mammals, especially in spider monkeys (*Ateles* spp) two-toed sloths (*Choloepus hoffmani*) and a porcupine (*Coendou rothschildi*),[143] as compared to ground-dwelling species. In studies in Panama, experimental infection in wildlife elicited similar antibody responses with VSI as with VSNJ virus, with the exception that five of eight bird species also developed antibodies.[152] As has been found with VSNJ, VSI has also infected laboratory animals.[51,116,140,141] Sandflies, especially *Lutzomyia trapidoi*, have been found to be naturally infected in the American tropics, and to transovarially transmit VSI virus to their progeny.[147] *Ae. aegypti* mosquitoes have been shown to transmit VSI following inoculation.[10,100,114] VSI virus has been shown to replicate in inoculated *Dr. melanogaster*[23,123] and in the leafhopper *Peregrinus maidis,* which is, interestingly, the natural vector of a plant rhabdovirus.[95]

The natural vertebrate hosts of COC appear to be tropical rodents of the genera *Herteromys, Zygodontomys, and Oryzomys.*[95,123] The Argentine COC isolate was from horses involved in a vesiclar disease outbreak.[48] Other domesticated animals (cattle and pigs)[48] and wildlife (bats)[44] have been infected experimentally with COC virus.

ALA virus was isolated from horses with vesicular disease.[48] Cattle were shown to be susceptible to inoculation with this virus.[48]

CHP virus has been isolated from human beings[11] and from two species of hedgehogs (*Atelerix spiculatus* and *A. albiventris*).[8] Antibodies in horses, cattle, sheep, and goats have indicated that they were also exposed to the virus in nature.[11] Mice and languir monkeys have been infected in the laboratory.[11]

PIR virus was isolated from a human being and from an opossum (*Philander opossum*), and serological evidence has been presented of infection of other marsupials, monkeys, edentates, rodents, bats, swine, and water buffaloes.[8,154] Mice, white rats, guinea pigs, and hamsters have been infected experimentally.[8]

ISF virus has only been recovered from *Phlebotomus papatasi,* but serological studies have indicated that natural infections of gerbils (*Rhombomys opimus* and *Tatera indica*) and human beings have occurred. Inoculated mice and guinea pigs have responded with antibody production.[153]

Transmission

Despite intensive study for more than 30 years, most notably in the tropical rain forests of Panama, the epidemiology and maintenance of VS viruses in nature are not clearly understood. In Panama, phlebotomine sandflies (Figure 2) have been shown to play an important role both as vectors and as reservoirs of VSI virus. VSI virus has been repeatedly isolated from sandflies, particularly *Lutzomyia trapidoi,*[122,150] and sandflies have experimentally transmitted the virus from infected hamsters to mice.[148] The virus has been demonstrated to replicate in sandflies, and in a series of classical experiments, was shown to be transovarially transmitted to their progeny.[147,149] Infected progeny transmitted the virus by bite.[147] In nature, occurrence of virus appeared to be seasonal, with most isolations having been made from sandflies captured from October to March.[55] Transovarial transmission was not 100% efficient, however, and virus had to be acquired horizontally, or sandfly infection rates would eventually have declined to zero. It was demonstrated that wild vertebrates, especially arboreal mammals, had high antibody prevalence rates,[81,143,151] but, when experimentally infected with VSI virus developed little or no viremia.[152] Similarly, experimentally infected cattle, horses, or swine did not develop viremia either.[48,56] Sandflies were experimentally shown to take a very small volume of blood, and blood levels of virus of 10^4/mℓ were required to infect them,[147] a far greater level of viremia than that observed in wild vertebrates. Alternative sources of virus available to sandflies have not been identified.

Human infections, as indicated by high antibody prevalence, have occurred in areas where sandflies are abundant.[127] Cattle and human antibody prevalence rates have been high in moist areas of Central America,[81] but have not appeared to be related to rainfall distribution pattens[36]

VSNJ epidemiology in the tropics has been less well studied than that of VSI. In contrast to VSI, insect vectors have not been implicated in transmission of VSNJ. Wild vertebrates, bats, carnivores, and rodents have commonly shown serological evidence of infection. High prevalence of antibodies has been detected in people, especially in areas of low rainfall and at altitudes of 350 to 649 m.[36] Both serological and clinical evidences of bovine infections have been reported.

In Colombia, one of the most ecologically diverse countries in the world, VSI and VSNJ infections both occur annually in cattle. Epidemics have been reported from the hot, humid lowlands (mean temperature 28°C) to the cool, high altiplanos (mean temperature 8°C and 2700 m altitude).[57] These outbreaks have been seasonal with 88% of the VSNJ and 82% of the VSI outbreaks occurring from July through December.[57] VSNJ was isolated from *Simulium* black flies during one epidemic in dairy cattle in northwestern Colombia,[154] but it was not determined whether the black flies were mechanical or biological vectors.

VSI and VSNJ viruses have caused numerous epidemics in the U.S. Mechanisms of spread and maintenance during interepidemic periods have not been elucidated. Epidemics have often appeared essentially simultaneously within a broad area.[107] Incidence within populations has been very irregular. Outbreaks have often started in animals on pasture[83] in bottom lands and flood plains,[107] and then spread unevenly through the populations, sparing some individuals, pastures and entire farms, within the affected area for no apparent reason.[71,85] Spread has not appeared to follow human or animal routes of movement,[67,107] nor has there been any evidence to suggest that outbreaks have resulted from introduction of infected animals into the area.[107] VS may have been spread within milking herds via virus-contaminated milking machines or milkers' hands.[47,110] There is, however, no evidence to suggest that direct animal to animal contact spread in the field had taken place.[83] Experimentally, transmission of VSNJ has taken place when infected swine have been housed with swine with foot lacerations.[120] Transmission of VS virus has also been accomplished by feeding susceptible porcine meat scraps contaminated with VSNI virus.[120] The sudden occurrence of VS in cattle and horses, and patchy spread, have suggested transmission by insect vectors from some unrecognized reservoir.[129] VSI was isolated from *Culex sp.* mosquitoes during an epidemic of VSI in New Mexico,[146] and has been shown to replicate in insects. VS epidemics have invariably stopped with the onset of cold weather; this also suggests insect transmission. However, isolations of viruses from insects during epidemics have been rarer than would have been expected if arthropods were important vectors. Essentially unsuccessful attempts to transmit VS viruses with northern hematophagous diptera have also suggested that, although occasional mechanical transmission may have occurred, these insects have not served as vectors in the field.[52]

Endemic VSNJ has been reported in the southeastern U.S. In contrasts to epidemic VS, the endemic VSNJ has regularly infected pigs, including a high percentage of feral swine[68,87,107] as well as cattle.[64] The disease in cattle has appeared to spread from foci.[64] The high antibody prevalence in swine and in wildlife, like deer and racoons[87,88] that inhabit low-lying swampy areas, has suggested that these are the areas of virus maintenance, perhaps in the lower forms of life upon which these animals feed.[68]

The epidemiology of VSI and VSNJ viruses has remained enigmatic. Cases in the field have occurred as though transmission were via arthropod vectors. Both VSI and VSNJ viruses have replicated well in insects and their cells in culture, but only VSI in the tropics has been shown to be arthropod-borne. Both viruses have infected a remarkably wide range of vertebrates and have been shown to do so in nature; yet very few vertebrates have been shown to develop a viremia sufficient to infect arthropod vectors. It has been proposed that VS viruses may be plant viruses[64] with double envelopes that are noninfectious for vertebrates.[81] These viruses may be ingested by insects (by aphids sucking plant juices or sandflies imbibing nectar), replicate in the arthropods, and mature to one-enveloped forms infectious for vertebrates.[81] Vertebrate infections may result from ingestion of virus-containing arthropods through contamination of small wounds of the lips or oral mucosa, or may result from bites by VS virus-infected arthropods.

The epidemiology of COC virus infections in the tropics has not been well studied. The virus has been shown to infect small rodents,[84-86] and has been recovered from one of their ectoparasites, *Gigantolaelaps* sp. mites,[84,85] and from *Culex* sp. mosquitoes.[85] Rodents have been considered to be unlikely sources of infectious blood meals for mites and mosquitioes[85] because viremias are of low magnitude and short duration.[86] The virus has been isolated from healing wounds and crusts in one,[86] but not in subsequent[152] experiments. Antibody prevalence in rodents has been highest following rainy seasons.[85] Bats (*Myotis lucifugus*) have been shown to be susceptible to experimental infection, to develop high-titered viremias, and to serve as sources of infectious blood meals for *Aedes aegypti* mosquitoes which have then transmitted the virus by bite to suckling mice.[44] The role of bats in COC epidemiology in nature has remained unknown .

PIR virus has also been associated with small mammals. The virus has been isolated from an opossum, and serological evidence has indicated infection of several marsupial species, primates (including human beings), edentates, rodents, bats, swine, and water buffaloes in nature.[154] The importance of these vertebrates in maintenance of PIR virus in nature has remained unknown, but viremia and death have resulted from experimental infection of *Didelphis marsupialis* and *Philander* sp. opossums. No association of PIR virus with field-collected arthropods has been made, but this virus has been shown to replicate in inoculated *Ae. aegypti*[154] and in *Dr. melanogaster*.[24]

CHA virus has been isolated from *Phlebotomus* sp. sandflies and from people in India.[42] Serological evidence has indicated that large domestic animals have also been infected.[8] This virus has been isolated from hedgehogs in Africa, but no association with arthropods has been established there.[8] CHA virus has been experimentally transmitted from mouse to mouse by bites of *Ae. aegypti, Ae. albopictus, An. stephensi,* and *Culex taeniorhynchus*. Transmission has appeared to be inefficient,[126] and there has been no evidence presented to show that the virus replicated in these mosquitoes. CHA virus did multiply in inoculated *Dr. melanogaster*.[24]

CONTROL

Prevention and Treatment

Effective and economical control of VS is difficult without a clear understanding of the epidemiology of these infections. Live VSNJ[96-98] and formalin-inactivated VSNJ and VSI[38] vaccines have been developed for use in dairy cattle, and have appeared to be successful in preventing clinical cases of disease. The live VSNJ vaccine has been administered intramuscularly. This vaccine has been shown to elicit no febrile response, reduction of milk production, mastitis, udder inflammation, vesicle formation, anorexia, virus shedding, or spread to unvaccinated controls in the herds.[99] The live vaccine has been labile, and stabilizers have been required to maintain adequate viability.[97,108]

Noninfectious T particles or subcomponents have shown some promise for use as vaccines. Defective interfering T particles have been noninfectious and antigenically active.[75] They have been the predominant particle produced by some cell cultures, as gecko lung cells,[102] and have been separated from infectious virions by sucrose density gradient centrifugation.[60] The spike-like projections of the virions have been shown to be antigenic[25,27] and have been purified by density gradient centrifugation and on Sephadex® G200 column.[17,25,27] The feasibility of spike or other subcomponent[17-19] antigens for use as vaccine in cattle, horses, or swine has not been explored.

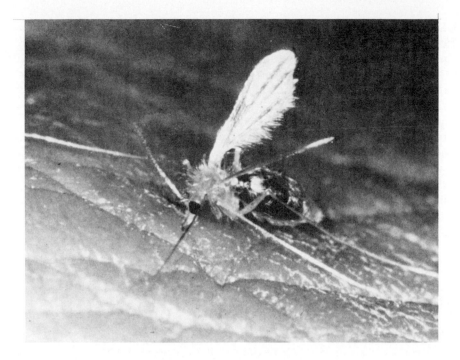

FIGURE 2.   A phlebotamine sandfly vector of vesicular stomatitis Indiana, *Lutzomyia trapidoi*, taking a blood meal. (Photograph by Dr. R. E. Tesh.)

Pre- or post-exposure chemotherapy of human beings, cattle, horses, or swine against VS disease has not yet been attempted. Ammonium 5-tungsto-2-antimoniate administered to mice shortly before VS virus infection was protective.[161] Mice have also been protected from disease by two polyanionic interferon inducers, polyinosinic/polycytidylic acid and maleic acid/divinyl ether copolymer[41] administered 4 hours before inoculation with VS virus. The effectiveness of these compounds in natural hosts, and under field conditions is unknown.

Good sanitary practices have helped to limit the spread of the disease among dairy cattle. Thorough hand and milking-machine washing has been recommended to control mechanical spread within milking herds. Susceptible animals should be stabled well-separated from infected animals and not be permitted to contact forage or water which infected animals have contacted. The effects of the disease have been reduced by control of secondary infections. Erosions should be kept clean, and antibiotics administered if signs of secondary infections are observed.

A number of chemicals have been effectively used to inactivate VS viruses, and can be employed as disinfectants. These have included calcium hypochlorite (50%) at 1 to 1000, benzalkonium chloride (10%) at 1 to 200, polyethoxy polypropoxy ethanol-iodine complex (7.75%) with nonyl phenyl ether of polyethylene glycoiodine complex (3.75%) at 1 to 200, cresylic acid and soap at 1 to 200, formalin (as 36.3% dissolved gas) at 1 to 100, hexachlorophene (0.75% as 2% of soap) at 1 to 50, phenols, quaternary ammonium, commercial bleach, and several other compounds at lesser concentrations.[119,162] Soda ash (sodium carbonate) at 2% or less did not inactivate VS viruses.[119]

PUBLIC HEALTH ASPECTS

Estimates of economic losses caused by VS epidemics have been made on a limited basis. In 1964, VSI occurred on 151 farms during one outbreak and the estimated loss was $30,631 1964 U.S. dollars, subdivided as $19,598 in dairy, $4,268 in beef and $6,599 in equine animals.[1] In a later VSNJ outbreak, milk production in dairy cattle declined 30%, but returned to normal in about 20 to 25 days, excluding animals that developed mastitis.[107] Beef cattle lost an average of 59 kg each.[107] In another VSNJ outbreak in dairy cattle, milk production declined 2.7 kg per cow per day for 17 days.[99]

Surveillance

Serological monitoring of livestock in endemic areas to assess their relative risk to VS infection has not been without difficulty. Neutralizing antibodies in convalescent animals have fluctuated, and have appeared to be an unreliable measure of an individual's return to susceptibility.[12,31,45,72,142,157] However, serum protection indices of approximately 1.7 or greater or titers of 1:100 or greater in the metabolic inhibition test have indicated resistance to experimental VSNJ challenge.[31,32]

REFERENCES

1. **Acree, J. A., Hodgson, D. R., and Page, R. W.,** Epicootic Indiana vesicular stomatitis in Southwestern United States, in *Proc. U.S. Livestock Sanit. Assoc.,* 68, 1964, 375.
2. **Arstila, P.,** Hemagglutinins of vesicular Stomatitis Virus, Dissertation, Medical Faculty, University of Turku, Finland, 1973, 1.
3. **Arstila, P.,** Quantitative studies on adsorption, elution, and haemagglutination of vesicular stomatitis virus, *Arch. Virol.,* 51, 51, 1976.
4. **Arstila, P., Halonen, P., and Salmi, A.,** Hemagglutinin of vesicular stomatitis virus, *Arch. Gesamte Virusforsch.,* 27, 198, 1969.
5. **Artsob, H. and Spence, L.,** Growth of vesicular stomatitis virus in mosquito cell lines, *Can. J. Microbiol.,* 20, 329, 1974.
6. **Artsob, H. and Spence, L.,** Persistent infection of mosquito cell lines with vesicular stomatitis virus, *Acta. Virol. Engl. Ed.,* 18, 331, 1974.
7. **Baxt, B. and Bablanian, R.,** Mechanisms of vesicular stomatitis virus-induced cytopathic effects II. Inhibition of macromolecular synthesis induced by infectious and defective-interfering particles, *Virology,* 72, 383, 1976.
8. **Berge, T. O., Ed.,** *International Catalogue of Arboviruses,* Publ. No. (CDC) 75-8301, Public Health Service, U.S. Department of Health, Education and Welfare, Atlanta, 1975.
9. **Bergold, G. H. and Munz, K.,** Ultrastructure of cocal, Indiana and New Jersey serotypes of vesicular stomatitis virus, *J. Ultrastruct. Res.,* 17, 233, 1967.
10. **Bergold, G. H., Suarez, O. M., and Munz, K.,** Multiplication in and transmission by *Aedes aegypti* of vesicular stomatitis virus, *J. Invest. Pathol.,* 11, 406, 1968.
11. **Bhatt, P. N. and Rodrigues, F. M.,** Chandipura: a new arbovirus isolated in India from patients with febrile illness, *Indian J. Med. Res.,* 55, 1295, 1967.
12. **Boulanger, P.,** Complement fixation tests on swine serum. I. In the diagnosis of vesicular stomatitis, *Can. J. Comp. Med. Vet. Sci.,* 19, 37, 1955.
13. **Boulanger, P. and Bannister, G. L.,** A modified direct complement-fixation test for the detection of antibodies in the serum of cattle previously infected with vesicular stomatitis virus, *J. Immunol.,* 85, 368, 1960.
14. **Bradish, C. J. and Kirkham, J. B.,** The morphology of vesicular stomatitis virus (Indiana C) derived from chick embryos or cultures of BHK 21/13 cells, *J. Gen. Microbiol.,* 44, 359, 1966.
15. **Brandly, C. A., Hanson, R. P., and Chow, I. I.,** Vesicular stomatitis with particular reference to the 1949 Wisconsin epizootic, in Proc. 88th Annu. Meet. Am. Vet. Med. Assoc., 1951, 61.
16. **Brody, J. A., Fischer, G. F., and Peralta, P. H.,** Vesicular stomatitis virus in Panama. Human serologic patterns in cattle raising area, *Am. J. Epidemiol.,* 86, 158, 1967.
17. **Brown, F. and Cartwright, B.,** The antigens of vesicular stomatitis virus: II. The presence of two low molecular weight immunogens in virus suspensions, *J. Immunol.,* 97, 612, 1966.
18. **Brown, F., Cartwright, B., and Almeida, J. D.,** The antigens of vesicular stomatitis virus. I. Separation and immunogenicity of three complement-fixing components, *J. Immunol.,* 96, 537, 1966.

19. **Brown, F., Cartwright, B., and Smale, C. J.,** The antigens of vesicular stomatitis virus: III. Structure and immunogenicity of antigens derived from the virion by treatment with Tween and ether, *J. Immunol.,* 99, 171, 1967.

20. **Burge, B. W. and Huang, A. S.,** Comparison of membrane protein glycopeptides of Sinbis virus and vesicular stomatitis virus, *J. Virol.,* 6, 176, 1970.

21. **Burton, A. C.,** Stomatitis contagiosa in horses, *Vet. J.,* 73, 234, 1917.

22. **Bussereau, F.,** Etude du symptome de la sensibilité au CO_2 produit par le virus de la stomatite vésiculaire chez *Drosophila melanogaster.* I. VSV de serotype New Jersey et le virus cocal. A study of CO_2 sensitivity produced by vesicula stomatis virus in *Drosophila melanogaster.* I. The effect of New Jersey and coccal strains of virus, *Ann. Inst. Pasteur, Paris,* 121, 223, 1971.

23. **Bussereau, F.,** Etude du symptome de la sensibilite au CO_2 produit par les virus de la stomatite vésiculaire chez *Drosophila melanogaster:* II. VSV de serotype Indiana. Studies on CO_2 sensitivity in *Drosophila melanogaster* after infection with vesicular stomatitis virus. II. VSV Indiana serotype. *Ann. Inst. Pasteur, Paris,* 122, 1029, 1972.

24. **Bussereau, F.,** The CO_2 sensitivity induced by two rhabdoviruses, Piry and Chandipura, in *Drosophila melanogaster, Ann. Microbiol, (Paris),* 126B, 389, 1975.

25. **Bussereau, F., Cartwright, B., Doel, T. R., and Brown, F.,** A comparative study of the surface projections of different strains of vesicular stomatitis virus, *J. Gen. Virol.,* 29, 189, 1975.

26. **Cartwright, B. and Brown, F.,** Serological relationships between different strains of vesicular stomatitis virus, *J. Gen. Virol.,* 16, 391, 1972.

27. **Cartwright, B., Smale, C. J., and Brown, F.,** Surface structure of veiscular stomatitis virus, *J. Gen. Virol.,* 5, 1, 1969.

28. **Cartwright, B., Smale, C. J., and Brown, F.,** Dissection of vesicular stomatitis virus into the infective ribonucleoprotein and immunizing components, *J. Gen. Virol.,* 7, 19, 1970.

29. **Cartwright, B., Smale, C. J., Brown, F., and Hull, R.,** Model for veiscular stomatitis virus, *J. Virol.,* 10, 256, 1972.

30. **Cartwright, B., Talbot, P., and Brown, F.,** The proteins of biologically active subunits of vesicular stomatitis virus, *J. Gen. Virol.,* 7, 267, 1970.

31. **Casteñeda, J., and Hanson, R. P.,** Complement-fixing antibodies as a measure of immunity of cattle to the virus of vesicular stomatitis New Jersey, *Am. J. Vet. Res.,* 27, 963, 1966.

32. **Casteñeda, G. J., Lauerman, L. H., and Hanson, R. P.,** Evaluation of virus neutralization tests and association of indices to cattle resistance, in *Proc. U.S. Livestock Sanit. Assoc.,* 68, 1964, 455.

33. **Center for Communicable Diseases,** *Vet. Public Health Notes,* 2, 5, 1965.

34. **Chow, T. L., Hanson, R. P., and McNutt, S. H.,** The pathology of vesicular stomatitis in cattle, in *Proc. Book Am. Vet. Med. Assoc.,* 1951, 119.

35. **Chow, T. L., and McNutt, S. H.,** Pathological changes of experimental vesicular stomatitis of swine, *Am. J. Vet. Res.,* 14, 420, 1953.

36. **Cline, B. L.,** Ecological associations of vesicular stomatitis virus in rural Central America and Panama, *Am. J. Trop. Med. Hyg.,* 25, 875, 1976.

37. **Cooper, P. D. and Bellett, A. J. D.,** A transmissible interfering component of vesicular stomatitis virus preparations, *J. Gen. Microbiol.,* 21, 485, 1959.

38. **Correa, W. M.,** Prophylaxis of vesicular stomatitis: a field trial in Guatemalan dairy cattle, *Am. J. Vet. Res.,* 25, 1300, 1964.

39. **Crick, J. and Brown, F.,** Interference as a measure of cross-relationship in the vesicular stomatitis group of rhabdoviruses, *J. Gen. Virol.,* 18, 79, 1973.

40. **David-West, T. S. and Labzoffsky, N. A.,** Electron microscopic studies on the development of vesicular stomatitis virus, *Arch. Gesamte Virusforsch.,* 23, 105, 1968.

41. **DeClercq, E. and Merigan, T. C.,** Local and systemic protection by synthetic polianionic interferon inducers in mice against intranasal vesicular stomatitis virus, *J. Gen. Virol.,* 5, 359, 1968.

42. **Dhanda, V., Rodrigues, F. M., and Gosh, S. N.,** Isolation of chandipura virus from sandflies in Aurangabad, *Indian J. Med. Res.,* 58, 179, 1970.

43. **Dimopoullos, G. T., Fellowes, O. N., Callis, J. J., Poppensiek, G. C., Tessler, J., and Hess, W. R.,** Heat-inactivated vesicular stomatitis virus (VSV) as antigen in the complement-fixation test, *Am. J. Vet. Res.,* 18, 688, 1957.

44. **Donaldson, A. I.,** Bats as possible maintenance hosts for vesicular stomatitis virus, *Am. J. Epidemiol.,* 92, 132, 1970.

45. **Earley, E., Peralta, P. H., and Johnson, K. M.,** A plaque neutralization method for arboviruses, *Proc. Soc. Exp. Biol. Med.,* 125, 741, 1967.

46. **Edelman, R. and Wheelock, E. F.,** Specific role of each human leukocyte type in viral infection. I. Monocyte as host cell for vesicular stomatitis virus replication, *In Vitro,* 1, 1139, 1967.

47. **Ellis, E. M. and Kendall, H. E.,** The public health and economic effects of vesicular stomatitis in a herd of dairy cattle, *J. Am. Vet. Med. Assoc.,* 144, 377, 1964.

48. **Federer, K. E., Burrows, R., and Brooksby, J. B.,** Vesicular stomatitis virus: the relationship between some strains of the Indiana serotype, *Res. Vet. Sci.,* 8, 103, 1067.

49. **Fellowes, O. N.,** Comparison of cryobiological and freeze-drying characteristics of foot and mouth disease virus and of vesicular stomatitis virus, *Cryobiology,* 4, 223, 1968.

50. **Fellowes, O. N., Dimopoullos, G. T., and Callis, J. J.,** Isolation of vesicular stomatitis virus from an infected laboratory worker, *Am. J. Vet. Res.,* 16, 623, 1955.

51. **Fellowes, O. N., Dimopoullos, G. T., Tessler, J., Hess, W. R., Vardman, T. H., and Callis, J. J.,** Comparative titrations of vesicular stomatitis in various animal species and in tissue culture, *Am. J. Vet. Res.,* 27, 799, 1956.

52. **Ferris, D., Hanson, R. P., Dicke, R. J., and Roberts, R. H.,** Experimental transmission of vesicular stomatitis by diptera, *J. Infect. Dis.,* 96, 184, 1955.

53. **Fields, B. N. and Hawkins, K.,** Human infection with the virus of vesicular stomatitis during an epizootic, *N. Engl. J. Med.,* 277, 989, 1967.

54. **Gaidamovich, S. Ya., Uvarov, V. N., and Alekseeva, A. A.,** Isolation of the vesicular stomatitis virus from a patient, *Vop. Virusol.,* 11, 77, 1966.

55. **Galindo, P., Srihongse, S., Rodaniche, E., and Greyson, M. A.,** An ecological survey for arboviruses in Almirante, Panama, 1959—1962, *Am. J. Trop. Med. Hyg.,* 15, 385, 1966.

56. **Geleta, J. N. and Holbrook, A. A.,** Vesicular stomatitis — patterns of complement-fixing and serum-neutralizing antibody in serum of convalescent cattle and horses, *Am. J. Vet. Res.,* 22, 713, 1961.

57. **Gonzalez, G.,** Studies On Strains of VSV From Colombia, Ph.D. thesis, University of Wisconsin — Madison, 1977.

58. **Griffin, T. P., Hanson, R. P., and Brandly, C. A.,** The effect of environmental temperature on susceptibility of the mouse to vesicular stomatitis viruses, in Proc. 91st. Annu. Meet. Am. Vet. Med. Assoc., 1954, 192.

59. **Guierrez, B. E., Ramirez Rocha, J., Cardona, U. A., Ulloa Valendia, J., and Torres Gutierrez, A.,** Cultivos celulares en el aislamiento de enfermedades vesiculares. Cell cultures in the isolation of viruses of vesicular diseases. *Rev. Inst. Colomb. Agropecu.,* 8, 31, 1973.

60. **Hackett, A. J., Schaffer, F. L., and Madin, S. H.,** The separation of infectious and autointerfering particles in vesicular stomatitis virus preparations, *Virology,* 31, 114, 1967.

61. **Halonen, P. E., Murphy, F. A., Fields, B. N., and Reese, D. R.,** Hemagglutinin of rabies and some other bullet-shaped viruses, *Proc. Soc. Exp. Biol. Med.,* 127, 1037, 1968.

62. **Halonen, P. E., Toivanen, P., and Nikkari, T.,** Non-specific serum inhibitors of activity of haemagglutinins of rabies and vesicular stomatitis viruses, *J. Gen. Virol.,* 23, 309, 1973.

63. **Hanson, R. P.,** The natural history of vesicular stomatitis virus, *Bacteriol. Rev.,* 16, 179, 1952.

64. **Hanson, R. P.,** Discussion of the natural history of vesicular stomatitis, *Am. J. Epidemiol.,* 87, 264, 1968.

65. **Hanson, R. P.,** Vesicular stomatitis, in *Diseases of Swine,* Dunne, H. W. and Leman, A. D., Eds., Iowa State Univ. Press, Ames, Iowa, 1975, 308.

66. **Hanson, R. P., and Brandly, C. A.,** Epizootiology of vesicular stomatitis. *Am. J. Public Health,* 47, 205, 1957.

67. **Hanson, R. P. and Karstad, L.,** Further studies on vesicular stomatitis, in *Proc. U.S. Livestock Sanit. Assoc.,* 61, 300, 1957.

68. **Hanson, R. P. and Karstad, L.,** Feral swine as a reservoir of vesicular stomatitis virus in Southeastern United States, in *Proc. U.S. Livestock Sanit. Assoc.,* 62, 1958, 309.

69. **Hanson, R. P., Rasmussen, A. F., Brandly, C. A., and Brown, J. W.,** Human infection with the virus of vesicular stomatitis, *J. Lab. Clin. Med.,* 36, 754, 1950.

70. **Heggers, J. P.,** Quantitative studies on the infectivity of vesicular stomatitis virus (Indiana serotype) in "L" cells, *J. Am. Med. Technol.,* 30, 479, 1968.

71. **Heinz, E.,** Vesicular stomatitis in cattle and horses in Colorado, *North Am. Vet.,* 26, 726, 1945.

72. **Holbrook, A. A.** Duration of immunity and serologic patterns in swine convalescing from vesicular stomatitis, *J. Am. Vet. Med. Assoc.,* 141, 1463, 1962.

73. **Hopkins, S. R. and Janney, G. C.,** The fluorescent antibody technique applied to vesicular stomatitis virus using serum fractionated with ethodin, *Am. J. Vet. Res.,* 23, 603, 1962.

74. **Howatson, A. F,** Vesicular stomatitis and related viruses, in *Advances in Virus Research,* Smith, K. M., Lauffer, M. A., and Barg, E. B., Eds., Academic Press, New York, 1970, 195.

75. **Huang, A. S., Greenawalt, J. W., and Wagner, R. R.,** Defective T particles of vesicular stomatitis virus: I. Preparation, morphology, and some biologic properties, *Virology,* 30, 161, 1966.

76. **Huang, A. S. and Wagner, R. R.,** Comparative sedimentation coefficients of RNA extracted from plaque-forming and defective particles of vesicular stomatitis virus, *J. Mol. Biol.,* 22, 381, 1966.

77. **Jenney, E. W.,** Vesicular stomatitis in the United States during the last five years (1963—1967), in *Proc. U.S. Livestock Sanit. Assoc.,* 71, 1967, 371.

78. **Jenney, E. W. and Mott, L. O.**, Serologic studies with the virus of vesicular stomatitis II. Typing of vesicular stomatitis convalescent serum by direct complement fixation, *Am. J. Vet. Res.*, 24, 874, 1963.

79. **Jenney, E. W., Mott, L. O., and Traub, E.**, Serological studies with the virus of vesicular stomatitis. I. Typing of vesicular stomatitis by complement fixation, *Am. J. Vet. Res.*, 19, 993, 1958.

80. **Jensen, M. M. and Rasmussen, A. F.**, Stress and susceptibility to viral infections. II. Sound stress and susceptibility to vesicular stomatitis virus, *J. Immunol.*, 90, 21, 1963.

81. **Johnson, K. M., Tesh, R. B., and Peralta, P. H.**, Epidemiology of vesicular stomatitis virus: some new data and a hypothesis for transmission of the Indiana serotype, *J. Am. Vet. Med. Assoc.*, 155, 2133, 1969.

82. **Johnson, K. M., Vogel, J. E., and Peralta, P. H.**, Clinical serological response to laboratory-acquired human infection by Indiana type vesicular stomatitis virus (VSV), *Am. J. Trop. Med. Hyg.*, 15, 244, 1966.

83. **Jonkers, A. H.**, The epizootiology of the vesicular stomatitis virus: reappraisal, *Am. J. Epidemiol.*, 86, 286, 1967.

84. **Jonkers, A. H., Shope, R. E., Aitken, T. H. G., and Spence, L.**, Cocal virus, a new agent in Trinidad related to vesicular stomatitis, type Indiana, *Am. J. Vet. Res.*, 25, 236, 1964.

85. **Jonkers, A. H., Spence, L., and Aitken, T. H. G.**, Cocal virus epizootiology in Bush Bush forest and the Narvia swamp, Trinidad, W. I.: further studies, *Am. J. Vet. Res.*, 26, 758, 1965.

86. **Jonkers, A. H., Spence, L., Coakwell, C. A., and Thornton, J. J.**, Laboratory studies with wild rodents and viruses native to Trinidad, *Am. J. Trop. Med. Hyg.*, 13, 613, 1964.

87. **Karstad, L. H., Adams, E. V., Hanson, R. P., and Ferris, D. H.**, Evidence for the role of wildlife in epizootics of vesicular stomatitis, *J. Am. Vet. Med., Assoc.*, 129, 95, 1956.

88. **Karstad, L. and Hanson, R. P.**, Vesicular stomatitis in deer, *Am. J. Vet. Res.*, 18, 162, 1957.

89. **Karstad, L. and Hanson, R. P.**, Primary isolation and comparative titrations of five field strains of vesicular stomatitis virus in chicken embryos, hogs, and mice, *Am. J. Vet. Res.*, 19, 233, 1958.

90. **Kelley, R. K. and Loh, P. C.**, Some properties of an established fish cell line from *Xiphophorus helleri* (red swordtail), *In Vitro*, 9, 73, 1973.

91. **Klenk, H. D., Compans, R. W., and Choppin, P. W.**, An electron microscopic study of the presence or absence of neuraminic acid in enveloped viruses, *Virology*, 42, 1158, 1970.

92. **Knudson, D. L.**, Rhabdoviruses, *J. Gen. Virol.*, 20, 105, 1973.

93. **Kowalczyk, T. and Brandly, C. A.**, Experimental infection of dogs, ferrets, chinchillas, and hamsters with vesicular stomatitis virus, *Am. J. Vet. Res.*, 15, 98, 1954.

94. **Kowalczyk, T., Hanson, R. P., and Brandly, C. A.**, Infectivity and pathogenicity of vesicular stomatitis virus for ferrets, *Am. J. Vet. Res.*, 58, 180, 1955.

95. **Lastra, J. R. and Esparza, J.**, Multiplication of vesicular stomatitis virus in the leafhopper *Peregrinus maidis* (Ashm.) a vector of a plant rhabdovirus, *J. Gen. Virol.*, 32, 139, 1976.

96. **Lauerman, L. H. and Hanson, R. P.**, Field trial vaccination against vesicular stomatitis in Georgia, in *Proc. U.S. Livestock Sanit. Assoc.*, 67, 1963, 473.

97. **Lauerman, L. H. and Hanson, R. P.**, Field trial vaccination against vesicular stomatitis in Panama, in *Proc. U.S. Livestock Sanit. Assoc.*, 67, 1963, 483.

98. **Lauerman, L. H., Kuns, M. L., and Hanson, R. P.**, Field trial of live virus vaccination procedure for prevention of vesicular stomatitis in dairy cattle. I. Preliminary immune response, in *Proc. U.S. Livestock Sanit. Assoc.*, 66, 1962, 365.

99. **Liebermann, H., Hahnefeld, H., and Hahnefeld, E.**, Einige chemischphysikalische und biologische eigenschaften des virus der stomatitis vesicularis (typ Indiana). Some chemico-physical and biological properties of vesicular stomatitis virus (type Indiana), *Arch. Exp. Veterinaermed.*, 20, 839, 1966.

100. **Liu, I. K. M. and Zee, Y. C.**, The pathogenesis of vesicular stomatitis virus, serotype Indiana, in *Aedes aegypti* mosquitoes. I. Intrathoracic injection, *Am. J. Trop. Med. Hyg.*, 25, 177, 1976.

101. **Lozano Pardo, J.**, La estomatitis vesicular, su importancia en el problema de la profilaxis de la fiebre aftosa, Vesicular stomatitis and its importance in the problem of prophylaxis in hoof and mouth disease, *Vet. Zootecn.*, 13, 37, 1961.

102. **Lunger, P. D. and Clark, H. F.**, Host effect on vesicular stomatitis virus morphogenesis and "T" particle formation in reptilian, avian, and mammalian cell lines, *In Vitro*, 11, 239, 1975.

103. **McClain, M. E. and Hackett, A. J.**, A comparative study of the growth of vesicular stomatitis virus in five tissue culture systems, *J. Immunol.*, 80, 356, 1958.

104. **McSharry, J. J. and Wagner, R. R.**, Lipid composition of purified vesicular stomatitis viruses, *J. Virol.*, 7, 59, 1971.

105. **McSharry, J. J. and Wagner, R. R.**, Carbohydrate composition of vesicular stomatitis virus, *J. Virol.*, 7, 412, 1971.

106. **Mengeling, W. L. and Van der Maaten, M. J.**, Identification of selected animal viruses with fluorescent antibodies prepared from multivalent antiserums, *Am. J. Vet. Res.*, 32, 1825, 1971.

107. **Meyer, N. L., Moulton, W. M., Jenney, E. W., and Rodgers, R. J.,** Outbreaks of vesicular stomatitis in Oklahoma and Texas, in *Proc. U.S. Livestock Sanit. Assoc.*, 64, 1960, 324.

108. **Michalski, F., Parks, N. F., Frantisek, S., and Clark, H. G.,** Thermal inactivation of rabies and other rhabdoviruses: stabilization by the chelating agent ethylenediamine tetraacetic acid at physiological temperatures, *Infect. Immun.*, 14, 135, 1976.

109. **Miyoshi, K., Harter, D. H., Hsu, K. C.,** Neuropathological and immunofluorescence studies of experimental vesicular stomatitis virus encephalitis in mice, *J. Neuropathol. Exp. Neurol.*, 30, 266, 1971.

110. **Mohler, J. R.,** Vesicular stomatitis in Horses and Cattle, Bull. No. 662, in U.S. Department of Agriculture, Washington, D.C., 1930.

111. **Mudd, J. A., Leavitt, R. W., Kingsbury, D. T., and Holland, J. J.,** Natural selection of mutants of vesicular stomatitis virus by cultured cells of *Drosophila melanogaster, J. Gen. Virol.*, 20, 341, 1973.

112. **Murphy, F. A.,** Evolution of rhabdovirus tropisms, in *Viruses, Evolution and Cancer,* Kurstak, E. and Maramorosch, K., Eds., Academic Press, New York, 1973, 699.

113. **Murphy, F. A., Harrison, A. K., and Bauer, S. P.,** Experimental vesicular stomatitis virus infection: ultrastructural pathology, *Exp. Mol. Pathol.*, 23, 426, 1975.

114. **Mussgay, M. and Suarez, O.,** Multiplication of vesicular stomatitis virus in *Aedes aegypti* (L) mosquitoes, *Virology,* 17, 202, 1962.

115. **Myers, W. L. and Hanson, R. P.,** Immunodiffusion studies on the antigenic relationships within and between serotypes of vesicular stomatitis virus, *Am. J. Vet. Res.,* 23, 896, 1962.

116. **Myers, W. L. and Hanson, R. P.,** Studies on the response of rabbits and guinea pigs to inoculation with vesicular stomatitis virus, *Am. J. Vet. Res.,* 23, 1078, 1962.

117. **Nishiyama, Y., Yasuhiko, I., Kaoru, S., Yoshinobu, K., and Ikuya, N.,** Polykaryocyte formation induced by VSV in mouse L cells, *J. Gen. Virol.,* 32, 85, 1976.

118. **Orenstein, J., Johnson, L., Shelton, E., and Lazzarini, R. A.,** The shape of vesicular stomatitis virus, *Virology,* 71, 291, 1976.

119. **Patterson, W. C., Holbrook, A. A., Hopkins, S. P., and Songer, J. R.,** The effect of chemical and physical agents on the viruses of vesicular stomatitis and vesicular exanthama, in *Proc. U.S. Livestock Sanit. Assoc.,* 62, 1953, 294.

120. **Patterson, W. C., Jenny, E. W., and Holbrook, A. A.,** Experimental infections with vesicular stomatitis in swine. I. Transmission by direct contact and feeding infected meat scraps, in *Proc. U.S. Livestock Sanit. Assoc.,* 59, 1955, 368.

121. **Patterson, W. C., Mott, L. O., and Jenny, E. W.,** A study of vesicular stomatitis in man, *J. Am. Vet. Med. Assoc.,* 133, 57, 1958.

122. **Peralta, P. H. and Shelokov, A.,** Isolation and characterization of arboviruses from Almirante, Republic of Panama, *Am. J. Trop. Med. Hyg.,* 15, 369, 1966.

123. **Printz, P.,** Adaptation du virus de la stomatite vesiculaire a *Drosophila melanogaster.* Adaptation of the virus of vesicular stomatitis to *Drosophila melanogaster. Ann. Inst. Pasteur, Paris,* 119, 520, 1970.

124. **Proctor, S. J. and Sherman, K. C.,** Ultrastructural changes in bovine lingual epithelium infected with vesicular stomatitis virus, *Vet. Pathol.,* 12, 362, 1975.

125. **Rabinowitz, S. G., Dal Canto, M. C., and Johnson, T. C.,** Comparison of central nervous system disease produced by wild-type and temperature-senstive mutants of vesicular stomatitis virus, *Infect. Immun.,* 13, 1242, 1976.

126. **Ramachandra, R., Singh, K. R. P., Dhanda, V., and Bhatt, P. N.,** Experimental transmission of Chandipura virus by mosquitoes, *Indian J. Med. Res.,* 55, 1306, 1967.

127. **Shelokov, A. and Peralta, P. H.,** Vesicular stomatitis virus, Indiana type: an arbovirus infection of tropical sandflies and humans? *Am. J. Epidemiol.,* 86, 149, 1967.

128. **Ribelin, W. E.,** The cytopathogenesis of vesicular stomatitis virus infection in cattle, *Am. J. Vet. Res.,* 19, 66, 1958.

129. **Roberts, R. H., Dicke, R. J., Hanson, R. P., and Ferris, D. H.,** Potential insect vectors of vesicular stomatitis in Wisconsin, *J. Infect. Dis.,* 98, 121, 1956.

130. **Rosenthal, L. J. and Sheckmeister, I. L.,** Comparison of microtiter procedures with the plaque technique for assay of vesicular stomatitis virus, *Appl. Microbiol.,* 21, 400, 1971.

131. **Sabin, A. B. and Olitsky, P. K.,** Influence of host factors on neuroinvasiveness of vesicular stomatitis virus. I. Effect of age on the invasion of the brain by virus instilled in the nose, *J. Exp. Med.,* 66, 15, 1937.

132. **Sabin, A. B. and Olitsky, P. K.,** Influence of host factors on neuroinvasiveness of vesicular stomatitis virus. II. Effect of age on the invasion of the peripheral and central nervous system by virus injected into leg muscles or the eye, *J. Exp. Med.,* 66, 35, 1937.

133. **Sabin, A. B. and Olitsky, P. K.,** Influence of host factors on neuroinvasiveness of vesicular stomatitis virus. IV. Variations in neuroinvasiveness in different species, *J. Exp. Med.,* 67, 229, 1938.

134. **Schaffer, F. L. and Soergel, M. E.**, Molecular weight estimates of vesicular stomatitis virus ribonucleic acids from virions, defective particles, and infected cells, *Arch. Gesamte Virusforsch.*, 39, 203, 1972.

135. **Schloemer, R. H. and Wagner, R. R.**, Mosquito cells infected with vesicular stomatitis virus yield unsialylated virions of low infectivity, *J. Virol.*, 15, 1029, 1975.

136. **Seibold, H. R. and Sharp, J. B., Jr.**, A revised concept of the pathologic changes of the tongue in cattle with vesicular stomatitis, *Am. J. Vet. Res.*, 21, 35, 1960.

137. **Shahan, M. S., Frank, A. H., and Mott, L. O.**, Studies of vesicular stomatitis with special reference to a virus of swine origin, *J. Am. Vet. Med. Assoc.*, 108, 5, 1946.

138. **Shelokov, A., Peralta, P. H., and Galindo, P.**, Prevalence of human infection with vesicular stomatitis virus, *J. Clin. Invest.*, 40, 1081, 1961.

139. **Singh, K. R. P., Goverdhan, M. K., and Bhat, U. K. M.**, Susceptibility of *Aedes w-albus* and *Anopheles stephensi* cell lines to infection with some arboviruses, *Indian J. Med., Res.*, 61, 1134, 1973.

140. **Skinner, H. H.**, The virus of vesicular stomatitis in small experimental hosts. I. White mice, cotton rats, chick embryos and young chickens, *J. Comp. Pathol. Ther.*, 67, 69, 1957.

141. **Skinner, H. H.**, The virus of vesicular stomatitis in small experimental hosts. II. Guinea pigs and rabbits, *J. Comp. Pathol. Ther.*, 67, 87, 1957.

142. **Sorensen, D. K., Chow, T. L., Hanson, R. P., Kowalczyk, T., and Brandly, C. A.**, Persistence in cattle of serum neutralizing antibodies of vesicular stomatitis virus, *Am. J. Vet. Res.*, 19, 74, 1958.

143. **Srihongse, S.**, Vesicular stomatitis virus infections in Panamanian primates and other vertebrates, *Am. J. Epidemiol.*, 90, 69, 1969.

144. **Stone, S. S. and Delay, P. D.**, A rapid complement-fixation test for identification of vesicular stomatitis virus in cattle, *Am. J. Vet. Res.*, 24, 1060, 1963.

145. **Strozzi, P. and Ramos-Saco, T.**, Teat vesicles as primary and almost exclusive lesions in an extensive outbreak of vesiclar stomatitis (New Jersey strain) in milking cows, *J. Am. Vet. Med. Assoc.*, 123, 415, 1953.

146. **Sudia, W. D., Fields, B. N., and Calisher, C. H.**, The isolation of vesicular stomatitis virus (Indiana strain) and other viruses from mosquitoes in New Mexico, 1965, *Am. J. Epidemiol.*, 86, 598, 1967.

147. **Tesh, R. B. and Chaniotis, B. N.**, Transovarial transmission by phlebotomine sandflies, *Ann. N.Y. Acad. Sci.*, 266, 125, 1975.

148. **Tesh, R. B., Chaniotis, B. N., and Johnson, K. M.**, Vesicular stomatitis virus, Indian serotype: multiplication and transmission by experimentally infected phlebotomine sandflies (*Lutzomyia trapidoi*), *Am. J. Epidemiol.*, 93, 1971.

149. **Tesh, R. B., Chaniotis, B. N., and Johnson, K. M.**, Vesicular stomatitis virus (Indiana serotype): transovarial transmission by phlebotomine sandflies, *Science*, 175, 1477, 1972.

150. **Tesh, R. E., Chaniotis, B. N., Peralta, P. H., and Johnson, K. M.**, Ecology of viruses isolated from Panamanian phlebotomine sandflies, *Am. J. Trop. Med. Hyg.*, 23, 258, 1974.

151. **Tesh, R. B., Peralta, P. H., and Johnson, K. M.**, Ecologic studies of vesicular stomatitis virus I. Prevalence of infection among animals and humans living in an area of endemic VSV activity, *Am. J. Epidemiol.*, 90, 255, 1969.

152. **Tesh, R. B., Peralta, P. H., and Johnson, K. M.**, Ecologic studies of vesicular stomatitis virus. II. Results of experimental infection in Panamanian wild animals, *Am. J. Epidemiol.*, 91, 216, 1970.

153. **Tesh, R., Saidi, S., Javadian, E., Loh, P., and Nadim, A.**, Isfahan virus, a new vesiculovirus, *Am. J. Trop. Med. Hyg.*, 26, 299, 1977.

154. **Theiler, M. and Downs, W. G.**, *The Arthropod-Borne Viruses of Vertebrates,* Yale University Press, New Haven, 1973, 281.

155. **Thormar, H.**, A comparison of cocal and vesicular stomatitis virus, serotypes New Jersey and Indiana, *Virology*, 31, 323, 1967.

156. **Tilles, J. G.**, Enhancement of vesicular stomatitis virus following adsorption with poly-L-ornithine *Proc. Soc. Exp. Biol. Med.*, 131, 76, 1969.

157. **Vadlamudi, S. and Hanson, R. P.**, The neutralization test for vesicular stomatitis virus in chicken embryos and tissue cultures, *Cornell Vet.*, 53, 16, 1963.

158. **Valle, M.**, Factors affecting plaque assay of animal viruses with special reference to vesicular stomatitis and vaccinia virus, *Acta Pathol. Microbiol. Scand.*, 219, 69, 1971.

159. **Wagner, R. R., Prevec, L., Brown, F., Summers, D. F., Sokol, F., and MacLeod, R.**, Classification of rhabdovirus proteins: a proposal, *J. Virol.*, 10, 1228, 1972.

160. **Warren, J. and Cutchins, E. C.**, General characteristics and viral susceptibility of bovine embryonic tissue cultures, *Virology*, 4, 297, 1957.

161. **Werner, G. H., Jasmin, C., and Chermann, J. C.**, Effect of ammonium 5-tungsto-2-antimoniate on encephalomyocarditis and vesicular stomatitis virus infections in mice, *J. Gen. Virol.*, 31, 59, 1976.

162. **Wright, H. S.**, Inactivation of vesicular stomatitis virus by disinfectants, *Appl. Microbiol.*, 19, 96, 1970.

163. **Yang, Y. J., Stoltz, D. B., and Prevec, L.,** Growth of vesicular stomatitis virus in a continuous culture line of *Antheraea eucalypti* moth cells, *J. Gen. Virol.,* 5, 473, 1969.
164. **Yunker, C. E. and Cory, J.,** Infection of Grace's *Antheraea* cells with arboviruses, *Am. J. Trop. Med. Hyg.,* 17, 889, 1968.

ARBOVIRAL ZOONOSES IN CANADA

WESTERN EQUINE ENCEPHALOMYELITIS (WEE)

H. Artsob

NAME AND SYNONYMS

Western equine encephalomyelitis is commonly used as the name for the disease in horses. In people it is commonly called western equine encephalitis or simply western encephalitis.

HISTORY

Forage poisoning, cerebro-spinal meningitis, corn-stalk disease, sleeping sickness, and blind staggers were all used to describe a disease in horses, which was very likely WEE, in western Canada prior to 1935. The first definite recognition of WEE viral infection in Canada was in 1935. During horse outbreaks in Manitoba and Saskatchewan, WEE virus was isolated from horse brains.[12]

ANIMAL INFECTION

From a veterinary aspect, WEE is the most important arboviral infection in Canada. At least 17 major horse epidemics have been documented from 1935 to the present, as shown in Table 1. Between 1935 and 1938, over 60,000 horse cases were recorded in Manitoba and Saskatchewan provinces.[8,12,30] Following the introduction of vaccination of horses in 1938, morbidity and mortality both reduced rapidly, but the virus remains endemic in the western provinces and small outbreaks still occur.[7,9,10,17,20,21,26,32]

In studies on animals other than horses, Yuill et al.[36] reported evidence that WEE epidemics in snowshoe hares (*Lepus americanus*) in 1963 and 1965 were followed by increased snowshoe hare mortality rates.

HUMAN INFECTION

Human infections with western equine encephalitis were first reported in 1938 in Manitoba[11] and Saskatchewan.[13] In 1941 a large epidemic occurred in the prairie provinces with 509 cases in Manitoba,[11] 543 cases in Saskatchewan[8] and 42 cases in Alberta.[22] Subsequent outbreaks have occurred in the prairie provinces, especially in 1947,[9,32] 1953,[10] 1963,[9,25] 1965,[29] and 1975.[35] Human encephalitis cases due to western equine encephalitis have also been recognized in British Columbia,[16,17] and one case has been serologically diagnosed in eastern Canada.[27]

EPIDEMIOLOGY

Occurrence

Since the isolation of WEE virus from a horse in Saskatchewan in 1935,[12] the virus has been found to be endemic in the three prairie provinces — Manitoba, Saskatchewan, and Alberta. In 1971 and 1972, WEE virus activity was demonstrated in British Columbia.[16,17] Serological evidence of WEE activity has been presented in Quebec province in 1955[27] and in western Ontario in 1975.[20]

Table 1
EPIDEMICS OF WESTERN EQUINE ENCEPHALOMYELITIS IN HORSES IN CANADA

Year	Province	Comments	Ref.
1935	Manitoba and Saskatchewan	Large WEE outbreak; first isolation of WEE in Canada from horse brain	12
1937	Manitoba	Large outbreak involving approximately 12,000 horses with 27% mortality rate	30
	Saskatchewan	Extensive outbreak involving all sections of Saskatchewan except the extreme northwest	12
1938	Manitoba	WEE outbreak extending into northwestern Manitoba	30
	Saskatchewan	Estimate 52,500 horse cases with over 15,000 deaths	8
1941	Prairie provinces	250 — 350 cases in each province with low mortality rate	7
1953/4	Saskatchewan	76 reported cases in southeastern Saskatchewan	10
1963	Manitoba	173 clinical cases	20
	Saskatchewan	279 cases with 47 deaths	10
1964	Manitoba	73 clinical cases	20
1965	Manitoba	75 horse cases with 9 deaths	32
	Alberta	63 serologically diagnosed and 73 presumptive positives; also 5 WEE isolations from brain	36
1966	Manitoba	51 equine cases	21
1967/9	Manitoba	8 cases in 1967, 14 cases in 1968, 41 cases in 1969	20
1971	British Columbia	60 cases in Okanagan Valley with 15 deaths	17
1975	Ontario	Serological evidence for up to 4 cases in northwestern Ontario	20
	Manitoba	261 clinically suspect cases; 65 confirmed and 80 presumptive positive	20

Reservoirs

Burton et al.,[6] in studies on Saskatchewan birds in 1962 and 1963, obtained 25 isolations of WEE virus including 23 isolates from English sparrows and one isolate each from a Swainson's hawk and a mourning dove. The virus from the mourning dove was obtained early in the year (May 19), suggesting latent infection.

Virus neutralizing antibodies against WEE virus have been detected in many birds in the prairie provinces, including Brewer's blackbird, common red-wing, crow, rock dove, Swainson's hawk, Franklin's gull, ring-billed gull, magpie, robin, English sparrow, sharptailed grouse, barn swallow, starling, ruffed grouse, chicken, and turkey.[4,6,15] In addition, several wild duck species have been found to possess neutralizing antibodies to WEE virus and oral infection of ducks has been experimentally achieved.[3] Hemagglutination inhibiting antibodies were found in English sparrows taken in Essex County, Ontario in 1975 and 1976, in two catbirds captured at Prince Edward Point, Ontario in 1976, and in white-crowned sparrows and catbirds captured at Long Point, Ontario in 1977[11a]

In studies on wild mammals, WEE virus has been isolated frequently from Richardson's ground squirrels,[6,14,18] and this host has been postulated as playing an important role in the natural history of WEE virus in the Canadian prairies.[18,19] Neutralizing antibodies have been found in other mammals, including Franklin ground squirrel, snowshoe hare, red fox, skunk, pig, bison, moose, and pronghorn sheep.[2,4,15,34,36]

Reptiles and amphibians have also been implicated as potential reservoirs of WEE virus in the prairie provinces following virus isolations from and demonstration of virus neutralizing antibodies in garter snakes and leopard frogs.[5,28,32]

Transmission

Western equine encephalitis virus has been isolated from mosquitoes of at least nine species,[23] including members of the *Aedes, Culex,* and *Culiseta* genera.[24,31] *Culex transalis* is the principal epidemic transmitter, but it is believed that other species contribute to the maintenance of the endemic status of the disease in the prairies[24] and in more northerly parts of Canada where *Cx. tarsalis* is absent.[4] Also, *Cu. inornata* may be a significant transmitter of the virus during horse epidemics.[24]

CONTROL

A vaccine is available to protect horses, but not the human population. Therefore, an early warning system designed for the prediction and prevention of epidemics is used as the basic line of defense.

Annual studies of the immunity of host populations and determination of the prevalence of virus both by studying the infection rates in birds (sentinel chickens or nestling birds) and by determining the numbers of vector mosquitoes are used in the endemic prairie provinces.[23] Such careful monitoring for WEE activity provided a warning of extensive virus activity in Manitoba in 1975, and was the basis for an immediate application of insecticides to avert a potential epidemic.[1]

REFERENCES

1. **Anon.,** Western encephalomyelitis, *Can. J. Public Health,* 67(Suppl. 1), 1976.
2. **Barrett, M. W. and Chalmers, G. A.,** A serologic survey of pronghorns in Alberta and Saskatchewan, 1970—1972, *J. Wildl. Dis.,* 11, 157, 1975.
3. **Burton, A. N., Connell, R., Rempel, J. G., and Gollop, J. B.,** Studies on western equine encephalitis associated with wild ducks in Saskatchewan, *Can. J. Microbiol.,* 7, 295, 1961.
4. **Burton, A. N. and McLintock, J.,** Further evidence of western encephalitis infection in Saskatchewan mammals and birds and in reindeer in northern Canada, *Can. Vet. J.,* 11, 232, 1970.
5. **Burton, A. N., McLintock, J., and Rempel, J. G.,** Western equine encephalitis virus in Saskatchewan garter snakes and leopard frogs, *Science,* 154, 1029, 1966.
6. **Burton, A. N., McLintock, J. R., Spalatin, J., and Rempel, J. G.,** Western equine encephalitis in Saskatchewan birds and mammals 1962—1963, *Can. J. Microbiol.,* 12, 133, 1966.
7. **Cameron, G. E. W.,** Western equine encephalitis, *Can. J. Public Health,* 33, 383, 1942.
8. **Davison, R. O.,** Encephalomyelitis in Saskatchewan, 1941, *Can. J. Public Health,* 33, 388, 1942.
9. **Dillenberg, H.,** Human western equine encephalomyelitis (WEE) in Saskatchewan *Can. J. Public Health,* 56, 17, 1965.
10. **Dillenberg, H. O., Acker, M. S., Belcourt, R. J. P., and Nagler, F. P.,** Some problems in the epidemiology of neurotropic virus infections, *Can. J. Public Health,* 47, 6, 1956.
11. **Donovan, C. R. and Bowman, M.,** Some epidemiological features of poliomyelitis and encephalitis, Manitoba, 1941, *Can. J. Public Health,* 33, 246, 1942.
11a. **Dorland, R., Mahdy, M. S., Artsob, H., and Prytula, A.,** Wild bird surveillance in the study of arboviral encephalitis, in *Arboviral Encephalitides in Ontario With Special Reference to St. Louis Encephalitis,* Mahdy, M. S., Spence, L., and Joshua, J. M., Eds., Ontario Ministry of Health, Toronto, 1979, 208.
12. **Fulton, J. S.,** A report of two outbreaks of equine encephalomyelitis in Saskatchewan, *Can. J. Comp. Med.,* 2, 39, 1938.
13. **Gareau, U.,** Clinical aspects of an epidemic of human encephalomyelitis in Saskatchewan in 1938, *Can. J. Public Health,* 32, 1, 1941.
14. **Gwatkin, R. and Moynihan, I. W.,** Search for sources and carriers of equine encephalomyelitis virus, *Can. J. Res.,* 20, 321, 1942.
15. **Hoff, G. L., Yuill, T. M., Iversen, J. O., and Hanson, R. P.,** Selected microbial agents in snowshoe hares and other vertebrates of Alberta, *J. Wildl. Dis.,* 6, 472, 1970.
16. **Kettyls, G. D. M. and Bowmer, E. J.,** Western equine encephalitis, in *Epidemiol. Bull.,* 19, 24, 1975.
17. **Kettyls, G. D., Verrall, V. M., Wilton, L. D., Clapp, J. B., Clarke, D. A., and Rublee, J. D.,** Arbovirus infections in man in British Columbia, *Can. Med. Assoc. J.,* 106, 1175, 1972.

18. **Leung, M. L., Burton, A., Iversen, J., and McLintock, J.,** Natural infections of Richardson's ground squirrels with western equine encephalomyelitis virus, Saskatchewan, Canada, 1964—1973, *Can. J. Microbiol.,* 21, 954, 1975,

19. **Leung, M.-K., Iversen, J., McLintock, J., and Saunders, J. R.,** Subsutaneous exposure of the Richardson's ground squirrel (*Spermophilus richardsonii* Sabine) to western equine encephalomyelitis virus, *J. Wildl. Dis.,* 12, 237, 1976.

20. **Lillie, L. E., Wong, F. C., and Drysdale, R. A.,** Equine epizootic of western encephalomyelitis in Manitoba, 1975, *Can. J. Public Health,* 67 (Suppl. 1), 21, 1976.

21. **MacKay, J. F. W., Stackiw, W., and Brust, R. A.,** Western encephalitis (W.E.) in Manitoba — 1966, *Manit. Med. Rev.,* 48, 56, 1968.

22. **McGugan, A. C.,** Equine encephalomyelitis (western type) in humans in Alberta, 1941, *Can. J. Public Health,* 33, 148, 1942.

23. **McLintock, J.,** The arbovirus problem in Canada, *Can. J. Public Health,* 67(Suppl. 1), 8, 1976.

24. **McLintock, J., Burton, A. N., McKiel, J. A., Hall, R. R., and Rempel, J. G.,** Known mosquito hosts of western encephalitis virus in Saskatchewan, *J. Med. Entomol.,* 7, 446, 1970.

25. **Morgante, O., Barager, E. M., and Herbert, F. A.,** Central nervous system disease in humans due to simultaneous epidemics of echovirus type 9 and western encephalomyelitis virus infection in Alberta, *Can. Med. Assoc. J.,* 98, 1170, 1968.

26. **Morgante, O., Vance, H. N., Shemanchuk, J. A., and Windsor, R.,** Epizootic of western encephalomyelitis virus infection in equines in Alberta in 1965, *Can. J. Comp. Med.,* 32, 403, 1968.

27. **Pavilanis, V., Wright, I. L., and Silverberg, M.** Western equine encephalomyelitis: report of a case in Montreal, *Can. Med. Assoc. J.,* 77, 128, 1957.

28. **Prior, M. G. and Agnew, R. M.,** Antibody against western equine encephalitis virus occurring in the serum of garter snakes (Colubridae: Thamnophis) in Saskatchewan, *Can. J. Comp. Med.,* 35, 40, 1971.

29. **Rozdilsky, B., Robertson, H. E., and Chorney, J.,** Western encephalitis: report of eight fatal cases: Saskatchewan epidemic, 1965, *Can. Med. Assoc. J.,* 98, 79, 1968.

30. **Savage, A.,** Note on the prevalence of encephalomyelitis in Manitoba horses prior to 1941, *Can. J. Public Health,* 33, 258, 1942.

31. **Shemanchuk, J. A. and Morgante, O.,** Isolation of Western encephalitis virus from mosquitoes in Alberta, *Can. J. Microbiol.,* 14, 1, 1968.

32, **Snell, E.,** Preventive medicine-selective topics of current interest, *Manit. Med. Rev.,* 46, 23, 1966.

33. **Spalatin, J., Connell, R., Burton, A. N., and Gollop, B. J,.** Western equine encephalitis in Saskatchewan reptiles and amphibians, 1961—1963, *Can. J. Comp. Med.,* 28, 131, 1964.

34. **Trainer, D. O. and Hoff, G. L.,** Serologic evidence of arbovirus activity in a moose population in Alberta, *J. Wildl. Dis.,* 7, 118, 1971.

35. **Waters, J.,** An epidemic of western encephalomyelitis in humans — Manitoba, 1975, *Can. J. Public Health,* 67 (Suppl. 1) 28, 1976.

36. **Yuill, T. M., Iversen, J. O., and Hanson, R. P.,** Evidence for arbovirus infections in a population of snowshoe hares: a possible mortality factor, *Bull. Wildl. Dis. Assoc.,* 5, 248, 1969.

EASTERN EQUINE ENCEPHALOMYELITIS (EEE)

H. Artsob

NAME AND SYNONYMS

Eastern equine encephalomyelitis is commonly used as the name for the disease in horses. In people, it is commonly called eastern equine encephalitis or simply eastern encephalitis.

HISTORY

Eastern equine encephalitis was first recognized in Canada in 1938 when the virus was isolated from the blood of a horse in St. George, Ontario.[5]

ANIMAL INFECTION

Two documented horse outbreaks of EEE have occurred in Canada. The first occurred in Ontario in 1938 with twelve cases and two deaths in the St. George area and six or seven apparent cases in the St. Catharines area.[5] Virus was isolated from horse blood and histopathological changes characteristic of encephalitis were observed. In 1972 an epidemic occurred in the eastern townships of Quebec. Approximately 25 horses died and virus was isolated from the brains of five horses.[1b]

HUMAN INFECTION

No clinical cases of eastern equine encephalitis have been diagnosed in Canada. A survey of 208 human sera from north-central Alberta showed no evidence of neutralizing antibodies.[3] However, three of 4706 human sera collected from Quebec province between 1971 and 1974 possessed hemagglutination inhibiting antibodies to EEE.[1]

EPIDEMIOLOGY

Occurrence

EEE virus has been isolated from horses in Quebec[1b] and from horses[5] and a migratory bird[4] in Ontario. In addition, two virus isolates have been reported from snowshoe hares in Alberta.[7] Neutralizing antibodies have been reported in snowshoe hares in Alberta and in pronghorn sheep in Alberta and Saskatchewan.[1a]

Reservoir

EEE virus has been isolated from a migratory bird at Long Point, Ontario[4] illustrating a possible means for yearly introduction of virus into Canada.

Transmission

No virus isolations have been made from mosquitoes in this country. However, two potential vectors of EEE virus, *Culiseta melanura* and *Coquillettidia perturbans* are present in Quebec.[2] The Canadian distribution of *Culex perturbans* extends from Nova Scotia to British Columbia.[6]

CONTROL

A horse vaccine is in use in some provinces. No specific mosquito control measures have been undertaken in Canada.

REFERENCES

1. **Artsob, H., Spence, L., Th'ng, C., and West, R.,** National Arbovirus Reference Service, Toronto, unpublished data, 1977.
1a. **Barrett, M. W. and Chalmers, G. A.,** A serologic survey of pronghorns in Alberta and Saskatchewan, 1970—1972, *J. Wildl. Dis.,* 11, 157, 1975.
1b. **Bellavance, R., Rossier, E., LeMaitre, M., and Willis, N. G.,** Eastern equine encephalomyelitis in Eastern Canada, *Can. J. Public Health,* 64, 189, 1972.
2. **Harrison, R. J., Rossier, E., and Lemieux, B.,** The first Canadian case of eastern equine encephalitis observed in the Eastern Townships, Quebec, *Ann. Soc. Ent. Que.,* 20, 27, 1975.
3. **Hoff, G. L., Yuill, T. M., Iversen, J. O., and Hanson, R. P.,** Selected microbial agents in snowshoe hares and other vertebrates of Alberta, *J. Wildl. Dis.,* 6, 472, 1970.
4. **Karstad, L.,** Surveillance for arbovirus infections in migrating birds at Long Point, Ontario, 1961—62, *Ont. Bird Banding,* 1, 1, 1965.

5. Schofield, F. W. and Labzoffsky, N., Report on cases of suspected encephalomyelitis occurring in the vicinity of St. George, *Rep. Ont. Dept. Agric.*, 29, 25, 1938.
6. Steward, C. C. and McWade, J. W., The mosquitoes of Ontario (Diptera: Culicidae) with keys to the species and notes on distribution, *Proc. Entomol., Soc. Ont.*, 91, 121, 1960.
7. Yuill, T. M., Iversen, J. O., and Hanson, R. P., Evidence for arbovirus infections in a population of snowshoe hares: a possible mortality factor, *Bull. Wildl. Dis. Assoc.*, 5, 248, 1969.

ST. LOUIS ENCEPHALITIS (SLE)

H. Artsob

NAME AND SYNONYMS

St. Louis encephalitis is the name of the disease in human patients. Avian and lower mammalian infections are considered to be entirely subclinical.

HISTORY

The first definite recognition of SLE virus in Canada was in 1971 when the virus was isolated from a pool of *Culex tarsalis* collected in the Weyburn area of southern Saskatchewan.[1]

ANIMAL INFECTION

No evidence is available to suggest clinical infection of wild or domestic animals in Canada due to SLE virus. A variety of nestling and juvenile wild birds are considered to act as amplifying hosts, and a variety of mammals are probably infected but act as dead-end hosts.

HUMAN INFECTION

The first diagnosed cases of St. Louis encephalitis in Canada were recognized in 1975, with 66 cases in Ontario and one case each in Quebec and Manitoba.[3,12,14] The 1975 outbreak in Ontario involved the southern part of the province in the Windsor-Sarnia-Chatham area, the Niagara region, and the city of Toronto. Four patients who died showed typical histological features of viral encephalitis with perivascular cuffing and microglial proliferation at necropsy; virus was recovered from the brain of one.[14] Human SLE infections were again recognized in 1976; four cases were diagnosed in southern Ontario.[2] No cases of SLE were diagnosed in Ontario from 1977 to 1979. However, two SLE cases were reported in Manitoba in 1977.[17]

EPIDEMIOLOGY

Occurrence

Human infections due to SLE virus have been diagnosed in Quebec,[3] Ontario,[2,14] and Manitoba.[12] Neutralizing antibodies to the virus have been found in residents of Saskatchewan,[10] Alberta,[4] and British Columbia.[6-9] SLE virus has been isolated from mosquitoes in southern Saskatchewan.[1]

Reservoir

High prevalence of antibodies against SLE virus was observed in English sparrows collected in southern Ontario following the 1975 outbreak,[3a] providing suggestive evidence that these birds were reservoirs of the virus during the outbreak. In 1961 and 1962, a low prevalence of antibody was detected in migratory birds collected at Long Point, Ontario.[5] Subsequently, hemagglutination-inhibiting antibodies to SLE virus were found in 12.8% of migratory birds taken at Prince Edward Point and Long Point, Ontario in 1976.[3a] Neutralizing antibodies to SLE virus were also detected in three nonmigratory birds collected near Penticton, British Columbia in 1970.[6]

Neutralizing antibodies have been detected in rodent[7,8] sera collected in British Columbia, in snowshoe hare[4] sera collected in Alberta and in one moose,[16] and two bull snakes[13] trapped in Alberta.

Transmission

St. Louis encephalitis virus has been isolated from *Cx. tarsalis* mosquitoes collected in western Canada.[1] No isolations were made from a limited number of mosquito pools collected following the 1975 outbreak in southern Ontario.[18] It is considered that *Culex* spp., particularly *Cx. pipiens,* were primary vectors during the outbreak. These mosquitoes are fairly common in southern Ontario but not in central or northern Ontario.[15] In 1976, two isolates of SLE virus were obtained from mixed pools of Cx. pipiens-restuans collected from Essex County in southern Ontario.[15a]

CONTROL

Following the 1975 outbreak, many Ontario municipalities, particularly those located within the epidemic zone, established or enlarged larviciding programs. Adulticiding procedures were used in 1975 and 1976 in areas of Ontario where there was evidence of virus activity. Public education campaigns were undertaken and an information pamphlet concerning mosquito control was distributed by the province. Physicians and medical officers were alerted to be vigilant for all possible arboviral infections, and laboratory testing of all suspected SLE patients was stressed.[11] Special encephalitis kits were made available to physicians to use in collecting of specimens.

PUBLIC HEALTH ASPECTS

A sentinel chicken surveillance program was established in Ontario in 1976, using flocks placed in strategic areas of southern Ontario. Mosquito trapping was also undertaken to determine species counts and for virus isolations. This surveillance system has been extended in 1977 to include weekly collections of house sparrows for serological monitoring of SLE viral activity.

REFERENCES

1. **Burton, A. N., McLintock, J., and Francy, D. B.,** Isolation of St. Louis encephalitis and Cache Valley viruses from Saskatchewan mosquitoes, *Can. J. Public Health,* 64, 368, 1973.
2. **Community Health Protection Branch,** in Weekly Bulletin, Epidemiology Service, Ontario Ministry of Health, Toronto, Oct. 8, 1976.
3. **Davidson, W. B., Snell, E., Joshua, J. M., and West, R.,** Human arboviral infection in Canada — 1975, *Can. Dis. Wk. Rep.,* 81, 21, 1976.
3a. **Dorland, R., Mahdy, M. S., Artsob, H., and Prytula, A.,** Wild bird surveillance in the study of arboviral encephalitis, in *Arboviral Encephalitides in Ontario With Special Reference to St. Louis Encephalitis,* Mahdy, M. S., Spence, L., and Joshua, J. M., Eds., Ontario Ministry of Health, 1979, 208.

4. **Hoff, G. L., Yuill, T. M., Iversen, J. O., and Hanson, R. P.**, Selected microbial agents in snowshoe hares and other vertebrates of Alberta, *J. Wildl. Dis.*, 6, 472, 1970.
5. **Karstad, L.**, Surveillance for arbovirus infections in migrating birds at Long Point, Ontario — 1961—62, *Ont. Bird Banding*, 1, 1, 1965.
6. **McLean, D. M., Bergman, S. K. A., Goddard, E. J., Graham, E. A., and Purvin-Good, K. W.**, North-south distribution of arbovirus reservoirs in British Columbia, 1970, *Can. J. Public Health*, 62, 120, 1971.
7. **McLean, D. M., Chernesky, M. A., Chernesky, S. J., Goddard, E. J., Ladyman, S. R., Peers, R. R., and Purvin-Good, K. W.**, Arbovirus prevalence in the East Kootenay region, 1968, *Can. Med. Assoc. J.*, 100, 320, 1969.
8. **McLean, D. M., Crawford, M. A., Ladyman, S. R., Peers, R. R., and Purvin-Good, K. W.**, California encephalitis and Powassan virus activity in British Columbia, 1969, *Am. J. Epidemiol.*, 92, 266, 1970.
9. **McLean, D. M., Ladyman, S. R., and Purvin-Good, K. W.**, Westward extension of Powassan virus prevalence, *Can. Med. Assoc. J.*, 98, 946, 1968.
10. **McLintock, J.**, The arbovirus problem in Canada, *Can. J. Public Health*, 67, (Suppl. 1), 8, 1976.
11. **Rhodes, A. J., Smith, H. B., and Spence, L.**, Laboratory tests in diagnosis of St. Louis encephalitis, *Ont. Med. Rev.*, 43, 229, 1976.
12. **Sekla, L. H. and Stackiw, W.**, Laboratory diagnosis of western encephalomyelitis, *Can. J. Public Health*, 67(Suppl. 1), 33, 1976.
13. **Spalatin, J., Connell, R., Burton, A. N. and Gallop, B. J.**, Western equine encephalitis in Saskatchewan reptiles and amphibians, 1961—1963, *Can. J. Comp. Med.*, 28, 131, 1964.
14. **Spence, L., Artsob, H., Grant, L., and Th'ng, C.**, St. Louis encephalitis in southern Ontario: laboratory studies for arboviruses, *Can. Med. Assoc. J.*, 116, 35, 1977.
15. **Steward, C. C. and McWade, J. W.**, The mosquitoes of Ontario (Diptera: Culicidae) with keys to the species and notes on distribution, *Proc. Entomol. Soc. Ont.*, 91, 121, 1960.
15a. **Thorsen, J., Artsob, H., Surgeoner, G., Helson, B., Spence, L., and Wright, P.**, Virus isolations from mosquitoes in southern Ontario in 1976 and 1977, in *Arboviral Encephalitides in Ontario with Special Reference to St. Louis Encephalitis*, Mahdy, M. S., Spence, L., and Joshua, J. M., Eds., Ontario Ministry of Health, Toronto, 1979, 199.
16. **Trainer, D. O. and Hoff, G. L.**, Serological evidence of arbovirus activity in a moose population in Alberta, *J. Wildl. Dis.*, 7, 118, 1971.
17. **Waters, J. R.**, Encephalitis surveillance — Manitoba, 1977, *Can. Dis. Wk. Rep.*, Health and Welfare Canada, 81, 2, 1978.
18. **Wright, R. E. and Artsob, H.**, National Arbovirus Reference Service, Toronto, unpublished data, 1976.

CALIFORNIA ENCEPHALITIS (CE)

H. Artsob

NAME AND SYNONYMS

California encephalitis is the group name under which the disease is reported. Locally the several viruses of the group are used to identify infections.

HISTORY

The first Canadian isolation of a member of the California group of arboviruses was made in 1963 when snowshoe hare virus was isolated from indicator rabbits placed at Richmond, Ontario.[12] A second member of the California encephalitis group, Jamestown Canyon virus, was subsequently isolated from mosquitoes in pools collected in Alberta in 1964 and 1965.[7] In addition, the trivittatus serotype was isolated from mosquitoes collected in southern Ontario in 1976.[30a]

ETIOLOGY

Classification

The California encephalitis virus group belongs to the *Bunyavirus* genus of the family Bunyaviridae.[4]

DEFINITION

The California encephalitis group of viruses is maintained in nature by an amplification cycle involving small vertebrates and woodland *Aedes spp.* mosquitoes. No specific disease has been recognized in animal hosts with any of the viruses in the group, although increased mortality associated with infection has been suggested.[34] Human infections by snowshoe hare and Jamestown Canyon viruses have been recognized only by serological surveys.

ANIMAL INFECTION

No clinical infections of mammals due to California encephalitis viruses have been recognized in Canada. However, Yuill, et al., in studies on population dynamics and antibody rates to California encephalitis virus in snowshoe hares, *Lepus americanus* in Alberta from 1961 to 1967, provided evidence that mortality was higher among hares with California encephalitis antibodies than those without.[34]

HUMAN INFECTION

The first clinical cases of disease due to California group encephalitis viruses to be diagnosed in Canada were encountered in 1978 when three cases of encephalitis were detected in boys from Quebec,[3a] and one case was diagnosed in an adult male suffering from aseptic meningitis in Ontario.[1a] In all instances, snowshoe hare virus appeared to be the infecting serotype. Antibodies to California encephalitis virus have been detected in human sera in Quebec,[1] Ontario,[13,29,30] Manitoba,[13] Alberta,[6,8] and British Columbia.[10,11]

EPIDEMIOLOGY

Occurrence

California encephalitis virus has been isolated in Quebec,[32] Ontario,[1b,12] Manitoba,[31a] Saskatchewan,[9,26] Alberta,[5,7,27] and British Columbia,[14] as well as in the Yukon,[6,22,23] and Northwest Territories.[31] In addition, neutralizing antibodies to California encephalitis virus have been detected in Nova Scotia.[3]

Most isolations made in Canada have been of the snowshoe hare subtype. However, isolations of Jamestown Canyon virus have been made in Saskatchewan[9] and Alberta.[5,7] Type identification is still pending on the California group isolates from Quebec province.[32]

Reservoir

The primary reservoir for California encephalitis virus in Canada appears to be the snowshoe hare, *L. americanus*. Snowshoe hare virus has been isolated from the blood of a young hare in Alberta,[5] and high antibody rates have been found in hares caught in Nova Scotia,[3] Quebec,[2] Ontario,[19,21,25,28,29] Alberta,[5,6,33,34] British Columbia,[15,24,28] and the Yukon.[16-18,22] Squirrels also appear to be important reservoirs for California encephalitis viruses in Canada. Neutralizing antibodies have been detected in ground squirrels, *Citellus undulatus*[16-18,22] and *C. franklinii*,[6] and in the red squirrel, *Tamiasciurus hudsonicus*.[6,15-18,24] McLean, et al.[16] presented evidence to suggest that in the summer of 1974 *C. undulatus* was the main natural reservoir for California encephalitis virus in the Yukon in the virtual absence of snowshoe hares. Neutralizing antibodies have been detected in other mammals in Canada including marmots (*Marmota monax*[29] and *M. flaviventris*,[15,20,24] porcupines,[6,29] raccoons,[29] chipmunks,[20] lynx,[6] coyotes,[6] cattle,[6] and moose.[6]

Transmission

Virus isolations in eastern Canada have included two isolates of California encephalitis group viruses from *Aedes communis* mosquitoes in Quebec,[32] and isolates of snowshoe hare virus from *Ae. fitchii* and *Ae. triseriatus, Ae. dorsalis,* and *Culex* spp mosquitoes in Ontario.[1b,30a] In addition, trivittatus virus has been isolated from Ae. trivittatus taken in Essex County of southern Ontario.[30a] Isolations of snowshoe hare and Jamestown Canyon viruses have been made from *Ae. fitchii* gr., *Ae. punctor* gr., *Ae. cataphylla,* and *Ae. excrucians* mosquitoes collected in north-central Saskatchewan,[9] Snowshoe hare virus has also been isolated from *Ae. implicatus* mosquitoes collected near Macdowall, Saskatchewan.[26] In Alberta, snowshoe hare virus has been isolated from *Culiseta inornata,*[27] *Ae. communis* gr.,[5,7] and *Ae. stimulans* gr.[5,7] mosquitoes, while Jamestown Canyon virus has been obtained from *Ae. communis gr.,*[5,7] and from *Aedes* spp. gr.[5,7] mosquitoes. Snowshoe hare virus isolations have been made in British Columbia from a mixed pool of *Ae. vexans* and *Ae. canadensis*[14] mosquitoes, in the Northwest Territories from *Ae. hexodontus-punctor* gr.[31] mosquitoes, in the Yukon from *Ae. canadensis*[16,17,22] *Ae. cinereus*[16,17] and *Cu. inornata*[16,17] mosquitoes, and in Manitoba from *Ae. communis.*[31a] The snowshoe hare subtype has also been isolated from *Aedes* spp. larvae and pupae collected in the Yukon in 1974[16] and from *Aedes* spp. larvae collected in the Yukon in 1975,[23] as well as from *Ae. implicatus* reared from larvae collected in Saskatchewan,[26] strongly suggesting the possibility of virus overwintering by transovarial transfer.

CONTROL

No specific mosquito control measures had been undertaken in Canadaprior to 1978.

PUBLIC HEALTH ASPECTS

No public health implications of California group infections had been documented in Canada prior to 1978.

REFERENCES

1. **Artsob, H., Spence, L., Th'ng, C., and West, R.,** Serological Survey for human arbovirus infections in the province of Quebec, *Can. J. Public Health,* (Abstr.), 69, 75, 1978.
1a. **Artsob, H. and Spence, L.,** Human arboviral infections in Canada, 1976—1979, *Can. Dis. Wk. Rep.,* 5, 2, 1980.
1b. **Artsob, H., Wright, R., Shipp, L., Spence, L., and Th'ng, C.,** California encephalitis virus activity in mosquitoes and horses in southern Ontario, 1975, *Can. J. Microbiol.,* 24, 1544, 1978.
2. **Belloncik, S., Artsob, H., Trudel, C., and Spence, L.,** unpublished data, 1975.

3. Embree, J. E., Rozee, K. R., and Embil, J. A., Antibodies to California encephalitis and Powassan viruses in the snowshoe hare *(Lepus americanus)* population of Nova Scotia, 44th Annu. Mtg. Canadian Public Health Assoc., Montreal, Abstr., Dec. 1—3, 1976.

3a. Fauvel, M., Artsob, H., Calisher, C. H., Davignon, L., Chagnon, A., Skvorc-Ranko, R., and Belloncik, S., California group virus encephalitis in three children from Quebec: clinical findings and serodiagnosis, *Can. Med. Assoc. J.,* 122, 60, 1980.

4. Fenner, F., The classification and nomenclature of viruses, *Intervirology,* 6, 1, 1975—76.

5. Hoff, G. L., Yuill, T. M., Iversen, J. O., and Hanson, R. P., Snowshoe hares and the California encephalitis virus group in Alberta, 1961—1968, *Bull. Wildl. Dis. Assoc.,* 5, 254, 1969.

6. Hoff, G. L., Yuill, T. M., Iversen, J. O., and Hanson, R. P., Selected microbial agents in snowshoe hares and other vertebrates of Alberta, *J. Wildl. Dis.,* 6, 472, 1970.

7. Iversen, J., Hanson, R. P., Papadopoulos, O., Morris, C. V., and DeFoliart, G. R., Isolation of viruses of the California encephalitis virus group from boreal Aedes mosquitoes, *Am. J. Trop. Med. Hyg.,* 18, 735, 1969.

8. Iversen, J. O., Seawright, G., and Hanson, R. P., Serologic survey for arboviruses in central Alberta, *Can. J. Public Health,* 62, 125, 1971.

9. Iversen, J. O., Wagner, R. J., deJong, C., and McLintock, J., California encephalitis virus in Saskatchewan: isolation from boreal Aedes mosquitoes, *Can. J. Public Health,* 64, 590, 1973.

10. Kettyls, G. D., Verrall, V. M., Hopper, J. M. H., Kokan, P., and Schmitt, N., Serological survey of human arbovirus infections in southeastern British Columbia, *Can. Med. Assoc. J.,* 99, 600, 1968.

11. Kettyls, G. D., Verrall, V. M., Wilton, L. D., Clapp, J. B. Clarke, D. A., and Rublee, J. D., Arbovirus infections in man in British Columbia, *Can. Med. Assoc. J.,* 106, 1175, 1972.

12. McKiel, J. A., Hall, R. R., and Newhouse, V. F., Viruses of the California encephalitis complex in indicator rabbits, *Am. J. Trop. Med. Hyg.,* 15, 98, 1966.

13. McKiel, J. A., Hall, R. R., Valentine, G. H., and Tusz, L. J., Incidence of human infection with California encephalitis virus in Ontario and Manitoba, 20th. Annu. Mtg. Canadian Society of Microbiologists, Abstr., Halifax, June 2—4, 1970.

14. McLean, D. M., California encephalitis virus isolations from British Columbia mosquitoes, *Mosq. News,* 30, 144, 1970.

15. McLean, D. M., Bergman, S. K. A., Goddard, E. J., Graham, E. A., and Purvin-Good, K. W., North-south distribution of arbovirus reservoirs in British Columbia, 1970, *Can. J. Public Health,* 62, 120, 1971.

16. McLean, D. M., Bergman, S. K. A., Gould, A. P., Grass, P. N., Miller, M. A., and Spratt, E. E., California encephalitis virus prevalence throughout the Yukon Territory, 1971—1974, *Am. J. Trop. Med. Hyg.,* 24, 676, 1975.

17. McLean, D. M., Gergman, S. K. A., Graham, E. A., Greenfield, G. P., Olden, J. A., and Patterson, R. D., California encephalitis virus prevalence in Yukon mosquitoes during 1973, *Can. J. Public Health,* 65, 23, 1974.

18. McLean, D. M., Clarke, A. M., Goddard, E. J., Manes, A. S., Montalbetti, C. A., and Pearson, R. E., California encephalitis virus endemicity in the Yukon Territory, 1972, *J. Hyg.,* 71, 391, 1973.

19. McLean, D. M., Cobb, C., Gooderham, S. E., Smart, C. A., Wilson, A. G., and Wilson, W. E., Powassan virus: persistence of virus activity during 1966, *Can. Med. Assoc. J.,* 96, 660, 1967.

20. McLean, D. M., Crawford, M. A., Ladyman, S. R., Peers, R. R., and Purvin-Good, K. W., California encephalitis and Powassan virus activity in British Columbia, 1969, *Am. J. Epidemiol.,* 92, 266, 1970.

21. McLean, D. M., deVos, A., and Quantz, E. J., Powassan virus: field investigations during the summer of 1963, *Am. J. Trop. Med. Hyg.,* 13, 747, 1964.

22. McLean, D. M., Goddard, E. J., Graham, E. A., Hardy, G. J., and Purvin-Good, K. W., California encephalitis virus isolations from Yukon mosquitoes, 1971, *Am. J. Epidemiol.,* 95, 347, 1972.

23. McLean, D. M., Grass, P. N., Judd, B. D., Cmiralova, D., and Stuart, K. M., Natural foci of California encephalitis virus activity in the Yukon Territory, *Can. J. Public Health,* 68, 69, 1977.

24. McLean, D. M., Ladyman, S. R., and Purvin-Good, K. W., Westward extension of Powassan virus prevalence, *Can. Med. Assoc. J.,* 98, 946, 1968.

25. McLean, D. M., Smith, P. A., Livingstone, S. E., Wilson, W. E., and Wilson, A. G., Powassan virus: vernal spread during 1965, *Can. Med. Assoc. J.,* 94, 532, 1966.

26. McLintock, J., Curry, P. S., Wagner, R. J., Leung, M. K., and Iversen, J. O., Isolation of snowshoe hare, virus from *Aedes implicatus* larvae in Saskatchewan, *Mosq. News,* 36, 233, 1976.

27. Morgante, O. and Shemanchuk, J. A., Virus of the California encephalitis complex: isolation from *Culiseta inornata, Science,* 157, 692, 1967.

28. Newhouse, V. F., Burgdorfer, W., McKiel, J. A., and Gregson, J. D., California encephalitis virus. Serologic survey of small wild mammals in northern United States and southern Canada and isolation of additional strains, *Am. J. Hyg.,* 78, 123, 1963.

29. **Newhouse, V. F., McKiel, J. A. and Burgdorfer, W.,** California encephalitis, Colorado tick fever and Rocky Mountain spotted fever in eastern Canada, *Can. J. Public Health,* 55, 257, 1964.

30. **Spence, L., Artsob, H., Grant, L., and Th'ng, C.,** St. Louis encephalitis in southern Ontario: laboratory studies for arboviruses, *Can. Med. Assoc. J.,* 116, 35, 1977.

30a. **Thorsen, J., Artsob, H., Surgeoner, G., Helson, B., Spence, L., and Wright, R.,** Virus isolations from mosquitoes in southern Ontario 1976 and 1977, in *Arboviral Encephalitides in Ontario With Special Reference to St. Louis Encephalitis,* Mahdy, M. S., Spena, L., and Joshua, J. M., Eds., Ontario Ministry of Health, 1979.

31. **Wagner, R. J., deJong, C., Leung, M. K., McLintock, J., and Iversen, J. O.,** Isolations of California encephalitis virus from tundra mosquitoes, *Can. J. Microbiol.,* 21, 574, 1975.

31a. **Wagner, R. J., Leung, M. K., McLintock, J. J. R., and Iverson, J. O.,** On the natural occurrence of snowshoe hare virus in Manitoba, *Mosq. News,* 39, 238, 1979.

32. **Woodall, J. P. and Grayson, M. A.,** personal communication, 1977.

33. **Yuill, T. M. and Hanson, R. P.,** Serologic evidence of California encephalitis and western equine encephalitis virus in snowshoe hares, *Zoonoses Res.,* 3, 153, 1964.

34. **Yuill, T. M., Iversen, J. O. and Hanson, P.,** Evidence for arbovirus infections in population of snowshoe hares: a possible mortality factor, *Bull. Wildl. Dis. Assoc.,* 5, 248, 1969.

COLORADO TICK FEVER (CTF)

H. Artsob

NAME AND SYNONYMS

Colorado tick fever is the name of the human disease. Animal infections with CTF virus are considered to be entirely subclinical in nature.

HISTORY

Colorado tick fever was first recognized in Canada in 1952 when virus was isolated from *Dermacentor andersoni* ticks collected in Banff National Park.[2]

ANIMAL INFECTION

In Canada, neutralizing antibodies were detected in five of forty-nine snowshoe hares (*Lepus americanus*) caught near Richmond, Ontario in 1962.[6]

HUMAN INFECTION

No clinical cases of CTF have been diagnosed in Canada. However, complement fixing and neutralizing antibodies have been detected in sera of residents of British Columbia.[4,5]

EPIDEMIOLOGY

Colorado tick fever virus has been isolated from *D. andersoni* ticks collected in Alberta[1,2] and in southeastern British Columbia.[3] In addition, the demonstration of neutralizing antibodies against CTF from British Columbia and Ontario has indicated that the virus is being transmitted over a wider area.

REFERENCES

1. **Brown, J. H.,** Colorado tick fever in Alberta, *Can. J. Zool.,* 33, 389, 1955.
2. **Eklund, C. M., Kohls, G. M., and Brennan, J. M.,** Distribution of Colorado tick fever and virus-carrying ticks, *JAMA,* 157, 335, 1955.
3. **Hall, R. R., McKiel, J. A., and Gregson, J. D.,** Occurrence of Colorado tick fever virus in *Dermacentor andersoni* ticks in British Columbia, *Can. J. Public Health* 59, 273, 1968.
4. **Kettyls, G. D., Verrall, V. M., Hopper, J. M. H., Kokan, P., and Schmitt, N.,** Serological survey of human arbovirus infections in southeastern British Columbia. *Can. Med. Assoc. J.,* 99, 600, 1968.
5. **Kettyls, G. D., Verrall, V. M., Wilton, L. D., Clapp, J. B., Clarke, D. A., and Rublee, J. D.,** Arbovirus infections in man in British Columbia, *Can. Med. Assoc. J.,* 106, 1175, 1972.
6. **Newhouse, V. F., McKiel, J. A., and Burgdorfer, W.,** California encephalitis, Colorado tick fever and Rocky Mountain spotted fever in eastern Canada. Serological evidence, *Can. J. Public Health,* 55, 257, 1964.

VESICULAR STOMATITIS (VS)

H. Artsob

NAME AND SYNONYMS

Vesicular stomatitis is the name of the infection for both animals and people.

HISTORY

Mohler[2] in 1904 in the U.S., described a disease strongly resembling VS which was recognized as occurring at irregular intervals in both the U.S. and Canada. It is likely that the disease was scattered throughout North America in the nineteenth century.

ANIMAL INFECTION

Outbreaks of VS were observed in cattle and horses in Manitoba in 1937 and 1949.[1] It was estimated that 500 horses and cattle were affected during the 1949 outbreak.

HUMAN INFECTION

No human cases of VS have been diagnosed in Canada.

EPIDEMIOLOGY

VS outbreaks in cattle and horses in 1937 and 1947 in Manitoba during late summer 1937 and 1949 resulted from the northward movement of the virus from Minnesota and Wisconsin where VS outbreaks were widespread earlier in those years.[1] Both outbreaks were confined primarily to wooded areas east of the Red River and along Lake Manitoba and Lake Winnipeg, and did not spread to livestock on farms on the open plain. It is considered that the New Jersey serotype was involved in the 1949 outbreak.

REFERENCES

1. **Hanson, R. P.,** The natural history of vesicular stomatitis, *Bacteriol. Rev.,* 16, 179, 1952.
2. **Mohler, J. R.,** Mycotic stomatitis of cattle, *U.S. Bur. Animal Ind. Circ.,* 51, 1904.

POWASSAN ENCEPHALITIS

H. Artsob

NAME AND SYNONYMS

Powassan encephalitis is the name applied to the human disease. Clinical disease has not been demonstrated in lower animals infected with Powassan virus in nature.

HISTORY

Powassan virus was first isolated from the brain of a boy who died of acute encephalitis in Powassan, Ontario in 1958.[12] Three additional human cases were serologically diagnosed in Canada in 1975 and 1976.[1,20,21] Powassan virus was recovered from ticks (*Ixodes marxi*) in 1963,[14] and from wild mammals (woodchucks) in 1964.[18] The virus has been recovered from ticks and small wild mammals in the U.S. since 1960.[23]

ETIOLOGY

Classification
Powassan virus is classified in the *Flavivirus* genus of the family Togaviridae.[3]

DEFINITION

Powassan encephalitis is an acute disease of children varying clinically from undifferentiated febrile illness to encephalitis. Human beings are believed to be dead-end hosts. Small wild mammals are believed to serve as reservoir hosts, with transmission by Ixodid ticks.

ANIMAL INFECTION

Animal infections in nature have not been associated with clinical disease, but fatal encephalitis has been produced experimentally in suckling and weanling laboratory mice. Virus isolations have been made from woodchucks (*Marmota monax*), red squirrels (*Tamias-ciuriss hudsonicus*), deer mice (*Peromuscus spp.*), foxes (*Vulpes fulva*), and spotted skunks (*Spilogale putorius*).[8,10,13,14,17,22] With the exception of skunks which have not been surveyed, all of these mammals plus *M. flaviventris* woodchucks, *T. hudsonicus* red squirrels, meadow mice (*Microtus* sp.), chipmunks (*Eutamicus* sp.), and raccoons (*Procyon loton*), have shown neutralizing antibodies in 13 to 89% of the animals sampled.[9,11,13,17,22]

HUMAN INFECTION

Six human cases of Powassan infection have been diagnosed in Canada, with two from Quebec and four from Ontario. The first recorded case was in a five-year-old boy from Powassan, Ontario, who developed acute encephalitis and died.[12] At necropsy, typical perivascular cuffing was observed in the brain, and virus was recovered from brain tissue. A second, and also severe, case of encephalitis occurred in 1972 in an eight-year-old boy.[21] The patient survived, but suffered moderate sequelae. In 1975, a case of Powassan encephalitis was diagnosed in a three and a half year-old boy from western Quebec[1] with encephalitis and symptoms of upper cervical cord lesions resulting in involvement of the shoulder girdle muscles. Some residual sequelae were observed. A fourth case of Powassan infection was diagnosed in a 15-year-old girl in Ontario in 1976.[20] Symptoms were mild and no sequelae were observed. Two additional Powassan cases have been reported. In 1977, a 14-month-old girl near Kingston, Ontario suffered meningoencephalitis due to Powassan virus,[24] and in 1979 an 18-year-old girl experienced a severe case of Powassan encephalitis following a visit to a cottage near Lower Buckhorn Lake in Ontario.[5a]

EPIDEMIOLOGY

Occurrence

Powassan virus has been isolated in Ontario from human brain,[12] ticks,[8,14,17] red squirrel,[14] woodchuck,[18] porcupine,[18] and groundhog blood.[8] In addition, serological evidence has been found of natural occurrence of Powassan virus in woodchucks, porcupines, groundhogs, red squirrels, chipmunks, and snowshoe hares in British Columbia[7,9,11,12] in Canada. In the U.S., virus has been isolated from ticks, woodchucks, and foxes in New York; ticks and deer mice in South Dakota; ticks in Colorado; and spotted skunk in California.[19a,22,23] Serological evidence of infection has been obtained in foxes and raccoons in New York and deer mice, meadow mice, and chipmunks in South Dakota.[22]

Reservoir

Neutralizing antibodies to Powassan virus have been found in numerous small mammals. Powassan virus has been isolated from *I. marxi* ticks collected from one red squirrel, *T. hudsonicus,* and from the blood of another squirrel.[14] Isolations of Powassan virus, as well as high antibody prevalence in squirrels and ground hogs in the North Bay-Powassan region of Ontario, have led to the consideration of these animals as important reservoirs in the maintenance cycle of Powassan virus.[8,10,14,17]

Transmission

Ixodid ticks are believed to be the natural vectors of Powassan virus. Isolations have been obtained from *I. marxi* and *I. cookei*[8,10,17] ticks. *I. cookei* ticks are also found in southern Ontario[6] and in the eastern townships of Quebec where they may have been associated with one human case.[4,21] In the U.S., Powassan virus has been recovered from *I. cookei* ticks in New York, *I. spinipalpus* ticks in South Dakota, and *Dermacentor andersoni* ticks in South Dakota and Colorado.[23]

CONTROL

No vaccine is available, and no specific tick control measures have been undertaken as yet.

REFERENCES

1. **Conway, D., Rossier, E., Spence, L., and Artsob, H.,** Powassan virus encephalitis with shoulder girdle involvement, *Can. Dis. Wk. Rep.,* 85, 2, 1976.
2. **Embree, J. E., Rozee, K. R., and Embil, J. A.,** Antibodies to California encephalitis and Powassan viruses in the snowshoe hare (*Lepus americanus*) population of Nova Scotia, in 44th Annu. Mtg. Canadian Public Health Association, Abstr. Montreal, Dec. 1—3, 1976.
3. **Fenner, F.,** The classification and nomenclature of viruses, *Intervirology,* 6, 1, 1975/76.
4. **Harrison, R. J., Rossier, E., and Lemieux, B.,** Prémier cas d'encephalomyelite de Powassan au Quebec, *Ann. Soc. Entomol. Que.,* 20, 48, 1975.

5. **Hoff, G. L., Yuill, T. M., Iversen, J. O., and Hanson, R. P.,** Selected microbial agents in snowshoe hares and other vertebrates of Alberta, *J. Wildl. Dis.*, 6, 472, 1970.

5a. **Joshua, J. M., Crapper, D. R., Spence, L., Artsob, H., and Surgeoner, G. A.,** A case of Powassan encephalitis—Ontario, *Can. Dis. Wk. Rep.*, 129, 5, 1979.

6. **Ko, R. C.,** Biology of *Ixodes cookei* Packard (Ixodidae) of groundhogs (*Marmota monax* Erxleben), *Can. J. Zool.*, 50, 433, 1972.

7. **McLean, D. M., Bergman, S. K. A., Goddard, E. J., Graham, E. A., and Purvin-Good, K. W.,** North-south distribution of arbovirus reservoirs in British Columbia, 1970, *Can. J. Public Health*, 62, 120, 1971.

8. **McLean, D. M., Best, J. M., Mahalingam, S., Chernesky, M., and Wilson, W. E.,** Powassan virus: summer infection cycle, 1964, *Can. Med. Assoc. J.*, 91, 1360, 1964.

9. **McLean, D. M., Chernesky, M. A., Chernesky, S. J., Goddard, E. J., Ladyman, S. R., Peers, R. R., and Purvin-Good, K. W.,** Arbovirus prevalence in the East Kootenay region, 1968, *Can. Med. Assoc. J.*, 100, 320, 1969.

10. **McLean, D. M., Cobb, C., Gooderham, S. E., Smart, C. A., Wilson, A. G., and Wilson, W. E.,** Powassan virus: persistence of virus activity during 1966, *Can. Med. Assoc. J.*, 96, 660, 1967.

11. **McLean, D. M., Crawford, M. A., Ladyman, S. R., Peers, R. R., and Purvin-Good, K. W.,** California encephalitis and Powassan virus activity in British Columbia, 1969, *Am. J. Epidemiol.*, 92, 266, 1970.

12. **McLean, D. M. and Donohue, W. L.,** Powassan virus: isolation of virus from a fatal case of encephalitis, *Can. Med. Assoc. J.*, 80, 708, 1959.

13. **Mclean, D. M., Ladyman, S. R., and Purvin-Good, K. W.,** Westward extension of Powassan virus prevalence, *Can. Med. Assoc. J.*, 98, 946, 1968.

14. **McLean, D. M. and Bryce Larke, R. P.,** Powassan and Silverwater viruses: ecology of two Ontario arboviruses, *Can. Med. Assoc. J.*, 88, 182, 1963.

15. **McLean, D. M., MacPherson, L. W., Walker, S. J., and Funk, G.,** Powassan virus: surveys of human and animal sera, *Am. J. Public Health*, 50, 1539, 1960.

16. **McLean, D. M., McQueen, E. J., Petite, H. E., MacPherson, L. W., Scholten, T. H., and Ronald, K.,** Powassan virus: field investigations in northern Ontario, 1959 to 1961, *Can. Med. Assoc. J.*, 86, 971, 1962.

17. **McLean, D. M., Smith, P. A., Livingstone, S. E., Wilson, W. E., and Wilson, A. G.,** Powassan virus: vernal spread during 1965, *Can. Med. Assoc. J.*, 94, 532, 1966.

18. **McLean, D. M., Vos, A., and Quantz, E. J.,** Powassan virus: field investigations during the summer of 1963, *Am. J. Trop. Med. Hyg.*, 13, 747, 1964.

19. **McLean, D. M., Walker, S. J., MacPherson, L. W., Scholten, T. H., Ronald, K., Wyllie, J. C., and McQueen, E. J.,** Powassan virus: investigations of possible natural cycles of infection, *J. Infect. Dis.*, 109, 19, 1961.

19a. **Main, A. J., Carey, A. B., and Downs, W. G.,** Powassan virus in *Ixodes cookei* and Mustelidae in New England, *J. Wildlife Dis.*, 15, 585, 1979.

20. **Rossier, E.** Powassan encephalitis — Ontario, *Can. Dis. Wk. Rep.*, 202, 2, 1976.

21. **Rossier, E., Harrison, R. J., and Lemieux, B.,** A case of Powassan encephalitis, *Can. Med. Assoc. J.*, 110, 1173, 1974.

22. **Whitney, E.,** Serological evidence of group A and B arthropod-borne virus activity in New York State, *Am. J. Trop. Med. Hyg.*, 12, 417, 1963.

23. **Whitney, E. and Jamnback, H.,** The isolation of Powassan virus in New York State, *Proc. Soc. Exp. Biol. Med.*, 119, 432, 1965.

24. **Wilson, M. S., Wherrett, B. A., and Mahdy, M. S.,** Powassan virus meningoencephalitis: a case report, *Can. Med. Assoc. J.*, 121, 320, 1979.

ARBOVIRAL ZOONOSES IN SOUTH AMERICA

MAYARO FEVER

F. P. Pinheiro

NAME AND SYNONYMS

Mayaro virus is the causative agent for the febrile illness in human beings known as "Mayaro fever". There are no other known names for this illness.

HISTORY

The first isolations of the Mayaro Fever (MAY) virus were made from the blood of five febrile patients in Trinidad in 1954.[1] In the following year, an outbreak of Mayaro fever was recognized in a rural community 120 miles east of Belém, Brazil.[8] Uruma virus, which was isolated from sick persons during an outbreak of fever that occurred in Bolivia in 1954 to 1955,[31] is now considered as a strain of Mayaro virus. The agent has also been recovered from human patients in Surinam.[23] Serological surveys have indicated the occurrence of human infections of Mayaro fever in Guyana,[12,33] Colombia,[14] Peru,[22] Panama,[34] and Costa Rica.[13] In addition, the virus has been isolated from mosquitoes in Trinidad, Colombia, and Brazil,[2,16a,17,35] from lizards and a marmoset in Brazil[16a,35] and from a wild bird in southern U.S.[6]

ETIOLOGY

Mayaro virus belongs to the genus *Alphavirus* of the family Togaviridae. The virions are spherical enveloped particles, have cubic symmetry and 32 capsomeres 2 to 4 nm in diameter. The size of the Mayaro virions as estimated by electron microscopy is 40 ± nm.[30] Serologically the agent is a member of the group A arboviruses, antigenically closely related to Semliki Forest virus.[7] These two agents show some crossreaction by the hemagglutination inhibition (HI) and complement-fixation (CF) tests, but they can be readily separated by these methods.[7] They are closely related by the mouse intraperitoneal neutralization (N) test;[7] however, they are quite distinct by the plaque-inhibition and plaque reduction neutralization tests.[20,28] The virus contains a hemagglutinin which can be extracted from brains of inoculated infant mice by sucrose-acetone. With certain strains, the hemagglutinin may be demonstrated in suckling mouse serum, but not in suckling mouse brains. The hemagglutinin is active against chicken and goose erythrocytes at a pH range of 6.0 to 6.8, with an optimal pH of 6.2 to 6.4 at +4°C. A low titering hemagglutinin can also be obtained from infected hamster kidney cell cultures.[11]

Mayaro virus will replicate and produce cytopathic effect and plaques in BHK-21, Vero, and HeLa cell lines, in primary cultures of Pekin duck or rhesus monkey kidney cells, and in chicken or mouse embryo fibroblasts.[5,16,25] Two Brazilian strains of Mayaro virus produce small and large plaques, respectively, in overlaid cultures of chicken embryo cells. Although antigenically similar, the large plaque variant causes more intense lesions in the connective tissue of infant mice. Only the small variant can produce cytopathic effects in chick embryo cultures maintained under fluid medium.[26]

DEFINITION

Mayaro fever is an acute, benign, nonfatal febrile human illness caused by an arthropod-borne virus which lends its name to the disease.

ANIMAL INFECTION

Clinical

No disease has been reported in naturally infected animals. Infant, but usually not adult, mice succumb within 2 to 4 days when inoculated intracerebrally or intraperitoneally with the virus, although a few strains cause death of adult mice when injected intracerebrally.[2] The Uruma strain is also pathogenic to newborn hamsters and to embryonating hens' eggs.[31] An experimental *Cebus* monkey inoculated subcutaneously with Mayaro virus had viremia for at least 3 days, leukopenia, and developed neutralizing antibodies in high titer.[9] The marmoset *Callithrix argentata* also becomes viremic when experimentally infected with the virus.[16a]

Pathology

In experimentally infected mice, Mayaro virus produces an encephalitis with lytic necrosis of the neurons, but with no cell infiltrates or any peculiar distribution in the brain. In addition, the agent damages the connective tissue of the animals, especially periosteal, perichondrial, subcutaneous, pulmonary, and cardiac interstitial tissues. The dental pulp is moderately damaged. The lesions consist of necrotic foci of the connective cells with residual chromatin fragments.[10,35]

Diagnosis

The diagnosis depends on the isolation and identification of the virus, or, retrospectively, on serological findings. Whole blood, serum, plasma, or visceral organs from suspected patients are inoculated into infant mice or suitable cell cultures. Virus identification can be confirmed by the CF or HI tests, using the brains or serum of sick mice inoculated with the suspect tissue as a source of antigen and specific antiserum or mouse immune ascitic fluid. The HI or N test can also be used, especially when the agent is isolated in cell cultures. Mosquitoes to be assayed for virus using pools of 50 or fewer insects of the same species may be triturated, suspended in phosphate buffered saline containing 0.75% bovine albumin, and processed as above. Specimens which cannot be inoculated on day of collection should be kept in liquid nitrogen or in electrical freezers at $-60°$C or less.

HUMAN INFECTION

Clinical

Until recently, descriptions of Mayaro disease in man were based on the observation of some 12 patients from Trinidad, Brazil, and Bolivia.[1,8,31] According to these reports, the disease was a febrile illness accompanied by headache, epigastric pain, backache, pains all over the body, chills, nausea, and photophobia in most patients. In some of the Brazilian cases light icterus was noted.[8] In one patient from Trinidad, a swollen finger was noted, and rash was observed in the single case in Bolivia from whom Mayaro virus was isolated. During the 1978 outbreak of Mayaro virus disease in Belterra, Brazil, fever, arthralgia and exanthema were commonly observed among 43 laboratory-proven cases of Mayaro.[27a] Over 70% of the patients reported headache, myalgias, and chills. Dizziness, eye pain, nausea, vomiting, and photophobia were referred to less frequently. The fever may reach 40°C and the headache is severe. Arthralgia was present in all cases and affected predominantly the wrists, fingers, ankles and toes. Swelling of the affected joints was present in about 20% of the cases. Inguinal lymphadenopathy was observed in half of the patients. Rash consisted of either maculopapular or micropapular, isolated lesions which sometimes formed small areas of confluence. Rash was more prominent on the chest, back, arms, and legs with the face and hands less affected. Occasionally, the rash was generalized. Rash usually appeared on the fifth day of illness and lasted about 3 days. Clinical manifestations persisted from 2 to 5 days, which the exception of the arthralgia, which lasted in some patients for 2 months, and caused a temporary incapacity for work in some persons. Hepatomegaly or splenomegaly was not found. Although no deaths have been recorded, some cases required hospitalization. Leukopenia was a common finding within the first week of illness and white cell counts as low 2500/mm^3 were observed. White cell counts reach normal values after the second week postonset. Moderate lymphocytosis is the only abnormality observed in the differential counts. The platelet counts may be slightly decreased in some cases. No changes are seen in levels of serum bilirrubin and glutamic-pyruvic transaminase, but a moderate increase in the level of serum glutamic-oxaloacetic transaminase may occur, usually less than 100 units per 100 mℓ of serum.

Pathology

No lesions have been described in human patients.

Diagnosis

The diagnosis depends either on isolation and identification of the virus or on the demonstration of a rise in the antibody titer during the course of the disease. Virus isolations may be performed in suckling mice or appropriate cell cultures. For serological tests, paired serum samples should be obtained from patients, one during the acute phase of the illness and the other 2 or 3 weeks later. The HI, N, and CF tests are all applicable for detection of antibodies. The techniques for performing the tests and interpretation of results can be found elsewhere.[15]

EPIDEMIOLOGY

Serological Evidence

Mayaro virus infections are widespread among forest dwellers of certain tropical areas of the Americas. Not only has the virus been isolated from a number of patients in Brazil, Trinidad, Bolivia, and Surinam, but a high antibody prevalence rate has been found among certain populations of these countries, as well as in Guyana, Colombia, Peru, and Panama.[12,14,22,33,34] In a study in 1953, 9.6% of 551 adult residents of 17 localities in the Amazon basin of Brazil had neutralizing antibodies against Semliki Forest virus, probably representing actual Mayaro infections.[35] Recent serological surveys in the same region using HI tests indicated an antibody prevalence up to 60%. From 20 to 47% of Brazilian Indians in the Amazon basin appear to be immune to the agent. In a study of military recruits in central-western Brazil, 6% had HI antibodies to the agent in 1965.[24] Infections caused by Mayaro virus have been detected among Dutch military personnel stationed in Surinam.[18,21] So far, three large epidemics have been described, two in Brazil and one in Bolivia[8,21a,27a,31] among persons with close contact with the forest. Both Brazilian epidemics took place in the Amazon region. The first one was in a small settlement of the Guamà River, in 1955, during which about 50 persons were infected.[8] In the other one, which occurred in Belterra in 1978, some 800 persons of a population of 4000 were affected by the virus.[21a] The clinically apparent attack rate for Mayaro virus infection in Belterra was estimated to be 80% or greater.[21a] In Bolivia the agent was responsible for 10 to 15% of some 200 cases of jungle fever among Okinawan settlers in 1954—1955. None of the 15 deaths that occurred during the epidemic could be attributed to Mayaro virus.[31]

Mayaro virus seems to be maintained in nature in a cycle involving mammals, birds, and arthropods. Monkeys and marmosets have been implicated as natural reservoirs, since they have high prevalence of antibodies against Mayaro virus both in the Amazon region of Brazil and in Trinidad.[1,16a,27,35] Low prevalence of antibodies are found in most wild bird populations of the Amazon forest, except in *Columbigallina* spp. which show a high HI antibody rate. HI antibodies have also been found in wild rodents and marsupials, although no neutralization test surveys have been performed in these animals to confirm the specificity of the immunity.[35] The only isolations of Mayaro virus obtained from wild animals have been from two lizards and a marmoset in Brazil[16a,35] and from a wild bird captured in southern U.S.[6]

Aedes scapularis, Ae. serratus, Culex quinquefasciatus, Mansonia arribalzagai, Coquillettidia venezeulensis, M. wilsoni, and *Psorophora ferox* harbor the virus for about 12 days when inoculated parenterally, but only *Ae. scapularis* transmitted the agent to a chick by bite.[1a,1b]

The agent has been recovered many times from *Haemagogus* spp. mosquitoes,[16a,17,35] and one or more species are considered to be the vectors of the virus. A single strain of Mayaro virus has been obtained from *Coquillettidia venezuelensis* in Trinidad,[2] two strains have been isolated from *Sabethes* spp. and one each from *Culex* spp. and from *Gigantolaelaps* spp. in Brazil.[17,35]

Thus it seems that several wild animals may serve as vertebrate hosts for the agent and that numerous arthropods are involved in its transmission. The bulk of the evidence, however, supports the existence of monkey *Haemagogus* monkey transmission as the reservoir cycle.

CONTROL

There is no specific treatment for Mayaro fever. An experimental vaccine prepared by formalin inactivation of virus propagated in WI-38 human diploid cells has produced a satisfactory antibody response in weanling mice.[29]

PUBLIC HEALTH ASPECTS

Since Mayaro fever has affected mainly forest laborers, it can be considered as an occupational disease. Although the infection is endemic in some areas of the tropical Americas, it has caused no serious impact on human health.

No special surveillance regulations have been devised for Mayaro fever.

REFERENCES

1. **Anderson, C. R., Downs, W. G., Wattley, G. H., Ahin, N. W., and Reese, A. A.,** Mayaro virus: a new human disease agent. II. Isolation from blood of patients in Trinidad, B. W. I., *Am. J. Trop. Med. Hyg.,* 6, 1012, 1957.

1a. **Aitken, T. H. G.,** Virus transmission studies with Trinidadian mosquitoes, *West Indian Med. J.,* 6, 229, 1957.

1b. **Aitken, T. H. G., and Anderson, C. R.,** Virus transmission studies with Trinidadian mosquitoes. II. Further observations, *Am. J. Trop. Med. Hyg.,* 8, 41, 1959.

2. **Aitken, T. H. G., Downs, W. G., Anderson, C. R., and Spence, L.,** Mayaro virus isolated from a Trinidadian mosquito, *Mansonia venezuelensis, Science,* 131, 986, 1960.

3. **Bergold, G.H. and Mazzali, R.,** Plaque formation by arboviruses, *J. Gen. Virol.,* 2, 273, 1968.

4. Black, F. L., Hierholzer, W. J., Pinheiro, F. P., Evans, A. S., Woodall, J. P., Opton, E. M., Emmons, J. E., West, B. S., Edsall, G., Downs, W. G., and Wallace, G. D., Evidence for peristence of infectious agents in isolated human populations, *Am. J. Epidemiol.,* 100, 230, 1974.

5. Buckley, S. M., Applicability of the HeLa (Gey) strain of human malignant epithelial cells to the propagation of arboviruses, *Proc. Soc. Exp. Biol. Med.,* 116, 354, 1964.

6. Calisher, C.H., Gutiérrez, E., Maness, K. S. C., and Lord, R. D., Isolation of Mayaro virus from a migrating bird captured in Louisiana in 1967, *Bol. Of. Sanit. Panam.,* 8, 243, 1974.

7. Casals, J. and Whitman, L., Mayaro virus: a new human disease agent. I. Relationship to other arboviruses, *Am. J. Trop. Med. Hyg.,* 6, 1004, 1957.

8. Causey, O. R. and Maroja, O. M., Mayaro virus: a new human disease agent. III. Investigation of an epidemic of acute febrile illness on the River Guamá in Pará, Brazil, and isolation of Mayaro virus as causative agent, *Am. J. Trop. Med. Hyg.,* 6, 1017, 1957.

9. Causey, O. R., cited by Woodall, J. P., Virus Research in Amazônia, in *Atas Simpósio Biota Amazônica,* Vol. 6, Lent, H., Ed., Conselho Nacional de Pesquisas, Rio de Janiero, 1967, 31.

10. Dias, L. B., personal communication, 1977.

11. Diercks, F. H., Kundin, W.D., and Porter, T.J., Arthropod-borne virus hemagglutinin production by infected hamster kidney-cell cultures, *Am. J. Hyg.,* 73, 164, 1961.

12. Downs, W. G. and Anderson, C. R., Distribution of immunity to Mayaro virus infection in the West Indies, *West Ind. Med. J.,* 7, 190, 1958.

13. Fuentes, L. G. and Mora, J. A., Encuesta serólogica sobre arbovirus en Costa Rica, *Rev. Latinoam. Microbiol.,* 13, 25, 1971.

14. Groot, H., Estudios sobre virus transmitidos por artropodos en Colombia, *Rev. Acad. Colomb. Cienc. Exactas Fis. Nat.,* 12, 197, 1964.

15. Shope, R. E. and Sather, G. E., Arboviruses, in *Diagnostic Procedures for Viral, Rickettsial and Chlamidial Infections,* 5th ed., Lennette, E. H. and Schmidt, N. J., Eds., American Public Health Association, New York, 1979, 767.

16. Henderson, J. R. and Taylor, R. M., Propagation of certain arthropod-borne viruses in avian and primate cell cultures, *J. Immunol.,* 84, 590, 1960.

16a. Hoch, L. A., Peterson, N. E., LeDuc, J. W., Travassos da Rosa, J. F. S., and Travassos da Rosa, A. P. A., An outbreak of Mayaro virus disease in Belterra, Brazil. III. Vectors and vertebrate host studies, *Am. J. Trop. Med. Hyg.,* in press, 1981.

17. Berge, T. O., Ed., *International Catalogue of Arboviruses, including certain other Viruses of Vertebrates,* 2nd ed., Publ. No. (CDC) 75-8301, Public Health Service, U.S. Department of Health, Education and Welfare, Atlanta, 1975, 471.

18. Jonkers, A. H., Spence, L., and Karbaat, J., Arbovirus infections in Dutch military personnel stationed in Surinam. Further studies, *Trop. Geogr. Med.,* 20, 251, 1968.

19. Karabatsos, N. and Buckley, S. M,. Susceptibility of the baby-hamster kidney-cell line (BHK-21) to infection with arboviruses, *Am. J. Trop. Med. Hyg.,* 16, 99, 1967.

20. Karabatsos, N., Antigenic relationship of group A arboviruses by plaque reduction neutralization testing, *Am. J. Trop. Med. Hyg.,* 24, 527, 1975.

21. Karbaat, J., Jonkers, A. H., and Spence, L., Arbovirus infections in Dutch military personnel stationed in Surinam. A preliminary study, *Trop. Geogr. Med.,* 4, 370, 1964.

21a. LeDuc, J. W., Pinheiro, F. P., and Travassos da Rosa, A. P. A., An outbreak of Mayaro virus disease in Belterra, Brazil. II. Epidemiology, *Am. J. Trop. Med. Hyg.,* in press, 1981.

22. Madalengoitia, J., Flores, W., and Casals, J., Arbovirus antibody survey of sera from residents of eastern Peru, *Bull. PAHO,* 7, 25, 1973.

23. Metselaar, D., Isolation of arboviruses of group A and group C in Surinam, *Trop. Geogr. Med.,* 18, 137, 1966.

24. Niederman, J. C., Henderson, J. R., Opton, E. M., Black, F. L., and Skvrnova, K., A nationwide serum survey of Brazilian military recruits, 1964. II. Antibody patterns with arboviruses, polioviruses, measles and mumps, *Am. J. Epidemiol.,* 86, 319, 1967.

25. Pinheiro, F. P., unpublished data, 1968.

26. Pinheiro, F. P. and Dias, L. B., Virus Mayaro e Una: estudo de variantes produzindo grandes a pequenas placas, in *Atas Simposia Biota Amazonica,* Vol. 6, Lent, H., Ed., Conselho National de Pesquisas, Rio de Janiero, 1967, 211..

27. Pinheiro, F. P., Bensabath, G., Andrade, A. H. P., Lins, Z. C., Fraiha, H., Tang, A. T., Lainson, R., Shaw, J. J., and Azevedo, M. C., Infectious diseases along Brazil's trans Amazon highway: surveillance and research, *Bull. PAHO,* 8, 111, 1974.

27a. Pinheiro, F.P., Freitas, R. B., Travassos da Rosa, J. F. S., Gabbay, Y. B., Mello, W. A., LeDuc, J. W., and Oliva, O. F. P., An outbreak of Mayaro virus disease in Belterra, Brazil, I. Clinical and virological findings, *Am. J. Trop. Med. Hyg.,* in press.

28. **Porterfield, J. S.,** Cross-neutralization studies with group A arthropod-borne viruses, *Bull. WHO,* 24, 735, 1961.
29. **Robinson, D. M., Cole, F. E., Jr., McManus, A. T., and Pedersen, C. E., Jr.,** Inactivated Mayaro vaccine produced in human diploid cell cultures, *Mil. Med.,* 141, 163, 1976.
30. **Saturno, A.,** The morphology of Mayaro virus, *Virology,* 21, 131, 1963.
31. **Schaeffer, M., Gajdusek, D. C., Lema, A. B., and Eichenwald, H.,** Epidemic jungle fevers among Okinawan colonists in the Bolivian rain forest. I. Epidemiology, *Am. J. Trop. Med. Hyg.,* 8, 372, 1959.
32. **Sellers, R. F.,** The use of a line of hamster kidney cells (BHK-21) for growth of arthropod-borne viruses, *Trans. R. S. Trop. Med. Hyg.,* 57, 433, 1963.
33. **Spence, L. and Downs, W. G.,** Virological investigations in Guyana 1956—1966, *West Ind. Med. J.,* 17, 83, 1968.
34. **Srihongse, S., Stacy, H. G., and Gauld, J. R.,** A survey to assess potential human disease hazards along proposed sea level canal routes in Panama and Colombia. IV. Arbovirus surveillance in man, *Mil. Med.,* 138, 422, 1973.
35. **Woodall, J. P.,** Virus research in Amazônia, *Atas Simpôsia Biota Amazônica,* Vol. 6, Lent, H., Ed., Conselho Nacional de Pesquisas, Rio de Janiero, 1967, 31.

MUCAMBO FEVER

F. P. Pinheiro

NAME AND SYNONYMS

The name Mucambo fever is used to describe illness in human beings caused by Mucambo virus. No synonyms are used for the disease.

HISTORY

The first strain of Mucambo (MUC) virus was isolated in 1954 from the blood of a sentinel monkey exposed in the Oriboca forest near Belém, Para, Brazil.[4] Subsequently, many strains of the agent have been recovered from sentinel mice, wild rodents, and mosquitoes in Brazil and in Trinidad. Although the virus appears to be endemic in wildlife in certain areas of these countries, there is no evidence that it causes disease in animals under natural conditions. Antibodies against the agent have been found in people in Brazil, Surinam, and French Guiana, and the virus has been isolated from blood samples from febrile patients in Brazil and Surinam.[4,13] However, no epidemics have been reported.

ETIOLOGY

Mucambo virus is a group A arbovirus, placed in the genus *Alphavirus* of the family Togaviridae. It was initially considered to be a strain of Venezuelan equine encephalomyelitis (VEE) virus.[4] Although the two agents are antigenically closely related, they have been shown to be distinct from each other by the neutralization (N), hemagglutination inhibition (HI) and complement-fixation (CF) tests.[15] By HI kinetic studies,[21] Mucambo virus is classified as type 3 of the VEE complex. It possesses a hemagglutinin which can be prepared from brains of infected mice extracted by sucrose-acetone, and which is active against goose erythrocytes at a pH of 6.0 to 6.2 with an optimum pH of 6.2 at 37°C. A laboratory hemagglutinin can be prepared from serum of young hamsters inoculated intracerebrally with the virus.[18]

The virus may be replicated in a wide variety of cell culture systems. Plaques are produced in primary cultures of chicken, turkey, or mouse embryos and in BHK-21 and Vero cell lines under agar overlay.[3,14] Cytopathic effect is produced in GMK (green monkey kidney), H.Ep. 2[14] and HeLa cell lines.[15] Chick embryo and BHK-21 cultures have been found to be as, or more, sensitive than suckling mice for virus isolation. Plaques appear within 2 to 3 days after inoculation and the titers reach 10^9 PFU/mℓ.[14] No electron microscopic studies have been conducted on Mucambo virions. Based on studies of the 1B strain of VEE virus by thin section electron microscopy,[8] it can be speculated that the virus particles have a size of 60 nm, are enveloped, have a diameter of 46 nm, and a capsid diameter of 30 nm.

DEFINITION

Mucambo fever is an acute, benign, febrile human illness, produced by an arbovirus of the VEE complex. The virus, which is endemic in rodents in certain areas in northern South America, is classified as VEE type 3.

ANIMAL INFECTION

Clinical

The agent has not been associated with natural disease in any kind of domestic animals, in contrast to the epidemic strains of VEE virus which are highly pathogenic to horses. A 10-month-old horse inoculated intramuscularly with a high dose of Mucambo virus developed viremia which persisted for 3 days, fever beginning 24 hr after injection, and a persistent leucopenia.

In laboratory animals, infant mice inoculated intracerebrally (i.c.) or intraperitoneally (i.p.) die in 1 or 2 days. Adult mice inoculated i.c. usually die within 6 days with some animals showing hind leg paralysis, but following i.p. inoculation, only a few succumb. The virus titer in the brains of suckling mice inoculated either i.c. or i.p. usually reaches 10^9 LD$_{50}$/0.02 mℓ, but only 10^7 to 10^8 LD$_{50}$ in adult mice inoculated by the i.c. route. Adult hamsters succumb when infected either by i.c. or subcutaneous (s.c.) routes;[17] guinea pigs survive when inoculated i.p.[15] A *Cynomolgus* spp. monkey inoculated i.c. with the agent developed viremia, fever, slight paresis, and encephalitis.[19]

Pathology

Histopathological studies in mice have revealed mild lesions in the liver with the presence of fatty infiltration and frequently binucleation in the hepatocytes, occasional foci of necroses in these cells, and hyperplasia of the Kupffer cells, the latter in animals which survive for a longer period of time. The kidneys show hemorrhagic glomerulitis with some glomeruli showing increased cellularity variably, accompanied by epithelial proliferation in the capsule, and by capillary congestions. Intense and widespread lesions are observed in the brain with neuronal destruction, proliferation of glial cells, and perivascular infiltration of mononuclear cells.[6] In livers of infected mice, electron microscopy reveals perichromatin granuli, filaments, and tubular structures in the cell nuclei. In addition, nonspecific alterations such as enlargement of the nucleoli presence of fat droplets, fat vesicles, and empty vesicles may be observed. Numerous phagosomes may be seen in the Kupffer cells. Capillary occlusion and obliteration of the Bowman spaces of the kidneys by swelling of the podocytes and herniation of the tubular epithelium may occur. Swelling of the epithelium of the proximal tubules may lead to necrotic ruptures and formation of cylinders of cytoplasmatic and nuclear debris. The renal alterations are thought to be caused by intoxication secondary to the viral hepatitis and encephalitis.[1,2]

Diagnosis

Diagnosis of Mucambo virus infections is based on virus isolation and serological findings. Samples of serum, plasma, whole blood, and visceral organs are used for virus isolation attempts. These materials are inoculated i.c. into infant mice, and the animals are observed for signs of illness. Brains of sick mice are used as a source of antigen against specific immune serum or immune ascitic fluid in CF tests. In areas where a great variety of arboviruses may be present, it is recommended that CF tests against representative antigenic groups of arboviruses found in the region be employed initially with hyperimmune ascitic fluid or sera.

Mucambo virus may be isolated in cell cultures able to support its replication either by plaque techniques or in cells maintained under fluid medium. Plaques usually appear in 2 to 3 days after the cultures have been inoculated. Cells from the plaque periphery may be aspirated with Pasteur pipets and emulsified in phosphate buffer containing 0.75% of bovine albumin. Fluids may be harvested from cell cultures maintained under liquid medium when the cells show 3 to 4+ cytopathic effect. The cell emulsions or harvested fluids may be used in neutralization tests with Mucambo antiserum or immune ascitic fluid. In sentinel monkey studies, periodic sera should be collected and compared for development of titers demonstrable by HI, CF, or neutralization tests. A fourfold increase in titer (or more) between any two samples is considered definitive for infection. By neutralization indices, convalescent samples should have an index of 1.7 logs or greater than earlier samples. Caution should be observed in interpretating results in areas where several group A arboviruses may be present.

HUMAN INFECTION

The incubation period is unknown. The disease has been mild, with moderate fever lasting about 3 days, headache and dizziness, nausea, photophobia, and muscle pain of low intensity in the arms, legs, and back. None of the patients diagnosed in Brazil required hospitalization or were absent from work during the period of illness. Two persons who acquired laboratory infections developed severe fever with headache and other pains, severe pharyngitis, and some involvement of the central nervous system. One of the patients had previously received VEE vaccine.[5]

Pathology

No lesions have been reported in human patients.

Diagnosis

Laboratory diagnosis is described in the previous section.

EPIDEMIOLOGY

The virus is endemic in certain areas of the Amazon basin of Brazil, Trinidad, Surinam, and French Guiana, and has been detected near Sao Paulo (south Brazil) in sentinel mice.[12] In different localities in the Amazon basin in Brazil, HI antibody prevalence rates have varied from 0 to 34%,[14,20] with an overall rate around 6%, but no outbreaks of human illness due to Mucambo virus have been observed in this area.

Five febrile cases in Parà State,[20] and two cases in Surinam[13] have been diagnosed by viral isolation. Six per cent of Dutch soldiers stationed in Surinam in 1962 to 1963 acquired HI antibodies to Mucambo virus.[10]

The virus is maintained in nature by a silent sylvatic cycle which involves rodents and mosquitoes. It has been frequently isolated from *Oryzomys capito* and *Proechimys guyannensis* in Brazil, and from *Oryzomys laticeps, Zygodontomys brevicauda,* and *Heteromys anomalus* in Trinidad.[11,20] A single isolate was obtained from *Nectomys squamipes* and five strains from marsupials in Brazil and Trinidad. In addition, one strain was isolated from a bird, *Pipra erythrocephala.*[9] The virus has been recovered many times from *Culex (Melanoconium) portesi* as well as from other *Culex* spp. mosquitoes and from *Aedes, Mansonia, Haemagogus, Sabethini, Wyeomyia,* and *Psorophora* spp. in Brazil, Trinidad, French Guiana, and Surinam.[7,11,20] Transmission of the agent to mice by naturally infected *Culex (M) portesi* and by laboratory infected *Aedes aegypti* has been demonstrated.[9,13]

Antibodies to the agent are commonly found in wild rodents and in certain species of marsupials in the forests near Belém, Brazil.[20] The virus has been isolated more often from *Oryzomys capito* than from other wild animals in the area. Since these rodents also develop high levels of viremia,[16] and because there is a positive correlation between Mucambo virus transmission and the abundance of nonimmune *O. capito* in an area,[16] it is considered that they are important reservoir hosts for the virus. Other rodent species as well as marsupials may be infected, but they have not been shown to play a reservoir role. Human exposure is believed to occur during crepuscular hours when *Culex (Melanoconium)* spp. mosquitoes are active.

CONTROL

Since the clinical course of Mucambo fever is generally mild, only antipyretic drugs are recommended, and no specific measures have been devised for its control. Should serious outbreaks occur, general measures applicable to mosquito-borne viruses should be followed.

PUBLIC HEALTH ASPECTS

Mucambo fever seems to have no serious impact on human health.

REFERENCES

1. Araújo, R., Dias, L. B., and Huth, F. Veränderungen von Mäusenieren nach experimenteller infektion mit Mucambo virus, *Virchows Arch. B.,* 354, 312, 1972.
2. Arújo, R., Dias, L. B., and Huth, F., Alteracões ultra-estruturais do figado de camundongos albinos após inoculacão experimental com arbovírus Mucambo (Tipo An 10967), *Rev. Inst. Med. Trop. S. Paulo,* 15, 377, 1973.
3. Bergold, G. H. and Mazzali, R., Plaque formation by arboviruses, *J. Gen. Virol.,* 2, 273, 1968.
4. Causey, O. R., Causey, C. E., Maroja, O. M., and Macedo, D. G., The isolation of arthropodborne viruses, including members of two hitherto undescribed serological groups, in the Amazon region of Brazil, *Am. J. Trop. Med. Hyg.,* 10, 227, 1961.
5. De Mucha-Macias, J. and Sánchez-Spindola, I., Two human cases of laboratory infection with Mucambo virus, *Am. J. Trop. Med. Hyg.,* 14, 475, 1965.
6. Dias, L. B., Duarte, F., and Paola, D., Lesões pouco usuais na histopatologia experimental de arbovírus Amazônicos, *Rev. Soc. Bras. Med. Trop.,* 6, 135, 1972.
7. Haas, R. A. and Arron-Leeuwin, A. E. F., Arboviruses isolated from mosquitos and man in Surinam, *Trop. Geogr. Med.,* 27, 409, 1975.
8. Berg, T. O., Ed., *International Catalogue of Arboviruses, Including Certain Other Viruses of Vertebrates,* 2nd ed., Pub. No. (CDC) 75-8301, Public Health Service, U.S. Department of Health, Education and Welfare, Atlanta, 1975, 738.

9. **Berg, T. O., Ed.,** *International Catalogue of Arboviruses, Including Certain Other Viruses of Vertebrates,* 2nd ed., Pub. No. (CDC) 75-8301, Public Health Service, U.S. Department of Health, Education and Welfare, Atlanta, 1975, 503.

10. **Jonkers, A. H., Spence, L., and Karbaat, J.,** Arbovirus infections in Dutch military personnel stationed in Surinam. Further Studies, *Trop. Geogr. Med.,* 20, 251, 1968.

11. **Jonkers, A.H., Spence, L., Downs, W. G., Aitken, T. H. G., and Worth, C. B.,** Arbovirus studies in Bush-Bush forest, Trinidad, W. I., September 1959—December 1964. VI. Rodent-associated viruses (VEE and agents of Groups C and Guama): isolations and further studies, *Am. J. Trop. Med. Hyg.,* 17, 285, 1968.

12. **Lopes, O. S. and Sacchetta, L. A.,** Isolation of Mucambo virus, a member of the Venezuelan equine encephalitis virus complex in the State of São Paulo, Brazil, *Rev. Inst. Med. Trop. S. Paulo,* 20(2), 82, 1978.

13. **Metselaar, D.,** Isolation of arboviruses of group A and group C in Surinam, *Trop. Geogr. Med.,* 18, 137, 1966.

14. **Pinheiro, F. P.,** unpublished data, 1968.

15. **Shope, R. E., Causey, O. R., Andrade, A. H. P., and Theiler, M.,** The Venezuelan equine encephalomyelitis complex of group A arthropod-borne viruses, including Mucambo and Pixuna from the Amazon region of Brazil, *Am. J. Trop. Med. Hyg.,* 13, 723, 1964.

16. **Shope, R. E., and Woodall, J. P.,** Ecological interaction of wildlife, man, and a virus of the Venezuelan equine encephalomyelitis complex in a tropical forest, *J. Wildl. Dis.,* 9, 198, 1973.

17. **Srihongse, S. and Johnson, K. M.** Hemagglutinin production and infectivity patterns in adult hamsters inoculated with group C and other new world arboviruses, *Am. J. Trop. Med. Hyg.,* 18, 273, 1969.

18. **Travassos da Rosa, A. P. A.** personal communication, 1968.

19. **Verlinde, J. D.,** Susceptibility of Cynomolgus monkeys to experimental infection with arboviruses of group A (Mayaro and Mucambo), group C (Oriboca and Restan) and an unidentified arbovirus (Kwatta) originating from Surinam, *Trop. Geogr. Med.,* 20, 385, 1968.

20. **Woodall, J. P.,** Virus research in Amazônia, in *Atas Simposia Biota Amazônica,* Vol. 6, Lent, H., Ed., Conselho Nacional de Pesquisas, Rio de Janiero, 1967, 31.

21. **Young, N. A.and Johnson, K. M.,** Antigenic variants of Venezuelan equine encephalitis virus: their geographic distribution and epidemiologic significance, *Am. J. Epidemiol.,* 89, 286, 1969.

BUSSUQUARA FEVER

F. P. Pinheiro

SYNONYMS

Bussuquara fever is the name used to describe the human disease caused by Bussuquara virus.

HISTORY

Bussuquara (BSQ) virus has been frequently isolated from sentinel and wild animals, and from mosquitoes in Brazil, Panama, and Colombia.[8] A single isolation has been obtained from a human patient.[12] The prototype strain of the virus was recovered from the blood of a sentinel monkey (*Alouatta beelzebul*) exposed in a forest near Belém, Brazil.[5] Bussuquara virus has not been associated with epidemics in human or other animal populations.

ETIOLOGY

Bussuquara virus belongs to the group B arboviruses and is placed in the genus *Flavivirus* of the family Togaviridae. It crossreacts with Ilhéus, St. Louis encephalitis, bat salivary gland, and other flaviviruses by hemagglutination inhibition (HI), complement-fixation (CF), and neutralization (N) tests, although they are also separable by these tests.[5] A hemagglutinin can be extracted from infected mouse brains by acetone-ether and sucrose-acetone or by treating brain crude suspension with protamin.[8] The hemagglutinin is active against goose erythrocyte cells at an optimal pH of 6.8 at 27°C and against 1-day-old chicken erythrocytes. The agent produces plaques in primary cultures of Pekin duck kidney[7] and chicken and turkey embryos,[9] and in BHK-21, Vero, rhesus monkey kidney MA 104, LLC-MK2,[1,13] and in MA-111 line of continuous newborn rabbit kidney[3] cell lines. In addition, it causes cytopathic effect in Vero and HeLa cell lines.[2,9] The infectivity titer in the Vero cell line is about 1 log lower than in infant mice inoculated intracerebrally (i.c.)[1,9]

The virions are 20 to 50 nm in diameter, possess a lipoprotein envelope, and contain ribonucleic acid. They are heat-labile and sensitive to sodium deoxycholate.

DEFINITION

Bussuquara fever is an acute febrile benign illness of human beings caused by an arbovirus which gives its name to the virus.

ANIMAL INFECTION

No disease has been reported in domestic animals. With the exception of the sentinel monkey, which died about 2 weeks after the prototype virus was detected in his blood, no disease has been associated with infection in wild animals. It causes death of infant Swiss mice following i.c. or i.p. inoculation. Adult mice die after i.c. inoculation, but they survive and produce antibody following i.p. inoculation. Adult hamsters inoculated either i.c. or i.p., and adult *Proechimys* spp. infected by the i.p. route produce antibodies but no signs of illness.[8,11]

Pathology

Histopathological lesions compatible with a diagnosis of yellow fever (YF) were reported in the liver of the sentinel howler monkey from which the original isolation of Bussuquara virus had been obtained[5] about 2 weeks earlier. Attempts to obtain hepatic lesions in howler monkeys by experimental infection with two strains of Bussuquara virus, one of which was the prototype strain, failed to reveal anything significant.

Diagnosis

Virus isolation and identification are the usual laboratory methods for the diagnosis of the infection. Samples of whole blood, plasma, serum, or visceral organs are inoculated i.c. into infant mice and the animals are observed for signs of illness. The CF test is employed for virus identification using brain suspensions obtained from sick mice and an immune or hyperimmune to Bussuquara virus mouse ascitic fluid. In view of the antigenic relationships of the group B arboviruses, it is advisable to include in the test immune ascitic fluids to the other members of this group that are known to occur in the region. In order to recover the agent from arthropods, the insects are pooled by species, triturated in a buffer solution containing bovine albumin or rabbit serum, and inoculated into mice. The isolates are identified in the manner described above.

Table 1
CLINICAL SYMPTOMS OF 234 PATIENTS EXAMINED AT THE EMERGENCY HOSPITAL OF ITANHAÉM, FROM APRIL TO JUNE 1975

Symptoms	No. patients	%
Headache	219	93.6
Fever	212	90.6
Vomit	120	51.3
Weakness	106	45.3
Anorexia	55	23.5
Abdominal pain	49	20.9
Nausea	45	19.3
Conjunctival congestion	37	15.8
Myalgia	11	4.7

Table 2
NEUROLOGICAL SYMPTOMS OF 234 PATIENTS EXAMINED AT THE EMERGENCY HOSPITAL OF ITANHAÉM, FROM APRIL TO JUNE 1975

Symptoms	No. patients	%
Mental confusion	122	51.0
Meningeal irritation	134	57.3
Kernig	32	13.7
Brudzinski	29	12.4
Motor impairment		
Walking disturbance	116	49.6
Equilibrium disturbance	67	28.6
Cerebellar syndrome	32	13.7
Reflex disturbance		
Hyper	59	25.2
Hypo	32	13.7
No reflex	16	6.8
Muscular disturbance		
Hypotonic	30	12.8
Hypertonic	28	12.0
Speech disturbance	24	10.3
Convulsion	4	1.7

15 years of age, females have assumed indoor duties and have appeared to be definitely protected. Clinically recognized infections have not occurred in babies under 2 years of age.[9-11] This pattern is similar to that of sylvan yellow fever in South America.

Environment

Rocio virus infections have occurred in sea level plains areas with high rainfall (>4000 mm yearly) and high humidity (average 85%). Mosquito density is high in such areas during summer and fall months and these have been the seasons of highest inci-

Table 3
DISTRIBUTION OF HUMAN CASES OF ENCEPHALITIS BY SEX AND AGE GROUPS COMPARED WITH THE POPULATION UNDER RISK IN AN EPIDEMIC AREA IN THE STATE OF SÃO PAULO, BRAZIL, 1975

Ages	Patients			Population under risk		
	Males	Females	M/F[a]	Males	Females	M/F[a]
0-15	70	60	1.1	2592	2545	1.0
15-30	125	34	3.6	1526	1391	1.1
+ 30	95	48	2.0	1784	1541	1.1
Total	290	142	2.0	5902	5477	1.0

[a]   Male/female ratio

Table 4
OCCUPATIONS OF 217 ENCEPHALITIC PATIENTS IN PERUÍBE AREA, SÃO PAULO STATE, 1975

Occupation	No. patients	%
Children and students	68	31.5
Farm hands	56	25.9
Houseworkers	42	19.5
House builders	29	13.4
All others	22	9.7
Totals	217	100.0

dence of infections, with declines or disappearance of the disease in winter. This pattern is similar to that of St. Louis, Japanese, Murray Valley, and other flaviviral encephalitides.[3]

CONTROL

Prevention and Therapy

There is no specific therapy for encephalitis caused by Rocio virus infections. Supportive hospital care measures as nursing care and symptomatic treatment have helped to reduce mortality rates.[11] No isolation measures have been considered necessary. There is no available vaccine. Vector control should be considered as a control measure but its effectivity can only be postulated as no vectors have been identified.

Epidemic Measures

During outbreaks, people should be warned not to enter epidemic areas. During the 1975 epidemics, at least 12 known patients were visitors to Peruibe and Itanhaem. Suspected patients should be hospitalized as early in the clinical course of the disease as possible, even before definitive central nervous system manifestations appear.

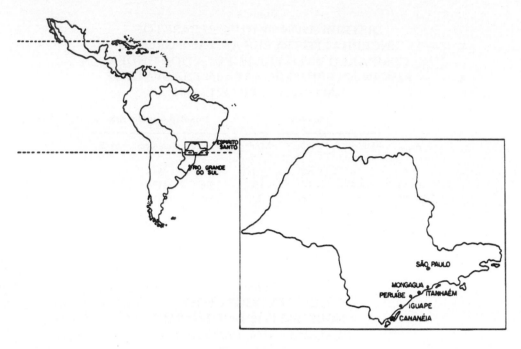

FIGURE 1.   Map showing epidemics of human encephalitis which occurred in the coastal areas of São Paulo State Brazil.

PUBLIC HEALTH ASPECTS

Economic and Social Impact

Rocio viral encephalitis epidemics characterized by high morbidity and mortality rates have seriously disrupted activities in affected communities. Adult male patients who have been unable to work during the acute phase of the illness and who have frequently remained incapacitated due to sequelae have been unable to support their families. The epidemics have occurred in coastal tourist areas and have profoundly affected the local tourist trades.

Reporting

Rocio virus infections are not reported in Brazil except during epidemics.

Surveillance

Systematic surveillance for Rocio virus activity is being done through the examination of sera from wild birds captured in the risk areas[4,9] and by serological diagnosis of human encephalitis occurring in the epidemic region.

REFERENCES

1. **Berge, T. O.,** Ed., *International Catalogue of Arboviruses,* 2nd ed., Pub. No. (CDC) 75-8301, Public Health Service, U.S. Department of Health, Education and Welfare, Atlanta, 1975.
2. **Casals, J.,** Immunological techniques for animal viruses, in *Methods in Virology,* Vol. 3, Maramorosh, K. and Koprowsky, H., Eds., Academic Press, New York, 1967, 113.
3. **Clarke, D. H. and Casals, J.,** Arboviruses, group B, in *Viral and Rickettsial Infections of Man,* Horsefall, F. L. and Tamm, I., Eds., J. B. Lippincott Co., Philadelphia, 1965, 606.
4. **Lord, R. D., Calisher, C. H., Chappell, A., Metzger, W. R., and Fischer, G. W.,** Urban St. Louis encephalitis surveillance through wild birds, *Am. J. Epidemiol.,* 99, 360, 1974.

5. Monath, T. P., Wilson, D. C., and Casals, J., The 1979 yellow fever epidemic in Okwoga District, Benue Plateau State, Nigeria. 3. Serological responses in persons with and without pre-existing heterologous group B immunity, *Bull. WHO*, 49, 235, 1973.
6. Monath, T. P., Kemp, G. E., Cropp, C. B., and Bowen, G. S., Experimental infection of house sparrow (*Passer domesticus*) with Rocio virus, *Am. J. Trop. Med. Hyg.*, 27, 1255, 1978.
7. Rosenberg, S., Neuropathological study of a new viral encephalitis. The encephalitis of Sao Paulo south sea coast (preliminary report), *Rev. Inst. Med. Trop.*, 19, 280, 1977.
8. Souza Lopes, O., Coimbra, T. L. M., Sacchetta, L. A., and Calisher, C., Emergence of a new arbovirus disease in Brazil. I. Isolation and identification of the etiological agent, Rocio Virus, *Am. J. Epidemiol.*, 108 (5), 394, 1978.
9. Souza Lopes, O., Sacchetta, L. A., Coimbra, T. L. M., Pinto, G. H., and Glasser, C. M., Emergence of a new arbovirus disease in Brazil. II. Epidemiological studies on 1975 epidemics, *Am. J. Epidemiol.*, 108 (5), 394, 1978.
10. Souza Lopes, O., Sacchetta, L. A., France, D. B., Jakob, W. L., and Calisher, C. H., Emergence of a new arbovirus disease in Brazil. III. Isolation of Rocio virus from Psorophora ferox (Humboldt, 1819), *Am. J. Trop. Med. Hyg.*, in press.
11. Tiriba, A. C., Miziara, A. M., Lorenzo, R. et al., Encefalite humana primaria epidemica por arbovirus observada no litoral sul do Estado de Sao Paulo, *Rev. Assoc. Med. Brasil*, 22, 415, 1976.

OROPOUCHE FEVER

F. P. Pinheiro

NAME AND SYNONYMS

Oropouche fever is the name given to the illness caused by Oropouche virus. It is also known as Febre de Mojuí in the Santarém area of north Brazil, where an epidemic of the illness occurred first in the village of Mojuí dos Campos in 1975, and subsequently throughout the area.

HISTORY

The initial isolation of the Oropouche (ORO) virus was made in Trinidad in 1955 from the blood of a febrile forest worker.[1] In 1960 the virus was isolated from a pool of *Coquillettidia venezuelensis* in Trinidad.[1,17] The first isolations of the agent in Brazil were made in 1960 from a *Bradypus tridactylus* sloth captured at a forested area located along the Belém-Brasília Highway, and from a pool of *Aedes serratus* mosquitoes caught near the same site.[13] The following year, an epidemic of Oropouche fever occurred in Belém, Brazil during which some 11,000 people were infected.[15d] From 1967 to 1975, other extensive outbreaks have occurred, all in urban centers of the Amazon region. No deaths have been attributed to this febrile illness.[15,15a]

ETIOLOGY

Serologically, Oropouche virus is 1 of at least 16 viruses included in the Simbu group of the Bunyamwera supergroup of the family Bunyaviridae.[8,10] Although these viruses can be differentiated by complement-fixation (CF) tests, they have some cross reaction. Based upon the physico-chemical properties of its members, the viruses in the Simbu group have spherical, enveloped virions 90 to 100 nm in diameter, containing segmented ribonucleic acid, and with helical capsid symmetry.[7,10] They may be inactivated by ether or sodium deoxycholate. Oropouche virus contains a hemagglutinin which may be prepared by sucrose extraction of brains of infected suckling mice, followed by sonication and trypsin treatment.[3] The hemagglutinin is active against goose erythrocytes at an optimum pH of 6.0. Acetone extracted serum of infected hamsters also constitutes an excellent hemagglutinin.[18]

The agent multiplies in primary chick embryo, Vero (green monkey kidney), and BHK-21 (baby hamster kidney) clone 13-cell cultures under fluid medium with cell destruction.[9,12] It also forms plaques in monolayers of these cultures, and of MA 111 (rabbit kidney) and LLC-MK2 (simian kidney) cell lines overlaid with agar.[4,16]

DEFINITION

Oropouche fever is a benign, febrile human illness often accompanied by headache, chills, myalgia, arthralgia, photophobia, and dizziness. Epidemiological evidence suggests that the agent is transmitted among persons through the bites of *Culicoides* spp. midges.[6,15a,15c] Experimentally, these midges can transmit Oropouche virus by bite from hamster to hamster,[15b] but the vectors and reservoir hosts of the sylvatic cycle remain unknown.

ANIMAL INFECTION

There is no evidence as yet that Oropouche virus can produce disease in naturally infected animals. The only isolation of the agent obtained from wild animals came from four sloths of the species *Bradypus tridactylus* captured in the Amazon region of Brazil which manifested no visible signs of illness,[15a] and the virus has not been recovered from domestic animals. Experimentally, it produces lethal infection in 3-day-old Swiss mice and 3-week-old Syrian hamsters when inoculated by intracerebral (i.c.), intraperitoneal (i.p.), or subcutaneous (s.c.) routes. The virus has been readily demonstrated by electron microscopy in the blood of infected hamsters.[11] Infected suckling mice show irritability, prostration, and death 2 to 3 days after i.c. inoculation. Adult mice develop fatal infections following i.c. injection of virus, but survive after i.p. and s.c. inoculations. Chickens 1 to 45 days of age have shown no signs of illness when inoculated with low or high doses of the virus by s.c. and intramuscular i.m. routes. In addition, they have failed to develop viremia, or to serologically convert. No disease was observed in *Saimiri, Cebus,* and *Alouatta* spp. monkeys following s.c. injection of the virus. However, the animals developed viremia for 3 or more days reaching $10^{4.5}$ suckling mouse $LD_{50}/0.02$ mℓ, followed by appearance of antibodies.[15a] Experimentally infected *Bradypus tridactylus* circulate the virus up to 6 days, but no signs of illness were observed in the animals.[15a] Adult white rats and rabbits inoculated i.p. with high doses of virus manifested no signs of illness and developed only a low level viremia. Rabbits inoculated i.c. did not become sick. In addition to laboratory animals, the agent can be propagated serially in embryonated chicken eggs inoculated by yolk-sac and amniotic-sac routes; embryo mortality becomes regular with serial yolk sac passages.[1]

Pathology

Infected mice have developed encephalitis characterized by interstitial edema and neuronal destruction by colliquative and coagulation necrosis.[5] Infected hamsters have demonstrated minimal lesions in the brain and marked hepatitis characterized by initial focal lesions which later become diffused. Necroses of coagulation predominates, accompanied by destruction of the trabeculae, sinusal congestion and hemorrhage, with very little mesenchymal reaction.

Cellular changes are observed by electron microscopy in livers of hamsters as early as 6 hr after inoculation.[2] The changes in hepatocytes consist of diminution in ribosomes, foci of endoplasma reticular dilation with appearance of fingerprint type images, focal cytoplasmic degeneration, and presence of multilammelar bodies. Progressive margination of chromatin is observed in nucleii followed by collapse of membranes, shrinkage, and necrosis. The Kupffer cells show hyperplasia with their nuclei exhibiting tubular forms and reduced chromatin.

Diagnosis

Virus isolation can be achieved by intracerebral inoculation of suckling mice, weaned hamsters, Vero cell line cultures, or primary cultures of chicken embryo cells with whole blood or serum, or with homogenates of animal visceral organs. Suspensions of infected mouse brains in veronal buffer may be used as an antigen in CF virus identification against an Oropouche hyperimmune mouse ascitic fluid. Neutralization tests may be performed in mice or in cell cultures by the plaque reduction method, or in a microneutralization test using Vero cells under fluid medium. The last method is recommended for its reliability, economy, and simplicity.

HUMAN INFECTION

The onset of the disease is usually abrupt. Fever, headache, myalgia, arthralgia, chills, dizziness, and photophobia are most common clinical findings. Nausea, vomiting, diarrhea, and conjunctival congestion, epigastric pain or burning sensations in various parts of the body may also occur. Cough and coryza may be primary symptoms, but may also be due to an intercurrent infection. The fever is high, reaching 40°C in some patients. Headache is severe and the muscle pains are generalized, but most are in the neck and back. Moderate leukopenia is usually observed, although slight leucocytosis can be present in certain patients. No abnormalities have been encountered in the urine. No rash, jaundice, hepatomegaly, splenomegaly, and lymph node enlargement have been observed. Although some patients become severely ill, occasionally to the point of prostration, no fatalities or sequelae have been attributed to the disease. The illness lasts from 2 to 7 days, but a proportion of patients complain of asthenia which can persist up to a few weeks. A significant number of persons have reported one or more recurrences of the same symptoms present during the initial onset or, simply suffer headache, myalgia, and asthenia occurring up to 10 or more days after initial recovery.[15]

The laboratory diagnosis may be based on virus isolation or on the demonstration of a rise in antibody titer to the agent in paired serum samples. Serum or whole-blood samples are used in virus isolation. HI and neutralization tests are used in serological diagnosis.

EPIDEMIOLOGY

Oropouche virus has been isolated only in Trinidad and northern Brazil, but the presence of neutralizing antibodies in monkeys captured in the Magdalena valley in Colombia[8] has suggested its occurrence in a wider area. No human epidemics have been recorded in Trinidad, and the antibody prevalence rate among forest workers of this island has been low.[1] In Brazil, seven large epidemics have been recorded in six areas in the Amazon basin.[15,15a] The first laboratory-confirmed epidemic occurred in 1961 in Belém, the capital of Pará state. The subsequent epidemics have occurred in the Bragança area in 1967, in Belém again in 1968, in the Santarém area in 1975, and in the towns of Baião and Itupiranga in 1972 and in 1975, respectively, and in the Tomé-Acú area in 1978. In Belém, it was estimated that 11,000 people were infected in the suburbs of the city during the 1961 epidemic. The 1968 epidemic lasted about 6 months, and 101 strains of Oropouche virus were isolated from the sera of 658 febrile cases. There was no marked sex distribution in the cases. Most cases occurred in the 6- to 30-year-old age group. The distribution of cases through the city was markedly uneven, with 80% being confined to one district. In the Bragança area, 29% of the population of about 30,000 showed antibody titers after the epidemic was over. In the Santarém epidemic, about 17,000 persons living in the county seat and in three small towns were infected.[15a]

There is strong epidemiological evidence that Oropouche virus is maintained in nature by a wild cycle involving monkeys, sloths, birds, and possibly other animals. In Trinidad, a high prevalence of antibodies has been found in *Alouatta* and *Cebus* spp. monkeys.[1] Antibodies to Oropouche virus have been found in most monkey and wild bird populations surveyed in the Amazon basin.[14,15a] The fact that Oropouche virus has been recovered from sloths on four occasions suggests that these animals can play a role as vertebrate hosts for the virus. Sloths also become viremic when experimentally infected with the agent.[15a] Nevertheless, only 1 (4.1%) of 24 sloths captured in the Amazon region had HI antibodies to Oropouche virus.[15a] The birds of the Formicariidae family have usually presented the highest antibody prevalence rates.[15,15a] Surprisingly, none of 51 sloths or 15 monkeys captured in the forests of the Santarém area during the 1975 outbreak had antibodies to the agent, although about 5% of the wild and domestic birds sampled in the epidemic foci had HI antibodies to Oropouche virus.[15]

The vector(s) of Oropouche virus in nature are still unknown. The virus has been isolated from one pool each of *Coquillettidia venezuelensis* in Trinidad and *Aedes serratus* in Brazil, and multiplication of the virus in experimentally inoculated *Aedes serratus, Aedes scapularis, Culex quinquefasciatus,* and *Psorophora ferox* has been demonstrated.[1] No transmission, however, was obtained when the infected mosquitoes were allowed to bite 2-day-old mice or hamsters.[1] Three isolations have been obtained from over 30,000 *Culex quinquefasciatus* Say mosquitoes collected during urban epidemics. One came from a pool of engorged mosquitoes; the other two were from nonengorged specimens. *Culicoides* midges have been abundant in epidemic sites, and eight strains of Oropouche virus were isolated from some 90,000 *Culicoides paraensis* collected during the outbreak of Santarém and Tomé-Açu area epidemics.[12,15] Successful transmission of Oropouche virus from hamster to hamster by *C. paraensis* has been demonstrated in the laboratory.[15b] There has been no evidence of direct human-to-human transmission, and no virus has been demonstrated in throats of viremic patients. Those findings, together with the fact that no virus can be demonstrated in the throat of viremic patients, suggests that *C. paraensis* may be the main vectors during urban epidemics.

CONTROL

The treatment of patients is symptomatic. Antipyretic and analgesic drugs are indicated, and patients should observe bed rest.

No specific control measures can be taken to stop urban epidemics until the mechanisms of the transmission may be elucidated. *Culicoides* midge control may be attempted, but more information on the biology of these midges and their susceptibility to insecticides is required before any extensive vector control programs can be adopted.

PUBLIC HEALTH ASPECTS

Epidemics of Oropouche fever have had severe impacts on the communities where they have occurred. Despite the benign nature of the human disease, many patients have required hospitalization. With its high attack rates, a large segment of a community may be immobilized at one time creating temporary, but considerable loss, of manpower.

Surveillance for increases in febrile illnesses of nonmalaria origin, followed by laboratory confirmation of their bunyaviral etiology, are the measures to be undertaken. Prompt and extensive reporting by physicians and readily available laboratory assistance are needed.

REFERENCES

1. **Anderson, C. R., Spence, L., Downs, W. G., and Aitken, T. H. G.**, Oropouche virus: a new human disease agent from Trinidad, West Indies, *Am. J. Trop. Med. Hyg.*, 10, 574, 1961.
2. **Araújo, R., Dias, L. B., Araújo, M. T. F., Pinheiro, F. P., and Oliva, O. F. P.**, Alteracoes ultraestruturais no fígado de hamsters após inoculação experimental com arbovírus Oropouche (tipo BeAn 19991), *Rev. Inst. Med. Trop. São Paulo*, 20(1), 45, 1978.
3. **Ardoin, P., Clarke, D. H., and Hannoun, C.**, The preparation of arbovirus hemagglutinins by sonication and trypsin treatment, *Am. J. Trop. Med. Hyg.*, 18, 592, 1969.
4. **Bergold, G. H. and Mazzali, R.**, Plaque formation by arboviruses, *J. Gen. Virol.*, 2, 273, 1968.
5. **Dias, L. B.**, personal communication, 1977.
6. **Dixon, K. E., Travassos da Rosa, A. P. A., Travassos da Rosa, J. F., and Llewellyn, C. R.**, Oropouche virus. II. Epidemiological observations during an epidemic in Santarém, Pará, Brazil, in 1975, *Am. J. Trop. Med. Hyg.*, in press, 1981.
7. **Holmes, I. H.**, Morphological similarity of Bunyamwera supergroup viruses, *Virology*, 43, 708, 1971.
8. **Berge, T. O.**, Ed., *International Catalogue of Arboviruses, Including Certain Other Viruses of Vertebrates*, 2nd ed., Pub. No. (CDC) 75-8301, Public Health Service, Department of Health, Education, and Welfare, Atlanta, 1975.
9. **Karabatsos, N., and Buckley, S. M.**, Susceptibility of the baby-hamster kidney-cell line (BHK-21) to infection with arboviruses, *Am. J. Trop. Med. Hyg.*, 16, 99, 1967.
10. **Murphy, F. A., Harrison, A. K., and Whitfield, S. G.**, Bunyaviridae: morphologic and morphogenetic similarities of Bunyamwera serologic supergroup viruses and several other arthropod-borne viruses, *Intervirology*, 1, 297, 1973.
11. **Araújo, R., Araújo, M. T. F., Dias, L. B., Pinheiro, F. P., Peters, D., Muller, G., Nielsen, G., and Schmetz, C.**, unpublished observations, 1976.
12. **Pinheiro, F. P.**, unpublished data, 1966.
13. **Pinheiro, F. P., Pinheiro, M., Bensabath, G., Causey, O. R. and Shope, R. E.**, Epidemia de vírus Oropouche em Belém, *Rev. Serv. Espec. Saúde Pública*, 12, 15, 1962.
14. **Pinheiro, F. P., Bensabath, G., Andrade, A. H. P., Lins, Z. C., Frahia, H., Tang, A. T., Lainson, R., Shaw, J. J., and Azevedo, M. C.**, Infectious diseases along Brazil's trans Amazon highway: surveillance and research, *Bull. PAHO*, 8, 111, 1974.
15. **Pinheiro, F. P., Travassos da Rosa, A. P. A., Travassos da Rosa, J. F., and Bensabath, G.**, An outbreak of Oropouche virus disease in the vicinity of Santarém, Pará, Brazil, *Tropenmed. Parasitol.*, 27, 213, 1976.
15a. **Pinheiro, F. P., Travassos da Rosa, A. P. A., Travassos da Rosa, J. F., Ishak, R., Freitas, R. B., Gomes, M. L. C., Oliva, O. F. P., and LeDuc, J. W.**, Oropouche virus. I. A review of clinical, epidemiological and ecological findings, *Am. J. Trop. Med. Hyg.*, in press, 1981.
15b. **Pinheiro, F. P., Hoch, A. L., Gomes, M. L. C., and Roberts, D. R.**, Oropouche virus. IV. Laboratory transmission by *Culicoides paraensis*, *Am. J. Trop. Med. Hyg.*, in press, 1981.
15c. **Roberts, D. R., Hoch, A. L., Dixon, K. E., and Llewellyn, C. R.**, Oropouche virus. III. Entomological observations from three epidemics in Pará, Brazil, 1975, *Am. J. Trop. Med. Hyg.*, in press, 1981.
15d. **Shope, R. E. and Andrade, A. H. P.**, cited in Woodall, J. P., Virus research in Amazônia, *Atas Simpósia Biota Amazônica*, Vol. 6, Lent, H., Ed., Conselho Nacional de Pesquisas, Rio de Janiero, 1967, 31.
16. **Stim, T. B.**, Arbovirus plaquing in two simian kidney cell lines, *J. Gen. Virol.*, 5, 329, 1969.
17. **Theiler, M. and Downs, W. G.**, Oropouche: the story of a new virus, *Yale Sci.*, 37(6), 1963.
18. **Travassos da Rosa, A. P. A.**, personal communication, 1969.

GROUP C BUNYAVIRAL FEVERS

F. P. Pinheiro

NAME AND SYNONYMS

The individual names of the different members of the Bunyamwera supergroup of arboviruses are used to describe their respective diseases in people, e.g., Apeu fever, Caraparu fever, Marituba fever, etc.

HISTORY

The group C arbovirus classification was established in 1961 to assemble several serologically interrelated viruses isolated from wild and sentinel anir. ls, mosquitoes, and people.[9,14] The first recognized member of the group C viruses, Marituba virus, was isolated in 1954 from the blood of a sentinel monkey exposed in the Oriboca forest located about 20 km east of Belém, Brazil,[10] and hundreds of strains of six antigenic types have been recovered from sentinel mice and monkeys, rodents, marsupials, Culicine mosquitoes, and human beings in the Amazon basin of Brazil.[10]

ETIOLOGY

The group C viruses belong to the Bunyamwera supergroup of the family Bunyaviridae.[21] They comprise 11 members which show immunological relationships.[9] The seven antigenic types which occur in Brazil are Apeu, Caraparu, Marituba, Murutucu, Oriboca, Itaqui, and Nepuyo. The virions have a mean diameter of approximately 100 nm, membrane-like margins, and surface projection layers. In the infected cells, virus particles are seen forming by budding from Golgi and endoplasmic reticular membranes and inside of the cisternae of these organelles. In the hemagglutination-inhibition test (HI) and neutralization (N) test, three pairs of viruses can be distinguished. The three viruses of each pair exhibit close relationships by HI and N tests, and they are three closely related pairs, Apeu-Caraparu, Marituba-Murutucu and Oriboca-Itaqui. However, complement fixation (CF) tests reveal three different groupings, Marituba-Apeu, Murutucu-Oriboca and Caraparu-Itaqui viruses.[27]

All group C viruses found in Brazil produce a hemagglutinin which may be acetone-extracted from sera of infected suckling mice or adult hamsters.[14,29] A hemagglutinin can also be prepared for most strains from sucrose-acetone extracted livers of infected mice. The liver hemagglutinin reacts poorly with immune serum in the HI test[9] unless it is further extracted by sonication and subsequent absorption onto calcium phosphate followed by stepwise elution.[1] Workable hemagglutinin can also be obtained from fluids of inoculated HeLa cell cultures extracted by acetone and rehydrated to 1/10 of the original volume.[6] The hemagglutinin is active against goose erythrocytes at an optimum pH of 6.0. Most viruses hemagglutinate at an optimal temperature of 27°C, but Nepuyo antigen agglutinates best at 4°C. A good CF antigen may be prepared from infected mouse livers.[9]

All Brazilian group C viruses multiply in a variety of cell culture systems, producing cytopathic effect in HeLa, HeLa S3, Detroit 6, H.Ep. 1, H.Ep. 2, human embryonic intestine, BHK-21, and Vero cell lines,[5,7,18,23] and plaques in overlaid cultures of primary Rhesus monkey kidney cells, and in BHK-21, Vero, and LLC-MK2 cell lines.[4,13,30]

DEFINITION

Group C viral fevers are benign, febrile illnesses of human beings caused by any of the agents belonging to the group C arboviruses.

ANIMAL INFECTION

Virological and/or serological evidence indicate that inapparent group C viral infections may occur in a variety of species of wild rodents, marsupials, and possibly other sylvatic animals. The viruses have been isolated many times from sentinel monkeys with no visible signs of illness.

In laboratory animals, 1- to 4-day-old Swiss mice inoculated by the intracerebral (i.c.) or intraperitoneal (i.p.) routes become viremic and die. Caraparu, Murutucu, and Oriboca viruses readily kill adult mice after inoculation by these routes as well, but Apeu, Marituba, Itaqui, and Nepuyo viruses cause few or no deaths in adults. Caraparu, Oriboca, and Itaqui viruses are lethal to hamsters following i.c. or subcutaneous (s.c.) inoculation.[29] Viremia is observed irregularly in rhesus monkeys and *Oryzomys laticeps* and *Zygodontomys brevicauda* rodents inoculated by the s.c. route.[2,15] Subcutaneous inoculation of Marituba virus in four sloths of the genus *Bradypus* resulted in viremia and three deaths.[14]

Pathology

The histopathologic lesions in experimentally infected mice and naturally infected sentinel mice are encephalitic and hepatic.[11] In the brain, hydropic swelling, nuclear vacuolation, clasmatodendrosis, chromatolysis, shrinking, and neuronal necrosis with occasional areas of spongiosis and encephalomalacia involving the gray and the white matter, have been observed but without neuronophagia. Lesions have been most frequent in the gray matter (cerebral cortex), followed by lesions in the basal ganglia, hippocampus, spinal cord, and cerebellum. Capillary congestion and perivascular cellular infiltration by lymphocytes and plasma cells has been found infrequently in the meninges. Hepatic lesions have been most marked in animals infected with Caraparu, Itaqui, Murutucu, and Itaqui viruses, and have been characterized by acidophilic and hyaline degeneration of the liver cells, presence of corpuscular structures of the Councilman type, and necrosis of the liver cells, but with minimal mesenchymal reaction. The distribution of the lesions has at times been irregular, without conforming to lobular patterns, and in other animals has involved the entire liver parenchyma while characteristically preserving the centro-lobular section.

Diagnosis

Virus isolation can be accomplished by inoculating suckling mice intracerebrally with blood, serum, plasma, or visceral organs from animals. Vero and other susceptible cell cultures may also be used for attempted virus isolation. A method devised for the rapid identification of isolates belonging to group C viruses is recommended for identification.[27]

HUMAN INFECTION

Clinical

The group C viruses cause a benign, febrile human illness. Fever may reach 40.8°C and persist for 4 to 5 days. Clinical manifestations commonly include severe headache, malaise, and sensation of chills, with some patients experiencing muscle and joint pains, vertigo, nausea, conjunctival injection, and photophobia. Incapacitation begins with the onset of fever, and the disease may be severe to the point of prostration with weakness persisting for several weeks after the acute symptoms have subsided. No neurological abnormalities have been observed. The symptoms are accompanied by low or normal white blood cell counts.[10,12,20]

All cases of group C disease have been registered among forest laborers and laboratory personnel working with the viruses.

Pathology

No lesions have been reported in human patients infected with group C viruses.

Diagnosis

Laboratory confirmation of diagnosis is based on isolation and identification of virus from serum or whole blood samples collected from patients during the first 3 days of illness when viremia occurs. Serological diagnosis is based on significant antibody changes between acute and convalescent serum samples but the interpretation of results is often difficult due to heterologous antibody responses.[12,27]

EPIDEMIOLOGY

Occurrence

Group C arboviruses have been found in South, Central, and North America. Seven antigenic types have been identified in Brazil, and excluding Nepuyo virus, have been isolated from febrile patients in the Amazon basin. Surveys for HI antibodies have revealed prevalence rates as high as 15% in some communities of the Brazilian Amazon basin,[33] but complete absence in other communities in the same region, including populations of certain Indian villages.[23,24] A survey conducted in Belem, Brazil in 1960 showed that 11.4% of the population had antibodies to Caraparu virus and 0.41% and 3.5% were seropositive to Murutucu and Oriboca viruses, respectively,[3] with highest prevalence rates in persons living in sections of the city bordered by forest. No HI antibodies to Caraparu and Marituba viruses have been detected in military recruits from various parts of Brazil outside the Amazon basin.[22] Apeu and Itaqui viruses have been isolated exclusively in Brazil.

Outside Brazil, Caraparu and Oriboca viruses have also been recovered from patients in Surinam,[20] and Nepuyo virus from one patient in Guatemala.[26] Approximately 2.1% of 374 Dutch soldiers stationed in Surinam for 1 year acquired HI antibodies to Caraparu-like virus.[16] HI antibodies to Caraparu virus has been reported in 15% of inhabitants of eastern Peru.[19] In the eastern hemisphere, HI antibodies have been found to group C viruses in sera of residents of South and West Africa and of the U.S.S.R.,[31] but it is believed that these have resulted from infections by other viruses of the Bunyamwera supergroup.

Other members of the group have been found in several countries of the western hemisphere with Caraparu and Oriboca viruses recovered in Trinidad, Surinam, and French Guiana, and Caraparu virus in Panama.[14] Murutucu virus has been isolated in French Guiana.[14] Isolation of Marituba, Caraparu-Apeu, and Oriboca-Itaqui viruses have been reported in Peru.[25] Nepuyo virus, first isolated in Trinidad and Brazil,[28] has also been found in Panama, Mexico, Honduras,[14] and Guatemala.[26]

Reservoirs

Wild rodents and marsupials have been implicated as the main vertebrate hosts for the group C viruses. Caraparu, Murutucu, Oriboca, and Itaqui viruses have been recovered repeatedly from blood samples from *Proechimys guyannensis, Oryzomys capito,* and *Nectomys squamipes* rodents captured in the forests near Belém, Brazil. In the same area, but less frequently, marsupials have yielded Murutucu, Oriboca, and Itaqui viruses. Apeu and Marituba viruses have been isolated from viremic marsupials, but not from rodents. Nepuyo virus has been isolated once each from *Proechimys* spp. and *Nectomys* spp. in Brazil,[14] and twice from *Artibeus* spp. bats in Honduras.[8] High antibody prevalence rates to group C agents have been found in rodents and in marsupials. Rodents have exhibited higher HI antibody prevalence rates to Caraparu and Itaqui viruses than have marsupials, but the opposite has occurred to Apeu and Marituba viruses.[33]

Observations in Trinidad have indicated that *O. laticeps* and *Zygodontomys brevicauda* rodents may be commonly infected with Caraparu or Caraparu-like viruses, producing high levels of viremia.[15] These rodent populations show a high prevalence of antibodies to the Trinidad strains, and a marked seasonal fluctuation in the antibody prevalence rates.[17]

It seems probable that some group C viruses, such as Caraparu and Itaqui viruses, are rodent-associated terrestrial viruses. Others, such as Apeu and Marituba viruses seem to be maintained in an arboreal cycle in nature involving marsupials as vertebrate hosts. The two isolations of Nepuyo virus from bats in Honduras[8] raises the possibility that these animals may be vertebrate hosts for this and perhaps other group C viruses. Although no group C virus isolates have been obtained from bats in Brazil, neutralizing antibodies to Caraparu virus were found in four bat sera.[14]

Transmission

Numerous strains of the group C viruses have been obtained from *Culex* mosquitoes, and they are believed to be major vectors. Of 27 strains of Caraparu virus isolated from insects in Brazil, 13 were from *Cx. (M) vomerifer,* 3 were from *Cx. (Melanoconium) portesi* and 11 from other *Culex* spp.[14] Of 29 mosquito isolates of Caraparu or Caraparu-like strains isolated in Trinidad, 19 were from *Cx. (M) portesi.*[17] In Brazil, most arthropod isolates of Itaqui and Oriboca viruses have been obtained from *Cx. (M) portesi* and *Cx. (M) vomerifer.* Five isolates of Apeu virus have been made from *Cx. aikenii* and other *Culex* spp. Naturally infected *Cx. (M) portesi* have transmitted Marituba and Oriboca viruses to mice in the laboratory,[14,32] and transmission of Nepuyo virus to laboratory mice through bites of naturally infected *Culex* spp. has also been reported.[14] In addition to isolates from *Culex* spp. mosquitoes, isolates have also been obtained from one pool each of *Aedes arborealis* and *Ac. septemstriatus.*

CONTROL

There is no specific treatment for the group C arboviral infections. Bed rest and the administration of antipyretic drugs are recommended.

PUBLIC HEALTH ASPECTS

No firm assessment has been made of the public health impact caused by the group C viruses. In endemic areas, they may become a hazard for immigrants.

REFERENCES

1. **Ardoin, P. and Clarke, D. H.,** The use of sonication and of calcium-phosphate chromatography for preparation of Group C arbovirus hemagglutinins, *Am. J. Trop. Med. Hyg.,* 16, 357, 1967.
2. **Allen, W. P., Belman, S. G., and Borman, E. R.,** Group C arbovirus infections in Rhesus monkeys, *Am. J. Trop. Med. Hyg.,* 16, 106, 1967.

3. **Bensabath, G. and Andrade, A. H. P.,** Anticorpos para arbovírus no soro de residentes na cidade de Belém, Pará, *Rev. Serv. Espec. Saúde Publica.,* 12, 61, 1962.
4. **Bergold, G. H. and Mazzali, R.,** Plaque formation by arboviruses, *J. Gen. Virol.,* 2, 273, 1968.
5. **Buckley, S. M. and Shope, R. E.,** Comparative assay of arthropod-borne group C virus antibodies by tissue culture neutralization and hemagglutination-inhibition tests, *Am. J. Trop. Med. Hyg.,* 10, 53, 1961.
6. **Buckley, S. M., Pinheiro, F. P., and Clarke, D. H.,** Hemagglutinin formation by group C viruses in HeLa (Gey) cells, *An. Microbiol.,* 11, Parte A, 183, 1963.
7. **Buckley, S. M.,** Applicability of the HeLa (Gey) strain of human malignant epithelial cells to the propagation of arboviruses, *Proc. Soc. Exp. Biol. Med.,* 116, 354, 1964.
8. **Calisher, C. H., Chappell, W. A., Maness, K. S. C., Lord, R. D., and Sudia, W. D.,** Isolations of Nepuyo virus strains from Honduras, 1967, *Am. J. Trop. Med. Hyg.,* 20, 331, 1971.
9. **Casals, J. and Whitman, L.,** Group C, a new serological group of hitherto undescribed arthropod-borne viruses. Immunological studies, *Am. J. Trop. Med. Hyg.,* 10, 250, 1961.
10. **Causey, O. R., Causey, C. E., Maroja, O. M., and Macedo, D. G.,** The isolation of arthropod-borne viruses, including members of two hitherto undescribed serological groups, in the Amazon region of Brazil, *Am. J. Trop. Med. Hyg.,* 10, 227, 1961.
11. **De Paola, D.,** Pathology of the arboviruses, *An. Microbiol.,* 11, 187, 1963.
12. **Gibbs, C. J., Jr., Bruckner, E. A., and Schenker, S.,** A case of Apeu virus infection, *Am. J. Trop. Med. Hyg.,* 13, 108, 1964.
13. **Henderson, J. R. and Taylor, R. M.,** Propagation of certain arthropod-borne viruses in avian and primate cell cultures, *J. Immunol.,* 84, 590, 1960.
14. **Berge, T. O., Ed.,** *International Catalogue of Arboviruses, Including Certain Other Viruses of Vertebrates,* 2nd ed., Pub. No. (CDC) 75-8301, Public Health Service, Department of Health, Education and Welfare, Atlanta, 1975.
15. **Jonkers, A. H., Spence, L., Downs, W. G., and Worth, C. B.,** Laboratory studies with wild rodents and viruses native to Trinidad. II. Studies with the Trinidad Caraparu-like agent TRVL 34053-1, *Am. J. Trop. Med. Hyg.,* 13, 728, 1964.
16. **Jonkers, A. H., Spence, L., and Karbaat, J.,** Arbovirus infections in Dutch military personnel stationed in Surinam. Further studies, *Trop. Geogr. Med.,* 20, 251, 1968.
17. **Jonkers, A. H., Spence, L., Downs, W. G., Aitken, T. H. G., and Worth, C. B.,** Arbovirus studies in Bush Bush forest, Trinidad, W. I., September 1959-December 1964. VI. Rodent-associated viruses (VEE and agents of groups C and Guamá): isolations and further studies, *Am. J. Trop. Med. Hyg.,* 17, 285, 1968.
18. **Karabatsos, N., and Buckley, S. M.,** Susceptibility of the baby-hamster kidney-cell line (BHK-21) to infection with arboviruses, *Am. J. Trop. Med. Hyg.,* 16, 99, 1967.
19. **Madalengoitia, J., Flores, W. and Casals, J.,** Arbovirus antibody survey of sera from residents of Eastern Peru, *Bull. PAHO,* 7, 25, 1973.
20. **Metselaar, D.,** Isolation of arboviruses of group A and group C in Surinam, *Trop. Geogr. Med.,* 18, 137, 1966.
21. **Murphy, F. A., Harrison, A. K., and Whitfield, S. G.,** Bunyaviridae: morphologic and morphogenetic similarities of Bunyamwera serologic supergroup viruses, and several other arthropod-borne viruses, *Intervirology,* 1, 297, 1973.
22. **Niederman, J. C., Henderson, J. R., Opton, E. M., Black, F. L., and Skvrnova, K.,** A nationwide serum survey of Brazilian military recruits, 1964. II. Antibody patterns with arboviruses, polioviruses, measles and mumps, *Am. J. Epidemiol.,* 86, 319, 1967.
23. **Pinheiro, F. P.,** unpublished data, 1968.
24. **Pinheiro, F. P., Bensabath, G., Andrade, A. H. P., Lins, Z. C., Fraiha, H., Tang, A. T., Lainson, R., Shaw, J. J., and Azevedo, M. C.,** Infectious diseases along Brazil's Trans Amazon Highway: surveillance and research, *Bull. PAHO,* 8, 111, 1974.
25. **Scherer, W. F., Madalengoitia, J., Flores, W., and Acosta, M.,** Los primeros aislamientos de arbovirus de encefalitis del este y de grupos C y Guama en la region Amazonica del Peru, *Bol. Of. Sanit. Panam.,* 78, 485, 1975.
26. **Scherer, W. F., Dickerman, R. W., Ordonez, J. V., Seymour, C., III, Kramer, L. D., Jahrling, P. B., and Powers, C. D.,** Ecologic studies on Venezuelan encephalitis virus and isolations of Nepuyo and Patois viruses during 1968-1973 at a marsh habitat near the epicenter of the 1969 outbreak in Guatemala, *Am. J. Trop. Med. Hyg.,* 25, 151, 1976.
27. **Shope, R. E. and Causey, O. R.,** Further studies on the serological relationships of group C arthropod-borne viruses and the application of these relationships to rapid identification of types, *Am. J. Trop. Med. Hyg.,* 11, 283, 1962.
28. **Shope, R. E. and Whitman, L.,** Nepuyo virus, a new group C agent isolated in Trinidad and Brazil. II. Serological studies, *Am. J. Trop. Med. Hyg.,* 15, 772, 1966.

29. **Srihongse, S. and Johnson, K. M.,** Hemagglutinin production and infectivity patterns in adult hamsters inoculated with group C and other new world arboviruses, *Am. J. Trop. Med. Hyg.,* 18, 273, 1969.

30. **Stim, T. B.,** Arbovirus plaquing in two simian kidney cell lines, *J. Gen. Virol.,* 5, 329, 1969.

31. **Theiler, M. and Downs, W. G., Eds.,** *The Arthropod-Borne Viruses of Vertebrates,* 1st ed., Yale University Press, London, 1973, 227.

32. **Toda, A. and Shope, R. E.,** Transmission of Guama and Oriboca viruses by naturally infected mosquitoes, *Nature (London),* 208, 304, 1965.

33. **Woodall, J. P.,** Virus research in Amazônia, in *Atas Simpósio Biota Amazônica,* Vol. 6, Lent, H., Ed., Conselho Nacional de Pesquisas, Rio de Janiero, 1967, 31.

PIRY FEVER

F. P. Pinheiro

NAME AND SYNONYMS

The name of the etiological agent, Piry virus, is used to name the causative agent in human illness. There are no synonyms for Piry fever.

HISTORY

Piry virus is known to occur only in Brazil. The virus was isolated in 1960 from visceral organs of a marsupial *Philander opossum* captured in a forest near Belém.[8] No other strains have been recovered from naturally infected human beings, animals or insects, but several human cases of Piry virus infection have resulted from laboratory exposures. The virus was isolated from one patient; the other diagnoses have been serologically confirmed.[5] Serological evidence has indicated that Piry virus is endemic among human and wildlife populations in several areas of Brazil.[5,7]

ETIOLOGY

Piry virus is classified in the family Rhabdoviridae on the basis of its physico-chemical properties. Bullet shaped virions have been demonstrated by electron microscopy in sections of infected mouse brains and in infected BHK-21 and *Aedes albopictus* cell cultures.[2] The virions measure 155 × 62 nm, and are found budding from membranes of endoplasmic cysterns or marginal cytoplasmic membranes in the infected cells. Spherical and disc-shaped particles have been observed in infected BHK-21 cells by negative staining, and both the spherical and bullet-shaped particles have been observed in sections of cardiac muscle of infected mice.[1]

Piry virus belongs to the vesicular stomatitis (VS) antigenic group of arboviruses. It crossreacts by neutralization (N) test with the other four members of the group, especially with Chandipura virus.[5] A slight crossreaction is observed by complement-fixation (CF) test between Piry and Chandipura viruses, but not between Piry and VS New Jersey, VS Indiana or Cocal viruses.[5] The agent is readily inactivated by sodium deoxycholate. A hemagglutinin has been obtained from supernatant fluids of infected Vero cell cultures centrifuged at 40,000 rpm for 1 hr.[5] It is active against goose erythrocytes at an optimum pH of 6.2 at 4°C. However, no hemagglutinin has been obtained from brains, livers, or sera of infected mice treated with acetone, protamin, or freon-*n*-heptane[5].

The virus produces plaques in BHK-21 and GMK cell lines, and in embryonic cultures of chicken, turkey, and mouse cells overlaid with agar.[5] Several characteristic plaque sizes have been observed in embryo cell cultures infected with different strains of Piry virus.[6] It causes cytopathic effect (CPE) in Vero cells maintained under fluid medium.

DEFINITION

Piry fever is an acute, benign, febrile human illness caused by a virus of the VS group of the arboviruses.

ANIMAL INFECTION

Natural disease caused by Piry virus has not been reported in wild or domestic animals. Infant and adult Swiss mice succumb within 1 to 2 days after inoculation with high doses of the virus, either by the intracerebral (i.c.) or intraperitoneal (i.p.) routes. Adult white rats and guinea pigs survive after being infected by the i.p. route and produce antibodies against the agent. Adult hamsters develop a fatal infection when inoculated by the i.p. route. Viremia reaching as high as $10^{4.5}$ suckling mouse $LD_{50}/$ 0.02 mℓ and persisting at least 4 days before death have followed inoculation of marsupials *Didelphis spp.* and *Philander spp.* by the intramuscular (i.m.) and subcutaneous (s.c.) routes with high doses of virus.

Pathology
Experimental pathological studies in mice have shown basic damage in connective tissue, especially young connective tissue, from perichondrium, periosteum, dental germ, interstitia of skeletal muscles, myocardium, lungs and kidneys, and mesenchymal cells of liver. Lesions consist of necrotic foci of connective cells with karyorrhexis in edematous areas.[3] Electron microscopic studies have revealed cardiac alterations beginning in the mitochondria of the muscle fibers.[1] Tumefaction, cytolysis and rarefaction of the matrices of mitochondria may be observed concurrently with foci of hyperplasia of undamaged mitochondria. Later the heart fibers show tumefaction of the sarcoplasma, stretching of the myofibrilles and rupture of the myofilaments evolving to colliquative necrosis. Viral particles are observed in the cardiac fibers particularly in the endoplasmic reticula and in the vesicles located in the areas of mitochondrial hyperplasia.[1]

Diagnosis
Laboratory diagnosis of Piry virus infection depends upon the isolation and identification of the agent. For virus isolation, infant mice may be inoculated by the i.c. route with whole blood, serum, plasma, or visceral organs obtained from the animals, brains of sick mice harvested and suspended in veronal buffer, and the viral antigen identified by CF test using specific antisera or mouse hyperimmune ascitic fluid. Vero and other cell cultures susceptible to the virus may also be used for virus isolation.[4]

HUMAN INFECTION

Clinical features of Piry fever described here are based on the observations of four cases of laboratory infection which occurred in Belém, probably acquired by inhalation of aerosolized virus. Rapid onset beginning with back pain, chills, headache, and fever was followed by generalized muscular and joint pains, photophobia and congestion of the oropharynx. Fever, reaching to 38.8°C, persisted 1 to 2 days. The white blood cell counts remained within the normal limits. Recovery was uneventful following several days incapacitation.

Pathology

No lesions have been reported in human patients infected with the virus.

Diagnosis

Laboratory diagnosis is based on virus isolation and serological tests. The virus may be isolated by inoculation of patients' blood or serum i.c. into infant mice or susceptible cell lines as Vero or BHK-21. Virus isolation has been difficult to achieve, even when specimens have been collected within the first 2 days of illness. For serological diagnosis, paired acute and 2 to 3-week convalescent serum samples may be tested by CF or N tests in suckling mice or cell cultures.

EPIDEMIOLOGY

Serological surveys conducted in Brazil and other South American countries have indicated that human infections are limited to several areas of Brazil. Neutralizing antibodies to Piry virus have been detected in 4 to 17% of residents in communities surveyed in the Amazon basin.[7] Antibody prevalence rates from 13% in children below 9 years of age to 90% in persons above 50 years of age have been found in colonists from southern Brazil who were examined before moving into new settlements in the Amazon basin, suggesting that the Piry or an antigenically related virus is endemic in certain areas of southern Brazil as well.[7]

Although the prototype strain of Piry virus was isolated from the marsupial *P. opossum,* limited serological surveys have not demonstrated the presence of antibodies in opossums in the Amazon basin of Brazil. Neutralizing antibodies have, however, been found in sera of other marsupial species, in monkeys, edentates, and rodents in the Amazon basin.[5] A low antibody prevalence rate has been reported in water buffaloes and swine, but antibodies were not detected in a small number of horses and cattle tested in this area.[5] It is postulated that the virus is maintained in the Amazon basin in a sylvatic host-vector cycle, but the importance of various suspected mammalian hosts and the possible vectors have yet to be determined. Only serological evidence for Piry, or an antigenically related virus, has been reported in southern Brazil, and no studies on its ecology there have been conducted.

CONTROL

No specific treatment or vaccine is available for Piry fever.

Due to the high risk of infection among laboratory personnel, care should be taken by persons handling the virus. Preferrably, laboratory studies should be performed under aseptic hoods and wearing masks and gloves.

PUBLIC HEALTH ASPECTS

No information is available on a possible public health impact caused by the agent.

REFERENCES

1. **Araújo, R., Dias, L. B., Araújo, M. T. F., Pinheiro, F. P., and Moutinho, E. R. C.,** Miocardite experimental em camundongos albinos por virus Piry (Be An 24232). Estudo anatomo-patologico em microscopia otica e em microscopia electronica com demonstracão de particula viral, *Rev. Inst. Med. Trop. S. Paulo,* 20(2), 102, 1978.
2. **Bergold, G. H. and Munz, K.,** Characterization of Piry virus, *Arch. Gesamte Virusforsch.,* 31, 152, 1970.
3. **Dias, L. B.,** personal communication, 1977.
4. **Hammon, W. M. and Sather, G. E.,** Arboviruses, in *Diagnostic Procedures for Viral and Rickettsial Infections,* 4th ed., Lennette, E. H. and Schmidt, N. J., Eds., American Public Health Association, Inc., New York, 1969, 227.
5. **Berge, T. O., Ed.,** *International Catalogue of Arboviruses, Including Certain Other Viruses of Vertebrates,* 2nd ed., Pub. No. (CDC) 75-8301, Public Health Service, Department of Health Education and Welfare, Atlanta, 1975.
6. **Pinheiro, F. P.,** unpublished data, 1966.
7. **Pinheiro, F. P., Bensabath, G., Andrade, A. H. P., Lins, Z. C., Fraiha, H., Tang, A. T., Lainson, R., Shaw, J. J., and Azevedo, M. C.,** Infectious diseases along Brazil's Trans Amazon highway: surveillance and research. *Bull. PAHO,* 8, 111, 1974.
8. **Woodall, J. P.,** Virus research in Amazônia, in *Atas Simpósio Biota Amazônica,* Vol. 6, Lent, H., Ed., Conselho Nacional de Pesquisas, Rio de Janeiro, 1967, 31.

LOUPING ILL

C. E. G. Smith and M. G. R. Varma

NAME AND SYNONYMS

Louping ill is named after one or more of its clinical signs in sheep: affected animals may show nervous hyperactivity, leaping (louping, Scottish dialect) off the ground when startled, and in the ataxic stage, may have a "leaping" gait. Muscular twitching or tremors are common, and the disease is also called "trembling." This term has been confused in early French veterinary textbooks with la tremblante, a synonym for scrapie, a slow virus disease of sheep. The disease is also called *thwarter-ill,* a derivative of thorter-ill, probably referring to the distortion or twisting of the neck in the disease.

HISTORY

Experiments and observations published in 1897[56] by Williams showed, almost beyond doubt, that louping ill was transmitted to sheep by ticks (*Ixodes spp.*) He described the death from louping ill of 40 of 183 sheep when moved from a hill pasture onto a partially wooded one with an exceptionally high tick population. The relevant tick species and their behavior in relation to transmission were described by Wheler in 1899.[52] In 1930, Pool et al.[31] described serial transmission in the laboratory from sheep to sheep, and from sheep to swine by intracerebral inoculation of brain tissue from two naturally affected sheep. In 1931, Greig et al.[16] showed that a filterable virus was the cause of the disease, and that sheep which survived following subcutaneous inoculation were subsequently refractory to intracerebral challenge. MacLeod and Gordon, in 1932,[24] demonstrated transmission to sheep by nymphs and adults of *Ixodes ricinus* which, in their previous stage, had engorged on affected sheep. The early literature on louping ill has been reviewed by Pool.[32] The host relationships of *I. ricinus* have been exhaustively described by Milne,[28] and the ecology of the tick by MacLeod.[26] During large scale field trials of formalinized louping ill vaccine in sheep in 1935, it was recognized that scrapie virus could be a contaminant of louping ill vaccine stocks, and could remain infectious through the inactivation process.[17,57]

ETIOLOGY

Louping ill virus is antigenically very closely related to Russian spring-summer encephalitis virus complex,[1] and is classified in the tick-borne virus subgroup of the genus *Flavivirus* (group B arboviruses) of the family Togaviridae. The virions measure 22 to 27 nm. They are inactivated by ether or sodium deoxycholate. The optimal conditions for hemagglutination are at pH 6.4 and at 22 and 37° C. The virus produces paralysis and death in 3 to 4 days in suckling mice and in 7 days in adult mice inoculated intracerebrally (i.c.). Plaques are produced in porcine kidney cells (PS) and monkey kidney (Vero; LLC-MK$_2$) cell lines.

DEFINITION

Louping ill is a biphasic meningoencephalomyelitis principally affecting sheep, but also affecting cattle, red grouse (*Lagopus scoticus*), and less frequently, human beings in areas of rough hill pasture in Scotland, Northern England, Wales, and Ireland. Its seasonal occurrence is determined by the spring and autumn activity peaks of its tick host, *I. ricinus.* The virus has been isolated from a number of small mammal species, but their significance as reservoir hosts of the virus remains undetermined. The infection may be wholly maintained in a sheep-tick or sheep-tick-grouse cycle. Most recorded human infections have followed laboratory exposure. Transmission to human beings by ticks have been rare because the vector ticks only infrequently bite people, usually being limited to high contact persons as shepherds and abbattoir workers.

ANIMAL INFECTION

Sheep

Clinically, louping ill in sheep is typically a biphasic disease. The initial or viremic phase is characterized by fever, dullness, and a tendency to lie down. The second phase starts with a transient stage of excitability in which the animals tremble all over, lips and nostrils twitch, and if disturbed unexpectedly, the animals may suddenly leap into the air. Cerebellar ataxia follows with unsteady gait, staggering, and inability to maintain standing balance. There is often frothing at the nostrils and ropy saliva drooling from the mouth. Affected sheep become prostrate, and paddle violently with their feet, sometimes turning around on the ground, making characteristic depressions in the turf which are readily recognized by shepherds in endemic areas. Progressive paralysis follows, and infected sheep usually die within a short period. Sheep which recover from the second phase often remain unthrifty and may have wry necks or other residual paralysis.

In experimental studies,[33,34] 22 of 33 six-month-old sheep inoculated subcutaneously (s.c.) with 10^7 mouse LD_{50}, or cell culture plaque-forming unit (p.f.u.) doses of virus, were moribund within 6 to 11 days (mean 8 days). Ataxia rapidly progressed to complete flaccid paralysis within 3 to 5 hr. Two of eleven which survived were "chronically debilitated". Viremia was detected within 24 hr following inoculation, lasting until day 5 in those which survived, and longer in those which died. Viremia titer reached 10^3 to 3×10^7 p.f.u./0.2 mℓ on days 3 and 4, with the high levels recorded in those animals which died. Hemagglutination-inhibiting (HI) antibodies appeared by day 5 in sheep which survived, and by day 6 in those which died; maximum HI antibody titers were reached around day 8 in both groups. Initial antibody rises were IgM which persisted until wholly replaced by IgG around day 16. Neutralizing (N) antibodies were detected as early as day 3, and reached high levels by day 5, with highest titers in sheep which survived.

In other experiments, strain differences in virulence for sheep has been demonstrated with field virus. Sheep of all ages appear to be uniformly susceptible to subcutaneous inoculation. The incidence of encephalomyelitis in louping ill infection has been shown to be enhanced by concurrent tick-borne fever, an *Ehrlichia* infection also transmitted by *I. ricinus*,[13,15] by stress such as movement by truck from one pasture to another,[15] by poor nutritional state,[12,43] and possibly by cold and exertion.[43]

The outcome of infections in lambs has been demonstrated in a typical outbreak in Ayrshire[43] in spring of 1960. An approximate 80% clinical attack rate with a mortality of 62.5%, and an antibody prevalence rate in survivors of 60% were recorded. Mortality tended to diminish with age: in an outbreak in southern Eire,[48] 50 of 120 sheep, from an uninfected area exposed in an infected one, died of louping ill in the autumn. When these 50 were replaced, 50 of the flock of 120 died in the following autumn of louping ill.

Louping ill is often readily diagnosed by experienced shepherds, especially in outbreaks, by its seasonal occurrence, its association with tick-infested pastures, and its well-known clinical features. In individual cases, differential diagnosis is required from other sporadic tick-borne infections. Tick-borne fever may resemble the febrile phase of louping ill and tick pyemia[13] characterized by abscesses, especially in the central nervous system may cause paralysis. Diagnosis can be confirmed by histological examination of the brain, by virus isolation from brain or blood, or by serological tests. Characteristic lesions may be observed in the central nervous system, histologically as a typical arboviral meningoencephalomyelitis. The changes include congestion and infiltration of the meninges, perivascular cuffing, and neuronal degeneration in the cerebrum, cerebellum, and medulla. These are readily distinguishable from lesions of other central nervous system diseases of sheep in the British Isles. The virus may be readily isolated by i.c. inoculation of mice or inoculation of susceptible cell cultures. Neutralizing antibody titers may be measured in mice,[30] or in cell cultures;[34] HI antibody titers are measured by standard techniques.[30,34] Comparisons of paired sera taken early and late in the infection are desirable, but early specimens are often unavailable. Recent infections may usually be inferred from a high antibody titer appearing soon after the disease, and declining significantly over a following 4-week period.[30]

Cattle

There is no published information on the disease in cattle. Roberts has described sporadic cases of fatal illness in cattle confirmed histologically as louping ill in Wales.* Scattered observations have suggested that occasional cases may occur in cattle throughout the area where the disease is endemic in sheep.

Grouse

On a number of occasions, red grouse have been found sick or dead on the moors, and louping ill virus has been isolated from their brains.[36,49,55] In one case in a captive bird, infected ticks were believed to have been introduced in heather set out for feed for the bird.[45] Clinical descriptions are limited to experimental infections;[37,55] 2 to 8 days after inoculation in the tarsal pads, such birds have shown depression, anorexia, muscular weakness, and regurgitation of crop contents on handling, but no identifiable neurological signs have been recorded. In one study of 37 experimentally infected grouse, viremia was detected within 24 hr, lasted 6 to 7 days, and reached a peak of 10^4 to $10^{6.9}$ p.f.u./0.2 mℓ) on days 3 to 5. HI antibodies appeared by days 5 to 6, and maximum titers by days 8 to 10. A total of 29 birds died.[37] Lesions of the central nervous system[5] were characterized by perivascular cuffing in the meninges and superficial brain substance, and a small number of degenerated neurons, mainly in the anterior brainstem and basal ganglia. In birds dying between the 5th and 7th days of disease, changes were seen mainly in the cerebrum and optic lobes; in birds dying later, changes were more severe and generalized.

In a field survey, antibodies were detected in 17 of 181 apparently healthy shot birds.[55] However, Hardy, Scherer, and Warner[20] have shown that nonspecific neutralizing substances may appear in the blood of shot small birds, probably as a result of trauma to abdominal and thoracic viscera, so the significance of these findings remains in doubt.

HUMAN INFECTION

Human infections have most frequently been reported following needle prick or aerosol exposure in the laboratory. The human disease was first described in a laboratory-exposed patient.[38] Two cases occurred in persons engaged in skinning carcasses of non-

---

*   Roberts, H. E., Divisional Veterinary Officer, Aberystwyth, Wales, personal communication, 1977.

tick-infested sheep.[12] One infection followed a dental operation.[53] At least 26 laboratory acquired human cases have been reported.[12,35,38] Nine naturally acquired human cases have been described,[2,9,22,23] five of them probably exposed to tick bites, and four in which the source of infection could not be determined. One person had been skinning tick-infested sheep prior to his onset of illness.[22] Serological evidence exists of subclinical human infections.[12,22,38]

The disease in human patients is characteristically biphasic, closely resembling the biphasic meningoencephalitis caused by the very closely related Central European tick-borne encephalitis virus which is also transmitted by *I. ricinus*. After an incubation period estimated as 4 to 7 days, the first "influenzal" phase lasts 2 to 11 days, followed by an asymptomatic interval of 5 to 15 days (usually 5 or 6 days), and then by the second meningoencephalomyelitis phase, with a febrile period lasting 4 to 10 days. Either phase may be completely inapparent, or so mild as to go unrecognized.

The first phase is characterized by fever, headache (sometimes severe), weakness, and anorexia with various combinations of muscle or joint pains or tenderness (often lumbar, also legs, neck), retro-orbital pain, photophobia, conjunctivitis, diplopia, excessive sweating (sometimes without fever), insomnia, drowsiness, nausea, vomiting (sometimes projectile), and tender lymphadenitis (cervical except in one case where axillary glands were also involved), with or without pharyngitis.

After the symptomless interval, the second phase is characterized by severe headache, fever, vomiting, bradycardia, drowsiness (which may develop into coma), confusion, and sometimes delirium, tremors, nystagmus, or ataxia. Some patients develop diplopia, blurred vision, slurred speech, and excessive sweating in the absence of fever. Other less commonly seen symptoms include papular abdominal rash, vesicles on the palate, subconjunctival hemorrhages, deafness, severe diarrhea, and incontinence. Paralysis may involve one or both lower limbs or may be limited to ptosis of one eyelid or strabismus. Like the symptoms, physical signs have been highly variable, including neck stiffness, Kernig's sign, loss of reflexes, papilloedema, retrobulbar neuritis, ataxia, and pyramidal signs.

Clinical laboratory findings have included a mild leucopenia in the first phase, and often a leucocytosis in the second. The cerebrospinal (CSF) abnormalities are typical of aseptic meningitis with 50 to 800 cells (polymorphs initially predominating, lymphocytes later) and increased protein (reaching 200 mg/100 mℓ in one case at the 52nd day of disease). There may be a paretic Lange curve. In the second phase, electroencephalography may show diffuse changes predominantly on one side. Differential diagnoses, which must be considered in the second phase cases, include cerebral tumors or abscesses, tuberculous meningitis, and various types of aseptic meningitis.

After the 4 to 10 day febrile period, signs and symptoms disappear rapidly, although patients have been unable to return to work for 4 to 17 weeks after the second phase. Sequelae have been slight, but have included minor paresis and ataxia. CSF abnormalities have persisted up to 1 year following clinical recovery. Treatment is symptomatic, but dramatic improvement was observed in one near-comatose patient administered intravenous hydrocortisone.[50] All known human patients have survived.

In a review of the reported human cases of louping ill, in four of the nine naturally acquired cases, no initial phase was recognized. In all of the laboratory acquired cases, a first phase was described probably because the patients were under closer observation and some, or their attending physicians, would have been aware of the biphasic nature of the disease. Sixteen of the twenty-four laboratory cases had no recognized second phase. It is likely that such cases would remain undiagnosed outside the laboratory situation.

One aberrant laboratory case[8] appeared to have been limited to the first phase but without headache. The patient had injected conjunctiva, redness and edema of the oral mucous membranes, pharyngeal injection, ulceration of the soft palate, epistaxis, petechial hemorrhages on the face, neck, and forearms, and sinus tachycardia. Thrombocytopenia was associated with the hemorrhagic episodes. The clinical disease very closely resembled laboratory infections with the related Kyasanur Forest disease virus. Several cases in Northern Ireland which were retrospectively diagnosed as louping ill had been classed as poliomyelitis-like diseases.[23]

Laboratory diagnosis may be on the basis of virus isolation and identification, or on serological tests on paired sera. In the first clinical phase, virus may be isolated from the blood,[35] and early in the second phase from cerebrospinal fluid.[2] Neutralization,[34] HI, or complement fixation (CF) tests may be used in serological tests.[50] CF antibodies may be detectable as early as the onset of phase 2, usually rising by the end of the third week of disease, and reaching a maximum at 5 to 7 weeks. CF and N antibody titers rise more rapidly than do HI titers. Antibody titers may be measured in CSF as well, with titers generally lower than in sera; the ratio of serum/CSF titers compared with the ratio of titers characteristic for other viral encephalitides, as poliomyelitis, may have some differential diagnostic value. Webb et al.[50] found significant reductions of the normal ratio (256:1 to 2048:1[7]), 5 to 12 weeks after onset in one case and between 6 weeks and 1 year after onset in another.

EPIDEMIOLOGY

Louping ill is distributed throughout the rough hill grazing areas of Scotland, northern England, Wales, and Ireland. Its distribution is patchy, varying from enzootic in sheep in some areas as in the eastern Scottish border counties, to periodically epizootic in others, as the western Scottish borders.[43]

The disease has not been recorded in other areas of the British Isles although both sheep and *I. ricinus* are widely distributed. The behavior and ecology of *I. ricinus* play a major role in the epidemiology of the disease. For survival, the ticks require resting places which have an ambient temperature of at least 15°C for a period long enough for development, and which have an almost saturated relative humidity when temperatures exceed 15°C.[26] The most common habitats are in areas where the soil remains damp throughout the summer as marsh, peat, or moss-covered areas, and where there is a thick and usually matted vegetation cover like heather, bracken, and old and matted bent- or moor-grass. Such conditions are widely distributed on poorly drained hill pastures in the British Isles, especially in the Grampians, the Border Uplands, the Cumbrian hills, the Pennines, the Yorkshire moors, north Wales, and over much of Ireland. In a comparison of two hill pastures in Ayrshire,[43] on one that was sloping and well-drained, the antibody conversion rate in sheep was 31%, and the incidence in sentinel 1-year-old sheep was 11%; on the other, with large areas of swampy ground with thick grass and rushes, the corresponding rates were 88% and 50 to 60% respectively during the same season.

The biting activities of *I. ricinus* are confined to periods when the average weekly temperature is between 7 and 18°C.[26] Transmission, therefore, occurs in spring and autumn, the precise timing in any year varying with altitude and latitude, and with the weather. As lambing on hill pastures is timed to coincide with favorable weather conditions and the growth of grass, and varies with these same tick biting factors, lambing often occurs at the spring periods of maximum tick activity. During years when tick activity precedes lambing by as much as 2 to 3 weeks, immunity in the ewes is boosted, and previously nonimmune ewes may develop sufficient antibody levels soon enough to protect their lambs by transfer of passive immunity through colostrum. When tick activity is late in relation to lambing, only lambs of ewes with a high level of immunity, following infection in the previous year or following vaccination, will be protected.

Although *I. ricinus* will feed on any bird or mammal exposed to it,[28] sheep may support over 90% of the vector tick populations in northwest England. In the absence of sheep,[25] other mammals and birds may play a role in maintaining tick populations, and determine the presence or absence of the vector. The more common wild mammals of hill pasture, which may support *I. ricinus,* include red deer (*Cervus elaphus*) in the highlands and islands, hares (the brown hare, *Lepus europaeus* and the Scottish mountain hare, *L. timidus scoticus*), the common shrew (*Sorex araneus*), the long-tailed field mouse (*Apodemus sylvaticus*), and the field vole (*Microtus agrestis*). On a farm with endemic louping ill in sheep in Ayrshire, 44% of the small mammals trapped were *S. araneus,* 27% *M. agrestis,* and 13% *A. sylvaticus.*[42] Red deer may carry very heavy tick loads (up to 3000 to 4000 adult females per animal[21]), and hares may be heavily infested with all stages. Because of their smaller size, shrews, field mice and voles have much smaller tick loads. In the study in Ayrshire, *S. araneus* carried an average of 2 to 4 larvae per animal, *M. agrestis* 2 to 4 larvae, and 1 to 2 nymphs per animal, and *A. sylvaticus* 2 to 7 larvae per animal.[47] Milne[28] pointed out that in general, infestation is proportional to "sweeping front" area, thus a wide shaggy adult sheep will have much more opportunity for infestation than a lamb or a hare. In northwest England he found infestation rates in small mammals of 67% of *S. araneus,* 43% of *M. agrestis,* 65% of *A. sylvaticus,* 100% of hedgehogs (*Erinaceus europaeus*), and 51% of rabbits (*Oryctolagus cuniculus*). Those species which fluctuate widely in population numbers as voles, rabbits, partridges (*Perdix perdix*), and red grouse,[27] have been shown to play a significant role in fluctuations in tick populations, because in high years they enable a higher proportion of immature stages of *I. ricinus* to feed and reach the next stages. Voles which show large population fluctuations[6] were incriminated in an epidemic in sheep the year following a peak in the population of voles in Ayrshire.[43] The red grouse may be heavily tick-infested, especially with immature stages; as many as 157 larvae and nymphs have been recorded on a single chick.[46]

While any vertebrate species is likely to be infected incidentally by ticks in an infected area, only those species which circulate enough virus in their blood to infect ticks will transmit the infection and thus could act as reservoir hosts. Louping ill virus has been isolated from the brains of *S. araneus, A. sylvaticus,*[42] and red grouse;[36,45,55] antibodies have been demonstrated in red deer.[10] The minimal blood concentration required to infect *I. ricinus* is not known, but species with high viremias may be more likely to infect ticks regularly than those with low viremias. Compared with the high viremias exhibited by sheep and red grouse,[33,37] viremia seems to be transient and of low level in voles (duration 4 days, maximum titer $< 10^{1.5}$ LD$_{50}$),[40,47] field mice,[47] and hedgehogs (maximum titer $10^{1.7}$ LD$_{50}$) following experimental infection).* No information is available about viremia in shrews. On the basis of available information, sheep and red grouse appear to be the major reservoir hosts of louping ill.

Where the infection is endemic in sheep over a long period, the annual incidence of disease varies widely, but cases occur each year. Smith et al.[43] were able to calculate that with a stable infection rate in ewes of 40 to 60% per annum, the mean louping ill rate in lambs of gimmers or two-year-old ewes having their first lambs (which usually make up 1/5 to 1/6 of the flock) would be about 25%, and about 12% in all lambs. If the infection rate in ewes were to reach 90%, less than 2% of lambs would suffer from the disease. Both levels of prevalence have been observed in the Scottish borders.

---

*   Varma, M. G. R. and Smith, C. E. G., London School of Hygiene and Tropical Medicine, London, U.K., unpublished data, 1977.

In endemic areas, lambs frequently become infected before protection from maternally-derived antibodies is lost, developing active immunity without disease, and yearly boosting this immunity by re-exposure. This is well recognized by farmers who call it "acclimatization", and when farms are traded in these areas, the sheep are sold with them. When sheep from noninfected areas are introduced on to such farms, mortality from louping ill is high.[48] In nonendemic areas, the infection may be introduced at intervals and cause typical epidemics in lambs,[43] followed by a number of endemic years during which the incidence of clinical infection decreases.

The role of louping ill in controlling grouse populations is undetermined. Watt et al.[49] described a moor on which the population of red grouse had been high 10 years earlier, but at the time of reporting, although good broods were hatching, birds 4 to 6 weeks old were commonly seen sick, and grouse numbers were steadily declining. No laboratory diagnoses were made.

Infections appear to be uncommon in human beings, believed to be because of infrequent exposure by ticks. Ross[39] tested 408 paired-serum samples from residents of western Scotland during a year when louping ill was prevalent in sheep; 374 were from aseptic meningitis patients, 10 from patients with poliomyelitis-like illnesses, and 24 of encephalitis or meningoencephalitis patients. The only positive finding was in a farmer with a history of meningoencephalitis. Walton and Kennedy[48] found antibodies in 3 of 11 human sera collected in an epidemic area.

CONTROL

Control of louping ill in sheep is primarily based on vaccination. Tick control by dipping contributes to reducing parasitizing tick populations, but alone has not been shown to have a marked effect on the incidence of the disease in sheep on hill pastures. Dipping is effective only against attached ticks, leaving the very considerable tick populations on pastures untouched. Most commonly used dips are organophosphorus compounds, dioxathion, coumaphos, and Dursban®, all of which are commercially available, have good immediate kill, and prevent reinfestation for up to a month. Field trials with a new diamidine compound in East Scotland have shown that it compares favorably with these standard products.[19] Other methods of environmental control, including pasture rotation, cutting or burning of long grass, bushes and bracken, and drainage are not usually economically feasible on hill pastures. In an area in southwest Scotland, ditching and drainage followed by forestation significantly reduced tick populations.

Vaccination

As early as 1924, Stockman[44] reported experimental premunition by injecting susceptible sheep with the blood of acutely ill animals. The hazard was "not serious" in sheep more than 6-months-old, but was "often very severe" in young lambs. In 1934, Gordon[14,15] described a vaccine prepared of formalinized brain, spinal cord, and spleen from infected sheep. Laboratory[11] and field studies[15] showed that this vaccine would protect sheep if 3 to 4 doses at 2-week intervals were used to stimulate production of protective levels of antibody. Although a single dose caused no detectable antibody response, and did not protect sheep from developing viremia following natural infection,[30,54] it was effective in the field in considerably reducing the incidence of disease in sheep and cattle.[15] Inactivated vaccines were widely used in this way until 1967 when it was decided that the human health hazards in their production were too great. In 1965, O'Reilley et al.[29] reported successful laboratory and field studies in the use of antigenically related Langat virus[41] as a live-virus vaccine for sheep. This virus was nonpathogenic to sheep and gave significant protection against louping ill, at least equal to that provided by the formalinized brain tissue vaccine then in current use. Grešiková et al.[18] has described an attenuated vaccine prepared from a strain of louping ill virus which was nonpathogenic and conferred protection in sheep.

In 1970, Brotherston and Boyce[3] described a vaccine made from virulent louping ill virus grown in sheep kidney-cell cultures, formalinized, then concentrated tenfold by methanol precipitation, and administered emulsified in mineral oil. Laboratory and field studies[4] showed that a single dose of this vaccine elicited an antibody response and protected both sheep and their lambs (by passive antibody transfer) for at least 1 year and probably for 2 to 3 years. This vaccine is now commercially available and in general use.

The risk to people outside laboratories, and possibly abattoirs where infected sheep are handled, is small, and justifies no control measures. Abattoir workers should obviously avoid tick bites. For persons in high risk of exposure, a vaccine suitable for human use is needed. A formalinized mouse brain tissue vaccine[12] used on an experimental basis affords some, but not complete protection.

PUBLIC HEALTH ASPECTS

Louping ill is important as a public health hazard to laboratory personnel working with it, and to a lesser extent, as an occupational hazard of shepherds, abattoir, and veterinary workers. It occurs very rarely, if at all, among sportsmen and others who frequent rough hill pastures for recreational purposes.

REFERENCES

1. **Berge, T. O.,** Ed., *International Catalogue of Arboviruses,* 2nd ed., Pub. no. (CDC) 75-8031, Public Health Service, U.S. Department of Health, Education and Welfare, Atlanta, 1975.
2. **Brewis, E. G., Neubauer, C., and Hurst, E. W.,** Another case of louping-ill in man. Isolation of the virus, *Lancet,* 1, 689, 1949.
3. **Brotherston, J. G. and Boyce, J. B.,** Development of a non-infective protective antigen against louping-ill (arbovirus group B). Laboratory experiments, *J. Comp. Pathol.,* 80, 377, 1970.
4. **Brotherston, J. G., Bannatyne, C. C., Mathieson, A. O., and Nicholson, T. B.,** Field trials of an inactivated oil-adjuvant vaccine against louping-ill (arbovirus group B), *J. Hyg.,* 69, 469, 1971.
5. **Buxton, D. and Reid, H. W.,** Experimental infection of red grouse with louping-ill virus (flavivirus group). II. Neuropathology, *J. Comp. Pathol.,* 85, 231, 1975.
6. **Chitty, D.,** Self regulation of numbers through changes in viability, *Cold Spring Harbor Symp. Quant. Biol.,* 22, 277, 1957.
7. **Clarke, J. K., Dane, D. S., and Dick, G. W. A.,** Viral antibody in the cerebrospinal fluid and serum of multiple sclerosis patients, *Brain,* 88, 953, 1965.
8. **Cooper, W. C., Green, I. J., and Fresh, J. W.,** Laboratory infection with louping-ill virus: a case study, *Br. Med. J.,* 2, 1627, 1964.
9. **Davison, G., Neubauer, C., and Hurst, E. W.,** Meningo-encephalitis in man due to the louping-ill virus, *Lancet,* 2, 453, 1948.
10. **Dunn, A. M.,** Louping-ill. The red deer (*Cervus elaphus*) as an alternative host of the virus in Scotland, *Br. Vet. J.,* 116, 284, 1960.
11. **Edward, D. G. ff.,** Methods for investigating immunization against louping-ill, *Br. J. Exp. Pathol.,* 28, 368, 1947.
12. **Edward, D. G. ff.,** Immunization against louping-ill. Immunization of man, *Br. J. Exp. Pathol.,* 29, 372, 1948.
13. **Foggie, A.,** Studies on tick pyaemia and tick-borne fever, *Symp. Zool. Soc. London,* 6, 51, 1962.
14. **Gordon, W. S.,** The control of certain diseases of sheep, *Vet. Rec.,* Ser. N., 14, 1, 1934.

15. **Gordon, W. S., Brownlee, A., Wilson, D. R., and MacLeod, J.,** The epizootiology of louping-ill and tick-borne fever with observations on the control of these sheep diseases, *Symp. Zool. Soc. London,* 6, 1, 1962.

16. **Greig, J. R., Brownlee, A., Wilson, D. R., and Gordon, W. S.,** The nature of louping-ill, *Vet. Rec.,* 11, 325, 1931.

17. **Greig, J. R.,** Scrapie in sheep, *J. Comp. Pathol.,* 60, 263, 1950.

18. **Grešíková, M., Albrecht, P., and Ernek, E.,** Studies of attenuated and virulent louping-ill virus. Biology of viruses of the tick-borne encephalitis complex, *Proc. Symp. Czech. Acad. Sci.,* Smolenice, 1960, Libikova, H., Ed., 1962, 294.

19. **Griffiths, A. J.,** *Proc. 8th British Insecticide and Fungicide Conference,* 1975, 557.

20. **Hardy, J. L., Scherer, W. F., and Warner, D. W.,** Arbovirus neutralizing substances in avian plasmas, *Am. J. Trop. Med. Hyg.,* 13, 867, 1964.

21. **Hendrick, J., Moore, W., and Morison, G. D.** The tick problem, *Vet. Rec.,* 50, 1534, 1938.

22. **Lawson, J. H., Manderson, W. G., and Hurst, E. W.,** Louping-ill meningoencephalitis. A further case and a serological survey, *Lancet,* 2, 696, 1949.

23. **Likar, M. and Dane, D. S.,** An illness resembling acute poliomyelitis caused by a virus of the Russian spring-summer encephalitis/louping-ill group in Northern Ireland, *Lancet,* 1, 456, 1958.

24. **MacLeod, J. and Gordon, W. S.,** Studies in louping-ill (an encephalomyelitis of sheep). II. Transmission by the sheep tick *Ixodes ricinus* L. *J. Comp. Pathol.,* 45, 240, 1932.

25. **MacLeod, J.,** The part played by alternative hosts in maintaining the tick population of hill pastures, *J. Anim. Ecol.,* 3, 161, 1934.

26. **MacLeod, J.,** Ticks and disease in domestic stock in Great Britain, *Symp. Zool. Soc. London,* 6, 29, 1962.

27. **Middleton, A. D.,** Periodic fluctuations in British game populations, *J. Anim. Ecol.,* 3, 231, 1934.

28. **Milne, A.,** The ecology of the sheep tick, *Ixodes ricinus* L. Host relationships of the tick. Part 2. Observations on hill and moorland grazings in northern England, *Parasitol.,* 40, 14, 1949.

29. **O'Reilly, K. J., Smith, C. E. G., McMahon, D. A., Wilson, A. L., and Robertson, J. M.,** Infection of sheep and monkeys with Langat virus: cross-protection against other viruses of the Russian spring-summer complex, *J. Hyg. Camb.,* 63, 213, 1965.

30. **O'Reilly, K. J., Smith, C. E. G., McMahon, D. A., Bowen, E. T. W., and White, G.,** A comparison of methods of measuring the persistence of neutralizing and haemagglutinin-inhibiting antibodies to louping-ill virus in experimentally infected sheep, *J. Hyg.,* 66, 217, 1968.

31. **Pool, W. A., Brownlee, A., and Wilson, D. R.,** The etiology of louping-ill, *J. Comp. Pathol.,* 43, 253, 1930.

32. **Pool, W. A.,** The etiology of louping-ill. A review of the literature, *Vet. J.,* 87, 222, 1931.

33. **Reid, H. W. and Doherty, P. C.,** Experimental louping-ill in sheep and lambs. I. Viraemia and the antibody response, *J. Comp. Pathol.,* 81, 291, 1971.

34. **Reid, H. W. and Doherty, P. C.,** Louping-ill encephalomyelitis in the sheep. I. The relationship of viraemia and the antibody response to susceptibility, *J. Comp. Pathol.,* 81, 521, 1971.

35. **Reid, H. W., Gibbs, C. A., Burrells, C., and Doherty, P. C.,** Laboratory infections with louping-ill virus, *Lancet,* 1, 592, 1972.

36. **Reid, H. W. and Boyce, J. B.,** Louping-ill virus in red grouse in Scotland, *Vet. Rec.,* 95, 150, 1974.

37. **Reid, H. W.,** Experimental infection of red grouse with louping-ill virus (flavivirus group), *J. Comp. Pathol.,* 85, 223, 1975.

38. **Rivers, T. M. and Schwentker, F. F.,** Louping-ill in man, *J. Exp. Med.,* 59, 669, 1934.

39. **Ross, C. A. C.,** Louping-ill in the west of Scotland, *Lancet,* 2, 527, 1961.

40. **Seamer, J. and Zlotnik, I.,** Louping-ill and Semliki Forest virus infections in the short-tailed vole, *Microtus agrestis* (L.), *Br. J. Exp. Pathol.,* 51, 385, 1970.

41. **Smith, C. E. G.,** A virus resembling Russian spring-summer encephalitis from an Ixodid tick in Malaya, *Nature (London),* 178, 581, 1956.

42. **Smith, C. E. G., Varma, M. G. R., and McMahon, D. A.,** Isolation of louping-ill virus from small mammals in Ayrshire, Scotland, *Nature (London),* 203, 992, 1964.

43. **Smith, C. E. G., McMahon, D. A., O'Reilly, K. J., Wilson, A. L., and Robertson, J. M.,** The epidemiology of louping-ill in Ayrshire: the first year of studies in sheep, *J. Hyg. Camb.,* 62, 53, 1964.

44. **Stockman, S.,** Louping-ill, *Trans. Highl. Agric. Soc., Scotl.,* 36, 1, 1924.

45. **Timoney, P. J.,** Recovery of louping-ill virus from the red grouse in Ireland, *Br. Vet. J.,* 128, 19, 1972.

46. **Varma, M. G. R.,** The acarology of louping-ill, *Acarologia, fasc. h.s., 1964,* 241, 1964.

47. **Varma, M. G. R. and Smith, C. E. G.,** The epidemiology of louping-ill in Ayrshire, Scotland. II. Ectoparasites of small mammals (Ixodidae), *Folia Parasitol. (Prague),* 18, 63, 1971.

48. **Walton, G. A. and Kennedy, R. C.,** Tick-borne encephalitis virus in Southern Ireland, *Br. Vet. J.,* 122, 427, 1966.
49. **Watt, J. A., Brotherston, J. G. and Campbell, J.,** Louping-ill in red grouse, *Vet. Rec.,* 75, 1151, 1963.
50. **Webb, H. E., Connolly, J. H., Kane, F. F., O'Reilly, K. J. and Simpson, D. I. H.,** Laboratory infections with louping-ill with associated encephalitis, *Lancet,* 2, 255, 1968.
51. **Wessemeier, K.,** *Arch. Klin. Med.,* 182, 451, 1938.
52. **Wheler, E. G.,** Louping-ill and the grass tick, *J. R. Agric. Soc. Engl.,* Ser. 3, 9, 5, 1899.
53. **Wiebel, H.,** Über Louping-ill beim Menschen, *Klin. Wochenschr.,* 16, 632, 1937.
54. **Williams, H. and Thorburn, H.,** The serological response of sheep to infection with louping-ill virus, *J. Hyg.,* 59, 437, 1961.
55. **Williams, H., Thorburn, H., and Zeffo, G. S.,** Isolation of louping-ill virus from the red grouse, *Nature (London),* 200, 193, 1963.
56. **Williams, P.,** Louping-ill. Further researches into the causation and prevention of louping-ill or trembling in sheep. Ixodic toxaemia, *Trans. Highl. Agric. Soc. Scot.,* 9, 278, 1897.
57. **Wilson, D. R., Anderson, R. D., and Smith, W.,** Studies in scrapie, *J. Comp. Pathol.,* 60, 267, 1950.

ARBOVIRAL ZOONOSES IN CENTRAL EUROPE

TICK-BORNE ENCEPHALITIS (TBE)

M. Grěsíková and G. W. Beran

NAME AND SYNONYMS

Tick-borne encephalitis is caused by a complex of group B arboviruses transmitted by ticks of the family Ixodidae. There are two recognized types, the Far Eastern, or Russian spring-summer encephalitis (RSSE), and the Central European, or western, type of the disease, also called Czechoslovak tick-borne encephalitis, biphasic meningoencephalitis, or diphasic milk fever. Epidemiologically, the Far Eastern type is generally transmitted by *Ixodes persulcatus* and the Central European type by *Ixodes ricinus* ticks. Human disease of the Far Eastern type is usually clinically more severe, and characterized by higher case-fatality rates than those caused by the Central European type.

HISTORY

In the U.K., louping ill, the first of the tick-borne encephalitides to be recognized, was described over a century ago as a disease of sheep. The etiological virus may be differentiated clinically, epidemiologically, and antigenically from the other viruses in the TBE complex, and is considered separately. The Far Eastern, or RSSE type, was first described in the U.S.S.R. in 1937.[53] The Central European type was first recognized in a human patient in Czechoslovakia in 1948[14] during an epidemic in central Bohemia. Subsequently, this type has been recognized in Poland, Austria, Bulgaria, Hungary, Yugoslavia, German Democratic Republic, German Federal Republic, Switzerland, Finland, Sweden, Denmark, France, and Rumania. It is anticipated that it will be identified in additional countries in the future.

ETIOLOGY

Classification

TBE virus is classified in the genus *Flavivirus* of the family Togaviridae. On the bases of close antigenic relationship and tick transmission, TBE virus belongs to the tick-borne encephalitis complex.[9] Cross reactions with other arboviruses of ʰhe *Flavivirus* group are observed in the hemagglutination-inhibition (HZ) tests. The tick-ᴗorne encephalitis complex consists of seven types: Pawassan, looping-ill tick-borne encephalitis (Central European and Far Eastern subtypes), OMSK hemorrhagic fever, Negishi, Kyasanur forest disease, and Langat viruses.

Characteristics

The TBE viruses contain single-stranded RNA genomes with molecular weights of 3×10^6 daltons. Electron photomicrographs of purified virus show round virions 70 to 80 nm in diameter with projecting surface spikes.[42] The CsCl density is 1.24 g/cm.[3] The virions contain lipids, are ether, desoxycholate- and trypsin-sensitive, and are inactivated in 15 min at 55°C in saline, or at 60°C in 10% rabbit serum saline. The optimal stability pH is 7.6 to 8.2.[19] TBE viruses share common hemagglutinating antigens which are active on day-old chicken and/or goose erythrocytes. The hemagglutinin may be extracted from infected suckling mouse brain tissue by acetone-ether, sucrose-acetone, or fluorocarbon techniques. The hemagglutinin is inactivated at pH 5 in 18 hr, and is unstable in 1 M MgCl$_2$, CsCl, and 0.1% sodium desoxycholate.[23] The virions are synthesized in the cytoplasm of infected cells. Chicken embryo (CE), human embryo, and porcine kidney (PK) primary cell cultures and HeLa, Detroit 6, Hep-2, FL, cynomologous monkey myocardial, and other cell lines are all susceptible to TBE viruses. Cytopathic effect is produced in HeLa[28] and PS cells, and plaques are formed in CE and PK cells overlaid with agar medium.

DEFINITION

Tick-borne encephalitis is used to identify a group of important infectious diseases of human beings and lower animals. The TBE viruses are classified on the basis of replication in the tissues of vector ticks, production of viremia in vertebrate hosts, and transmission to susceptible vertebrates by bites of infected ticks. Both transovarial and transstadial transmission has been demonstrated in ticks, and the virus survives during hibernation.[8,35]

ANIMAL INFECTION

Clinical

Louping ill virus is strongly pathogenic for sheep and red grouse in the U.K. The other TBE viruses commonly cause subclinical infections in animals, except occasionally in dogs[52] and lambs in nature. A very wide variety of domestic and wild mammals are infected in nature and develop viremias. In hibernating animals, viremias may persist for extended periods. Infected cows, nanny goats, and ewes regularly excrete virus in the milk, an important mechanism of direct exposure to the young of these species, as well as to human beings.

Experimental inoculation of adult sheep by the subcutaneous (s.c.) route produces viremia of up to 5 days duration, localization of infection in lymphatic organs,[29] excretion in the milk from the second through the seventh days.[16] The Hypr strain inoculated s.c. causes viremia and excretion of virus in the milk.[16] In lambs, TBE viruses cause viremia, encephalitis, and death within 5 to 6 days. Virus may be recovered from brain tissue.[19]

In the laboratory, TBE viruses infect a very wide variety of experimental animals. Mice are universally susceptible by parenteral routes, developing viremia and encephalitis following intracerebral (i.c.) intraperitoneal (i.p.) or s.c. inoculation. Virus inoculated s.c. has been shown to replicate mainly in the reticuloendothelial system.[29] Syrian hamsters have been shown to develop clinically inapparent infections demonstrable by development of complement fixing (CF) antibodies and histologic changes in the brain.[45] Cynomolgous monkeys are more susceptible than rhesus monkeys. By i.c. or intraspinal inoculation, clinical encephalitis with characteristic histologic lesions may be produced, but s.c. inoculation leads to subclinical infection with production of CF antibodies. In embryonating hens' eggs inoculated on the chorioallantoic membrane, TBE viruses form tiny lesions on the membranes and stunt, but do not kill, the embryos. Following inoculation into the yolk sac, death ensues in 4 to 7 days. Virulence is greatest to young embryos, and at an incubation temperature of 34.4°C. It is postulated that older embryos produce interferon and are thus more resistant.[43]

Pathology

Characteristically the central nervous system (CNS) shows diffuse meningoencephalitis, more pronounced in the grey than the white matter, with degeneration and necrosis of neurons, perivascular and leptomeningeal infiltration, and focal glial proliferation. Fluorescent antibody (FA) studies on experimentally infected mice have shown fluorescence in scattered sympathetic and parasympathetic ganglia, sometimes in striated muscle and in some parts of the CNS, beginning within 2 days postinoculation. Fluorescence in the peripheral nerve trunks appears 1 to 2 days later. One of the outstanding features of TBE viruses is their affinity for peripheral nerves.[1]

Diagnosis

Definitive diagnosis of TBE infections is based on laboratory isolation and identification of the causative strain from blood or postmortem tissues of animals or of whole ground ticks.

HUMAN INFECTION

Clinical

TBE is characterized by abrupt onset following a 7 to 14-day incubation period. There are no recognized sex differences, but clinical disease is usually more severe in children than in adults. Clinically, the Far Eastern infections are somewhat different from Central European infections. In the Far Eastern disease, prodromal symptoms include severe headache, anorexia, nausea and vomiting, weakness, hyperesthesia, and photophobia. These are variably followed by sensorial changes, blurring or disturbance of vision, and diplopia. Progressive development of meningeal irritation and encephalitis may be pronounced, with accompanying changes in the cerebrospinal fluid (CSF). Epileptiform convulsions, paresis, or paralysis, usually ascending, may develop. Fever, usually about 38.5°C lasts 2 to 7 days in the nonfatal cases. Death, when it ensues, may occur from 1 to 7 days after onset. Patients which survive may have protracted convalescence and often residual paralysis of the shoulders and arms. Case fatality rates may reach 20%.

The Central European disease is typically diphasic, but in nearly half of recognized cases, either the first or second phase may be inapparent. The first viremic phase is typically influenza-like and persists about a week, followed by general improvement for several days. The second phase appears abruptly, with a clinical course similar to, but commonly more mild than, the Far Eastern disease. Most cases develop into a benign meningoencephalitis, but severe illness with residual shoulder paralysis and even fatal outcome (1 to 5%) may occur.

Throughout areas where TBE occurs, clinically mild, abortive, and inapparent cases diagnosed by serological tests have been described. Four clinical types are generally described: abortive, meningeal, encephalitic, and encephalomyelitic.

Diagnosis

History of tick bite or drinking raw goat milk are of presumptive importance. Laboratory confirmation of diagnosis is based on virus isolation and/or demonstration of specific antibody responses. During the initial viremic phase, virus may be isolated from blood. Postmortem CNS tissues from patients dying early in the disease may yield virus. Virus isolation is more difficult from specimens or tissues collected later after onset. Specimens should be promptly inoculated into cell cultures or laboratory animals, or quickly frozen and held at −70°C or lower until thawed for inoculation. Sera and protein fractions used in diluting media should be tested for viral inhibiting action before use. Solid tissues should be triturated in buffered media at neutral to slightly alkaline pH containing 10% inactivated serum. Virus isolation may be done in suckling mice by i.c. inoculation, in embryonating hens' eggs by yolk sac and cho-rioallantoic membrane inoculation, and in several kinds of cell cultures, including chick embryo and porcine embryo cells. Cytopathic effect (cpe) is irregular, plaques are obtained by the use of special medium, and interferon may be produced.[20] Serotyp-ing of isolates is done by neutralization (N) tests, CF tests, or hemagglutination inhi-bition (HI) tests. Extensive cross-reactions among flaviviruses occur by HI tests, and among the tick-borne encephalitis viruses of the flavivirus group by all three tests. By NT and CF tests, homologous titers are generally distinguishable from heterologous titers. In serological diagnosis, a four-fold rise in antibody levels between acute and convalescent sera is considered minimal.

EPIDEMIOLOGY

Occurrence

Prior to World War II, tick-transmitted encephalitis was recognized as a public health problem only in louping ill endemic areas of Scotland, and in RSSE endemic areas of the U.S.S.R. The Central European strains of TBE were recognized in Czech-oslovakia in 1948.[24,38] The distribution of TBE correlates with the geographical distri-bution of Ixodid ticks.

Reservoirs

The virus circulates in nature between ticks and wild vertebrate hosts in endemic foci. At least ten species of forest rodents have shown high titering viremia with long duration. Hedgehogs, shrews, and moles which have relatively stable susceptible pop-ulations of antibody-free juveniles each year, are believed to be important reservoirs.[25] Overwintering has been shown in hibernating hedgehogs and dormice. Water birds and bats have been identified as alternate hosts.[7,12,33] Goats, sheep, and cattle are predom-inant domesticated animal hosts, although dogs may be infected.

Vectors

A variety of Ixodid ticks serve as both reservoirs and vectors of TBE viruses. *Ixodes persulcatus* in the east and *I. ricinus* in the west are the most noted vectors, but *Der-macentor silvarum, D. pictus, D. marginatus, Haemophysalis concinna, H. inermis,* and *H. japonica douglasi* have also been found to serve as vectors, especially in habi-tats unfavorable to the *Ixodes* spp. ticks.[21,34] The immature nymphal ticks may become infected in feeding on viremic animals and then following molting transmit the virus to a new host during feeding. Transovarial passage of TBE viruses also occurs through multiple generations. The extent to which endemicity may be maintained solely by transovarial transmission in ticks, and the extent to which vertebrate hosts are re-quired, has not been elucidated.[2,8,39] Experimentally, maintenance of infection in *I. ricinus* has been demonstrated for 3 years, with successful overwintering in starving nymphs and adults, and nonstarving larvae and nymphs.

Transmission

Transmission to susceptible animals appears entirely by tick bites. Neither vertical transmission nor direct contact transmission has been demonstrated, even though lac-tating goats, sheep, and cattle shed virus in their milk.[15-17] Transmission to human beings takes place by several mechanisms. Tick-bite transmission occurs principally when people disturb habitats with high tick populations for work, for settling of new areas, or for vacationing. In eastern U.S.S.R., the vector ticks are most active in spring and early summer, so that peak incidence of RSSE is in May and June. In Europe, tick activity is extended longer, and cases of Central European encephalitis occur from late spring until early autumn. Milk borne epidemics involving clusters of people of all ages in both rural and urban areas have been associated with drinking raw goat milk[4] in both the east[36,46] and west,[4,49] raw sheep milk in Europe,[22] but not from cows' milk, although virus is known to be shed by infected cattle. Milk-borne infections in Europe have been reported as more mild than tick-borne disease, but this has not been recorded in Far Eastern U.S.S.R. In experimentally infected goats, Grešíková recorded viremia between 6 hr and 5 days postinoculation, and milk borne virus 2 to 7 days postinoculation.[15] In sheep, she recorded viremia between 1 and 5 days, and shedding in milk between 2 and 7 days postinoculation.[16] The virus was shown to persist in milk at least 48 hr, and in butter and cheese curd at least 2 months.[18] A third mechanism of human exposure has been in laboratory work with TBE viruses. Both clinically severe and fatal laboratory infections have occurred.[19]

Human hosts

Human beings are aberrant hosts of TBE and human-to-human transmission has not been recorded. The course of human infection is usually benign with mild disease followed by complete recovery, and only a small proportion of infected people develop severe central nervous system (CNS) disease terminating in protracted recovery with serious neurological sequelae or death. In natural foci, a high proportion of people have antibodies against TBE viruses.[19,27]

CONTROL

Prevention and Therapy

Protection from exposure is the most effective preventive measure.[5] Tick-infected areas may be avoided where possible, or treated with insecticides. Agricultural measures which reduce tick infestations are applicable. Drinking of only pasteurized milk, especially goat milk in areas where milk borne exposure may occur, is very important. Vaccination of milk goats with an inactivated tissue vaccine has been used successfully in Czechoslovakia.[6] Seroprophylaxis with immune sera or globulin has been applied. Extensive human vaccine studies have been carried out. A formalin inactivated infected mouse brain vaccine was used in mass vaccination programs in U.S.S.R. prior to World War II.[47] More recently less hazardous vaccines have been prepared in embryonating hens' eggs and chick embryo cell cultures.[3,26] Experimental vaccines of naturally or laboratory attenuated strains are under test.[30]

Regulatory measures

In U.S.S.R. and countries of Europe, TBE is a reportable disease.

Epidemic Measures

Since most epidemics have been milk borne, attention to consuming only pasteurized milk and milk products is most important. Prevention of tick-borne exposure is based on avoiding tick infested areas, vaccination of the population at risk, and tick control. Control of tick populations have been feasible only in limited areas.

Health Education

Health education in protection from ticks, vaccination, and utilization of pasteurized or boiled milk products is of critical importance in areas of high risk. Urban residents must be informed of the source and safety of their milk.

PUBLIC HEALTH ASPECTS

Economic and Social Impact

TBE is being recognized as a public health problem of increasing importance in the U.S.S.R. and Europe. Prior to extensive serological surveillance and emphasis on reporting, the extent of infections was not appreciated. The opening of new areas for development, and the increase in outdoor vacationing have brought additional people into high risk areas. Similarly, the expansion of domestic animal production into new areas has modified the natural balances in these areas, often causing explosions in tick and/or rodent reservoir populations with resulting increases in human exposure.[19,27,40]

REFERENCES

1. **Albrecht, P.**, Pathogenesis of neurotropic arbovirus infection, *Curr. Top. Microbiol. Immunol.*, 43, 45, 1968.
2. **Benda, R.**, The common tick "*Ixodes ricinus* L." as a reservoir and vector of tick-borne encephalitis. I. Survival of the virus (strain B3) during the development of the tick under laboratory conditions, *J. Hyg. Epidemiol. Microbiol. Immunol.*, (Praha) 2, 314, 1958, (in Czech).
3. **Benda, R. and Danes, L.**, Study of the possibility of preparing a vaccine against tick-borne encephalitis, using tissue culture methods. V. Experimental data for the evaluation of the efficiency of formol treated vaccines in laboratory animals, *Acta Virol.*, 5, 37, 1961.
4. **Blaskovič, D., Ed.**, *The Epidemic of Encephalitis in the Rožňava Natural Focus of Infection*, Slovak Academy of Sciences, Bratislava, 1954, (in Slovak).
5. **Blaskovič, D.**, Tick-borne encephalitis in Europe. Aspects of the epidemiology and control of the disease, *Ann. Soc. Belge Med. Trop.*, 38, 867, 1958.
6. **Blaskovič, D., Ed.**, *The Importance of Deliberate Immunization of Domestic Animals for a Natural Focus of Tick-borne Encephalitis*, Slovak Academy of Sciences, Bratislava, 1962, (in Slovak).
7. **Bolotovskij, V. M.**, Birds as reservoirs of tick-borne encephalitis virus, *Vopr. Med. Virusol.*, 6, Izd. AMN ZSSR, Moskva, 1960, (in Russian).
8. **Chumakov, M. P.**, Studies on virus encephalitides. 6. Transmission of tick-borne encephalitis to the offspring in Ixodidae ticks and the question of natural reservoirs of this infection, *Med. Parazitol. Parisit. Bolezni*, 6, 38, 1944, (in Russian).
9. **Clarke, D. H.**, Antigenic relationship among viruses of the tick-borne encephalitis complex as studied by antibody adsorption and agar gel prepipitin techniques, in *Biology of Viruses of the Tick-borne Encephalitis Complex*, Libikova, H., Ed., Czechoslovak Academy of Science, Prague, 1962, 67.
10. **Clarke, D. H. and Casals, J.**, Techniques for hemagglutination and hemagglutination-inhibition with arthropod-borne viruses, *Am. J. Trop. Med. Hyg.*, 7, 561, 1958.
11. **Draganescu, N.**, The laboratory investigations on viral encephalitides with the determination of etiological agents, *Stud. Cercet. Inframicrobiol.*, 15, 349, 1964, (in Rumenian).
12. **Ernek, E.**, The garganey (*Anas querquedula* L., 1758) as possible reservoir of tick-borne encephalitis virus, *Vet. Čas.*, 8, 8, 1959, (in Slovak).
13. **Fornosi, F. and Molnar, E.**, Zeckenenzephalitis in Ungarn. Die Isolation und Eigenschaften des Virus, *Acta Microbiol. Acad. Sci. Hung.*, 1, 9, 1954, (in Russian).
14. **Gallia, F., Rampas, J., and Hollender, L.**, Laboratory infection with encephalitis virus, *Čas. Lék. Česk.*, 88, 224, 1949, (in Czech.)
15. **Grešíková, M.**, Elimination of the tick-borne encephalitis virus by goat's milk, *Vet. Cas.*, 6, 177, 1957, (in Slovak).
16. **Grešíková, M.**, Recovery of the tick-borne encephalitis virus from the blood and milk of subcutaneously infected sheep, *Acta Virol.*, 2, 113, 1958.
17. **Grešíková, M.**, Excretion of the tick-borne encephalitis virus in the milk of subcutaneously infected cows, *Acta Virol.*, 2, 188, 1957.
18. **Grešíková, M.**, Persistence of tick-borne encephalitis virus in milk and milk products, *Cs. Epidem.*, 8, 26, 1959, (in Slovak).
19. **Grešíková, M.**, Studies on tick-borne arboviruses isolated in Central Europe, *biological works*, Slovak Academy of Sciences, Bratislava, 18(2), 5, 1972.
20. **Grešíková, M., Kožuch, O., and Molnar, E.**, Human infection with tick-borne encephalitis virus in the Tribec region, *Bull. WHO*, 36 (Suppl. 1), 81, 1967.
21. **Grešíková, M. and Nosek, J.**, Isolation of tick-borne encephalitis virus from Haemaphysalis inermis ticks, *Acta Virol.*, 10, 359, 1966.

22. Grešiková, M., Sekeyová, M., Stupalová, S., and Mecas, S., Sheep milk-borne epidemic of tick-borne encephalitis in Slovakia, *Intervirology*, 5, 57, 1975.

23. Grešiková, M. and Vachálkova, A., Influence of pH, heat, deoxycholate and ether on arbovirus haemagglutinin, *Acta Virol.*, 15, 143, 1971.

24. Hloucal, L. and Gallia, F., An epidemic of neurotropic virus disease in the district of Strakonice, *Sb. Lek.*, 51, 374, 1949, (in Czech.).

25. Kožuch, O., Grešiková, M., Nosek, J., Lichard, M., and Sekeyová, M., The role of small rodents and hedgehogs in a natural focus of tick-borne encephalitis, *Bull. WHO*, 36 (Suppl. 1), 61, 1967.

26. Levkovich, E. N., Experimental and epidemiological bases of the specific prophylaxis of tick-borne encephalitis, in *Biology of Viruses of the Tick-borne Encephalitis Complex*, Libiková, H., Ed., Czechoslovak Academy of Sciences, Prague, 1962, 317.

27. Libiková, H., Grešiková, M., Reháček, J., Ernek, E., and Nosek, J., Immunological surveys in natural foci of the tick-borne encephalitis, *Bratisl. Lek. Listy*, 43, 40, 1963, (in Slovak).

28. Libiková, H. and Vilček, J., A simple neutralization test for viruses of the tick-borne encephalitis group, depending on a complete cytopathic effect in Hela cells. Preliminary report, *Acta Virol.*, 3, 181, 1959.

29. Malková, D., The lymphatic system in viral infection. An experimental study with tick-borne encephalitis virus in animals, *Rozpravy Cesk. Akad. Ved.*, 79(2), 1, 1969.

30. Mayer, V., A live vaccine against tick-borne encephalitis: integrated studies. I. Basic properties and behavior of the E5''14'' clone (Langat virus), *Acta Virol.*, 19, 209, 1975.

31. Moritsch, H. and Krausler, J., Tick-borne encephalitis in lower Austria 1956-1958, *Dtsch. Med. Wochenshr.*, 84, 1934, 1959.

32. Müller, W., Experimentelle Untersuchungen uber das Vorkommen von Arboviren in Unterfranken, *Zentralbl. Bakteriol. Parasitenkd. Infektionskr. Hyg. Abt. 1 Grig. A*, 214, 145, 1970.

33. Nosek, J., Grešiková, M., and Reháček, J., Persistence of TBE virus in hibernating bats, *Acta Virol.*, 5, 112, 1961.

34. Pavlov, P., Studies on tick-borne encephalitis of sheep and their natural foci in Bulgaria, *Zentralbl. Bakteriol. Parasitenkd. Infektionskr. Hyg. Abt. 1, Grig. A.*, 206, 360, 1968.

35. Pavlovskij, E. N., Ticks and tick-borne encephalitis, in *Parazitology of Far East*, Medgiz, Moskva, 1947, 212. (in Russian).

36. Pogodina, V. V., Epidemiology and prevention of alimentary infections of tick-borne encephalitis, *J. Hyg. Epidemiol. Microbiol. Immunol.*, 5, 75, 1961.

37. Przesmycki, F., Taytsch, Z., Semkov, R., and Walentynowitz-Stanczyk, R., Studies on tick-borne encephalitis, *Przegl. Epidemiol.*, 8, 205, 1954, (in Polish).

38. Rampas, J. and Gallia, F., The isolation of encephalitis virus from *Ixodes ricinus* ticks, *Čas. Lek. Česk.*, 88, 1179, 1949, (in Czech).

39. Reháček, J., Transovarial transmission of tick-borne encephalitis virus by ticks, *Acta Virol.*, 6, 220, 1962.

40. Sekeyová, M. and Grešiková, M., Haemagglutination-inhibiting antibodies against arboviruses in cattle sera, *J. Hyg. Epidemiol. Microbiol. Immunol.*, 11, 417, 1967, (Prague).

41. Sinnecker, H., Zeckenencephalitis in Deutschland, *Zbl. Bakt. Orig.*, 180, 12, 1960.

42. Slávik, I., Mayer, V., and Mrena, E., Morphology of purified tick-borne encephalitis virus, *Acta Virol.*, 11, 66, 1967.

43. Slonin, D. and Roslerova, V., Pathogenicity of tick-borne encephalitis virus for chicken embryo. I. Influence of chicken embryo age and incubation, temperature on the lethal activity of the virus, *Acta Virol.*, 9, 473, 1965.

44. Slonim, D., Šimon, J., and Závadová, H., Pathogenicity of tick-borne encephalitis virus. VII. Relation between infective and pathogenic activity for Rhesus monkeys, *Acta Virol.*, 10, 413, 1966.

45. Slonim, D., Závadová, H., and Šimon, J., Pathogenicity of tick-borne encephalitis virus. VI. Relation between infective and pathogenic activity for golden hamsters, *Acta Virol.*, 10, 336, 1966.

46. Smorodincev, A. A., Alekseyev, B. P., Gulamova, V. P., Drobyshevskaya, A. I., Ilyenko, V. I., Klenov, K. N., and Churilova, A. A., The epidemiologic characteristics of bi-phasic virus meningoencephalitis. Zh. Mikrobiol. Epidemiol. Immunobiol., 5, 54, 1953, (in Russian).

47. Smorodincev, A. A., Levkovich, E. N., and Dankowski, N. L., Experiments on the prevention of spring-summer encephalitis in the endemic centers by vaccinating the inhabitants with the dead vaccine, *Arkhiv Biol. Nauk.*, 59, 1, 92, 1940, (in Russian).

48. Svedmyr, A., von Zeipel, G., Holmgren, B., and Lindahl, J., Tick-borne meningoencephalomyelitis in Sweden, *Arch. Gesamte Virusforsch.*, 8, 565, 1958.

49. Tongeren, Van H. A. E., Wilterdink, J. B., Wyler, R., and Richling, E., Encephalitis in Austria. III. A serological survey followed up by an epidemiological study in the endemic region of Styria during the outbreak of 1954, *Arch. Gesamte Virusforsch.*, 6, 143, 1955.

50. **Vapcarov, I., Trpmanov, A., Spasov, Z., Nikov, D., and Dragiev, T.,** Zweiwellen-Meningocnce-phalitis in Sud-Bulgarien, *Sov. Med.,* 2, 86, 1954.

51. **Vesenjak-Zmijanac, J., Bedjanic, M., Rus, S., and Kmet, J.,** Virus meningoencephalitis in Slovenia. 3. Isolation of causative agent, *Bull. WHO,* 12, 513, 1955.

52. **Wandeler, A., Steck, F., Frankhauser, R., Kammermann, B., Grešíková, M., and Blaškovič, D.,** Isolierung des Virus der zentraleuropaischen Zeckenencephalitis in der Schweiz, *Pathol. Microbiol.,* 38, 258, 1972.

53. **Zilber, L. A. and Soloviev, V. D.,** Far Eastern tick-borne spring-summer (spring) encephalitis, *Am. Rev. Sov. Med.,* Special Suppl. 5, 1, 1946.

ŤAHYŇA VIRUS INFECTION

V. Bárdoš

NAME AND SYNONYMS

Ťahyňa virus infection usually has no synonyms. Lumbo virus originally isolated in Africa is a geographical variant of Ťahyňa virus. It is indistinguishable by laboratory tests from Ťahyňa virus.[30,32]

HISTORY

Five strains of an arbovirus were isolated from *Aedes caspius* and *Ae. vexans* during July and August in 1958 near the village of Ťahyňa Czechoslovakia.[10] Ťahyňa virus is the first mosquito-borne virus to be recognized in Central Europe.

ETIOLOGY

Classification

Ťahyňa virus belongs to the family Bunyaviridae, genus *Bunyavirus,* and is a member of the California serogroup.[43] The prototype Bárdoš 92 strain is related to, but not identical with, other strains of the California serogroup.[20]

Characteristics

Ťahyňa virions are spherical, enveloped, and have a diameter of 92 ± 4 nm with 15-nm spikes. They are sedimented in sucrose gradient density of 1.17 g/cm^3.[44] The genome is composed of noninfective RNA[6] in three segmented single strands of molecular weights, 2.9×10^6 daltons, 1 molecule of 2.0×10^6 daltons, and 3 molecules of 0.5×10^6 daltons, giving a total weight of 6.4×10^6 daltons.[19] Purified virus contains RNA-dependent polymerase.[17]

Freshly isolated Ťahyňa virus strains passed not more than 3 to 4 serial intracerebral (i.c.) mouse passages are thermoresistant, showing less than 1 log titer loss at 50°C for 15 min.[35] No changes in thermoresistance have been noted through 21 serial passages in hamster, GMK, or *Aedes albopictus* cell lines.[25] An extraneural variant of Ťahyňa virus was inactivated from a titer of $10^{3.57}$ LD$_{50}$/0.3 mℓ at 37°C for 24 hr, and from a titer of $10^{5.37}$ LD$_{50}$/0.03 mℓ at 56°C for 1 hr. The Bárdoš prototype strain "92" was inactivated at 4 to 6°C in 39 days, and at −15°C, a -log$_{10}$-titer loss was observed in 94 days.[3] Ťahyňa virus is sensitive to ether, chloroform, freon, sodium desoxycholate, trypsin, papain, and formalin. It is not stabilized by Ca^{++} and Mg^{++}

ions.[3,41] Suckling white mice and rats succumb to infection following i.c. or subcutaneous (s.c.) inoculation of virus, but fatal infections in adult white mice and young Syrian hamsters occur only following i.c. inoculation. Death occurs 3 to 7 days postinoculation, and the virus titer in brains is from $10^{6.0}$ to $10^{8.6}$ $LD_{50}/0.01$ ml in mice, or 0.03 ml in hamsters. Guinea pigs and rabbits infected by the i.c. route develop an inapparent immunizing infection. Ťahyně virus has been isolated from striated muscle, lungs, and brain of experimentally infected adult white mice both with and in the absence of viremia.[6] Replication of the virus has been shown in fragments of human embryo striated muscle, lungs, and brain in vitro.[45-48] The multiplication of Ťahyňa virus in neural, and many extraneural, tissues of experimentally infected suckling white mice has also been documented by fluorescent antibody (FA) technique.[60] Ťahyňa virus is lethal to embryonated hens' eggs inoculated in the yolk sac in 5 to 9 days.[9] Neuroadapted and cell-culture adapted strains cause cytopathic effect (CPE) in many cell cultures of human beings nonhuman primates, and other animal and avian origins, but the extraneurally passaged strain "236" produces cpe only in GMK cells.[42,49,51] Strains having no or only few i.c. mouse passages form predominantly large and medium-sized plaques, whereas strains with a high number of i.c. mouse passages form mostly small plaques.[36,39,50] Ťahyňa virus multiplies in cell culture of *Ae. aegypti, Ae. stephensi,* and *Ae. albopictus* mosquitoes at 28°C, but produce no cpe.[24,38,40] Human embryo organ cultures of lungs have supported Ťahyňa virus replication in vitro.[46, 47]

DEFINITION

Ťahyňa virus infection is a mosquito-borne viral infection characterized by an influenza-like febrile disease with pharyngitis, hyperemia of the conjunctiva, and in some patients, myalgia, central nervous system (CNS) involvement, or bronchopneumonia.[4] Animal infections are considered to be inapparent in nature.

ANIMAL INFECTION

Under natural conditions, no clinical manifestations have been described in Ťahyňa virus infected animals.[5] Virus has been isolated in nature from sentinel rabbits in Austria and Czechoslovakia. Naturally occurring antibodies have been demonstrated in hares, rabbits, ground squirrels, foxes, wild boars, deer, hedgehogs, horses, cattle, and swine in Czechoslovakia, Austria, and France. Experimentally, subclinical infections have been established in *Macaca rhesus, M. radiata,* and *Cercopithecus aethiops* monkeys injected subcutaneously with extraneurally passaged strain "236" of Ťahyňa virus. Chimpanzees infected with this strain either by subcutaneous injection or by allowing laboratory infected *Culiseta annulata* mosquitoes to bite them, developed not only viremia but clinical symptoms of disease similar to that recorded in human infections.[57,58] Death occurs in suckling mice inoculated by i.c. and intraperitoneal (i.p.) routes, weanling mice i.c., suckling rats i.c. and s.c., hamsters i.c., and embryonating hens' eggs by yolk sac inoculation. No illness has been observed in weanling mice inoculated by i.p. route, adult rats i.c., guinea pigs, i.c., or rabbits i.c.

HUMAN INFECTION

Clinical

Human illness with fever from 37.2 to 40.9 °C lasting 3 to 5 days has been observed, accompanied by headache, nausea, pharyngitis, and conjunctival hyperemia. Uncommonly observed have been meningoencephalitis or bronchopneumonia. In patients with CNS involvement, erythrocyte sedimentation rates have been accelerated, and pleocytosis of cerebrospinal fluid recorded. No residual sequela and no deaths have been recorded due to Ťahyňa virus infections.[4]

Pathology

Histologically, neuronal degeneration, glial cell proliferation, and perivascular infiltration have been recorded in experimentally infected mice.

Diagnosis

Ťahyňa virus infections are usually diagnosed serologically, testing paired sera in serum neutralization, complement fixation (CF), and hemagglutination inhibition (HI) tests. The plaque reduction neutralization test is the most specific serological test. Using local strains of Ťahyňa virus, HI and CF tests pose greater difficulties in preparing workable hemagglutinating antigens, and CF antibodies often appear late or remain completely absent. Virus isolation from the blood of patients has only recently been reported for the first time in Tahyna inflections for the whole California serogroup.[12,59]

EPIDEMIOLOGY

Occurrence

Ťahyňa virus isolations from mosquitoes and people and/or animals have now been reported from Czechoslovakia, Yugoslavia, France, Italy, Mozambique, Kenya, Austria, Federal Republic of Germany, U.S.S.R., Rumania, South Africa, and West Africa.[4,15] The Lumbo strain was reported from Mozambique.[30,32] Virus isolations of Ťahyňa virus from mosquitoes, and the presence of antibodies in the domestic population of some eastern regions of the U.S.S.R., have documented the presence of this virus in Asia.[33]

Serological surveys have documented that the highest prevalence of antibodies is in the population of central Europe, including Czechoslovakia, Hungary, and Austria, where rates reach 30 to 60%. In the northern, southern, western, and eastern countries of Europe, the overall percentages decrease to 5 to 15%,[15] but in villages situated near rivers, the prevalence of antibodies often reaches levels as high as in central Europe.[1,29] In localities where the infection is endemic, 50% of children at the age of 5 years may have antibodies, and by the age of 19 years 95% of the population may be positive.[16] In endemic foci during the arboviral season, July, August, and September[4,13] 1.8 to 36.8% of all hospitalized febrile patients have been serologically identified as Ťahyňa virus infections.[4] Bronchopneumonia was seen in 13.8%, and CNS involvement in 18.4 to 21.4% of patients in whom acute Ťahyňa virus infections were diagnosed.[4,22]

Reservoir

Wild mammals are the principal reservoir hosts of Ťahyňa virus. The highest prevalence of antibodies among species tested in endemic areas has been in hares 36.1%, rabbits 9.0 to 53.8%, and hedgehogs 13.1%.[5,29] Virus has also been isolated from sentinel rabbits exposed in nature. The virus was not found in 177 wild birds sampled in Czechoslovakia.[2,22,31] In surveys of domestic animals in endemic areas, the highest prevalence has been detected in horses (63.3%), swine (55.0%), and cattle (10.8%).[5] Domestic fowl have not been shown to be hosts of Tahyna virus.[52] In experimental animal infections, sufficiently high viremia was detected to infect the principal vector *Ae. vexans* in young hares and rabbits, young mice, hedgehogs, dormice, piglets, and 2- to 5-day-old colts.[7,8,34,37,53-56]

Transmission

Among the many species of mosquitoes from which Ťahyňa virus has been isolated, *Ae. vexans* has yielded the largest number of isolates, with infection rates from 0.14 to 2.2/1000 mosquitoes captured in endemic areas. It has a relatively low infection threshold of $10^{1.5}$ to $10^{1.8}$ mouse $LD_{50}/0.02$ mℓ, and a transmission rate of 60 to 90% following a 14-day extrinsic incubation period.[11,21, 26,28] Ťahyňa virus has also been recovered repeatedly from *Cu. annulata;* its infection threshold is greater than $10^{2.3}LD_{50}/0.02$ mℓ, and it gave a transmission rate of 54 to 100% after a 14-day extrinsic incubation period.[21,23,28] Ťahyňa virus has been detected in hibernating *Cu. annulata* 181 days after experimental feeding,[27] and has also been isolated from field-collected *Cu. annulata* larvae.[14] Other mosquitoes from which Ťahyňa virus has been isolated have been *Ae. caspius,* from which the prototype strain was obtained, *Ae. pembaensis, Anopheles hyrcanus,* and *Culex pipiens.*

Human Hosts

Human beings readily enter transmission cycles of Ťahyňa virus, but are considered aberrant hosts because viremic levels sufficient to infect the important vector *Ae. vexans* have not been recognized.[12,59]

CONTROL

Prevention and Treatment

No effective vaccines or specific immunoglobulins have been developed for prophylactic use. General mosquito control is appropriate, but the wide variety of vector species make specific control programs difficult. Health education to minimize contact with mosquitoes is appropriate. The public health impact of this infection remains largely undetermined.

REFERENCES

1. **Ackermann, R., Spithaler, W., Profittlich, W., and Spieckermann, D.,** The distribution of viruses of the California encephalitis group in the Federal Republik of Germany, *Dtsch. Med. Wochenschr.,* 95, 1057, 1970, (in German).
2. **Aspock, H., Graefe, G., and Kunz, C.,** Studies on the peiodicity of the occurrence of Tahyna and Calovo viruses, *Zentralbl. Bakteriol. Parisitenkd. Infektionskr. Hyg. Abt. 1: Orig. Reihe A.,* 217, 431, 1971, (in German).
3. **Bárdoš, V.,** The Tahyna virus. I. Study of its resistance to the action of some physical factors and chemical agents, *Acta Virol.,* 5, 50, 1961.
4. **Bárdoš, V.,** Recent state of knowledge of Tahyna virus infections, *Folia Parasitol. (Prague),* 21, 1, 1974.
5. **Bárdoš, V.,** The role of mammals in the circulation of Tahyna virus, *Folia Parasitol. (Prague),* 22, 257, 1975.
6. **Bárdoš, V.,** Tahyna virus in experimentally infected white mice, *Acta Virol.,* 9, 358, 1965.
7. **Bárdoš, V., Čupková, E., and Jakubik, J.,** Tahyna virus in foals, *Acta Virol.,* 9, 555, 1965.
8. **Bárdoš, V., Čupková, E., and Jakubik, J.,** Determination of the minimal Tahyna virus dose producing viraemia in suckling pigs, *Acta Virol.,* 10, 55, 1966.
9. **Bárdoš, V., Čupková, E., and Šefčovičová, L.,** The Tahyna virus. II. Characteristics and some biological properties and preliminary immunological classification, *Acta Virol.,* 5, 93, 1961.
10. **Bárdoš, V. and Danielová, V.,** The Tahyna virus — a virus isolated from mosquitoes in Czechoslovakia, *J. Hyg. Microb. Epidemiol. Mikrobiol. Immunol.,* 3, 264, 1959.
11. **Bárdoš, V. and Danielová, V.,** A study of Tahyna virus-Aedes vexans relationship under natural conditions, *Česk. Epidemiol. Mikrobiol. Immunol.,* 10, 389, 1961, (in Slovak).
12. **Bárdoš, V., Medek, M., Kania, V., and Hubalek, Z.,** Isolation of Tahyna virus from the blood of sick children, *Acta Virol.,* 19, 447, 1975.
13. **Bárdoš, V. and Rosický, B.,** A proposal for the evaluation of vertebrates as to their role in the circulation of arboviruses, *Folia Parisitol. (Prague),* 26, 89, 1979.

14. **Bárdoš, V., Ryba, J., and Hubalek, Z.,** Isolation of Tahyna virus from field collected Culiseta annulata (Schrk./larvae), *Acta Virol.,* 19, 446, 1975.

15. **Bárdoš, V. and Šefčovičová, L.,** The presence of antibodies neutralizing Tahyna virus in the sera of inhabitants of some European, Asian, African, and Australian countries, *J. Hyg. Microb. Epidemiol. Mikrobiol. Immunol.,* 5, 501, 1961.

16. **Bárdoš, V., Šefčovičová, L., Adamcová, J., and Červenka, J.,** Tahyna virus neutralizing antibodies in inhabitants of different age groups in an area of mass occurrence of mosquitoes, *Česk. Epidemiol. Mikrobiol. Immunol.,* 11, 238, 1962, (in Slovak).

17. **Bouloy, M., Colbere, F., Krams-Ozden, S., Vialat, P., Garapin, A. C., and Hannoun, C.,** Activite RNA polymerasique associee a bunyavirus (Lumbo), *C. R. Acad. Sci. Ser. D:,* 280, 213, 1975.

18. **Bouloy, M. and Hannoun, C.,** Effect de l'actinomycine D sur la multiplication du virus Tahyna, *Ann. Microbiol. (Paris),* 124B, 547, 1973.

19. **Bouloy, M., Krams-Ozden, Horodniceanu, F., and Hannoun, C.,** Three-segmented RNA genome of Lumbo virus (Bunyavirus), *Intervirology,* 2, 173, 1973-1974.

20. **Casals, J.,** Immunological relationship between Tahyna and California encephalitis viruses, *Acta Virol.,* 6, 140, 1962.

21. **Danielová, V.,** Quantitative relationship of Tahyna virus and the mosquito Aedes vexans, *Acta Virol.,* 10, 62, 1966.

22. **Danielová, V.,** To the seasonal occurrence of the Tahyna virus, *Folia Parasitol. (Prague),* 19, 189, 1972.

23. **Danielová, V.,** The vector efficiency of Culiseta annulata mosquito in relation to Tahyna virus, *Folia Parasitol. (Prague),* 19, 259, 1972.

24. **Danielová, V.,** Susceptibility of Aedes albopictus mosquito cell line to some arboviruses, *Acta Virol.,* 17, 249, 1973.

25. **Danielová, V.,** The property changes of two Tahyna virus strains by influence of serial passages in various environments, *Zentralbl. Bakteriol. Parasitkd. Infectionskr. Hyg. Abt. 1: Orig. Reihe A,* 229, 232, 1974.

26. **Danielová, V., Málková, D., Minař, J., and Ryba, J.,** Dynamics of the natural focus of Tahyna virus in southern Moravia and species succession of its vectors, the mosquitoes of the genus Aedes, *Folia Parasitol. (Prague),* 23, 243, 1976.

27. **Danielová, V. and Minař, J.,** Experimental overwintering of the Tahyna virus in mosquitoes Culiseta annulata (Schrk./Diptera, Culicidae), *Folia Parasitol. (Prague),* 16, 285, 1969.

28. **Danielová, V., Minař, J., and Ryba, J.,** Isolation of Tahyna virus from mosquitoes Culiseta annulata (Schrk. 1776), *Folia Parasitol. (Prague),* 17, 281, 1970.

29. **Hannoun, C., Panthier, R., and Corniu, R.,** Serological and virological evidence of the endemic activity of Tahyna virus in France, in *Arboviruses of the California Complex and the Bunyamwera Group,* Bardos, V., et al., Eds., Publishing House of the Slovak Academy of Sciences, Bratislava, 1969, 121.

30. **Kokernot, R. H., McIntosh, B. N., Worth, C. B., DeMorais, T., and Weinbren, M. P.,** Isolation of viruses from mosquitoes collected at Lumbo, Mozambique. I. Lumbo virus, a new virus isolated from Aedes (Skusea) pembaensis Theobald, *Am. J. Trop. Med. Hyg.,* 11, 678, 1962.

31. **Kolman, J. M., Danielová, V., Málková, D., and Smetana, A.,** The laboratory rabbit (Oryctolagus cuniculus L. var. domestica) as indicator of Tahyna virus in nature, *J. Hyg. Microb. Epidimol. Mikrobiol. Immunol.,* 10, 246, 1966.

32. **Kunz, C., Buckley, S. M., and Casals, J.,** Antibodies in man against Tahyna and Lumbo viruses determined by hemagglutination-inhibition and tissue-culture neutralization tests, *Am. J. Trop. Med. Hyg.,* 13, 738, 1964.

33. **Lvov, D. K., Gromashevsky, V. L., Sidorova, G. A., Tsirkin, Yu. M., Chervonsky, V. J., and Aristova, B. A.,** Isolation of Tahyna virus from Anopheles hyrcanus mosquitoes in Kyzylagach Preserve, Southeastern Azerbaijan, *Vopr. Virusol.,* 17, 18, 1972, (in Russian).

34. **Málková, D.,** The development of viraemia and neutralizing antibodies in the European suslik, fat dormouse and the common mole, experimentally infected with Tahyna virus, *Folia Parasitol. (Prague),* 17, 85, 1970.

35. **Málková, D.,** Thermosensitivity of Tahyna virus, *Acta Virol.,* 15, 309, 1971.

36. **Málková, D.,** Comparative study of two variants of Tahyna virus, *Acta Virol.,* 18, 407, 1974.

37. **Málková, D., Hodková, Z., and Chaturvedi, R.,** Overwintering of virus Tahyna in hedgehogs kept under natural conditions, *Folia Parasitol. (Prague),* 16, 245, 1969.

38. **Málková, D., and Marhoul, Z.,** Susceptibility of mosquito cell line Aedes aegypti to some arboviruses, in *Proc. III. Int. Coll. Invertebrate Tissue Culture,* Rehacek, J., Blaskovic, D., and Hink, W. F., Eds., Publ. House, SAV, Bratislava, 267, 1973.

39. **Málková, D. and Narender, Reddy G.,** Influence of early passages on the character of freshly isolated strains of Tahyna virus, *Acta Virol.,* 19, 333, 1975.

40. **Marhoul, Z.**, Multiplication of Tahyna, Calovo and Uukunicmi (strain Potepli) viruses in mosquito cell lines of Aedes aegypti and Anopheles stephensi, in *Proc. III. Int. Coll. Invertebrate Tissue Culture*, Rehacek, J., Blaskovic, D., and Hink, W. F., Eds., Publ. House, SAV, Bratislava, 275, 1973.

41. **Mayerová, A.**, Effect of pH, bivalent cations Mg^{++} and Ca^{++}, trypsin and papain on Tahyna virus, *Acta Virol.*, 10, 135, 1966.

42. **Porterfield, J. S.**, Studies with Tahyna virus, *Acta Virol.*, 5, 274, 1961.

43. **Porterfield, J. S., Casals, J., Chumakov, M. P., Gaidamovich, S. Ya., Hannoun, C., Holmes, I. H., Horzinck, M. C., Mussgay, M., Oker-Blom, N., and Russell, P. K.**, Bunyaviruses and Bunyaviridae, *Intervirology*, 6, 13, 1975/76.

44. **Samso, A., Bouloy, M., and Hannoun, C.**, Presence de ribonucleoproteines circulaires dans le virus Lumbo (Bunyavirus), *C.R. Acad. Sci. Ser. D.*, 280, 779, 1975.

45. **Schwanzer, V.**, Adsorption of Tahyna virus to some cell systems and tissue homogenates in vitro, in *Arboviruses of the California complex and the Bunyamwera group*, Bardos, V., et al., Eds., Publishing House of the Slovak Academy of Sciences, Bratislava, 1969, 249.

46. **Schwanzerová, I.**, Growth of California group viruses in tissue fragments, *Acta Virol.*, 17, 262, 1973.

47. **Schwanzerová, I.** Relationship of the Viruses of the California Group to the Fragments of Human Tissues in *Vitro*, CSc. thesis, Institute of Epidemiology and Microbiology, Bratislava, 1975, (in Slovak).

48. **Schwanzerová, I.**, Tahyna virus in tissue explants of experimentally infected suckling mice, *Acta Virol.*, 20, 73, 1976.

49. **Šefčovičová, L.**, Cultivation of Tahyna virus in stable cell lines, *Acta Virol.*, 9, 495, 1965.

50. **Šefčovičová, L.**, Tahyna virus: some biological properties of its strains, tested in vitro, *Biologia (Bratislava)*, 24, 210, 1969, Publ. House, SAV, Bratislava, (in Slovak).

51. **Šefčovičová, L. and Wallnerova, Z.**, Cytopathic activity of the extraneural variant of Tahyna virus in the GMK cell line, *Acta Virol.*, 11, 270, 1967.

52. **Šimková, A.**, Tahyna virus in birds, *Acta Virol.*, 6, 190, 1962.

53. **Šimková, A.**, Tahyna virus in rabbits, *Acta Virol.*, 6, 281, 1962.

54. **Šimková, A.**, Quantitative study of experimental Tahyna virus infection in potential reservoir animals, *Acta Virol.*, 7, 414, 1963.

55. **Šimková, A.**, Tahyna virus in hedgehogs, *Acta Virol.*, 8, 258, 1964.

56. **Šimková, A.**, Quantitative study of experimental Tahyna virus infection in hibernating hedgehogs, *J. Hyg. Epidemiol. Mikrobiol. Immunol.*, 10, 499, 1966.

57. **Šimková, A. and Bárdoš, V.**, Experimental Tahyna virus infections in primates, in *Arboviruses of the California complex and the Bunyamwera group*, Bárdoš, V., et al., Eds., Publishing House of the Slovak Academy of Sciences, Bratislava, 1969, 269.

58. **Šimková, A. and Danielová, V.**, Experimental infection of chimpanzees with Tahyna virus by Culiseta annulata mosquitoes, *Folia Parasitol. (Prague)*, 16, 255, 1969.

59. **Šimková, A. and Sluka, F.**, Isolation of Tahyna virus from the blood of a case of influenza-like disease, *Acta Virol.*, 17, 94, 1973.

60. **Wallnerová, Z.**, Fluorescent antibody technique in study of experimental Tahyna and La Crosse virus infection in suckling mice, in *Arboviruses of the California complex and the Bunyamwera group*, Bárdoš, V., et al., Eds., Publishing house of the Slovak Academy of Sciences, Bratislava, 1969, 237.

KEMEROVO VIRUS INFECTION

M. Grešíková

NAME AND SYNONYMS

The Kemerovo species of orbiviruses include the following subtypes: Kemerovo (isolated in Siberia), Tribeč (isolated in Western Slovakia), Chenuda (isolated in Egypt and S. Africa), Wad Modani (isolated in the Sudan, Malaysia, Jamaica, India, and Pakistan), Mono Lake (isolated in the U.S.), and Huacho (isolated in Peru).

HISTORY

In 1962, a scientific expedition by the U.S.S.R. Academy of Medical Sciences and the Institute of Virology of the Czechoslovak Academy of Sciences, Bratislava, investigated natural foci of tick-borne encephalitis (TBE) in the Kemerovo region of Western Siberia, U.S.S.R. The prototype Kemerovo virus was isolated by the group from *Ixodes persulcatus* ticks collected in the area. The Kemerovo virus produced cytopathic effect (cpe), and plaques in chick embryo cell cultures but was nonpathogenic for adult laboratory animals.[1,13] In 1963, Tribeč virus was isolated during an expedition of the group in the Western Tribeč Mountains of Slovakia.[5,7] The closely related Lipovník virus was isolated the same year from *Ixodes ricinus* ticks collected near Roznava in Eastern Slovakia.[14]

ETIOLOGY

Classification

Kemerovo viruses, of which there are 16 recognized subtypes, are classified in the genus *Orbivirus* of the family Reoviridae.

Characteristics

The virions are icosahedral in symmetry, enveloped, with diameter 64 ± 4 nm.[6] The genomes are double stranded, segmented, noninfectious RNA.[16,20] The infectivity of the virus decreases with increasing temperatures above 40°C, being inactivated by heating at 65°C for 30 min.[3,11,19] Tribeč virus is extremely sensitive to physical and chemical treatment, especially to acid and alkaline pH.[3,11,19]

DEFINITION

Kemerovo virus infection is an inapparent to clinically severe febrile illness of wild and domestic animals, birds, and human beings. It is transmitted by virus-infected ticks. Viruses of the closely related species have been isolated on 4 continents.

ANIMAL INFECTION

Clinical

Natural infections in goats, cattle, small feral mammals, and birds (predominantly *Turdus* spp.), have been recognized solely on the basis of serological findings. In experimental infections in laboratory animals, fatal encephalitis was produced by intracerebral (i.c.) inoculation of suckling mice or rats. In weanling mice, i.c. inoculation produced encephalitis with persistence of virus in the brain for 10 days but no detectable viremia or invasion of visceral organs.[8,9] Subcutaneous (s.c.) injection of suckling mice produced viremia but no clinical illness.[8,9] Intraperitoneal (i.p.) injection of juvenile mice led to antibody formation. Monkeys inoculated intrathalmically developed mild fever and central nervous system (CNS) inflammation, with virus in spinal fluid from 10 to 15 days postinoculation.[10,15]

Pathology

After i.c. inoculation in suckling mice, Tribeč or Kemerovo viruses cause progressive damage to glial cells and neurons, with widespread neuronal destruction by the time of death.[3,8,9,12] In monkeys inoculated with these viruses, meningitis, and choriomeningitis with perivascular infiltration of brain stem by 10 days, corpus striatum by 15 days, and thalmus by 20 days postinoculation were recorded.[10,15]

Diagnosis

Definitive diagnosis of infection by Kemerovo and Tribeč viruses is based on laboratory isolation and serological characterization of the virus. Blood and brain tissues are best for viral isolation, using inoculation of chick embryo or mouse L cell cultures,[3] or i.c. injection into suckling mice. Tribeč virus shows a high affinity to these cell cultures, with rapid adsorption of virus and short reproduction cycles ending in complete cpe of the cell monolayers. Viral isolates are identified by cross-CF and plaque neutralization tests with subtype specific antisera. Serological diagnosis in the absence of virus isolation may be difficult to interpret on single patients because of crossreactions among Kemerovo virus subtypes.

HUMAN INFECTION

Clinical

Kemerovo and Tribeč viruses were isolated from spinal fluid samples from patients with clinical meningoencephalitis[1] and meningitis,[3] but the role of this virus in human disease has not yet been clearly elucidated. In a serological survey of 100 sera from healthy persons in the area where Tribeč virus was isolated, 3% of the population were found to possess neutralizing antibodies to Tribeč virus. Blood and spinal fluid samples should be collected for laboratory assay.

EPIDEMIOLOGY

Occurrence

The occurrence of subtypes of Kemerovo virus is worldwide. Since 1962 and 1963, when Kemerovo and Tribeč, and Lipovnik viruses were isolated, many isolations of closely related viruses have been made in Azerbaijan, Canada, Egypt, India, Jamaica, Malaysia, Pakistan, Peru, Scotland, Sudan, U.S., and U.S.S.R. In addition to isolates from human patients, Kemerovo viruses have been recovered from naturally infected small mammals,[4,5,7] a sentinel goat,[2] and a bird in Egypt.[17]

Transmission

The Kemerovo viruses are, so far as is known, all tick-transmitted. Kemerovo subtype virus has been isolated from *Ixodes persulcatus* and *I. ricinus* ticks. In Central Europe, Tribeč and Lipovnik viruses have been isolated from *I. ricinus* ticks.[4,5,7,14] Tribec virus was also isolated in Rumania from *Haemaphysalis punctata* ticks; also ticks collected on sentinel goats which also yielded the virus.[2] Ochotskij virus from Tyuleniy Island, U.S.S.R. has been isolated from *I. putus* ticks. Other viruses of the Kemerovo species have been isolated from *Ornithodoros capensis, I. uriae (putus), Argas hermanni, Boophilus microplus, O. amblus, A. cooleyi, Rhipicephalus sanguineus, Hyalomma* spp., and *Amblyomma cajennense* in other *Ioxids* and *Argasids*.

Human Hosts

In the two reported cases of Kemerovo and Tribeč virus infection, the viruses were isolated from spinal fluid of patients with clinical diagnosis of meningoencephalitis and meningitis.[1,3]

CONTROL

Prevention and Therapy

There is no specific therapy for Kemerovo virus infections. Measures to reduce tick populations have not been practical in Central Europe. In selected areas of Siberia, direct application of DDT or HCH has given excellent control of some tick vectors. Health education for person protection from exposure are pertinent.

PUBLIC HEALTH ASPECTS

Economic and Social Impact

No clinical disease associated with animal infections by Kemerovo viruses have been reported. Diagnosed human cases have been rare so far and serological evidence of infection has not been widespread. Clinical human disease may, however, be serious.[1,3] At this time, surveillance studies for Kemerovo virus infections have still been limited.[3]

REFERENCES

1. **Chumakov, M. P., Karpovich, L. G., Sarmanova, E. S., Sergeeva, G. I., Bychkova, M. B., Tapupere, V. O., Libíkova, H., Mayer, V., Řeháček, J., Kožuch, O., and Ernek, E.,** Report of the isolation from Ixodes persulcatus ticks and from patients in Western Siberia of a virus differing from the agent of tick-borne encephalitis, *Acta Virol.,* 7, 82, 1963.
2. **Ernek, E., Kožuch, O., and Grešíková, M.,** Isolation of Tribeč virus from the blood of sentinel pastured goats in Tribeč region (Slovakia), *Acta Virol.,* 10, 367, 1966.
3. **Grešíková, M.,** Studies on Tick-borne Arboviruses Isolated in Central Europe, *Biological works,* Slovak Academy of Sciences, Bratislava, 2. XVIII., 5.
4. **Grešíková, M., Ernek, E., Kožuch, O., and Nosek, J.,** Some ecological aspects on Tribeč virus, *Folia Parasitol. (Prague),* 17, 379, 1970.
5. **Grešíková, M., Kožuch, O., Ernek, E., and Nosek, J.,** "Tribeč" a newly isolated virus from ticks Ixodes ricinus and small rodents, in Theoretical questions of natural foci of diseases, *Proc. Symp., Czechoslovak Acad. Sci.,* Prague, November 26, 1963, 439.
6. **Grešíková, M., Mrena, E., and Vachálková, A.,** Purification and morphology of Tribeč arbovirus, *Acta Virol.,* 13, 67, 1969.
7. **Grešíková, M., Nosek, J., Kožuch, O., Ernek, E., and Lichard, M.,** Study on the ecology of Tribeč virus, *Acta Virol.,* 9, 83, 1965.
8. **Grešíková, M. and Rajčáni, J.,** *Natural and Experimental Pathogenicity of Tick-borne Arboviruses (excluding group B), Isolated in Europe,* presented at the Int. Symp. Tick-Borne Arboviruses, (Excluding Group B), Smolenice, September, 1969.
9. **Grešíková, M. and Rajčani, J.,** Experimental pathogenicity of Tribeč arbovirus for mice, *Acta Virol.,* 13, 114, 1969.
10. **Grešíková, M., Rajčáni, J., and Hruzik, E.,** Experimental infection of rhesus monkeys with Uukuniemi virus, *Acta Virol.,* 14, 408, 1970.
11. **Grešíková, M., Vachálková, A., and Mrena, E.,** Some physicochemical properties of Tribeč arbovirus, Presented at the Int. Symp. Tick-Borne Arboviruses (Excluding Group B), Smolenice 1969.
12. **Libíkova, H., Ernek, E., and Albrecht, P.,** Pathogenicity and pathogenesis of Kemerovo virus and Kemerovo-like viruses in some laboratory and domestic mammals, *Acta Virol.,* 9, 423, 1965.
13. **Libíkova, H., Mayer, V., Kožuch, O., Rehacek, J., Ernek, E., and Albrecht, P.,** Isolation from Ixodes persulcatus ticks of cytophatic agents (Kemerovo virus) differing from tick-borne encephalitis virus and some of their properties, *Acta Virol.,* 8, 289, 1964.
14. **Libíkova, H., Řeháček, J., Grešíková, M., Kožuch, O., Somogyiova, J., and Ernek, E.,** Cytophatic viruses isolated from Ixodes ricinus ticks in Czechoslovakia, *Acta Virol.,* 8, 96, 1964.
15. **Libíkova, H., Tesařová, J., and Rajčáni, J.,** Experimental infection of monkeys with Kemerovo virus, *Acta Virol.,* 14, 64, 1970.
16. **Rosenbergová, M. and Slávik, I.,** Ribonuclease-resistant RNA of Kemerovo virus, *Acta Virol.,* 19, 67, 1975.
17. **Schmidt, J. R. and Shope, R. E.,** Kemerovo virus from a migrating common redstart of Eurasia, *Acta Virol.,* 15, 112, 1971.
18. **Topciu, V., Rosiu, N., Georgescu, L., Gherman, D., Arcan, P., and Csaky, N.,** Isolation of a cytophatic agent from the tick Haemaphysalis punctata, *Acta Virol.,* 12, 1968.
19. **Vachálková, A. and Grešíková, M.,** Some physico-chemical properties of Tribeč arboviruses, *Acta Virol.,* 13, 337, 1969.
20. **Žemla, J., Anderleová, A., and Grešíková, M.,** A study on the nature of the nucleic acid of arbovirus Tribeč, *Acta Virol.,* 12, 120, 1968.

ARBOVIRAL ZOONOSES IN AFRICA

ARBOVIRAL ZOONOSES IN SOUTHERN AFRICA

CHIKUNGUNYA FEVER

B. M. McIntosh and J. H. S. Gear

NAME AND SYNONYMS

The name chikungunya (CHIK), first used in the original outbreak in Tanzania, means in the local vernacular "that which bends up", and refers to the bent posture adopted by patients because of the severe joint pains. It is not a "place name" like the names of many other arboviruses. There are no synonyms, but the illness is sometimes described as being "denguelike" because of its clinical similarity to that disease.

HISTORY

Chikungunya (CHIK) fever was first identified as a clinical entity of viral origin during an epidemic in Tanzania in 1952 and 1953.[11,12] It is probable, however, that earlier outbreaks in Africa and elsewhere might have been confused with dengue. Virus was isolated from human beings and mosquitoes including *Aedes aegypti* during this outbreak, and shortly afterwards the virus was transmitted experimentally by *Ae. aegypti*. A strain of virus isolated during the outbreak was identified as a group A arbovirus (*Alphavirus*), and its etiological role confirmed serologically.[13] Human infection was subsequently recognized in several countries in tropical and subtropical Africa, and since 1958 it has been recognized as the cause of large epidemics in the Philippines, Thailand, Vietnam, and India. The fact that the virus has repeatedly been isolated from canopy-frequenting mosquito species, *Ae. africanus* in eastern and western Africa,[9,16] and the *Ae. furcifer-taylori* group in western and southern Africa,[10,14] has implicated wild primates as natural hosts. The virus has been isolated several times from wild primates (*Cercopithecus aethiops, Galago senegalensis, Papio papio*),[15] with antibody titers in wild populations and high levels of viremia in some instances. Since specific antibody titers have been demonstrated in wild populations, the involvement of at least some species of wild primates is now reliably established.[2,6]

ETIOLOGY

CHIK virus is classified in the genus *Alphavirus* within the family Togaviridae. Among alphaviruses, it is closest antigenically to O'nyong-nyong, Mayaro, and Semliki Forest viruses. In serological studies on human sera from Africa, the antibody response has been extremely difficult to differentiate from that caused by O'nyong-nyong virus. However, the viruses are readily separated by the low pathogenicity of the latter virus for suckling mice. CHIK virus is cultivated readily in the brains of suckling mice for which it is pathogenic, as well as in several cell lines. Wild-type virus is nonpathogenic for adult mice. A hemagglutinin is obtainable from the brains of suckling mice infected with the virus. There are slight antigenic differences between African and Asian CHIK virus strains.

DEFINITION

Chikungunya is a mosquito-borne illness in human beings characterized by fever, arthritis, rash, and mild hemorrhagic signs. It is caused by an alphavirus which is apparently transmitted in nature among wild primates by canopy-frequenting mosquitoes. How the virus persists in nature is not known, but there is evidence that bats may also be important natural hosts.

ANIMAL INFECTION

By experimental inoculation of virus, it has been shown that cattle, sheep, goats, horses, young chicks, seven species of wild birds, rabbits, guinea pigs, cats, and house rats are either nonsusceptible or produce only a low-level viremia.[1,5] Two species of African bats of the genera *Tadarida* and *Pipistrellus* circulated significantly high concentrations of virus after inoculation.[14] By the same means, it was shown that African rodents of the genera *Mastomys* and *Aethomys* responded to infection with low viremias, while *Mystromys* did so with high level viremia. Susceptibility studies also indicated that the baboon, *P. ursinus,* and monkeys of two species, *C. aethiops* and *Macaca radiata* produced high level viremias, but were otherwise largely asymptomatic.[5,8] On several occasions virus has been transmitted experimentally between monkeys by mosquitoes.

Virus has frequently been isolated from wild populations of mosquitoes of several species. Species found infected in Africa, and which are or might be important vectors, have been *Ae. aegypti, Ae. africanus,* members of *Ae. furcifer-taylori* group, and *Mansonia* species. Biological transmission has been demonstrated for *Ae. aegypti, Ae. furcifer, Ae. calceatus,* and *Mansonia africana.*[4,5,7,8,14]

HUMAN INFECTION

Clinical Features

In two accidental laboratory infections resulting from the bites of mosquitoes (*Ae. furcifer*) infected with an African strain of virus, the incubation periods were 22 and 80 hr. The onset of the illness is characteristically sudden, with the occurrence of intense pain in one or several joints, fever, myalgia, and sometimes nausea and vomiting. Headache, coryza, conjunctivitis, eye pain, photophobia, lymphadenopathy, and a maculopapular rash develop. The fever lasts 3 to 10 days and is often biphasic. The rash which develops between the 2nd and the 5th days of illness may be associated with purpuric spots, but generally the hemorrhagic signs seen in Asia have not been reported in Africa. Convalescence may be prolonged, with malaise and joint pain lasting several weeks or months. In convalescence, some patients develop periarticular nodules not unlike those seen in patients with rheumatoid arthritis.

Diagnosis

Clinically, the disease can be confused with O'nyong-nyong, dengue, Sindbis, and West Nile infections, and the diagnosis must be established by isolation and identification of virus and serologically. Virus is readily isolated from blood, often up to 6 days after onset. In Africa, a diagnosis based solely on antibody response is unreliable, as it is difficult or impossible to differentiate CHIK responses from those produced by O'nyong-nyong virus. However, these two viruses differ markedly in their pathogenicity for mice, so in order to establish the diagnosis it is important that virus isolation be attempted in all human infections, and the pathogenicity of the strains isolated be investigated in mice. In Africa, apart from O'nyong-nyong virus, the hemagglutin-ation-inhibition (HI) test will readily differentiate CHIK virus from other alphavirus infections.

EPIDEMIOLOGY

Past outbreaks and the results of serological surveys have revealed that human in-fection by CHIK virus is exceedingly common and widespread in tropical and subtrop-ical Africa. It is now evident that this virus is the predominant alphavirus infecting people in the warmer regions of Africa. In southern Africa the virus has been isolated from human patients in Zimbabwe and South Africa, and from mosquitoes of the *Ae. furcifer-taylori* group in South Africa.[14] In addition, its presence in Mozambique, Bot-swana, and Namibia has been revealed by serological surveys although, as stated pre-viously, confusion with O'nyong-nyong cannot be excluded. In southern Africa, where both tropical and temperate climates occur, the virus is present only in the tropical region, and its southern limits of distribution in this region appear to correlate with the 18°C midwinter isotherm.[2]

Recognized human infections in southern Africa have occurred infrequently, and have been interposed by lengthy interepidemic periods. The virus was first isolated in southern Africa in 1956 during a small rural epidemic in the Transvaal lowlands of South Africa. The next recognized outbreak was a large one in 1962 in the eastern lowlands of Zimbabwe.[3] The only other outbreaks have been in 1975 and 1976 in the same region of the Transvaal as the first outbreak.[14] All these outbreaks involved rural populations and occurred during very wet summers. Viral activity during interepidemic periods was only detected on one occasion, when evidence was found of recent infec-tion in a wild monkey population in South Africa.[2] Despite the irregularity in human infections, it seems probable that the virus is endemic in southern Africa.

Baboons and monkeys may circulate CHIK virus at levels that readily infect mos-quitoes, and antibodies have frequently been found in these wild primates, suggesting that they play an important role in the epidemiology of the disease. In a small, rural focus of intense human infection in the 1976 outbreak in South Africa, all of 76 ba-boons captured and tested shortly after the outbreak were found to have antibodies. Evidence of infection in baboons was also found after the outbreak in Zimbabwe. Observations in southern Africa have strongly suggested that wild primate infections have preceded or occurred concurrently with epidemics in the human population. In a population of vervet monkeys in South Africa, in which an immune rate of 54% was present initially, no further infection was detected during a 5-year period of interepi-demic surveillance,[2] indicating that this species was not strongly involved in mainte-nance of the virus. CHIK virus has frequently been isolated from canopy-frequenting species, *Ae. africanus* and *Ae. furcifer-taylori,* both of which probably utilize wild primates as preferential hosts. *Ae. furcifer-taylori* species have also been shown to be efficient vectors of the virus. There is much supportive epidemiological evidence that the latter species are the main vectors of both human and wild primate infection in southern Africa. These species breed in treeholes, coexist in the wooded savanna, and their geographical distribution in southern Africa correlates with that of the virus. They are prevalent in areas where human epidemics have occurred, and at the dormi-tory sites of wild primates. Although primarily arboreal feeders, they have been col-lected in large numbers off human bait at ground level, and so could readily transmit virus from wild primates to man. The experience in southern Africa has been that human epidemics have been largely rural and restricted to the wooded savanna, the endemic area of mosquitoes of *Ae. furcifer-taylori* species. Within the savanna, the large trees in riverine bush zones appear to favor virus transmission, as these trees are both prolific in larval habitats and utilized as dormitory sites by primates. Another habitat implicated in viral transmission, because of its use as a primate dormitory, is the high granite outcrops commonly present in the savanna of Zimbabwe and South Africa. The involvement of other animal species in the epidemiology of Chikungunya fever has been very inadequately studied. There is some evidence from Africa that bats may be involved. The virus has been isolated twice from the salivary glands of *Scotophilus* sp. in Senegal,[15] antibodies have been reported from bat populations, and some bat species have been shown to develop viremia.

CONTROL

No vaccine is available and it is doubtful whether immunization would be justified at present in Africa. Avoidance of mosquito contact is the most practical control measure, since the vectors involved in rural epidemics feed on people for only a limited period shortly after sunset, and are essentially sylvatic in habitats. Viremic patients should be protected from mosquitoes, particularly in urban environments where secondary epidemics transmitted by *Ae. aegypti* are likely. For the same reason, regular surveillance of mosquitoes in urban areas should be maintained. Epidemics in Africa in the past have not been a significant public health problem, but this favorable state of affairs could deteriorate in the future as a result of increasing urbanization giving rise to vast domestic populations of *Ae. aegypti.*

REFERENCES

1. **Bedekar, S. D. and Pavri, K. M.,** Studies with chikungunya virus. I. Susceptibility of birds and small mammals, *Indian J. Med. Res.,* 57, 1181, 1969.
2. **McIntosh, B. M.,** Antibody against chikungunya virus in wild primates in southern Africa, *S. Afr. J. Med. Sci.,* 35, 65, 1970.
3. **McIntosh, B. M., Harwin, R. M., Paterson, H. E., and Westwater, M. L.,** An epidemic of chikungunya in South-Eastern Rhodesia, *Cent. Afr. J. Med.,* 9, 351, 1963.
4. **McIntosh, B. M. and Jupp, P. G.,** Attempts to transmit chikungunya virus with six species of mosquito, *J. Med. Entomol.,* 7, 615, 1970.
5. **McIntosh, B. M., Paterson, H. E., Donaldson, J. M., and de Sousa, J.,** Chikungunya virus: viral susceptibility and transmission studies with some vertebrates and mosquitoes, *S. Afr. J. Med. Sci.,* 28, 45, 1963.
6. **Osterrieth, P. M. and Deleplanque-Liegeois, P.,** Presence d'anticorps vis-a-vis des virus transmis par arthropods chez le chimpanze (*Pan troglodites*). Comparaison de leur etat immunitair a celni de l'homme, *Ann. Soc. Belge Med. Trop.,* 41, 63, 1961.
7. **Paterson, H. E. and McIntosh, B. M.,** Further studies on the chikungunya outbreak in southern Rhodesia in 1962. II. Transmission experiments with *Aedes furcifer-taylori* group of mosquitoes and with a member of the *Anopheles gambiae* complex, *Ann. Trop. Med. Parasitol.,* 58, 52, 1964.
8. **Paul, S. D. and Singh, K. R. P.,** Experimental infection of *Macaca radiata* with chikungunya virus and transmission of virus by mosquitoes, *Indian J. Med. Res.,* 57, 802, 1969.
9. *Rapport Annuel,* Institut Pasteur Bangui, 1975.
10. *Report from Institut Pasteur Dakar,* Arthropod-borne virus information exchange, 31, 128, 1976.
11. **Robinson, M. C.,** An epidemic of virus disease in Southern Province, Tanganyika Territory, in 1952-53. I. Clinical features, *Trans. R. Soc. Trop. Med. Hyg.,* 49, 28, 1955.
12. **Ross, R. W.,** The Newala epidemic. III. The virus: isolation, pathogenic properties and relationship to the epidemic, *J. Hyg.,* 54, 177, 1956.
13. **Spence, L. P. and Thomas, L.,** Application of haemagglutination and complement-fixation techniques to the identification and serological classification of arthropod-borne viruses, *Trans. R. Soc. Trop. Med. Hyg.,* 53, 248, 1959.
14. **McIntosh, B. M.,** unpublished data, 1976.
15. **Robin, Y.,** unpublished data, 1962—1975.
16. **Weinbren, M. P., Haddow, A. J., and Williams, M. C.,** The occurrence of chikungunya virus in Uganda. I. Isolation from mosquitoes, *Trans. R. Soc. Trop. Med. Hyg.,* 52, 253, 1958.

SINDBIS FEVER

B. M. McIntosh and J. H. S. Gear

NAME AND SYNONYMS

Sindbis (SIN) fever is named for the village in the Nile Delta of Egypt where mosquitoes were collected from which the virus was first isolated. There are no synonyms.

HISTORY

Sindbis virus was first isolated in 1952 from *Culex univittatus* mosquitoes.[9] It was implicated as the cause of illness in human beings in Uganda in 1961,[10] and subsequently in South Africa,[4,8] and in Australia.[2] The virus was isolated from a crow, *Corvus corone* during the original studies in Egypt. This suggested an avian reservoir, a hypothesis that has subsequently been confirmed.

ETIOLOGY

SIN virus is the type species of the genus *Alphavirus* of the family Togaviridae.[1] Slight antigenic differences among strains from some countries have been observed. SIN virus is closer antigenically to western equine encephalitis virus than to other alphaviruses. It multiplies well in brains of suckling mice, and has been cultivated in several cell lines. Hemagglutinin is readily obtained from brains of infected suckling mice. Wild-type virus is nonpathogenic for adult mice inoculated intracerebrally.

DEFINITION

Sindbis fever is a mosquito-borne human disease caused by an Alphavirus, and characterized by arthralgia, rash, and malaise. The virus is maintained in wild birds by ornithophilic mosquitoes.

ANIMAL INFECTION

SIN virus is not known to cause illness or viremia in any domestic mammals. Antibodies have been found only rarely in sheep, goats, cattle, and horses in endemic areas in South Africa, indicating that these species are not significantly involved in transmission cycles. While adult chickens have developed only low-level viremias, very young chicks have circulated virus at high concentrations, and mortality has been recorded in such experimental infections. The virus was shown to circulate for about 3 days, and usually at high levels in 13 of 14 species of South African wild birds belonging to five families.[5] Antibody responses were detected in some of these birds; in others it could not be detected, or was transient.[7] *Culex univattatus* has been shown experimentally to be an efficient vector.[3] In one experiment, 23 out of 32 (72%, mosquitoes were infected when fed on a blood-virus mixture containing 5.1 logs of virus, and 12 out of 21 of these (57%) infected mosquitoes transmitted virus to chickens on the 18th day. It was also shown that virus concentrations as low as 1.7 logs will infect 10% of *Cx. univittatus* mosquitoes.

HUMAN INFECTION

Clinical Features

The incubation period is unknown. Low grade fever lasting a few days, lassitude, headache, joint pains, and generalized body aches and fatigue on slight exertion are early symptoms. Rash appears suddenly at the same time or 1 to 2 days later. The rash involves the trunk and limbs, being most common on the buttocks and legs, and may involve the palms and soles, but the face is usually not affected.[4,8] The lesions may appear in crops over a few days and last some 10 days, leaving brown stains. The spots are maculopapular, small, and show a tendency to vesiculate, especially when exposed to friction. Pruritis is sometimes present. Sore throat with mild inflammation and small ulcers may be observed. Pains in the small joints of the hands and feet are invariably present, and the larger joints of the limbs may also be affected. The tendons in the hands and feet may be painful. Lymphadenopathy is usually absent, but enlargement of the inguinal, occipital, and cervical nodes may occur. Signs of slight myocardial involvement have been reported. Acute illness is usually over within 10 days, although fatigue and tendon pains may persist for several weeks.

Diagnosis

The clinical picture is very similar to that seen in West Nile fever, so diagnosis must be established by isolation and identification of the virus or by serology. The virus may occasionally be isolated from blood samples collected in the early stages of the illness, but is more constantly isolated from vesicular fluid. In Africa, where there are no closely related viruses infecting people, diagnosis based on the hemagglutination-inhibition (HI) antibody response is reliable.

EPIDEMIOLOGY

SIN virus has been shown to be widely distributed in Africa, Europe, Asia, and Australia. It has been isolated in Egypt, Uganda, Mozambique, Nigeria, South Africa, Cameroon, Senegal, Central African Republic, Israel, Czechoslovakia, U.S.S.R., India, Philippines, Malaysia, Borneo, and Australia.

There is substantial evidence to indicate that the virus is maintained in wild birds of several species by ornithophilic mosquitoes. The virus has been isolated from wild birds in several different countries, and antibodies have frequently been found in wild avian populations. Sentinel domestic pigeons placed in endemic areas in South Africa have acquired natural infection by the virus under field conditions. A long-term study of infection in sentinel pigeons in South Africa suggested that avian infection only occurred during summer and autumn. It is not known how the virus passes through the dry winter season.

In South Africa, *Cx. univittatus* has been identified as the transmitting vector throughout the inland plaeau. This species from which the virus has frequently been isolated feeds primarily on birds, and its maintenance of transmission among birds is well substantiated.

Human infections and probably also avian infections are more frequent in the temperate, inland plateau than in the subtropical coastal lowlands of South Africa. Human infections in South Africa occur sporadically each year during the summer, probably because *Cx. univittatus* has a low feeding rate on people. Human infections on an epidemic scale were recorded in 1974 following very heavy rains,[6] when numbers of *Cx. univittatus* reached abnormally high levels, and there was considerable feeding on human beings by this species. Morbidity due to SIN virus was difficult to establish during this epidemic, as West Nile virus was causing human infections at the same time. Human viremias are negligible in SIN virus infections, making it probable that most human infections result from mosquito transmission to people from viremic birds. Human infection appears to be directly dependent upon avian infections, and widespread avian infections plus high vector mosquito populations appear to be necessary for human epidemics to occur.

CONTROL AND SIGNIFICANCE

Apart from the epidemic in 1974, Sindbis fever has not been recognized as a significant health problem in South Africa. It is possible that strains of virus from differnt countries may vary in their pathogenicity for people. As observed in South Africa, the illness can be fairly severe, yet clinical illness associated with infection in other countries has rarely been reported. The control of *Cx. univittatus* would be difficult, as its natural habitat, permanent ground pools with emergent vegetation is common in tropical areas. The control of avian populations would not be indicated with the present scale of human infection. Wild bird population control and maintenance of domestic fowl in screened enclosures do not appear to be feasible based on the presently recognized status of the public health problem. No vaccines are available for human or animal immunization.

REFERENCES

1. **Casals, J. and Brown, L. V.**, Haemagglutination with arthropod-borne viruses, *J. Exp. Med.*, 99, 429, 1954.
2. **Doherty, R. L., Bodey, A. S., and Carew, J. S.**, Sindbis virus infection in Australia, *Med. J. Aust.*, 2, 1016, 1969.
3. **Jupp, P. G. and McIntosh, B. M.**, Quantitative experiments on the vector capability of *Culex (Culex) univittatus* Theobald with West Nile and Sindbis viruses, *J. Med. Entomol.*, 7, 371, 1970.
4. **Malherbe, H., Strickland-Cholmley, M., and Jackson, A. L.**, Sindbis virus infection in man. Report of a case with recovery of virus from skin lesions, *S. Afr. Med. J.*, 37, 547, 1963.
5. **McIntosh, B. M., Dickinson, D. B., and McGillivray, G. M.**, Ecological studies in Sindbis and West Nile viruses in South Africa. V. The response of birds to inoculation of virus, *S. Afr. J. Med. Sci.*, 34, 77, 1969.
6. **McIntosh, B. M., Jupp, P. G., Dos Santos, I., and Meenehan, G. M.**, Epidemics of West Nile and Sindbis viruses in South Africa with *Culex (Culex) univittatus* Theobald as vector, *S. Afr. J. Sci.*, 72, 295, 1976.
7. **McIntosh, B. M., Madsen, W., and Dickinson, D. B.**, Ecological studies on Sindbis and West Nile viruses in South Africa. VI. The antibody response of wild birds, *S. Afr. J. Med. Sci.*, 34, 83, 1969.
8. **McIntosh, B. M., McGillivray, G. M., Dickinson, D. B., and Malherbe, H.**, Illness caused by Sindbis and West Nile viruses in South Africa. *S. Afr. Med. J.*, 38, 291, 1964.
9. **Taylor, R. M., Hurlbut, H. S., Work, T. H., Kingston, J. K., and Frothingham, T. E.**, Sindbis virus: a newly recognized arthropod-transmitted virus, *Am. J. Trop. Med. Hyg.*, 4, 844, 1955.
10. **Woodall, J. P., Williams, M. C., and Hewit, L. E.**, East African Virus Research Institute, *Annual Report*, 1961/62.

ARBOVIRAL ZOONOSES IN SOUTHERN AFRICA - WESSELSBRON FEVER

B. M. McIntosh and J. H. S. Gear

NAME AND SYNONYMS

Wesselsbron fever (WSL) is named for the town of Wesselsbron, South Africa, near which the epidemic in sheep occurred from which the virus was isolated. There are no synonyms.

HISTORY

Wesselsbron virus was first isolated in 1955 from a dead lamb during an outbreak of disease with abortion and high mortality in sheep, an episode suggestive of Rift Valley fever near Wesselsbron, South Africa.[7] A month later it was isolated at a second locality in South Africa over 500 miles away, from a febrile human being and from *Aedes circumluteolus* mosquitoes.[6] During early laboratory studies, the virus caused several infections in laboratory personnel. In subsequent years, the virus has been frequently isolated from mosquitoes in several countries in Africa, and its transmission by mosquitoes of several genera has been demonstrated.

ETIOLOGY

WSL virus is classified in the genus *Flavivirus* in the family Togaviridae.[1] It multiplies readily in the brains of suckling mice, in embryonating hens' eggs, in several cell lines, and in primary lamb kidney cell cultures. The diameter of the virion is estimated to be 45 nm.[3]

DEFINITION

Wesselsbron fever is a mosquito-borne disease of sheep and human beings caused by a Flavivirus and characterized mainly by abortion and lamb mortality in sheep; and fever, headache, muscular pains, and mild rash in human patients. In its predeliction for embryonic and hepatic tissues, and its epidemiology, the virus is remarkably similar to Rift Valley fever virus. The virus reservoir is unknown.

ANIMAL INFECTION

In newborn lambs, WSL fever is characterized by weakness, loss of appetite, and often by mortality. Adult sheep are more resistant and often show only a transient fever. Mortality in open ewes is usually low, but in pregnant animals it may reach 20%. Abortion may occur during the febrile phase in ewes or 6 to 14 days later. In the latter instance, virus can be isolated from the brains and livers of fetuses. In adult cattle, horses, and swine, experimental inoculation with WSL virus has mild to severe febrile responses. While outbreaks of disease in cattle have not been reported, the infection in newborn and pregnant animals has not been adequately studied. On one occasion, experimental inoculation of virus into a 2-month-old calf resulted in death. WSL virus was also isolated from an adult cow which had developed a naturally-acquired fatal illness. WSL virus has been isolated from a naturally infected gerbil *Des-

modillus auricularis in South Africa. Experimentally, viremia reaching 5.0 logs without signs of clinical illness has been shown to occur in this species. Experimental studies in five other species of South African rodents showed them to be nonsusceptible. Viremia has been demonstrated in two species of wild ducks and a coot.

In cattle and sheep of all ages, virus circulates at high concentrations in blood, and the duration of viremia can be up to 5 days. The lesions are mainly confined to the liver, and vary in severity, making histological diagnosis in mild cases unreliable. Lesions reported include diffuse fatty infiltration, bile pigmentation, and necrosis of hepatocytes, and inflammatory cell infiltration of the liver.[4] Intranuclear inclusion bodies sometimes occur in hepatocytes. These lesions require differentiation from those of Rift Valley fever and poisoning by *Tribulus* spp. plants.

WSL virus has been transmitted experimentally by *Aedes circumluteolus, Ae. caballus,* and *Culex zombaensis* mosquitoes in South Africa and by *Ae. aegypti* and *Cx. quinquefasciatus* in Thailand.[2,5]

HUMAN INFECTION

Clinical

In laboratory exposures, the incubation period has been 2 to 4 days, but in the field it is probably longer when transmitted by mosquito bites. The onset is characteristically sudden, with chills and pains in muscles, joints, and eyes, and fever. During the fever, which may last up to one week, patients often complain of hyperasthesia of the skin, and may develop an evanescent maculopapular rash. In severely ill patients there may be some signs of encephalitis, including photophobia, blurred vision, and mental impairment. Fatal cases have not been recognized. During convalescence, patients may complain of muscle pains persisting for several weeks. Blood counts show leucopenia and, clinical laboratory tests may show disorders of liver function.

Diagnosis

WSL virus can be isolated from blood or throat swabs during the acute illness. Serological diagnosis is possible in persons who have not had a previous flavivirus infection.

EPIDEMIOLOGY

In Africa, WSL virus has been isolated from animals and/or mosquitoes in South Africa, Zimbabwe, Cameroon, Nigeria, Uganda, Central African Republic, and Senegal. Serological surveys have also indicated its presence in Mozambique, Botswana, Namibia, and Madagascar. In Asia, WSL virus has been reported from Thailand.

WSL virus has been isolated on numerous occasions from a variety of mosquito species, and it seems likely that several species may act as vectors.

The frequency of isolation from *Aedes* spp., and the efficiency of transmission by mosquitoes of this genus have suggested that these mosquitoes are important vectors. In the sheep-rearing areas of South Africa the indications are that one or both members of the *Ae. caballus-juppi* group are the main vectors transmitting the virus among sheep. These species in the laboratory readily transmit virus after feeding on viremic sheep. During the rainy season when enormous populations of these mosquitoes appear, virus could rapidly be disseminated and maintained among sheep over large areas independent of any animal reservoir. These mosquitoes are short-lived as adults, however, and could not maintain transmission over long periods of time. Human exposure may result from bites of infected *Aedes* spp. mosquitoes, or in handling carcasses or tissues of animals which have died of the disease. A viremia of 4.0 logs has been recorded in a human patient, so transmission of virus from human beings to mosquitoes is likely.

No long-term reservoir hosts of WSL virus have been identified as yet. Isolation of the virus from a naturally infected gerbil has suggested the need for studies in field rodents.

CONTROL AND SIGNIFICANCE

Although antibody surveys have shown that human infection is widespread and common in the warmer regions of Africa, the significance of WSL infections to public health is difficult to assess. The extent to which infections are clinically apparent, mild, or subclinical is not known. No human epidemics have been identified, and it appears that human infections are mainly sporadic. Human exposures by handling infected tissues of domestic animals have been recorded, and may account for many infections in the sheep-rearing areas of South Africa. Protective clothing should be worn by persons handling suspected infected organs of domestic animals.

Since WSL virus was first identified in South Africa, several outbreaks in sheep have been identified, but it has been difficult to assess economic losses. Although antibody prevalence rates are high in cattle in subtropical coastal lowlands of South Africa, the extent of morbidity in these animals remains unknown. A vaccine prepared from a partially attenuated virus strain is available for immunization of adult sheep and lambs. This virus can cause fetal infection with meningo-encephalitis or abortion, so use of this vaccine in gestating sheep is not recommended.

REFERENCES

1. **Casals, J.,** The arthropod-borne group of animal viruses, *Trans. N.Y. Acad. Sci.,* 19, 219, 1957.
2. **Kokernot, R. H., Paterson, H. E., and de Meillon, B.,** Studies on the transmission of Wesselsbron virus by *Aedes (Ochlerotatus) caballus* (Theo), *S. Afr. Med. J.,* 32, 546, 1958.
3. **Lecatsas, G. and Weiss, K. E.,** Formation of Wesselsbron virus in BHK-21 cells, *Arch. Gesamte Virusforsch.,* 27, 332, 1969.
4. **Le Roux, J. M. W.,** The histopathology of Wesselsbron disease in sheep, *Onderstepoort J. Vet. Res.,* 28, 237, 1959.
5. **Simasathin, P. and Olson, L. C.,** Factors influencing the vector potential of *Aedes aegypti* and *Culex quinquefasciatus* for Wesselsbron virus, *J. Med. Entomol.,* 10, 587, 1973.
6. **Smithburn, K. C., Kokernot, R. H., Weinbren, M. P., and de Meillon, B.,** Isolation of Wesselsbron virus from a naturally-infected human being and from *Aedes (Bauksinella) circumluteolus* Theo, *S. Afr. J. Med. Sci.,* 22, 113, 1957.
7. **Weiss, K. E., Haig, D. A., and Alexander, R. A.,** Wesselsbron virus — a virus not previously described, associated with abortion in domestic animals, *Onderstepoort J. Vet. Res.,* 27, 183, 1956.
8. **Moore, D. L.,** personnal communication, 1969.
9. **Smith-Burn, K. C., Kokernot, R. H., Weinbren, M. P., and de Meillon, B.,** Studies on arthropod-borne viruses of Tongaland. IX. Isolation of Wesselsbron virus from a naturally infected human being and from *Aedes* (B), *Circumluteolus, S. A Afr. J. Med. Sci.,* 22, 113, 1957.
10. **Tomori, O.,** personal communication, 1972.
11. **Weiss, K. E., Haig, D. A., and Alexander, R. A.,** Wesselsbron virus — a virus not previously described, associated with abortion in domestic animals, *Onderstepoort J.,* 27, 183, 1956.

WEST NILE FEVER

B. M. McIntosh and J. H. S. Gear

NAME AND SYNONYMS

West Nile (WN) fever is named for the district of Uganda, East Africa where the virus was first isolated. There are no synonyms.

HISTORY

West Nile virus was first isolated in 1937 from the blood of a febrile human being.[9] The antigenic relationship of the virus to St. Louis encephalitis and Japanese encephalitis viruses was demonstrated shortly afterwards, and its characterization as a group B arbovirus (*Flavivirus*) was reported in 1954.[1] After the virus had been isolated from the blood of three children in Egypt in 1950, an ecological study on the viral fever was instituted in that country.[10] The main findings indicated that WN virus was the cause of a mild, endemic summer infection in children; the virus was maintained in birds by mosquitoes, mainly *Culex univittatus,* and possibly overwintered in retarded cyclical transmission in *Cx. pipiens.* WN virus has been the cause of epidemics from Israel,[2] through East Africa, to South Africa.[8]

ETIOLOGY

WN virus is classified in the genus *Flavivirus* of the family Togaviridae. Antigenically, it is a member of the St. Louis encephalitis complex within the flaviviruses, but except in Asia, it does not coexist geographically with other members of the complex that infect man. It multiplies readily in the brains of suckling and adult mice, as well as in several cell lines. It is also pathogenic for adult mice following intraperitoneal inoculation. Hemagglutinin can be obtained from the brains of infected suckling mice.

DEFINITION

West Nile fever is a mosquito-borne illness of human beings caused by a flavivirus and characterized by fever, headache, sore throat, muscular pain, rash, lymphadenopathy, and occasionally by meningoencephalitis. The virus is maintained in wild birds by ornithophilic mosquitoes.

ANIMAL INFECTION

Antibodies are common in cattle, but experimental infection of calves has failed to produce viremia. Antibodies have been found in horses, and natural cases of WN encephalitis in horses have been reported in France and Egypt. The predominant lesions in horses were in the ventral horns of the posterior spinal cord. Lesions in the brain were less severe, and consisted of meningeal edema and lymphocytic infiltration. Experimental infection of horses indicated that viremia levels were low, and probably these animals are not important sources of infection for mosquitoes. Several species of South African rodents have shown a low degree of susceptibility and the virus has been isolated twice from sentinel hamsters exposed in Mozambique. Experimental inoculations in 13 species of South African wild birds belonging to six families demonstrated clinically inapparent infections with viremias in 12 species.[5] Viremias lasted up to 4 days and rose to very high (6.0 logs) levels in some species. Inoculation of adult chickens produced only low viremia levels.

WN virus has been transmitted experimentally by several mosquito species, particularly *Culex* species. In South Africa, *Cx. univittatus* was shown to be an efficient vector.[4] A viremia level as low as 2.7 logs infected 80% of *Cx. univittatus,* and a transmission rate as high as 97% was obtained by feeding 4.1 to 4.6 logs of virus. Low temperatures and low infective doses were shown to decrease vector efficiency.[3] A reduction in the infecting dose from 5.0 to 2.6 logs reduced the transmission rate from 89 to 33%. A reduction in the holding temperature of infected mosquitoes from 26 to 18°C caused a drop in the transmission rate from 97 to 48%. The virus has been isolated occasionally from ticks, but experimental transmission studies have been unsuccessful or inconclusive. Aerosol transmission has been observed in several mammals and in human beings, and it seems likely that infection by ingestion may also occur.

HUMAN INFECTION

Clinical Features

The severity of human disease varies considerably, and is partially age-dependent, being mild in the young and increasing in severity with age, with encephalitis probably confined to the aged. The incubation is probably at least 3 but not more than 6 days. The onset is sudden with fever, which may persist for about 3 to 5 days. Headache, ocular pain, muscular pain, sore throat, nausea, and vomiting frequently occur. During the first 3 days, a maculopapular rash often appears, usually first on the trunk, then spreading to the face and extremities. Rash may persist for 5 to 7 days, then disappear without desquamation. Although arthralgia has not been frequently reported, it has been observed in South Africa. After subsidence, fever and other signs of illness may reappear for a few days. Signs of a meningoencephalitis may develop, but mortality is rare and permanent sequelae unknown. Convalescence is fairly rapid in children, although in adults it is somewhat prolonged and accompanied by weakness and lassitude.

Diagnosis

Clinically, the disease cannot be differentiated from Sindbis fever, and isolation of virus or detection of a specific antibody response are necessary for diagnosis. Although viremia levels are low, virus may persist for up to 6 days in the blood, and virus may usually be isolated from acute phase serum. Serological diagnosis is usually possible unless the patient has been infected previously by another flavivirus causing a broadly reactive antibody response and making interpretation of the test difficult or impossible.

EPIDEMIOLOGY

WN virus has been reported from Africa, Europe, and Asia. It has been isolated in Egypt, Uganda, Central African Republic, South Africa, Zaire, Mozambique, France, Cyprus, U.S.S.R., Israel, India, and Borneo. It is apparently well adapted for survival in temperate climates, and in South Africa human infections are actually more common in temperate than subtropical areas. There is substantial evidence from many countries indicating that a variety of species of wild birds and ornithophilic mosquitoes mainly of the genus *Culex* maintain the cycle of transmission of WN virus. The virus has frequently been isolated from *Culex* spp. mosquitoes and from a variety of avian species in several countries, and antibodies have been found in wild avian populations.

The exposure of sentinel pigeons in temperate areas of South Africa has demonstrated infection during every month in the summer and autumn, but no infections were recorded during the winter.[6] It is not known how the virus overwinters in temperate climates.

In the temperate areas of South Africa, *Cx. univittatus* has been identified as the maintaining vector.[7] It is primarily a bird-feeding mosquito. The virus has frequently been isolated from it, it possesses high vector capability, and has no difficulty transmitting WN virus after feeding on viremic birds. Observations of mosquitoes and other blood-sucking diptera feeding on sentinel pigeons has convincingly identified *Cx. univittatus* as the only important hematophagus parasite of the sentinel birds in the temperate areas in South Africa. Because of the low levels of viremia in chickens, these birds have not been considered to be epidemiologically significant sources of infection for mosquitoes. The presence of fowls in domestic environments may decrease human infections by diverting infected mosquitoes from human beings to poultry.

WN virus is considered the most common cause of arboviral infections in human beings in South Africa, and sporadic infections have been observed annually during summers since the presence of the virus was established. Immune rates in human populations have usually been between 2 to 25%, but rates of 50% have occasionally been recorded. Avian infections are common during summer, and the relatively low annual incidence of human infections in South Africa appears to be more because of the low feeding preference for people by *Cx. univittatus* than lack of sources of the virus. In 1974, however, a large epidemic infecting 50 to 80% of the human population occurred in the arid Karoo region of South Africa following exceptionally heavy rains.[8] It was demonstrated that because of its abnormally high population, a high rate of feeding by *Cx. univittatus* on human beings occurred. It is likely that this species is responsible for both sporadic and epidemic human infections.

Because of the low levels of viremia in human patients, the highest recorded being 1.8 logs of virus per mℓ and usually less than 1.0 logs, most human infections result from transmission by mosquitoes infected from viremic birds. In South Africa, an antibody survey of wild birds after the epidemic in 1974 showed very high immune rates, and it seems reasonably certain that an inapparent avian epidemic also occurred; indeed, without a high rate of avian infection it is unlikely that a human epidemic could eventuate. One consequence of the aberrant role of human infections is that high human-immune rates have no influence on the extent of viral transmission, but only on the incidence of overt human disease. High human-population immunity levels do not therefore decrease the incidence of disease among susceptible individuals.

CONTROL AND SIGNIFICANCE

As large epidemics of human infections have been infrequent in the past, and the illness is often mild, immunization of persons in populations at risk has not been indicated. During epidemics, avoidance of mosquito attacks and, where justified, control of the vector populations could be applied. Because of the relative severity of the disease in the aged, persons in this age category should exercise particular care in avoiding exposure to vectors. As poultry are frequently infected, handling their carcasses could be a source of infection for people working in poultry slaughter, processing, or research.

REFERENCES

1. **Casals, J. and Brown, L. V.,** Haemagglutination with arthropod-borne viruses, *Exp. Med.,* 99, 429, 1954.

2. **Goldblum, N., Sterk, V. V., and Jasinka-Klingberg, W.,** The natural history of West Nile fever. II. Virological findings and the development of homologous and heterologous antibodies in West Nile infection in man, *Am. J. Hyg.,* 66, 363, 1957.
3. **Jupp, P. G.,** Laboratory studies on the transmission of West Nile virus by *Culex (Culex) univittatus* Theobald; factors influencing the transmission rate, *J. Med. Entomol.,* 4, 455, 1974.
4. **Jupp, P. G. and McIntosh, B. M.,** Quantitative experiments on the vector capability of *Culex (Culex) univittatus* Theobald with West Nile and Sindbis viruses, *J. Med. Entomol.,* 7, 371, 1970.
5. **McIntosh, B. M., Dickinson, D. B., and McGillivray, G. M.,** Ecological studies on Sindbis and West Nile Viruses in South Africa. V. The response of birds to inoculation of virus, *S. Afr. J. Med. Sci.,* 34, 77, 1969.
6. **McIntosh, B. M. and Jupp, P. G.,** Infections in sentinel pigeons by Sindbis and West Nile viruses in South Africa, with observations on *Culex (Culex) univittatus* attracted to these birds, *J. Med. Entomol.,* 16, 234, 1979.
7. **McIntosh, B. M., Jupp, P. G., and Dos Santos, I.,** Infection by Sindbis and West Nile viruses in wild populations of *Culex (Culex) univittatus* Theobald (Diptera: Culicidae) in South Africa, *J. Entomol. Soc. South Afr.,* 41, 57, 1978.
8. **McIntosh, B. M., Jupp, P. G., Dos Santos, I., and Meenehan, G. M.,** Epidemics of West Nile and Sindbis viruses in South Africa with *Culex (Culex) univittatus* Theobald as vector, *S. Afr. J. Sci.,* 72, 295, 1976.
9. **Smithburn, K. C., Hughes, T. P., Burke, A. W., and Paul, J. H.,** A neurotropic virus isolated from the blood of a native of Uganda, *Am. J. Trop. Med. Hyg.,* 20, 471, 1940.
10. **Taylor, R. M., Work, T. H., Hurlbut, H. S., and Rizk, F.,** A study of the ecology of West Nile virus in Egypt, *Am. J. Trop. Med. Hyg.,* 5, 579, 1956.

RIFT VALLEY FEVER

B. M. McIntosh and J. H. S. Gear

NAME AND SYNONYMS

The term "enzootic hepatitis" used in the original description of the disease has fallen into disuse. Rift Valley fever (RVF) is named for the area of Kenya where the disease was first described.

HISTORY

Rift Valley fever virus was first isolated in 1930 from a sheep during an epidemic in sheep and cattle accompanied by abortion in the Rift Valley in Kenya.[1] At the time there was also illness in human beings. There was evidence that the virus was mosquito-borne, as there had been a suspected viral isolation from *Mansonia fuscopennata,* and the disease in sheep had ceased when they were protected from exposure to mosquitoes because of this suspicion. In 1944, several viral isolations were made from mosquitoes in Uganda, and the virus was transmitted by *Eretmapodites chryogaster,* one of the species implicated. From 1950 to 1956, several severe epidemics in South Africa, accompanied by human infection, were recognized in sheep and cattle. In 1953, the virus was isolated from *Aedes caballus* and *Culex theileri* during an outbreak in sheep. Wild-caught *Ae. caballus* were shown to transmit the virus to mice.[2] From 1969 to 1976, widespread outbreaks with severe economic losses occurred again in South Africa, as well as in Zimbabwe, Nambia, and Mozambique. During outbreaks in domestic animals in South Africa in 1975, several fatal infections in human beings were recognized.

ETIOLOGY

On morphological and morphogenetic grounds, RVF virus has provisionally been assigned to the family Bunyaviridae, although antigenically the virus has no known relations. The diameter of the virion is 94 nm. It matures in the cytoplasm, although intranuclear inclusions occur in vivo and in cell cultures. It multiplies readily in the liver and brain of mice, and in several cell lines. A hemagglutinin can be obtained from serum and liver of infected mice. The virus is inactivated when treated for 40 min at 56°C and by 1:1000 formalin. It is ether-sensitive. The virus appears to be very stable in serum, and has withstood 0.5% phenol for 6 months in the cold. There is evidence that the attenuated strain used for immunization is more labile.

DEFINITION

Rift Valley fever is a mosquito-borne virus disease of ungulates and human beings, characterized in ungulates by hepatitis and abortion, and in human patients by hepatitis accompanied in severe cases by hemorrhagic manifestations. People are usually infected by direct contact with infected domestic animals. The virus reservoir is unknown.

ANIMAL INFECTION

Rift Valley fever manifests itself most severely in sheep, although goats are reported to be almost as susceptible. The incubation period is 1 to 2 days. Infected animals show fever, weakness, loss of appetite, stiffness of gait or disinclination to move, vomiting, and sometimes a bloody nasal discharge and diarrhea. Death may occur within a day, and in young animals mortality can be as high as 90%. In adult sheep symptoms are less severe, but abortion followed by death of ewes is common. In cattle, abortion is the usual indication of infection, but subclinical infection is probably common. The main lesions are a necrotic hepatitis with extensive hemorrhages in the liver, kidneys, intestines, and body cavities. Cattle and sheep are viremic for about 4 days, and virus concentrations in the blood usually reach extremely high levels even in asymptomatic animals.

Clinically, the disease in animals is similar to Wesselsbron virus infection, so diagnosis is dependent upon isolation of the virus or by serology. Samples of serum or liver are the best source of virus. A serological diagnosis is reliable, since the virus is antigenically unique. Histologically, the lesions in RVF are mainly a focal necrosis with intranuclear inclusions of hepatocytes, but lesions are also present in the adrenal glands, spleen, kidneys, and lymph nodes.[5] It has been reported that the virus can infect buffaloes, camels, and antelopes, causing abortion and some mortality. Several species of wild rodents and monkeys have developed viremia after inoculation of virus. Horses, swine, cats, birds, rabbits, amphibians, and reptiles are either refractory to infection or show low susceptibility. Guinea pigs exposed experimentally may abort, and ferrets infected intranasally have developed fever and pulmonary consolidation.

RVF virus has been transmitted experimentally by several species of mosquitoes. Among the South African mosquito fauna *Culex theileri, Cx. zombaensis, Cx. neavei, Aedes juppi,* and *Eretmapodites quinquevittatus* have transmitted the virus.[4] Unsuccessful attempts to transmit virus have occurred with *Ae. caballus* mosquitoes and *Ornithodoros savignya* ticks. There is some doubt whether a 1953 report of transmission by *Ae. caballus* actually implicated this species, as what was formerly regarded as *Ae. caballus* has subsequently been found to consist of two species. *Ae. caballus* and *Ae. juppi*, Of the species tested, *Cx. theileri* proved to be the most efficient vectors. In tests using mice as recipient hosts, 11 out of 20 (55%) infected mosquitoes transmitted virus. This high transmission rate could not be confirmed in sheep in which 6 out of 23 (26%) infected *Cx. theileri* transmitted the virus to susceptible sheep.[3]

HUMAN INFECTION

The incubation period is from 3 to 7 days, most commonly about 4 days. The onset is sudden, with chills, muscle pains, especially in the back, joint pains, headache, which is often severe, and a biphasic fever which lasts about 1 week. After about 3 days, the temperature falls to normal and the patient feels well, but after further intervals of 1 to 2 days, recrudescence of the signs and symptoms and fever occurs, lasting about 2 additional days. Patients usually feel nauseous, often vomit, and on examination are noted to have flushed face, injected conjunctiva, and tenderness over the liver. Late in the course of the illness or early in convalescence, patients may complain of defective vision associated with retinitis with a typical cottonwool exudate on the macula. Occasionally both eyes are involved, and patients are severely handicapped by loss of vision. These lesions fortunately, gradually resolve and normal vision returns in most patients, but in some the defect may be more permanent. There may be the tendency to thrombosis in convalescence, and patients have developed coronary and deep vein thrombosis after attacks of Rift Valley fever. Recently cases have developed hemorrhagic diathesis with severe bleeding from mucous membranes, including epistaxis, hemetemesis and melena, and occasionally patients have developed cerebral hemorrhage with paraplegia. Several patients have died from profuse gastrointestinal hemorrhage, and on postmortem examination, the liver has shown extensive hemorrhage and marked necrosis of the parenchymal cells with typical eosinophilic degeneration of the cytoplasm and intranuclear eosinophilic inclusion bodies or granules. There is an initial leucocytosis followed by leucopenia, and in patients who develop a hemorrhagic state, a profound thrombocytopenia is associated with other marked disorders of coagulation. Tests show considerable disturbances of liver and kidney functions.

Diagnosis

Diagnosis is based on isolation and identification of virus from blood or, in fatal cases, from liver. Serological diagnosis is reliable, since the virus is antigenically unique. In human infections there is usually a history of contact with sick domestic animals which had aborted, but infections by RVF must be differentiated from Wesselsbron infections, which probably are also transmissible from animals to people.

EPIDEMIOLOGY

Until recently, RVF infections have been reported only in parts of Africa. Isolations of RVF virus have been reported from Kenya, Uganda, Nigeria, South Africa, Nambia, Zimbabwa, and Mozambique. Antibody surveys in human beings have shown that it is widely distributed in southern Africa, but with low prevalence rates. Immune persons have been found in Botswana and Angola, in addition to the countries in southern Africa from which virus has been isolated. Infections have been identified in a wide range of habitats from tropical forests to temperate grasslands, and severe epidemics have been recorded even in arid areas following heavy rains.

In southern Africa, RVF virus has usually appeared in extensive outbreaks in sheep and cattle following heavy rains during late summer and autumn. These outbreaks have been most prevalent in the sheep-rearing areas of South Africa and Nambia on the temperate inland plateau grasslands and arid habitats. The virus has been shown to be present in subtropical coastal lowlands of South Africa where sheep are scarce, but sporadic outbreaks and subclinical infections have been recorded in cattle. In sheep-rearing areas, the frequency of isolation during epidemics and of vector efficiency have indicated that *Cx. theileri* is probably the main epidemic vector, with other mosquito species also involved in a subsidiary role. Various biting flies have been suspected to have transmitted the virus mechanically among domestic animals during epidemics. The relative infrequency with which RVF virus has been isolated from naturally-infected mosquitoes, and the difficulty most mosquito species have in transmitting the virus, have suggested that the virus may not be mosquito-borne in its reservoir hosts.[6]

Human beings are readily infected by contact with organs of infected domestic animals and most human infections are probably acquired in this manner. Farming personnel and veterinarians have been most frequently infected and laboratory infections have also occurred. Virus is present in milk, and although this is a possible source of transmission to people, milk-borne infection has not been reported. Abattoirs may be another possible source of human exposure, as infection in animals is often subclinical.

CONTROL AND SIGNIFICANCE

During recent years, RVF has caused extremely severe economic losses in sheep and cattle in southern Africa. It is possible that some changes in the ecology of the virus have recently occurred resulting in an increase in infection of domestic animals. Human infection has, in consequence, also increased to the extent that protection of persons at high risk has had to be implemented. An inactivated vaccine for use in human beings has been used in South Africa, but its efficacy, even in multiple doses, has still to be assessed. Perhaps the most effective protection for people is large-scale immunization of domestic animals. This is difficult to ensure consistently, particularly if long interepidemic periods should intervene. Protective clothing should be worn by persons performing necropsies or gynecological manipulations on farm animals.

A live, attenuated virus vaccine is available for immunization of sheep and goats, but its use in pregnant animals can result in infection and abortion of fetuses. For immunization of pregnant sheep and goats, and for use in cattle, an inactivated wild-type virus vaccine is available. Valuable animals should be protected from exposure to mosquitoes and other biting flies during epidemics.

REFERENCES

1. **Daubney, R., Hudson, J. R., and Garnham, P. C.,** Enzootic hepatitis or Rift Valley fever. An undescribed virus disease of sheep, cattle and man from East Africa, *J. Pathol. Bacteriol.,* 34, 545, 1931.
2. **Gear, J., de Meillon, B., le Roux, A. F., Kofsky, R., Rose-Innes, R., Steyn, J. J., Olif, W. D., and Schutz, K. H.,** Rift Valley fever in South Africa. A study of the 1953 outbreak in the Orange Free State, with special reference to vectors and possible reservoir hosts, *S. Afr. Med. J.,* 29, 514, 1955.
3. **McIntosh, B. M. and Jupp, P. G.,** Dos Santos, I., and Barnard, B. J. H., Vector Studies on Rift Valley fever virus in South Africa, *S. Afr. Med. J.,* 58, 127, 1980.
4. **McIntosh, B. M., Jupp, P. G., Anderson, D., and Dickinson, D. B.,** Rift Valley Fever. 2. Attempts to transmit virus with seven species of mosquito, *J. S. Afr. Vet. Assoc.,* 44, 57, 1973.
5. **Schutz, K. C. A.** The pathology of Rift Valley fever or enzootic hepatitis in South Africa, *J. S. Afr. Vet. Med. Assoc.,* 22, 113, 1951.
6. **Smithburn, K. C., Haddow, A. J., and Lumsden, W. H. R.,** Rift Valley fever. Transmission of virus by mosquitos, *Br. J. Exp. Pathol.,* 30, 35, 1949.

BANZI FEVER, SPONDWINI FEVER, AND GERMISTON FEVER

B. M. McIntosh and J. H. S. Gear

Banzi fever — Banzi (BAN) virus, a flavivirus of the family Togaviridae, was isolated from the blood of a febrile child in South Africa in 1956.[1] The virus has since been isolated in Kenya and Mozambique. Antibodies have been found in surveys of human sera in Botswana, Nambia, and Angola, but the significance of the virus to human health is still unknown. It is closely related antigenically to Uganda S virus, and is maintained in wild rodents by *Culex rubinotus* mosquitoes.[2]

Spondweni fever — Spondweni (SPO) virus was first isolated in 1955 from a pool of *Mansonia uniformis* (Theo) mosquitoes collected in northern Zululand, South Africa.[3] It was shown to be a group B arthropod-borne or flavivirus. This virus has been isolated from several species of culicine mosquitoes. Recognized human cases have been limited to two laboratory workers who presumably contracted the infection in the course of work with the virus. They suffered generalized aches and pains, giddiness, severe headache, malaise, slight epistaxis, and nausea.[4] Antibody studies in the region have shown that this virus has caused human infections in northern Zululand.

Germiston fever — Germiston (GER) fever virus, a bunyavirus of the family Bunyaviridae was first recognized in 1958 in mosquitoes in South Africa.[5] During the initial studies on the virus two infections occurred in laboratory personnel, with fever, headache, muscular pains, and weakness. Antibody surveys have indicated that human infection has occurred in Botswana, Angola, and Nambia, and virus has been isolated in Uganda and Mozambique. The virus is maintained in wild rodents by *Culex rubinotus* mosquitoes.[2]

REFERENCES

1. **Smithburn, K. C., Paterson, H. E., Heymann, C. S., and Winter, P. A. D.,** An agent related to Uganda S virus from man and mosquitos in South Africa, *S. Afr. Med. J.*, 33, 959, 1959.
2. **McIntosh, B. M., Jupp, P. G., Dos Santos, I. S. L., and Meenehan, G. M.,** Culex (Eumelanomyia) rubinotus Theobald as vector of Banzi, Germiston and Witwatersrand Viruses. I. Isolation of virus from wild populations of *C. rubinotus, J. Med. Entomol.*, 12, 637, 1976.
3. **Kokernot, R. H., Smithburn, K. C., Muspratt, J., and Hodgson, B.,** Studies on arthropod-borne viruses of Tongaland. VIII. Spondweni virus, an agent previously unknown isolated from *Taeniorhynchus (mansonioides) uniformis* Theo, *S. Afr. J. Med. Sci.*, 22, 103, 1957.
4. **McIntosh, B. M., Kokernot, R. H., Paterson, H. E., and de Meillon, B.,** Isolation of Spondweni virus from four species of Culicine mosquitos and a report of two laboratory infections with the virus, *S. Afr. Med. J.*, 35, 647, 1961.
5. **Kokernot, R. H., Smithburn, K. C., Paterson, H. E., and McIntosh, B. M.,** Isolation of Germiston virus, a hitherto unknown agent, from Culicine mosquitos, and a report of infection in two laboratory workers, *Am. J. Trop. Med. Hyg.*, 9, 62, 1960.

ARBOVIRAL ZOONOSES IN EAST, CENTRAL AND WEST AFRICA

CHIKUNGUNYA FEVER

Y. Robin

NAME AND SYNONYMS

Chikungunya (CHIK) fever has no synonyms. It is named for the clinical characteristic of severe joint pains which cause the patients to "double up" in the Swahili language.

HISTORY

The first recorded outbreak of chikungunya fever was reported in the Newala district of southern Tanzania in 1952.[17,31] The virus has been isolated from human beings or mosquitoes in South Africa,[12] Uganda,[33] Zaire,[26] and Zimbabwe.[20] Serological surveys in Senegal showed antibody prevalence of 55% in the human population.[4] Human epidemics were reported in Senegal in 1966[29] in Nigeria in 1969,[24] and 1974[32] Since 1958, chikungunya infections have been associated with hemorrhagic fever in Southeast Asia[14] but such reports have not come from Africa.

ETIOLOGY

Chikungunya virus is classified in the genus *Alphavirus* of the family Togaviridae.[9] Serologically, it is very closely related to O'nyong nyong virus which caused explosive outbreaks of human disease in East Africa in 1959-1962.[13]

DEFINITION

Chikungunya fever is an acute dengue-like febrile illness characterized by relapsing joint pains and lasting 1 week or less. Nonhuman primates are the principal reservoir hosts and the virus is transmitted by a variety of mosquitoes.

ANIMAL INFECTION

Several African wild rodents, vervet monkeys, and baboons have developed viremias without clinical manifestations following experimental CHIK inoculation.[19,21] Rhesus monkeys have developed transient febrile illness following subcutaneous (s.c.) inoculation of infectious material.[33] Diagnosis of CHIK infections in animals is by isolation and identification of the virus from blood samples using suckling mice or cell culture techniques, or by demonstrating development of antibodies between acute and convalescent serum samples.[15]

HUMAN INFECTION

Clinical

The incubation period is considered to be 3 to 12 days. The onset of fever is characteristically sudden with no prodromal symptoms; headache is constant; excruciating joint pains often incapacitate the patient; asthenia is severe and anorexia total. The fever disappears within 2 to 3 days, and a maculopapular or scarlatiniform rash appears on the trunk and extensor surfaces of the limbs. Nausea and vomiting are frequently noted. The rash disappears within a few days, but joint pains may diminish slowly and asthenia and anorexia persist. In at least 50% of patients, apyrexial joint pains recur intermittently over a period up to 6 months, at times prostrating the patients. Hemorrhagic fever has not been reported in chikungunya fever patients in Africa. Fatalities have not been reported in Africa. Chikungunya appears to be the only arboviral infection causing severe residual articular pain.[6]

Diagnosis

During epidemics, clinical diagnoses are commonly definitive with fever, arthralgia, and exanthem found in almost all patients. Sporadic cases are more easily confused with malaria or influenza. Rashes may be difficult to recognize in black people, and arthralgia is frequently absent in children. Viral fevers caused by Ilesha, Tataguine, Bwamba, Orungo, or Zinga viruses may be confused with chikungunya fever. Definitive diagnosis is based on isolation of virus from acute phase blood samples collected within 2 to 3 days of onset, using suckling mice or cell cultures, or on serological findings in convalescence.

EPIDEMIOLOGY

Occurrence

Chikungunya virus has been reported from Africa, India, and Southeast Asia. In Africa, epidemics have been reported in Tanzania in 1952, in South Africa in 1956,[11] in northern Zimbabwe in 1959,[30] in Zaire in 1960,[27] in southern Zimbabwe in 1962,[9] in Senegal in 1966,[28,29] in Angola in 1970,[10] and in Nigeria in 1969[24] and 1974.[32] Serological surveys in West Africa have indicated that infections are widespread but of low incidence in forest areas, and of high incidence in savannas.[3]

Reservoirs

The existence of a sylvatic cycle was suggested as early as 1956, when CHIK virus was isolated from *Aedes africanus* mosquitoes collected in the canopy of the Zika forest of Uganda.[33] Serological evidences of infection in nonhuman primates were reported in Zaire in 1960[27] and Zimbabwe in 1964.[22] During the 1966 outbreak in Senegal, prevalence of antibody titers in *Erythrocebus patas* and *Cercopithecus aethiops* rose from 23%, 6 months before the outbreak, to 88% following the outbreak. Serological evidence of infection in nonhuman primates has been reported from Ethiopia,[1] Nigeria,[2] and Uganda.[18] Six isolations have been reported from wild animals collected in Senegal, two from salivary glands of *Scotophilus sp.* insectivorus bats, one from a *Galago senegalensis* bush baby, two from *Cercopethicus aethiops* vervet monkeys, and one from a *Papio papio* baboon. The rapidity with which primates develop antibodies following infection has led to considering them more as amplifying hosts than as reservoir hosts, except perhaps in forest canopy monkeys which appear to maintain a monkey-mosquito-monkey cycle.[18] Antibodies have been found in wild captured birds, rodents, bats, and reptiles.[8] Evidence has been obtained of viral activity in feral rodents 5 to 6 months before the human epidemic in Senegal in 1966. Three months after the epidemic, 1.8% of birds tested had antibodies.[8]

Transmission

Many mosquito species have been found infected in nature, and are considered to be at least potential vectors. Most incriminated in transmission have been *Ae. aegypti* in Tanzania, Senegal, Nigeria, and Angola,[8,10,17,24,25] *Culex pipiens fatigans* in northern Zimbabwe,[30] and *Ae. furcifer-taylori* in southern Zimbabwe.[20] CHIK virus has been isolated from numerous forest dwelling species, *Ae. africanus* and *Ae. opok* in Central African Republic, *Ae. africanus* in Ivory Coast and Uganda,[18] and *Ae. luteocephalus, Ae. dalzieli* and *Ae. furcifer-taylori* in Senegal.[16] The epidemiology of chikungunya fever in Africa shares many aspects in common with that of yellow fever. In West Africa, CHIK virus is maintained in the rain forest by monkey-*Ae. africanus*-monkey cycles. In the forest area of the Sudan, *Ae. luteocephalus,* which is more drought tolerant, replaces *Ae. africanus,* while in the savanna, *Ae. furcifer-taylori* serves as an amplifying vector during rainy seasons with *Ae. aegypti* transmitting the virus to people. In Senegal, it is suggested, based on the 1969 and 1975 epidemics, that the virus may have a 6-year periodicity.

Human hosts

As for yellow fever, two patterns of chikungunya infection appear, an epidemic chikungunya with interhuman transmission by *Ae. aegypti,* and a jungle chikungunya with transmission from canopy dwelling primates to people by forest mosquitoes. Human patients infected with CHIK virus have only short viremias and become immune for life; thus they play no maintenance role but may serve as sources of transmission in epidemics.

CONTROL

Prevention and therapy

No specific vaccines or therapeutic agents are applicable to chikungunya fever. Corticosteroids have been used in residual articular pains during convalescence. *Ae. aegypti* control on household and community levels is advocated in epidemic chikungunya fever. Avoidance of habitats of forest mosquitoes is the only applicable protection from jungle chikungunya fever.

Epidemic measures

Quick reduction of adult mosquito populations may be applicable in epidemic chikungunya fever. Household spraying and community fogging, or aerial spraying with ultra low volume insecticides may be applicable. Household and community efforts to eliminate, or empty and clean water-holding containers or treatment of water in containers with insecticides are applicable to larva control of *Ae. aegypti.*

Health education

Community education on the control of *Ae. aegypti.* mosquitoes can be highly effective in reducing populations of these mosquitoes. Education on personal protection from exposure by household or forest mosquitoes is very important.

PUBLIC HEALTH ASPECTS

Epidemics of chikungunya fever may involve thousands of patients, causing severe disruption and economic loss in affected communities. Although chikungunya fever is not a reportable disease, continuing surveillance is needed to elucidate its epidemiology and to aid in early recognition and institution of preventive measures in situations of potential epidemics.

REFERENCES

1. **Andral, L., Brès, P., Serié, C., Casals, J., and Panthier, R.,** Etudes sur la fièvre jaune en Ethiopie. 3 Etude sérologique et virologique de la faune selvatique, *Bull. Org. Mond. Santé,* 38, 855, 1968.
2. **Boorman, J. P. T. and Draper, G. C.,** Isolation of arboviruses in the Lagos area of Nigeria and a survey of antibodies to them in man and animals, *Trans. R. Soc. Trop. Med. Hyg.,* 62, 269, 1968.
3. **Brés, P.,** Données récentes apportées par les enquêtes serologiques sur la prévalence des arbovirus en Afrique avec reference spéciale a la fièvre jaune, *Bull. Org. Mond. Sante,* 43, 223, 1970.
4. **Brés, P., Lacan, A., Diop, I., Michel, R., Peretti, P., and Vidal, C.,** Les arbovirus au Senegal — enquete serologique, *Bull. Soc. Pathol. Exot.,* 56, 384, 1963.
5. **Brés, P., Williams, M. C., Simpson, D. H., and Santos, D. F.,** Identification of viruses isolated in Senegal, *E. Afr. Virus Res. Inst. Rep.,* 22, 1962/1963.
6. **Carey, D. E.,** Chikungunya and dengue: a case of mistaken identity? *J. Hist. Med. Allied Sci.,* 26, 243, 1971.
7. **Casals, J.,** Antigenic variants in arthropod-borne viruses. 10th Pacific Science Congress, Honolulu, (Abstr.) 458, 1961.
8. **Cornet, M., Taufflieb, R., and Chateau, R.,** Une epidemie d'arbovirose au Senegal (chikungunya). Premières donnèes épidémiologiques, in *Rapport de la 7eme Conference Technique de l'OCCGE, Bobo-Dioulasso,* 2, 895, 1967.
9. **Fenner, F.,** The classification and nomenclature of viruses, *Intervirology,* 6, 1, 1975/76.
10. **Filipe, A. R. and Pinto, M. R.,** Arbovirus studies in Luanda, Angola. 2. Virological and serological studies during outbreak of dengue like disease caused by the chikungunya virus, *Bull. Org. Mond. Sante,* 49, 37, 1973.
11. **Gear, J. H. S.,** Clinical aspects of chikungunya, *Ann. Microbiol.,* 11, 275, 1963.
12. **Gear, J. and Reid, F. P.,** The occurrence of a dengue like fever in the North Eastern Transvaal. 1. Clinical features and isolation of virus, *S. Afr. Med. J.,* 31, 253, 1957.
13. **Haddow, A. J., Davies, C. W., and Walker, A. J.,** O'nyong-nyong fever: an epidemic virus disease in East Africa, *Trans. R. Soc. Trop. Med. Hyg.,* 54, 517, 1960.
14. **Hammon, W. McD., Rudnick, A., and Sather, G. E.,** Viruses associated with epidemic hemorrhagic fever of the Philippines and Thailand, *Science,* 131, 1102, 1960.
15. **Hammon, W. McD. and Sather, G. E.,** Arboviruses, in *Diagnostic Procedures For Viral and Rickettsial Infections,* Schmidt, N. J. and Lenette, E. H., Eds., American Public Health Association, New York, 1969, 227.
16. **Institut Pasteur, Dakar, Centre Collaborateur OMS de Référence et de Recherche sur les arbovirus,** *Rapport Annuel,* 1976.
17. **Lumsden, W. H. R.,** An epidemic of virus disease in southern province Tanganyika territory in 1952-1953. 2. General description and epidemiology, *Trans. R. Soc. Trop. Med. Hyg.,* 49, 33, 1955.
18. **McCrae, A. W. R., Henderson, B. E., Kirya, B. G., Sempala, S. D. K.,** Chikungunya virus in the Entebbe area of Uganda: isolations and epidemiology, *Trans. R. Soc. Trop. Med. Hyg.,* 65, 152, 1971.
19. **McIntosh, B. M.,** Susceptibility of some african wild rodents to infection with various arthropod borne viruses, *Trans. R. Soc. Trop. Med. and Hyg.,* 55, 63, 1961.
20. **McIntosh, B. M., Harwin, R. M., Paterson, H. E., and Westwater, M. L.,** An epidemic of chikungunya in South Eastern Southern Rhodesia, *Cent. Afr. J. Med.,* 9, 351, 1963.
21. **McIntosh, B. M., Paterson, H. E., Donaldson, J. M., and de Sousa, J.,** Chikungunya virus: viral susceptibility and transmission studies with some vertebrates and mosquitoes, *S. Afr. J. Med. Sci.,* 28, 45, 1963.
22. **McIntosh, B. M., Paterson, H. E., McGillivray, G., and de Sousa, J.,** Further studies on the chikungunya outbreak in Southern Rhodesia in 1962. 1. Mosquitoes, wild primates and birds in relation to the epidemic, *Ann. Trop. Med. Parasitol.,* 58, 45, 1964.
23. **Moore, D. L., Causey, O. R., Carey, D. E., Reddy, S., Cooke, A. R., Akinkugbe, F. M., David-West, T. S., and Kemp, G. E.,** Arthropod borne viral infections of man in Nigeria, 1964-1970, *Ann. Trop. Med. Parasitol.,* 69, 49, 1975.

24. **Moore, D. L., Reddy, S., Akinkugbe, F. M., Lee, V. H., David-West, T. S., Cause, O. R., and Carey, D. E.,** An epidemic of chikungunya fever at Ibadan, Nigeria 1969, *Ann. Trop. Med. Parasitol.*, 68, 59, 1974.

25. Organisation Mondiale Santé, Ecologie des vecteurs et lutte antivecterielle en Santé Publique, Ser. Rapp. Tech. No. 561, 1975.

26. **Osterrieth, P. and Blandes-Ridaura, G.,** Recherches sur le virus chikungunya au Congo Belge. 1. Isolement du virus dans le Haut-Vele, *Ann. Soc. Belge. Med. Trop.*, 40, 199, 1960.

27. **Osterrieth, P., Deleplanque-Liegeois, P., and Renoirte, R.,** Recherches sur le virus chikungunya au Congo Belge. II. Enquete serologique, *Ann. Soc. Belge. Med. Trop.*, 40, 205, 1960.

28. **Robin, Y.,** Manifestation du virus chikungunya au Senegal — octobre novembre 1966, in *Rapport de la 7eme Conference Technique de l'OCCGE Bobo-Dioulasso*, 2, 891, 1967.

29. **Roche, S. and Robin, Y.,** Infections humaines par le virus chikungunya a Rufisque (Senegal), *Bull. Soc. Med. Afr. Noire. Lang. Fr.*, 12, 490, 1967.

30. **Rodger, L. M.,** An outbreak of suspected chikungunya fever in Northern Rhodesia, *S. Afr. Med. J.*, 35, 126, 1961.

31. **Ross, R. W.,** The Newala epidemic. III. The virus isolation, pathogenic properties and relationship to the epidemic, *J. Hyg.*, 54, 177, 1956.

32. **Tomori, O., Fagbami, A., and Fabiyi, A.,** The 1974 epidemic of chikungunya fever in children in Ibadan, *Trop. Geogr. Med.*, 24, 413, 1975.

33. **Weinbren, M. P., Haddow, A. J., and Williams, M. C.,** The occurrence of chikungunya virus in Uganda. 1. Isolation from mosquitoes, *Trans. R. Soc. Trop. Med. Hyg.*, 52, 253, 1958.

34. **Woodall, J. P.,** in *International Catalogue of Arboviruses Including Certain Other Viruses of Vertebrates*, 2nd ed., Pub. No. (CDC) 75-8301, Berge, T. O., Ed., Public Health Service, U.S. Department of Health, Education and Welfare, Washington, D.C., 1975, 216.

SEMLIKI FOREST VIRAL FEVER

Y. Robin

NAME AND SYNONYMS

Semliki Forest (SF) virus is not known to cause any clinical disease in nature. All pathological data on the infection has come from laboratory studies. There are no synonyms.

HISTORY

SF virus was first isolated in 1942 from *Aedes abnormalis* mosquitoes collected in Bwamba County, Uganda.[6] The virus has since been isolated from *Ae. argenteopunctatus* in Mozambique, *Mansonia africana* in Nigeria, *Eretmapodites grahami* in Cameroon, *Ae. vittatus* in Senegal, *Ae. palpalpis* group in Central African Republic, *Ae. dentatur* in the central plateau in Kenya, and *Anopheles funestus* in north Kenya.[3] The virus has also been isolated from naturally infected wild birds in Central African Republic and Nigeria, and from sentinel mice and a hedgehog in Nigeria.[1]

ETIOLOGY

SF virus is classified in the genus *Alphavirus* (group A arboviruses) of the family Togaviridae.[2] The virus is enveloped, spherical in shape, with an estimated diameter of 20 to 67 nm. The genome is single-stranded RNA.[7]

DEFINITION

Semliki Forest virus is an arbovirus of undetermined relationship to clinical disease. It has been isolated from a wide variety of mosquitoes and several avian and animal hosts in the absence of clinical disease. Serological studies, in addition to the virological findings, have indicated a widespread distribution in Africa and perhaps South Asia and southern Europe.

ANIMAL INFECTION

No overt disease has been recorded in conjunction with viremia in naturally infected birds and mammals. Laboratory animals have been experimentally infected by a variety of routes. Suckling and adult mice have developed fatal infection by intracerebral (i.c.) route and infection with variable mortality by intraperitoneal (i.p.), intranasal (i.n.) and oral routes. Rabbits, guinea pigs, monkeys, and chickens inoculated by various routes have developed inapparent, apparent, or even fatal infections, the last, only in mammals by i.c. injection. Virus isolation from blood samples, animal tissues, or mosquitoes may be made by i.c. injection into mice or inoculation in cell cultures. Identification of isolates by serological tests must be made on a basis of comparative titers against all alphaviruses present in the area.

HUMAN INFECTION

Clinically manifest disease has not been recognized, and SF virus has not been reported from infected persons, except in two cases of laboratory infection. Antibody prevalence rates up to 46% have been reported in several African surveys, and titers have been demonstrated in laboratory workers handling the virus. Antibody titers against SF virus have been reported from India, Malaysia, Vietnam, Thailand, Philippines, and Yugoslavia, but the specificity of the serological findings must await virological reports from these countries. Diagnosis of human infections must be based on isolation and identification of the virus.

EPIDEMIOLOGY

Occurrence
SF virus has been demonstrated to be widespread in East, Central, and West Africa and serological evidence indicates it may be as far south as Zaire and South Africa.

Reservoir
Both avian and mammalian infected hosts have been found in nature. Antibody titers have been demonstrated in rodents and domesticated animals in South Africa. In Senegal, during an episode of encephalitis in horses in Dara, antibody titers against SF virus were variably recorded in convalescent and contact animals, but no proof of association with the disease was made.[4]

Transmission
A wide variety of mosquitoes has been found infected in nature. In addition, experimental transmission has been demonstrated by *Ae. aegypti*, *Ae. togoi*, *An. albimanus*, and *An. quadrimaculatus*.

Human host

The role of human hosts in the transmission cycle is unknown.

CONTROL AND PUBLIC HEALTH ASPECTS

Since no disease caused by SF virus in animals or people is known in nature, no control measures have been pertinent and the virus has no known public health importance.

REFERENCES

1. Arbovirus Research Project, Ibadan, *Annual Report,* 1971-1972.
2. Fenner, F., The classification and nomenclature of viruses, *Intervirology,* 6, 1, 1975/76.
3. Institut Pasteur, Dakar, *Annual Report,* 1971.
4. Robin, Y., Bourdin, P., Le Gonidec, G., and Hème, G., Virus de la Forêt de Semliki et encéphalomyelites équines au Sénégal, *Ann. Microbiol. (Inst. Pasteur),* 125A, 235, 1974.
5. Smith, C. E. G. and Holt, D., Chromatography of arthropod borne viruses on calcium phosphate columns, *Bull. WHO,* 24, 749, 1961.
6. Smithburn, K. C. and Haddow, A. J., Semliki forest virus. Isolation and pathogenic properties, *J. Immunol.,* 49, 141, 1944.
7. Willems, W. R., Kaluza, G., Boschek, C. B., Bauer, H., Hager, H., Schutz, H. J., and Feister, H., *Science,* 203(4385), 1127, 1979.
8. Woodall, J. P., in *International Catalogue of Arboviruses Including Certain Other Viruses of Vertebrates,* 2nd ed., Berge, T. O., Ed., Pub. No. (CDC) 75-8301, Public Health Service, U.S. Department of Health Education and Welfare, Atlanta, 1975, 640.

SINDBIS FEVER

Y. Robin

NAME AND SYNONYMS

Sindbis (SIN) fever is the name of the disease caused by the Sindbis virus. There are no synonyms.

HISTORY

Sindbis virus was first isolated from mosquitoes collected at Sindbis, Egypt. No human or animal disease was associated, but serological surveys demonstrated antibodies in people in Egypt and the Sudan.[5] Since 1961, clinical disease has been identified in Uganda[3] and South Africa,[3] but not as yet in East or West Africa.

ETIOLOGY

SIN virus is the type species of the genus *Alphavirus* (group A arbovirus) of the family Togaviridae.[2] The virions are spherical enveloped particles averaging 32 nm diameter with single-stranded RNA genomes. They are sensitive to heat and to acid and lipid solvent treatment.[4]

DEFINITION

Sindbis fever is a mosquito-borne infection clinically varying from inapparent to overt disease with fever, generalized pains, and rash.

ANIMAL INFECTION

SIN virus has been isolated from birds in the Nile Delta and in South Africa,[5] and birds are considered to be reservoirs of the virus. The virus has not been isolated from animals but antibody titers have occasionally been recorded in domestic mammals.

HUMAN INFECTION

Clinical

Five cases of mild illness were seen in Uganda in 1961, characterized by fever, headache, generalized pains, and in two patients, mild icterus. Sindbis virus was isolated from blood samples of all five patients. A serological survey at Podor on the Senegal River showed a high prevalence of Sindbis and West Nile antibodies. Quite severe illness has been reported from South Africa, with SIN viral isolations from vesicular fluid from painful vesicles on the toes.

Diagnosis

Definitive diagnosis is based on virus isolation from blood or possibly vesicular fluid, or on specific antibody rises. Suckling mice or cell cultures are used for viral cultivation.

EPIDEMIOLOGY

Occurrence

In Africa, Sindbis virus has been reported on serological or virological bases from Egypt, Uganda, Mozambique, South Africa, Cameroon, Central African Republic, Nigeria, and Senegal. It has also been reported from Australia, India, Philippines, Malaysia, Israel, U.S.S.R., and Czechoslovakia.

Reserovir

Sindbis appears to be a virus of birds. The area of serological evidence of viral activity on the Senegal River is an area of heavy use by migratory birds.

Transmission

SIN virus is transmitted by infected mosquitoes of numerous species of *Anopheles, Aedes, Mansonia,* and especially *Culex* genera. In Senegal, the virus has been isolated from *An. brohieri, Ae. vittatus, Cx. perfuscus,* and *Cx. thalassius* mosquitoes.

Human host

Human infections appear to be tangential to the cycle of transmission in birds. Human infections play no role in maintaining viral activity.

CONTROL

Human infections appear to be uncommon and when they do occur, to be mild. Control by avoiding endemic areas of viral activity in birds or by personal mosquito control when in such areas is advised.

PUBLIC HEALTH ASPECTS

Sindbis fever is considered to be of minor public health importance at this time.

REFERENCES

1. East African Virus Research Institute, Annual Report, 1962.
2. **Fenner, F.,** The classification and nomenclature of viruses, *Intervirology,* 6, 1, 1975/76.
3. **Malherbe, M. and Strickland-Chomley, M.,** Sindbis virus infection in man, *S. Afr. Med. J.,* 37, 547, 1963.
4. **Taylor, R. M.,** in *International Catalogue of Arboviruses Including Certain Other Viruses of Vertebrates,* Ed., Berge, T. O., 2nd ed., Public Health Service, U.S., Department of Health, Education and Welfare, Washington, D.C., 1975, 656.
5. **Taylor, R. M., Hurlbut, H. S., Work, T. H., Kingston, J. R., and Frotingham, T. E.,** Sindbis virus: a newly recognized arthropod transmitted virus, *Am. J. Trop. Med. Hyg.,* 4, 844, 1955.

WESSELSBRON FEVER

Y. Robin

NAME AND SYNONYMS

Wesselsbron (WSL) fever is the name of the disease caused by Wesselsbron virus. There are no synonyms.

HISTORY

WSL virus was first described as the etiological agent of a newly recognized disease of sheep in South Africa.[11] Subsequently the virus was isolated from mosquitoes and from blood samples from human patients.[9] Serological surveys have indicated that human infections occur in West Africa.

ETIOLOGY

WSL virus is classified in the genus *Flavivirus* (group B arboviruses) of the family Togaviridae.[3] The virus has not been extensively characterized.[7] The size has been estimated at 45 nm diameter by electron microscopy. Hemagglutinin is produced in infected suckling mouse brains. The virus is sensitive to lipid solvents. A strain isolated from mosquitoes in the Cameroon is considered a subtype of WSL virus.[5]

DEFINITION

Wesselsbron fever is a mosquito-borne viral zoonosis causing abortion and occasionally death in gestating ewes, and death in newborn lambs. It causes an influenza-like febrile illness in human patients.

ANIMAL INFECTION

Animal disease has not been well studied in East or West Africa, but virological and serological evidence of the presence of WSL virus widely spread over the continent has been reported. It has been shown that previous Wesselsbron infection immunized monkeys against virulent yellow fever virus challenge.[4]

HUMAN INFECTION

Clinical

Natural human infections have not been recognized in East or West Africa. Laboratory-acquired infections have occurred in Ibadan, Nigeria[10] and in Dakar, Senegal.[1,5] Exposure was considered to be by inhalation of aerosolized virus. In one patient, the incubation period was fixed at 12 days. Onset of disease was abrupt, with fever reaching 39 to 40°C and severe headache, lower back pain, restlessness, anorexia, and cutaneous hyperesthesia in the upper trunk and arms. Patients recovered completely after 4 to 5 days.

Diagnosis

Virus isolation from blood may be made during the febrile period using suckling mice or cell culture techniques. Serological diagnosis is dependent on using adequate antigens to differentiate among flaviviruses present in the area.

EPIDEMIOLOGY

Occurrence

WSL virus has been isolated from human patients in South Africa, Zimbabwe, Cameroon, Uganda, Central African Republic, and in laboratory-acquired cases in Nigeria,[8,10] and Senegal.[6] No human epidemics have been reported.

Reservoir

Serological studies on domesticated animals in Senegal using hemagglutination-inhibition tests showed an antibody prevalence of 13.2% in cattle, 4.3% in sheep, and 6.4% in goats.[2] Of particular interest has been the isolation of WSL virus from a blood sample from a camel in Kano, Nigeria.[8] Natural outbreaks of clinical disease have been reported principally in sheep. The reservoir host of the virus remains unidentified.

Transmission

WSL virus has been isolated from numerous species of mosquitoes over Africa. Isolations were made from *Aedes dalzieli* and *Ae. minutus* mosquitoes collected at Kedougou, Senegal.[6]

CONTROL

Prevention of the disease in sheep has been the only area of concern. An attenuated live virus vaccine has been developed for immunization of ewes and lambs. Prevention of human infection is based largely on laboratory containment of the virus and on mosquito control in nature.

PUBLIC HEALTH ASPECTS

Outbreaks in sheep have had severe economic impact. The public health importance of the infection has been negligible.

REFERENCES

1. **Bres, P.,** Infection humaine a virus Wesselsbron par contamination de laboratoire, *Bull. Soc. Path. Exot.,* 58, 994, 1965.
2. **Chunikin, S. P., Karaseva, P. S., Taufflieb, R., Robin, Y., Cornet, M., and Camicas, J. L.,** Results of serological studies of circulation cycles of some arboviruses in the Republic of Senegal (West Africa), *Vopr. Virusol.,* 1, 52, 1971.
3. **Fenner, F.,** The classification and nomenclature of viruses, *Intervirology,* 6, 1, 1975/76.
4. **Henderson, B. E., Cheshire, P. P., Kirya, G. B., and Lile, M.,** Immunologic studies with yellow fever and selected African group B arboviruses in rhesus and vervet monkeys, *Am. J. Trop. Med. Hyg.,* 19, 110, 1970.
5. **Institut Pasteur de Dakar,** *Rapport Annuel,* 1974.
6. **Institut Pasteur de Dakar,** Centre Collaborateur OMS de Reference et de Recherche pour les arbovirus, *Rapport Annuel,* 1976.
7. **McIntosh, B. M.,** in *International Catalogue of Arboviruses Including Certain Other Viruses of Vertebrates,* 2nd ed., Pub. No. (CDC) 75-8301, Berge, T. O., Ed., Public Health Service, U.S. Department of Health, Education and Welfare, Atlanta, 1975, 754.
8. **Moore, D. L.,** personnal communication, 1969.
9. **Smith-Burn, K. C., Kokernot, R. H., Weinbren, M. P., and de Meillon, B.,** Studies on arthropod-borne viruses of Tongaland. IX. Isolation of Wesselsbron virus from a naturally infected human being and from *Aedes*(B), *Circumluteolus, S. Afr. J. Med. Sci.,* 22, 113, 1957.
10. **Tomori, O.,** personal communication, 1972.
11. **Weiss, K. E., Haig, D. A., and Alexander, R. A.,** Wesselsbron virus — a virus not previously described, associated with abortion in domestic animals, *Onderstepoort J.,* 27, 183, 1956.

WEST NILE FEVER

Y. Robin

NAME AND SYNONYMS

West Nile (WN) fever is the name of the disease caused by West Nile virus. There are no synonyms.

HISTORY

During investigations on yellow fever, a virus was isolated from a blood sample from a febrile woman in the West Nile province of Uganda.[6] The virus is serologically related to St. Louis encephalitis and Japanese encephalitis viruses.[5] Serological studies have indicated that the virus is widely distributed in Africa.

ETIOLOGY

WN virus is classified in the genus *Flavivirus* (group B arboviruses) of the family Togaviridae.[2] The virus is enveloped, spherical in shape, and with diameter 21 to 35 nm. The genome is single-stranded RNA. The virus is sensitive to the action of lipid solvents, ether, sodium deoxycholate, and chloroform, and of enzymes, trypsin, and papain. It is inactivated by formalin, p-chloromercuribenzoate, bisulfate, periodate, and heat. WN virus hemagglutinates goose, chick, and cock erythrocytes.[9]

DEFINITION

West Nile fever is an acute febrile dengue-like disease with rash and occasionally meningoencephalitis.

ANIMAL INFECTION

Clinical disease, characterized by encephalitis has been reported in horses and donkeys in Egypt and France, but overt WN infections have not been reported in animals in East and West Africa. WN virus has been isolated from *Dicrurus adsimilis* birds, *Arvicanthis niloticus* rodents, and a camel in Nigeria.[1]

HUMAN INFECTION

Clinical

West Nile infections in human beings, especially in children, are predominantly subclinical or mild abortive infections. In adults which develop clinical disease, the incubation period is about 3 days, followed by abrupt onset of fever and severe headache. Lymphadenitis, in some patients, rash, and, in some elderly patients, meningoencephalitis ensue. The duration of febrile illness is usually 3 to 5 days followed by rapid recovery, although in some patients convalescence is prolonged and characterized by marked asthenia. Severe infections have been reported in Senegal.[4]

Pathology

Fatal cases of WN fever have been characterized by meningoencephalitis with congestion and petechial hemorrhages. Histologically, all parts of the brain and anterior spinal cord were involved. Small hemorrhages and round cell cuffs were demonstrated perivascularly, and necrotic foci of nerve cells were reported in the grey matter.

Diagnosis

Clinical diagnosis is inconclusive except perhaps in recognized epidemics. Viral isolation is generally possible from blood samples collected between 2 days before and 4 to 5 days after onset of clinical illness. Serological diagnosis based on examination of acute and convalescent paired sera by hemagglutination inhibition, complement fixation, and neutralization tests is reliable only if multiple flavivirus antigens, including all of those which may be present in the area, are incorporated in the tests.

EPIDEMIOLOGY

In Africa, WN virus has been reported from Egypt, Uganda, Central African Republic, Nigeria, Senegal, Zaire, Mozambique, and South Africa. Serological studies have provided evidence that the virus is widespread in West Africa.

Reservoir

Intensive studies in Egypt have indicated that the principal vertebrate hosts are birds, and the principal vector is *Culex univittatus,* an ornithophilic mosquito.[7] Many isolations of WN virus have been reported from wild birds in Egypt, Nigeria, Central African Republic, South Africa, and in Asia, from Israel. In Senegal, a high prevalence of antibodies against WN and Sindbis virus has been demonstrated in people living along the Senegal River frequented by large numbers of migratory birds. WN virus has also been isolated from rodents and a camel in Nigeria.[1] The reservoir significance of these findings is unknown.

Transmission

WN virus had been isolated from a wide variety of mosquitoes, mostly of bird-feeding species. In Egypt and South Africa, the virus has been repeatedly recovered from ornithophilic *Cx. univittatus.* In Uganda, WN virus has been reported from *Mansonia metallica* and in Central African Republic, from *Cx. pruina* and *Cx. weishei,* all of which feed on birds.

Human host

Although human disease, even epidemic disease, is produced by WN infections, human involvement in the transmission cycle is tangential, and human patients are not considered to be sources of the virus to mosquitoes.

CONTROL

Preventive measures to avoid exposure to bird-feeding mosquitoes is advised[3,8] No specific therapy for human patients is known. In epidemics, population control of ornithophilic mosquitoes may be practical.

PUBLIC HEALTH ASPECTS

The impact of WN infections has been minor in East and West Africa, although it has been considered to be of greater importance in South Africa. Surveillance of the virus in birds and ornithophilic mosquitoes and population levels of these reservoir hosts and vectors are pertinent, especially in times of abnormally high rains or in areas newly opened to irrigation.

REFERENCES

1. Arbovirus Research Project, Ibadan, Annual Report, 1970.
2. Fenner, F., The classification and nomenclature of viruses, *Intervirology,* 6, 1, 1975/76.
3. **World Health Organization,** Ecologie des vecteurs et lutte antivectorielle en santé publique, *Ser. Rap. Tech. No.,* 561, 15, 1975.
4. **Robin, Y. and Ducloux, M.,** Arbovirose B à manifestations encéphalitiques prédominantes, *Bull. Soc. Med. Afr. Noire Lang Fr.,* 15, 419, 1970.
5. **Smithburn, K. C.,** Differentiation of the West Nile virus from the viruses of St. Louis and Japanese B Encephalitis, *J. Immunol.,* 44, 25, 1942.
6. **Smithburn, K. C., Hughes, T. P., Burke, A. W., and Paul, J. H.,** A neutropic virus isolated from the blood of a native of Uganda, *Am. J. Trop. Med. Hyg.,* 20, 471, 1940.
7. **Taylor, R. M., Work, T. H., Hurlbut, A. S., and Rizk, F.,** A study of the ecology of West Nile virus in Egypt, *Am. J. Trop. Med. Hyg.,* 5, 579, 1956.
8. Anon., Arboviruses and human disease, *WHO Tech. Rep. Ser.,* 369, 60, 1967.
9. **Woodhall, J. P.,** in *International Catalogue of Arboviruses Including Certain Other Viruses of Vertebrates,* 2nd Ed., Pub. No. (CDC) 75-8301, Berge, T. O., Ed., Public Health Service, U.S. Department of Health, Education and Welfare, Atlanta, 1975, 758.

ZIKA FEVER

Y. Robin

NAME AND SYNONYMS

Zika fever or Zika viral infection are names applied to the disease caused by Zika virus.

HISTORY

Zika virus was first identified in 1947 from the blood of a sentinel rhesus monkey in the Zika forest near Entebbe, Uganda.[2] Human infections were subsequently documented in Nigeria and Senegal,[4,6] and a laboratory acquired infection in Uganda.[7] Serological surveys have indicated widespread distribution in people in Africa and southern Asia. Numerous isolations have been made from mosquitoes in Africa and report made from Malaysia.

ETIOLOGY

Zika virus is classified in the genus *Flavivirus* (group B arboviruses) of the family Togaviridae.[3] The virions are spherical, enveloped, and of diameter 18 to 45 nm. The genomes are single-stranded RNA. Infectivity is retained for up to 6 months at 4°C in 50% glycerol, but is inactivated by ether, sodium deoxycholate, or chloroform. Hemagglutinin activity against goose and chick erythrocytes is present in infected suckling mouse brains.[8]

DEFINITION

Zika fever is mosquito-borne, inapparent to mild febrile infection with or without maculopapular rash in human beings, and is considered to be an inapparent infection in monkeys as well.

ANIMAL INFECTION

Naturally occurring animal infection has been recorded only in sentinel monkeys in Uganda. Experimentally infected donkeys developed subclinical viremias and antibody titers. Recognition of infection has been by virus isolation and identification. Suckling and adult mice inoculated intracerebrally (i.c.) or intraperitoneally (i.p.) develop fatal paralysis. Fatal encephalitis has been produced by i.c. inoculation of guinea pigs, but not rabbits. Serological surveys for natural infections in animals have been reported only in wild monkeys with 12.9% of 31 in Uganda showing neutralizing antibody titers.[1]

HUMAN INFECTION

Human Zika viral infections have been characterized by fever, malaise, and possibly maculopapular rash. Among five diagnosed human cases, one was laboratory acquired and one was in a mosquito collector for laboratory studies. Serological surveys have indicated up to a 50% antibody prevalence rate in Africa, India, and Southeast Asia.

Suckling mice inoculated by i.c. route, embryonating hens' eggs inoculated by various routes, and primary cell cultures of chicken embryo, duck embryo, or rhesus monkey kidney have been used in virus isolation. Hemagglutination inhibition (HI) and neutralization tests have been used in serological surveys.

EPIDEMIOLOGY

Occurrence

Zika virus isolations have been made from naturally infected human patients in Nigeria and Senegal, sentinel monkeys in Uganda, and *Aedes spp., Anopheles gambiae,* and *Mansonia uniformis* mosquitoes in Uganda, Central African Republic, Ivory Coast, Nigeria, and Senegal in Africa, and Malaysia in Asia. Serological surveys of human populations have shown 10.7% of 360 people in Uganda, 16.7% of 36 in Tanzania, 50% of 304 in Nigeria, up to 6% in Mozambique, 0.5% of 180 in Egypt, 33% of 440 in Senegal, 16.8% of 196 in India, 50.2% of 179 in Malaysia, 18% of 50 in Borneo, 12% of 153 in the Philippines, and 50% of 100 in Vietnam and Thailand to be seropositive, in all but the Senegal survey by neutralization tests. In addition, serological evidence of human infections has been reported from Ghana, Liberia, Ivory Coast, Cameroon, Zaire, and Ethiopia.[5,8]

RESERVOIR

The reservoir of Zika virus is unknown. Serological evidence of infection has been reported in West African monkeys.[1]

TRANSMISSION

Zika virus has been isolated from a wide variety of local mosquitoes in East, Central, and West Africa, plus from *Ae. aegypti* in Malaysia. The virus has been isolated in Uganda from *Ae. africanus,* in Central African Republic from *Ae. africanus* and *Ae. opok,* in Ivory Coast from *Ae. africanus,* in Senegal from *Ae. luteocephalus, Ae. vivittatus, Ae. dalzieli, Ae. furcifer-taylori* group, *An. gambiae,* and *M. uniformis,* and in Nigeria from *Ae. luteocephalus.* The epidemiological pattern of transmission may be very similar to that of yellow fever, with *Ae. africanus* transmitting the virus among monkeys in the forest canopy.

Human host

Human beings appear to enter the transmission cycle of Zika virus tangentially. Only a few human infections have been recognized, and they were benign febrile illncsses of short duration. It is considered that most human cases are subclinical or undifferentiated.

CONTROL AND PUBLIC HEALTH ASPECTS

Prevention of infection, if it has significance, is based on avoiding mosquito contact. The impact of this rather widespread infection appears to be negligible. Continuing surveillance of yellow fever will probably add to the knowledge of Zika fever as well.

REFERENCES

1. **Bernadou, J., Cornet, M., LeGonidec, G., Robin, Y., and Taufflieb, R.,** Rapport sur l'enquête sérologique fièvre jaune chez les singes d'Afrique Occidentale (2eme rapport) OCCGE-ORSTOM, Institut Pasteur de Dakar (doc polycopie,) 1973.
2. **Dick, G. W. A., Kitchen, S. F., and Haddow, A. J.,** Zika virus. 1. Isolation and serological specificity, *Trans. R. Soc. Trop. Med. Hyg.,* 46, 509, 1952.
3. **Fenner, F.,** The classification and nomenclature of viruses, *Intervirology,* 6, 1, 1975/76.
4. Institut Pasteur, Centre Collaborateur OMS de Référence et de Recherche pour les Arbovirus, *Rapport Annuel,* 1974 and 1976.
5. **Marchette, N. J., Garcia, R., and Rudnick, A.,** Isolation of Zika virus from *Aedes aegypti* mosquitoes in Malaysia, *Am. J. Trop. Med. Hyg.,* 18, 411, 1969.
6. **Moore, D. L., Causey, O. R., Carey, D. E., Reddy, S., Cooke, A. R., Akinkugbe, F. M., David-West, T. S., and Kemp, G. E.,** Arthropod borne viral infections of man in Nigeria, 1964-1970, *Ann. Trop. Med. Parasitol.,* 69, 49, 1975.
7. **Simpson, D. I. H.,** Zika virus infection in man, *Trans. R. Soc. Trop. Med. Hyg.,* 58, 335, 1964.
8. **Woodall, J. P.,** in *International Catalogue of Arboviruses Including Certain Other Viruses of Vertebrates,* 2nd ed., Pub. No. (CDC) 75-8301, Berge, T. O., Ed., Public Health Service, U.S. Department of Health, Education and Welfare, Atlanta, 1975, 782.

BUNYAMWERA FEVER

Y. Robin

NAME AND SYNONYMS

Bunyamwera (BUN) fever is the name of the infection caused by Bunyamwera virus. There are no synonyms.

HISTORY

The prototype BUN virus was isolated from a mixed pool of *Aedes* spp. mosquitoes collected in the Semliki Forest at Bunyamwera III, Bwamba County, Uganda in 1972.[8] Four isolations from human patients have been reported from South Africa, Nigeria Kenya, and Uganda.[1,4] The virus has been isolated from a variety of mosquitoes in Uganda, Cameroon, South Africa, Kenya, Nigeria, Senegal, and Central African Republic.[6] Only serological evidence of infection in animals has been reported.

ETIOLOGY

BUN is the type species of the genus *Bunyavirus* of the family Bunyaviridae. The virions are spherical, enveloped particles approximately 98 nm in diameter. The genome consists of a single strand of RNA in three pieces with total molecular weight 6 to 7×10^6 daltons. The virions develop in the cytoplasm of the host cells.[5] Hemagglutinin activity against goose and chick erythrocytes is produced in infected suckling mouse brains.[9]

DEFINITION

Bunyamwera fever is a mosquito-borne infection, varying from clinically inapparent to dengue-like, occurring widespread over Africa. Animal infections appear to be widespread but entirely subclinical.

ANIMAL INFECTION

Serological evidence of infection in animals has been reported in 33% of chimpanzees and 2.4% of monkeys tested in Zaire and Uganda, and in 15% of 406 domesticated animals, 0.4% of 245 rodents and 0.9% of 113 birds tested in South Africa by neutralization tests. Experimentally, paralysis and death follow injection by any route in mice of any age, although most strains kill adult mice only after serial passage in suckling mice or rhesus monkeys. Infection has been established, usually without clinical disease in albino rats, hamsters, rabbits, guinea pigs, rhesus and cercopithecus monkeys, lambs, and wild rodents with deaths only in hamsters and in one of three rhesus monkeys. Recognition of infection has been based on isolation and identification of the virus or neutralization serological tests.

HUMAN INFECTION

In the few clinically apparent human infections reported, the typical manifestations were headache, joint pains, malaise, and fever of 1 week or less duration. All recovered uneventfully. Specific diagnosis may be made by isolation of the virus in suckling mice by intracerebral inoculation or in human amnion, dog kidney, chick embryo, L929, HeLa or BHK_{21} cell cultures. The virus multiplies in embryonating hens' eggs, but embryonic deaths are variable. Serological tests must use multiple viral strains due to cross reactions with other related viruses, especially closely related Ilesha, Germiston, and Shokwe viruses.

EPIDEMIOLOGY

Occurrence
BUN virus has been isolated only in Africa south of the Sahara. Virus isolations from human patients or mosquito vectors have been reported from South Africa, Nigeria, Kenya, Uganda, Cameroon, Senegal, and Central African Republic. Serological survey evidence by neutralizing antibody titers has been reported from Zanzibar, South Africa, Zaire, Uganda, Guinea-Bissau, Mozambique, Liberia, Nigeria (7.2% of 97 sera), Tunisia (33% of 91 sera), and Tanzania (11.1% of 36 sera).[3] The specificity of all reported serological reactions cannot be fully assessed, and the possibility of cross-reactions with other bunyaviruses cannot be excluded. Seropositive human sera have been reported from Borneo (12.2% of 49 sera), Brazil (4.7% of sera), and Colombia (0.7% of 286 sera), but the specificity of these tests cannot be fully ascertained.

Reservoir
The possible reservoirs of BUN virus have not been identified. Serosurveys have indicated that a wide variety of domesticated and wild animals and birds become infected, but viremic animals have not been demonstrated in nature.[9]

Transmission
BUN appears to be entirely mosquito-borne. The virus has been isolated in Senegal in *Aedes dalziei* and *Ae. furcifer-taylori* group mosquitoes, in Nigeria from *Mansonia africanus,* in Uganda from *Aedes* spp., in Cameroon from *Aedes spp.,* in South Africa from *Ae. pembaensis* and *Ae. circumluteolus,* in Kenya from *Ae. pembaensis* and *M.*

uniformis, and in Central African Republic from *Culex spp.*[2,6,9] In addition, experimental infections by feeding BUN virus have been produced in *Ae. aegypti, Cx. fatigans, Anopheles quadrimaculatus,* and *Ae. circumluteolus,* and by intrathoracic inoculation in *Ae. canadensis* and *Ae. triseriatus.*

Human host

The role of human beings in the transmission cycle of BUN virus is not determined. The few documented human cases have been naturally or laboratory acquired.

CONTROL AND PUBLIC HEALTH ASPECTS

The health impact of this apparently widespread virus appears to be negligible. Avoiding mosquito contact is pertinent to preventing exposure to this and other mosquito-borne viruses. Precautions should be followed in laboratory operations to avoid exposure to this virus.

REFERENCES

1. **Bearcroft, W. G. C., Porterfield, J. S., and Sutton, R. N. P.,** The isolation and identification of Ukauwa, a Bunyamwera group virus from Nigeria, *Trans. R. Soc. Trop. Med. Hyg.,* 57, 308, 1963.
2. **Boorman, J. P. T. and Draper, C. C.,** Isolations of arboviruses in the Lagos area of Nigeria and a survey of antibodies to them in man and animals, *Trans. R. Soc. Trop. Med. Hyg.,* 62, 269, 1968.
3. **Brés, P.,** Données recentes apportées par les enquêtes sérologiques sur la prévalence des arbovirus en Afrique, avec rèférence spéciale a la fièvre jaune, *Bull. WHO,* 43, 223, 1970.
4. **Casals, J. and Clarke, D. H.,** Arboviruses other than groups A and B, in *Viral and Rickettsial Infections of Man,* Horsfall, F. L. and Tamm, I., Eds., J. B. Lippincott Philadelphia, 661, 1965.
5. **Fenner, F.,** The classification and nomenclature of viruses, *Intervirology,* 6, 1975/76.
6. Institut Pasteur de Dakar, Centre Collaborateur OMS de Rèférence et de Recherche pour les Arbovirus, *Rapport Annuel,* 1976.
7. **Anon.,** Ecologie des vecteurs et lutte antivectorielle en Santé Publique, *WHO Tec. Rep. Ser.,* 561, 1, 1975.
8. **Smithburn, K. C., Haddow, A. J., and Mahaffy, F.,** Neurotropic virus isolated from *Aedes* mosquitoes caught in Semlike forest, *Am. J. Trop. Med.,* 26, 189, 1946.
9. **Woodall, J. P.,** in *International Catalogue of Arboviruses Including Certain Other Viruses of Vertebrates,* 2nd ed., Pub. No. (CDC) 75-8301, T. O. Berge, Ed., Public Health Service, U.S. Department of Health Education and Welfare, Atlanta, 1975, 170.

BWAMBA FEVER

Y. Robin

NAME AND SYNONYMS

Bwamba (BWA) fever is the name of the disease caused by Bwamba virus. There are no synonyms.

HISTORY

BWA virus was first isolated from nine patients who had been working on a road construction project in the Bwamba forest of Uganda.[17] Subsequent isolations were made from patients with acute febrile illness in Cameroon and Nigeria, and with febrile illness with rash in Central African Republic.[5,6] The virus has been isolated from mosquitoes in Uganda, Nigeria, and Senegal.[2,9]

ETIOLOGY

BWA virus is classified in the genus *Bunyavirus* of the family Bunyaviridae. Serologically it is placed with Pongola virus in the Bwamba group.

ANIMAL INFECTION

In nature, BWA virus has not been isolated from any animals and has not been associated by seroconversion with any clinical disease. In South Africa, 1.0% of 94 wild birds[14] and 26.7% of 30 donkeys[10] surveyed were seropositive.[10,19] Seropositive monkeys have been reported from Uganda and Nigeria.[3,7,15] Experimentally, death is produced by intracerebral (i.c.) and subcutaneous (s.c.) inoculation in suckling mice, but only by i.c. inoculation in adult mice. Rhesus monkeys develop transient fever following i.c. or s.c. inoculation, but rabbits and dogs have been refractory to experimental inoculation. Recognition of infection would be by isolation and identification of the virus or by specific antibody rise between paired serum samples.

HUMAN INFECTION

Clinical

Virologically diagnosed clinical cases of Bwamba fever have been reported from Uganda, Nigeria, Cameroon, and Central African Republic.[5,6,13,17] Clinically, the infections have been characterized by high fever, headache, backache, general body ache, and variable sore throat and asthenia. In three patients reported in Central African Republic, micromaculopapular, slightly pruritic rash covering the entire body and lasting 1 to 2 days was reported. In all recognized cases, recovery has been uneventful, possibly with asthenia persisting a few days. Based on serological evidence, it is believed that most infections are subclinical or mild.

Diagnosis

The viremic phase during which virus may be isolated is typically brief. The virus may be isolated from blood samples by infection of suckling mice, inoculation of primary chick embryo or hamster kidney, BHK_{21}, Vero, or $LLC-MK_2$ cell cultures. In embryonating hens' eggs, viral multiplication occurs causing hemorrhagic lesions but not embryonic deaths. Hemagglutination inhibition (HI), complement fixation (CF), and neutralization tests are all used serologically.

EPIDEMIOLOGY

BWA virus has been isolated only in Africa, and limited serological surveys reported from other parts of the world have all been negative. In East, Central, and West Africa, serological data has indicated Bwamba infection to be the most common arboviral infection in the region.[7] In studies which have been reported, prevalence rates of 43% in Guinea-Bissau,[16] up to 97% in Tanzania and Uganda, and 37% in Mozambique were recorded. In several studies in Nigeria, rates of 77% in children 4 to 16 years old and 20.3% overall in western Nigeria,[12] 33% in northern Nigeria,[4] 4.4% in the Lagos area, and 52.2% in eastern Nigeria.[3] In a recent survey over Nigeria, 22% prevalence was recorded.[18]

Reservoir

Since the virus has never been isolated from naturally infected animals, little is known of reservoir hosts. Compared to antibody prevalence rates in people, relatively low rates have been reported in birds and animals.[3,7,10,14] A recent study in Nigeria found no positive sera among 502 animals and birds tested.[18]

Transmission

BWA virus is mosquito-borne. The virus has been isolated in Uganda from *Anopheles funestus*,[11] in Senegal from *An. gambiae*,[9] and in Nigeria from *An. funestus*,[1] *Aedes circumluteolus* in the Nujeko forest of the Northwestern State, *Ae. spp.*, *An. costani*, *An. coustani-paludis*, and *Mansonia uniformis*.[11,18] Based on studies in Nigeria, it has been suggested that *An. circumluteolus* is a major vector, but the high prevalence of antibody titers in people would stress that *Anopheles* spp. mosquitoes may also be important.

Environment

In serosurveys in the five ecological zones in Nigeria, prevalence rates of 68.2% were found in the southern guinea savanna zone, 40.6% in swamp forest, and 32.1% in rain forest areas.[18]

Human host

People appear to be important hosts of BWA virus. Susceptibility appears unrelated to sex or age.

CONTROL AND PUBLIC HEALTH ASPECTS

Human infections appear to be extremely common, but clinically inapparent or mild and of little public health significance. Further studies are needed to elucidate the transmission cycle of the virus. The epidemiological relationship of Bwamba virus to serologically related Pangola virus and the possible heterotypic reactions which may have occurred in serosurveys of the two viruses have not been fully assessed.

REFERENCES

1. Arbovirus Research Project, Ibadan, Annual Report, 1969.
2. Arbovirus Research Project, Ibadan, Annual Report, 1971-1972.
3. **Boorman, J. P. and Draper, C. C.,** Isolations of arboviruses in the Lagos area of Nigeria, and a survey of antibodies to them in man and animals, *Trans. R. Soc. Trop. Med. Hyg.,* 62, 1968.
4. **Casals, J.,** in Yale Arbovirus Research Unit, Annual Report, 1966, 22.
5. **Causey, O. R., Kemp, G. E., Madbouly, M. H., and Lee, V. H.,** Arbovirus surveillance in Nigeria 1964-1967, *Bull. Soc. Path. Exot.,* 62, 249, 1969.
6. **Chambon, L., Brés, P., Chippaux, Cl., Brottes, H., Salaun, J. J., and Digoutte, J. P.,** Rôle des arbovirus dans l'étiologie des fièvres exanthématiques en Afrique Centrale, *Med. Afr. Noire,* 16, 185, 1969.
7. **Dick, G. W. A.,** Epidemiological notes on some viruses isolated in Uganda, *Trans. R. Soc. Trop. Med. Hyg.,* 47, 13, 1953.
8. **Fenner, F.,** The classification and nomenclature of viruses, *Intervirology,* 6, 1, 1975/76.
9. **Institut Pasteur Dakar,** Centre Collaborateur OMS de Référence et de Recherche pour les Arbovirus, Rapport Annuel, 1976.
10. **Kokernot, R. H., Smithburn, K. C., and Kluge, E.,** Neutralizing antibodies against arthropod-borne viruses in the sera of domestic quadrupeds ranging in Tongaland, Union of South Africa, *Ann. Trop. Med. Parasitol.,* 55, 73, 1961.
11. **Lee, V. H., Monath, T. P., Tomori, O., Fagbami, A., and Wilson, D. C.,** Arbovirus studies in Napeko Forest, a possible natural focus of yellow fever virus in Nigeria. II. Entomological investigations and virus isolated, *Trans. R. Soc. Trop. Med. Hyg.,* 68, 30, 1974.

12. **Macnamara, F. N., Horn, D. W., and Porterfield, J. S.,** Yellow fever and other arthropod-borne viruses. A consideration of two serological surveys made in South-Western Nigeria, *Trans. R. Soc. Trop. Med. Hyg.,* 53, 202, 1959.
13. **Moore, D. L., Causey, O. R., Carey, D. E., Reddy, S., Cooke, A. R., Akinkugbe, F. M., David-West, T. S., and Kemp, G. E.,** Arthropod-borne viral infections of man in Nigeria, 1964-1970, *Ann. Trop. Med. Parasitol.,* 69, 40, 1975.
14. **Paterson, H. E., Kokernot, R. H., and Davis, D. H. S.,** Studies on arthropod-borne virus of Tongaland. IV. Birds of Tongaland and their possible role in virus disease, *S. Afr. J. Med. Sci.,* 22, 63, 1957.
15. **Pelissier, A. and Rousselot, R.,** Enquête sérologique sur l'incidence des virus neurotypes chez quelques singes de l'Afrique Equatoriale Francaise, *Bull. Soc. Path. Exot.,* 37, 228, 1954.
16. **Pinto, M. R.,** Survey for antibodies to arboviruses in the sera of children in Portuguese Guinea, *Bull. Org. Mond. Sante,* 37, 101, 1967.
17. **Smithburn, K. C., Mahaffy, A. F., and Paul, J. H.,** Bwamba fever and its causative virus, *Am. J. Trop. Med. Hyg.,* 21, 75, 1941.
18. **Tomori, O., Monath, T. P., Lee, V. H., Fagbami, A., and Fabiyi, A.,** Bwamba virus infection: a sero survey of vertebrate in five ecological zones in Nigeria, *Trans. R. Soc. Trop. Med. Hyg.,* 68, 461, 1974.
19. **Woodall, J. P.,** in *International Catalogue of Arboviruses Including Other Viruses of Vertebrates,* 2nd ed., Pub. No. (CDC) 75-8301, Berge, T. O., Ed., Public Health Service, U.S. Department of Health, Education and Welfare, Atlanta, 1975, 180.

DUGBE VIRAL FEVER

Y. Robin

NAME AND SYNONYMS

Dugbe (DUG) viral fever or Dugbe viral infection are names applied to the disease caused by Dugbe virus.

HISTORY

DUG virus was first identified in 1964 at Ibadan, Nigeria from *Amblyomma variegatum* ticks hand picked from infested cattle.[3] Numerous strains have been isolated in nature from people, cattle, one giant pouched rat, a variety of species of ticks, two pools of *Culicoides* spp. midges, and one pool of *Aedes aegypti* mosquitoes in Nigeria, from people and ticks in Central African Republic, and from ticks in Senegal and Cameroon.[1,5]

ETIOLOGY

DUG virus has been placed in the Nairobi sheep disease group of bunya-like viruses in the family Bunyaviridae. DUG and Ganjam viruses are serologically related to the Nairobi sheep disease virus. The virions are spherical, enveloped, and 90 to 100 nm in diameter. They are sensitive to sodium deoxycholate and chloroform. Some strains produce a low titering hemagglutinin in infected suckling mouse brains which is active against goose erythrocytes at 37°C at pH 6.6[2]

DEFINITION

Dugbe virus is considered to cause widespread and clinically inapparent infections in cattle, among which it is transmitted by local species of ticks. Human infections are tangential to the natural cycle of transmission, and are characterized by febrile illness, especially in children.

ANIMAL INFECTION

Natural infections in animals are considered to be entirely inapparent. Experimental infections in suckling mice cause paralysis and death only following intracerebral (i.c.) inoculation, and experimental infections in adult mice are entirely asymptomatic. Recognition of infection is by virus isolation and identification, or serologically by hemagglutination inhibition (HI) and complement fixation (CF) tests.

HUMAN INFECTION

Clinical

Human DUG viral infections have been reported from Nigeria and Central African Republic. The first recognized case was in a laboratory employee in Ibadan, Nigeria. After a 5-day incubation period following laboratory exposure, he developed fever, chills, nausea, and prostration. Leucopenia with 1700 leucocytes per mm[1] was recorded on the fifth day after onset, accompanied by drop in fever. Recovery was protracted with weakness, lassitude, and anorexia, but was complete without sequelae. All recognized naturally occurring cases have been in children.[7]

Three nonfatal DUG fever cases have been identified in Bangui, Central African Republic. Virus was recovered from a blood sample from a febrile child. A second adult patient suffering intense headache, vomiting, and diarrhea yielded virus in the cerebrospinal fluid. A third adult patient suffering headache, prostration, vomiting, diarrhea, and a maculopapular rash with pruritis yield virus in a blood sample.[8]

Diagnosis

Laboratory diagnosis is based on isolation and identification in i.c. inoculated suckling mice. Isolation may be made in BSC-1, Vero, and LLC-MK$_2$ cell lines in which the virus produces plaques. Serological responses are generally of a low level. HAI and CF tests are most reliable, with results of neutralization tests being quite inconclusive.

EPIDEMIOLOGY

Occurrence

DUG virus has been reported only from Africa, from Nigeria, Senegal, Cameroon, Uganda, and Central African Republic. The only reported serological survey showed 29% of 331 market cattle and 3.7% of 81 sheep and goats in Nigeria to be seropositive.

Reservoir

DUG virus has been frequently isolated from cattle in Nigeria, varying from 4 to 17% by month of sampling, with an average 7.4% of cattle tested yielding virus. It has been postulated that the continual introduction into Nigeria of cattle from the north provides a sufficient susceptible population to maintain endemicity.[6] The role of the giant pouched rat, *Cricetomys gambianus,* from which one isolation was made in Nigeria has not been delineated as yet.

Transmission

DUG virus was isolated from 358/4435 *Ixodes* spp., 106/850 *Amblyomma variega-*

tum, 4/864 *Boophilus decoloratus,* 67/663 *Hyalomma truncatum,* and 2/106 *H. rufipes* ticks studied in Nigeria, as well as from *A. variegatum* in Central African Republic and *A. lepidum* in Uganda.[9] The vector role of mosquitoes and *Culicoides* spp. midges found in Nigeria has only been speculated.

Human host

Serological surveys in Nigeria have been negative for antibodies against DUG virus.[4] The paucity of human cases, six in all, in comparison to the frequency of infection in cattle, has led to consideration that transmission to human beings is a relatively rare event and entirely tangential to the natural transmission cycle.[4]

CONTROL AND PUBLIC HEALTH ASPECTS

The relative rarity of human infections and the innocuous nature of infections in domesticated animals has led to placing minimal importance on the infection. Laboratory personnel working in laboratories where the virus is present should use precautions to avoid exposure.

REFERENCES

1. **Causey, O. R.,** Dugbe, *Am. J. Trop. Med. Hyg.,* 19, 1123, 1970.
2. **Causey, O. R.,** Dugbe, in *International Catalogue of Arboviruses Including Certain Other Viruses of Vertebrates,* 2nd ed., Berge, T. O., Ed., Public Health Service, U.S. Department of Health, Education, and Welfare, Atlanta, 1975, 252.
3. **Causey, O. R., Kemp, G. E., Casals, J., Williams, R. W., Madbouly, M. H.,** Dugbe virus a new arbovirus from Nigeria, *Nigerian J. Sci.,* 5, 41, 1971.
4. **David-West, T. S., Cooke, A. R., David-West, A. S.,** A serological survey of Dugbe virus antibodies in Nigerians, *Trans. R. Soc. Trop. Med. Hyg.,* 69, 358, 1975.
5. Institut Pasteur De Dakar, Centre Collaborateur OMS de Reference et de recherche pour les arbovirus, Rapport Annuel, 1976.
6. **Kemp, G. E., Causey, O. R., and Causey, C. E.,** Virus isolations from trade cattle, sheep, goats and swine at Ibadan, Nigeria, 1964—1068, *Bull. Epizoot. Dis. Afr.,* 19, 131, 1971.
7. **Moore, D. L., Causey, O. R., Carey, D. E., Reddy, S., Cooke, A. R., Akinkugbe, F. M., David-West, T. S., and Kemp, G. E.,** Arthropod-borne viral infections of man in Nigeria, 1964-1970, *Ann. Trop. Med. Parasitol.,* 69, 49, 1975.
8. **Sureau, P., Cornet, J. P., Germain, M., Camicas, J. L., and Robin, Y.,** Enquête sur les arbovirus transmis par les tiques en République Centrafricaine (1973-1974). Isolement des virus Dugbe, CHF-Congo, Jos et Bhanja, *Bull. Soc. Pathol. Exot.,* 69, 28, 1976.
9. **Tukei, P. M., Williams, M. C., Monkwaya, L. R., Henderson, B. E., Kaufuko, G. W., and McCrae, A. W. R.,** Virus isolations from Ixodid ticks in Uganda. Part 1. Isolation and characterization of ten strains of a virus not previously described from Eastern Africa, *East Afr. Med. J.,* 47, 265, 1970.

ZINGA FEVER

Y. Robin

NAME AND SYNONYMS

Zinga (ZGA) fever is the name of the disease caused by Zinga virus. There are no synonyms.

HISTORY

ZGA virus was first identified in 1969 from a pool of *Mansonia africana* mosquitoes collected on the banks of the Labaye River near its confluence with the Oubangui River in Central African Republic.[1] The virus has since been isolated from people in Central African Republic[2] and from people and mosquitoes in Senegal.[3] Serological studies in Central African Republic have indicated that the infection may occur in monkeys and larger wild mammals, but not in rodents and birds in nature.

ETIOLOGY

ZGA virus has not been classified or grouped. Very limited studies have indicated that the virus passes 0.22 μ pore diameter membrane filters, and is sensitive to ether, sodium deoxycholate, and chloroform. It is highly pathogenic to suckling and adult mice inoculated by intracerebral (i.c.) and intraperitoneal (i.p.) routes.

DEFINITION

Zinga fever is a mosquito-borne, dengue-like disease characterized by fever, headache, and joint pains with a benign course. Large wild mammals appear to be vertebrate hosts.

ANIMAL INFECTION

In nature, no clinical disease has been associated virologically or serologically with ZGA virus infections in animals, and evidence that it does infect animals has been entirely by prevalence of antibody titers. In Central African Republic 56% of 91 buffaloes, 26% of 73 wart hogs, 40% of 5 elephants, 50% of 4 monkeys, 43% of 21 hartebeest, and 21% of 47 other animals seropositive by hemagglutination inhibition (HI) test, but none of 2 bush pigs, 3 giant forest hogs, 123 feral rodents, or 113 wild birds. In addition, the virus was not recovered from 1400 feral rodents or 3500 wild birds sampled. In the laboratory, mice inoculated i.c. or i.p. died in 1 ½ to 2 days.

HUMAN INFECTION

Clinical
Onset of clinical disease has been sudden with fever, headache, and joint pains, especially in the ankles. The fever is often biphasic and accompanied by leucopenia. Recovery has been uneventful.

Diagnosis
Isolation and identification of the virus from acute phase blood samples into suckling mice has been the basis of diagnosis of reported cases. Serologically, neutralization tests have been considered to be more specific than HAI or complement fixation (CF) tests.

EPIDEMIOLOGY

Occurrence
At this time, ZGA virus has been isolated only from people and mosquitoes in Central African Republic and Senegal. Sero surveys have reported a 4.4% antibody prev-

alence rate in Central African Republic and 2.4% in Congo-Brazzaville among suburban and savannah residents.

Reservoir

ZGA virus has never been isolated from animals, but virological surveys of even modest size have only been reported in wild birds and rodents. Serological evidence indicates that infection in monkeys and larger mammals in nature may be common.[1]

Transmission

In Central African Empire, ZGA virus has been isolated from *Mansonia africana* collected in forest environment and from *Aedes* spp. of the palpalis group, both of which feed on large mammals. In Senegal, the virus has been isolated on three occasions from *Ae. dalzielli* collected by human bait techniques in the forest gallery at Kedougou Field Station. This mosquito feeds on both people and large mammals.

CONTROL AND PUBLIC HEALTH ASPECTS

The health impact of Zinga fever appears to be negligible. Infection has not been demonstrated in domesticated animals, and no clinical disease has been associated with infections in large wild mammals. The virus is, however, highly virulent in laboratory mice and its presence in nature does merit surveillance.

REFERENCES

1. **Digoutte, J. P., Cordellier, R., Robin, Y., Pajot, F. X., and Geoffroy, B.,** Le virus Zinga (Ar B 1976) nouveau prototype d'arbovirus isolé en République Centrafricaine, *Ann. Microbiol. (Institut Pasteur)*, 125B, 107, 1974.
2. **Digoutte, J. P., Jacobi, J. C., Robin, Y., Gagnard, V. J. M.,** Infection à virus Zinga chez l'homme, *Bull. Soc. Path. Exot.*, 67, 451, 1974.
3. Institut Pasteur Dakar, Centre Collaborateur OMS de Référence et de Recherche pour les Arbovirus, Rapport Annuel, 1976.

OTHER ARBOVIRAL ZOONOSES IN AFRICA

A. Fabiyi

Arboviruses in all recognized families as well as ungrouped have been reported from Africa. The presence of the following viruses has been virologically documented.

Family Togaviridae, genus *Alphavirus* (group A arboviruses): Chikungunya, O'nyong-nyong, Semliki Forest, Sindbis, Middleburg, and Ndumu. In the genus *Flavivirus* (group B arboviruses): Banzi, Bouboui, Dakar bat, Dengue 1, Dengue 2, Entebbe bat, Koutango, Kadam, Ntaya, Patiskum, Spondweni, Uganda S, Usutu, Wesselsbron, West Nile, Yellow fever, Zika and Saboya.

Family Bunyaviridae, genus *Bunyavirus:* Ingwavuma, Bunyamwera, Bwamba, Germiston, Ilesha, Pongola, Sabo, Sathuperi, Shamonda, Sango, Simbu, Shuni, Birao, Nola, Tahyna, Thimiri, Bahig, Tete, Matrih, and Butambi. In the bunyavirus-like group which are morphologically similar but serologically unrelated: Arumowot, Bhanja, Congo, Dugbe, Nairobi sheep disease, Rift Valley fever, Naples and Sicilian sandfly, Sudan, Tataguine, Thogoto, Witwatersrand (M'Poko and Yaba I), and Gordil.

Family Reoviridae, genus *Orbivirus:* Acado, African horse sickness, Bluetongue, Chenuda, Epizootic hemorrhagic disease of deer, Lebombo, Kemorovo, and Orungo (UgMP-359).

Family Rhabdoviridae, genus *Rhabdovirus:* Chandipura, Kamese, Mossuril and Bovine ephemeral fever.

Ungrouped arboviruses: Quaranfil, Chandipura, Jos, Somone, Zinga, Nyamanini, Oyo, Pretoria, Bandia, Qualyab, Botekor, Nyando, and African swine fever.

O'nyong-nyong viral infection — O'nyong-nyong fever was first identified in Uganda in 1959 from which it is believed to have spread to Kenya, Tanzania, and Malawi. The human disease is characterized by sudden onset with chills and epistaxis, pain and stiffness in the back and joints, headache, irritating rash, and prominent lymphadenitis.[10]

Dakar bat viral infection — The natural hosts of Dakar bat virus are believed to be bats. The virus has been identified in *Scotophilus nigrita* and *Tadarida condylura.*[1,2,16]

Dengue 1 and 2 viral infection — Serological evidence of dengue infections in galagos and monkeys has been reported from Nigeria.[9] The first descriptions of human dengue in Africa were reported in 1881 and 1883 during outbreaks of febrile disease in East Africa.[5,12] Dengue viruses types 1 and 2 were first isolated in Ibadan, Nigeria between 1964 and 1968.[4] The clinical disease is characterized by fever, headache, myalgia, abdominal pain, rash which may be petechial, lymphadenopathy, and variably, central nervous system involvement. Signs of dengue also include leucopenia and thrombocytopenia. The viruses are usually isolated from acute phase blood samples in suckling mice. Dengue hemorrhagic fever as diagnosed in Asia has not been recognized in Africa. Dengue fever in Africa is readily confused clinically with a wide variety of other arboviral infections.

In a recent serological survey of human beings and nonhuman primates in Nigeria, 45% of 1816 human sera had neutralizing antibodies against dengue 2 virus. The prevalence of antibody titers was higher in adults than in children. The highest prevalence, 63%, was in residents of lowland savannahs followed by those (42%) living in rain forests, and with the lowest prevalence in residents of the southern guinea and plateau savannas. Antibody prevalence in urban residents averaged 48% with 37% in rural residents.[9] In monkeys and galagos, an average of 48% of monkeys and 25% of galagos had antibody titers. In the Nupeko forest, at the confluence of the Kaduna and Niger Rivers, 74% of the monkeys had neutralizing antibodies. These findings were considered to establish the existence of a natural forest cycle of dengue involving nonhuman primates in Nigeria. Dengue 1 has only been isolated from human patients, but dengue 2 has been isolated from both naturally infected people and *Aedes aegypti* mosquitoes in Nigeria.[9]

Entebbe bat viral infection — The natural hosts from which Entebbe bat virus has been isolated have been *Tadarida limbata* and *T. condylura* bats. Experimentally infected mice have shown degenerative lesions without marked cellular infiltration in the hypocampus.

Koutango viral infection — Kontango virus has been identified in wild rodents in Senegal and Central African Republic.

Potiskum viral infection — Potiskum virus has been identified in wild rodents, *Cricetomys gambianus, Mostomys natalensis,* and *Arvicanthis nilothicus.*

Uganda S viral infection — Uganda S virus has been isolated from naturally infected wild monkeys. Encephalitis is produced in experimentally infected mice.[6,13]

Usutu viral infection — Usutu virus was reported from a naturally infected wild *Turdus bibonyanus* bird.

Ilesha viral infection — Ilesha virus was initially isolated from a human patient in

Nigeria, and has since been reported from Uganda, Cameroon, Central African Republic, and the West Nile District of Uganda. The primary vector is considered to be *Anopheles gambiae* mosquitoes.

Arumwot viral infection — Arumwot virus has frequently been isolated from wild rodents. In Nigeria, it has been identified in the absence of clinical disease from viremic *Crucidura* spp., *Tatera kempii, Arvicanthis niloticus,* and *Thamonomys macmillan.*

Bhanja viral infection — Bhanja virus has been isolated from sheep, cattle, birds (*Xerus erythropus,*) and hedgehogs (*Atelerix albiventris*).

Nairobi sheep disease — Nairobi sheep disease causes widespread disease in sheep, characterized by echymotic hemorrhages and fatal gastroenteritis. At necropsy, hyperplasia of mesenteric lymph nodes and tubular nephrosis are also observed. Clinical human infections with fever and arthralgia have occasionally been reported, and serological studies have indicated that subclinical human infections are sporadic. Animal infections have been reported from Nigeria, Uganda, Kenya, Central African Republic, Mozambique, and South Africa. Human disease has been recognized only in Uganda. The virus is transmitted by ticks and has been isolated from *Ripicephalus appendiculatus, Amblyomma variegatum, Boophilus decoloratus, Hyalomma rufipes, H. truncatum,* and *B. annulatus* ticks, and from *Culicoides* spp. midges collected in nature. The virus is serologically closely related to Dugbe and Ganjam viruses.

Tataguine viral infection — Tataguine virus was originally identified in a human patient in Senegal. It has subsequently been isolated from human patients in West and Central Africa.[3] In Nigeria, serological surveys showed a highest prevalence of antibody titers (16%) in residents in savanna and lowest on plateau regions.

Thogoto viral infection — Thogoto virus has been isolated from human patients with febrile illness characterized by optic neuritis and meningoencephalitis.

African horse sickness — African horse sickness virus has been reported in naturally infected horses, mules, and donkeys. The disease in horses is characterized by pulmonary hyperemia and edema, gastric and intestinal hyperemia, hydrothorax, hydroparidium, and edematous subcutaneous and intramuscular infiltrations.

Bluetongue — Bluetongue virus causes an important disease in small wild and domesticated ruminant animals, especially in sheep. Bluetongue in sheep is characterized by catarhal stomatitis, rhinitis, enteritis, and muscular paralysis. Abortion may occur in gestating ewes. In cattle, necrosis of oral mucous membranes and teat and udder epithelium has been observed. The virus has been isolated from *Crucidura* spp. rodents in Nigeria. Naturally-occurring human infections have not been documented. The virus is transmitted by *Culicoides* spp. midges.

Epizootic hemorrhagic disease in deer — The virus of epizootic hemorrhagic disease in deer has been isolated from *Culicoides* spp. midges in Nigeria, but no evidence of infection by this virus in deer or other hosts has been reported in Africa.

Orungo Viral Infection — Several epidemics of Orungo fever have been reported in Nigeria, characterized by nausea, vomiting, myalgia, fever lasting up to 7 days, headache, fine papular rash involving the face, chest and abdomen appearing about the third day of illness, conjunctivitis, skin tenderness, and leucopenia.[7,8] In a serosurvey in 17 localities in the 4 ecological zones of Nigeria, antibody titers were reported in 23% overall, with the highest prevalence in the Guinea savanna and lowest in rain forest zones. Serological evidence of infection in 24% of *Cercopithecus mona* and *Aethiops tantalus* monkeys, and 50% of sheep surveyed in Nigeria.[15] *Aedes dentatus* and *Anopheles* spp. mosquitoes have been identified as vectors of Orungo virus, and it has been suggested that both people and animals may enter actively in transmission cycles of the virus. In Uganda, where the virus was first isolated from mosquitoes, associated human infection has not been reported.

Chandipura viral infection — Chandipura virus has been identified in hedgehogs, *Atelerix spiculus* and *A. albiventris* in Nigeria.

Mossuril viral infection — Serological evidence of Mossuril viral infection has been reported in yellow baboons, *Papio cynocephalus* in Mozambique.

Bovine ephemeral fever — Serological evidence of bovine ephemeral fever has been reported in young calves at the Ibadan University Farm, Nigeria.

African swine fever — African Swine Fever virus circulated without associated clinical disease in a variety of wild wart hogs, *Phacochoerus aethiopicus,* bush pigs, *Potomochoerus* spp., and giant forest hogs, *Hylochoerus meinertzhageni* in East Africa. In domesticated swine, clinical disease characterized by fever, anorexia, cyanosis of the skin, enteritis, and uncoordination are observed. At necropsy, lymphoreticular destruction, vasculitis, widespread hemorrhage, and variable thrombosis and infarction are observed.[11,14] Neutralizing antibodies are not produced in any species, but complement fixation and agar gel immunodiffusion tests are applicable for serological tests. The virus has spread from Africa to Portugal, Spain, France, Italy, Cuba, Dominican Republic, Haiti, and Brazil in recent years, but extensive eradication efforts have been successful in France, Italy, and Cuba and are in progress in Dominican Republic and Brazil. African swine fever virus is not considered to infect human beings.

REFERENCES

1. **Bres, P. and Chambon, L.,** Isolement a partir de glandes salivaries de chauve — souris, *Ann. Institut Pasteur.,* 104, 705, 1963.
2. **Bres, P. and Chambon, L.,** Techniques pour l'etude de l'infection naturalle des chauves — souris par les arbovirus, *Ann. Institut Pasteur,* 107, 34, 1963.
3. **Bres, P., Williams, M. C., and Chambon, L.,** Isolement an Senegal d'un nouvean prototype d'arbovirus, la souche "Tataguine", *Ann. Inst. Pasteur Paris,* 3, 585, 1966.
4. **Carey, D. E., Causey, O. R., Reddy, S., and Cooke, A. R.,** Dengue viruses from febrile patients in Nigeria, 1964-1968, *Lancet,* 1, 105, 1971.
5. **Christie,** On the epidemics of dengue fever, their diffusion and etiology, *Glasgow Med. J.,* 16, 116, 1881.
6. **Dick, G. W. A. and Haddow, A. J.,** A hitherto unrecorded virus isolated from mosquitoes: I. Isolation and pathogenicity, *Trans. R. Soc. Trop. Med. Hyg.,* 46, 600, 1952.
6a. **De Tray, D. E.,** *Adv. Vet. Sci.,* 8, 299, 1963.
7. **Fabiyi, A., Tomori, O., and El-Bayoumi, M. S. M.,** Epidemic of a febrile illness associated with UgMP-359 virus in Nigeria, *West Afr. Med. J.,* 23, 9, 1975.
8. **Fabiyi, A., Tomori, O.,** unpublished data.
9. **Fagbami, A. H., Monath, T. P., and Fabiyi, A.,** Dengue virus infection in Nigeria, a survey for antibodies in monkeys and humans, *Trans. R. Soc. Med. Hyg.,* 71, 60, 1977.
10. **Haddow, A. J., Davies, C. W., and Walker, A. J.,** O'nyong-nyong fever: epidemic virus disease in East Africa: I. Introduction, *Trans. R. Soc. Trop. Med. Hyg.,* 54, 517, 1960.
11. **Heuschle, W. P. and Coggins, L.,** *Bull. Epizoot. Dis. Afr.,* 13, 255, 1965.
12. **Hirsch, A.,** *Handbook of Geographical and Historical Pathology,* 1, 55, 1883.
13. **Institut Pasteur, Bangui,** Annual Report, 1970.
14. **Montgomery, R. E.,** On a form of swine fever occurring in British East Africa (Kenya), *J. Comp. Path. Therap.,* 34, 151, 1921.
15. **Tomori, O. and Fabiyi, A.,** Neutralizing antibodies to Orungo virus in man and animals in Nigeria, *Trop. Geogr. Med.,* 28, 233, 1976.
16. Virus Research Laboratory, Annual Report, University of Ibadan, Nigeria, 1966.

CONGO FEVER IN AFRICA

Y. Robin

NAME AND SYNONYMS

Congo (CON) fever, Congo hemorrhagic fever and Crimean hemorrhagic fever (CHF) are considered to be caused by strains of bunya-like virus belonging to the CON-CHF serological group.

HISTORY

The viral etiology of Crimean hemorrhagic fever was demonsrated by Chumakov in 1945, but the CHF virus was not identified until 1967. The Congo virus was isolated in 1956 from the blood of a young patient with fever, headache, nausea and vomiting, backache, generalized joint pains, and photophobia in Kisangani, Zaire. The virus was subsequently isolated from blood samples from 11 febrile patients and 1 cow in Uganda,[12,18,20-22] cows, goats and hedgehogs in Nigeria,[11] a cow in Kenya, a goat in Senegal,[10] and from a variety of ticks in Nigeria, Senegal, and Central African Republic, and Uganda.[10,11] In 1970, the identity between CON and CHF viruses was reported by Casals.[3]

ETIOLOGY

CON-CHF viruses have been placed in a Crimean-Congo hemorrhagic fever group consisting of the Congo and Hazara strains in the family Bunyaviridae.[13,14] These strains are morphologically bunyavirus-like but are unrelated serologically to the Bunyamwera supergroup. The virions are spherical, enveloped, and 70 to 140 nm in diameter. The genomes consist of single stranded RNA. The viruses are sensitive to ether and chloroform, and produce a hemagglutinin in infected suckling mouse brains which is active against goose erythrocytes at 37°C at pH 7.2 to 7.3.[1,4]

DEFINITION

CON-CHF viral infection is a febrile dengue-like disease, occasionally with hemorrhagic manifestations in human patients and a clinically inapparent infection in a variety of animals, though possibly causing abortion in cattle. A variety of ticks are considered to be principal vectors.

ANIMAL INFECTION

No overt disease has been demonstrated in connection with viremia in most infected animals, though possible association with abortion in cattle has been reported. Subclinical infections have been produced experimentally in sheep and calves. In suckling and adult mice, paralysis and death follow intracerebral (i.c.) inoculation and in suckling mice by intraperitoneal (i.p.) inoculation as well. Recognition of current infection is based on isolation and identification of the virus and of retrospective infection by fluorescent antibody (FA) techniques or plaque reduction tests in a variety of cell cultures.[6]

HUMAN INFECTION

Clinical

Twelve human cases of CON fever were reported in Zaire and Uganda between 1956 and 1963, whereas hundreds of CHF patients have been reported from U.S.S.R.[5] Clinical disease in Africa has been characterized by fever, headache, generalized pains, photophobia, and prostration. Two laboratory-acquired infections have been described in detail. An animal attendant at the East African Virus Research Institute in Entebbe, Uganda was hospitalized with a temperature of 38°C, severe headache, joint pains, photophobia, and anorexia. He developed severe hematesis and died on the 4th day after onset. At necropsy, only multiple small ulcers in the gastric mucosa were recorded.[17] A virologist at the Institut Pasteur, Bangui, Central African Republic developed febrile illness with sudden onset after a 4-day incubation period. During the early clinical phase, fever fluctuated between 39 and 39.5°C with nausea, chills and sweating, neuralgia, asthenia, and anorexia. After 3 days, temperature returned to normal but stiffness, asthenia and anorexia persisted. Virus was isolated from a blood sample on the 2nd day after onset and sera collected on the 15th day showed antibodies by fluorescent antibody (FA) technique but not by the complement fixation (CF) test.[10] A serological survey in Nigeria showed neutralizing antibodies in 24 of 250 volunteers.[8] The specificity of these serological findings could not be fully confirmed.[23] Diagnosis is based on viral isolation and identification. FA techniques and plaque reduction tests using LLC-MK$_2$, Vero or BHK$_{21}$ cell lines have given most promising serological results. The agar-gel immunodiffusion test has not given adequately specific results and nonspecific virus neutralizing substances in sera have made results of neutralization tests difficult to interpret. The appearance of CF antibodies in convalescence has been variable.[16,23]

EPIDEMIOLOGY

Occurrence

In Africa, CON virus has been isolated in Zaire, Uganda, Kenya, Nigeria, Central African Republic, and Senegal. CHF virus has been isolated in western Crimea, the Kersh peninsula, the Rostov on the Don, and Astrakan regions of U.S.S.R. as well as in Bulgaria and Pakistan.

Reservoir

Virological and/or serological evidence of infection has been reported from Africa and U.S.S.R. in cattle, goats, hedgehogs, sheep, horses, and hares.[7,9,11] The role of these and/or other animals or birds in the maintenance of endemicity has not been ascertained.[7,9,11]

Transmission

CON-CHF viruses appear to be principally tick-borne although one isolation from *Culicoides* spp. midges has been reported from Nigeria. Ticks from which virus has been isolated in nature include *Hyalomma* spp. in Nigeria, Senegal, U.S.S.R., and Pakistan, *Amblyomma variegatum* in Nigeria, Senegal, Central African Republic, and Uganda, and *Boophilus decoloratus* in Nigeria, Senegal, and Central African Republic. Infected ticks appear to remain lifelong carriers, commonly 1 to 2 years, but transovarial transmission in ticks needs more investigation. Experimental transmission by injection of infected tick saliva has been effected.[9] The role of migratory birds in transporting infected ticks across U.S.S.R. and Africa has not been investigated. Much further study of the natural habitats and nidality of the vectors of CON-CHF viruses is needed.[2,19] Direct human-to-human transmission has occurred by contact with blood of hospitalized patients.

Human Host

Human infection is considered incidental in the natural cycle of transmission, with exposure occurring only when people enter natural foci and disturb the habitat or through laboratory exposure.

CONTROL

Prevention and Treatment

Prevention is largely based on personal measures to avoid tick infested areas where CON-CHF and other tick activities must be carried on in such areas, including wearing protective clothing and applying diethyltoluamide, dimethylphtalate, or other repellents. In areas where concentrations of cases may occur, tick control by clearing or application of insecticides may be appropriate. Health education is directed toward personal protective measures. Patients should be kept in strict isolation to prevent nosocomial transmission by contact with blood of viremic patients.

PUBLIC HEALTH ASPECTS

In Africa, CON virus infections have not been identified as a public health hazard of sufficient magnitude to merit control actions in people, animals, or ticks. In U.S.S.R., CHF is of much greater public health importance and tick infested areas should be avoided during spring and summer periods of maximal activity.

REFERENCES

1. **Ardoin, P., Clarke, D. H., and Hannoun, C.,** The preparation of arbovirus hemagglutinin by sonication and trypsin treatment, *Am. J. Trop. Med. Hyg.,* 18, 592, 1969.
2. **Audy, J. R.,** The localization of disease with special reference to the zoonoses, *Trans. R. Soc. Trop. Med. Hyg.,* 52, 308, 1958.
3. **Casals, J.,** Antigenic similarity between the virus causing Crimean hemorrhagic fever and Congo virus, *Proc. Soc. Exp. Biol. and Med.,* 131, 233, 1970.
4. **Casals, J. and Tignor, G. H.,** Neutralization and hemagglutination inhibition tests with Crimean hemorrhagic fever — Congo-virus, *Proc. Soc. Exp. Biol. Med.,* 145, 960, 1974.
5. **Chumakov, M. P. et al.,** Etiology, epidemiology and clinical manifestations of Crimean hemorrhagic fever and West-Nile fever, papers presented at a practical scientific conference in Astrakhan Oblast, May 21, 1968, *Institute of Poliomyelitis and Virus Encephalitides, Academy of Medical Sciences of the U.S.S.R., Astrakhan District Sanitary Epidemiological Service,* 1969, 6.
6. **Chumakov, M. P., Ed.,** *Viral Hemorrhagic Fevers,* Vol. 19, Institute of Poliomyelitis and Virus Encephalitides, Academy of Medical Sciences of the U.S.S.R., Moscow, 1971.
7. **Chunickin, S. P., Karaseva, A. P. S., Taufflieb, R., Robin, Y., Cornet, M., and Camicas, J. L.,** Results of serological study of circulation cycles of some arboviruses in the Republic of Senegal, West Africa, *Vopr. Virusol.,* 1, 52, 1971.
8. **David-West, T. S., Cooke, A. R., and David-West, A. S.,** Seroepidemiology of Congo virus (related to the virus of CHF) in Nigeria, *Bull. WHO,* 51, 543, 1974.
9. **Hoogstraal, H.,** Virus and ticks, in *Viruses and Invertebrates,* Gibbs, A. J., Ed., North-Holland Publishing, Amsterdam, 1972, 351.
9a. **Hoogstraal, H.,** The epidemiology of tick-borne Crimean-Congo hemorrhagic fever in Asia, Europe, and Africa, *J. Med. Epidemiol.,* 15, 307, 1979.
10. **Institut Pasteur de Dakar,** Centre Collaborateur OMS de Référence et de Recherche pour les arbovirus, *Rapport Annuel,* 1976.
11. **Kirya, B. G. and Kafuko, G. W.,** Congo, *Am. J. Trop. Med. Hyg.,* 19, 1141, 1970.
12. **Mason, J. P.,** Agents sent from other laboratories for identification agent 3011, *E. Afr. Virus. Res. Inst.,* Rep. No. 7, 25, 1956/57.

13. **Murphy, F. A., Harrison, A. K., and Whitefield, S. G.,** Bunyaviridae: morphologic and morphogenetic similarities of Bunyamwera serologic super group viruses and several other arthropod-borne viruses, *Intervirology,* 1, 297, 1973.

14. **Porterfield, J. S., Casals, J., Chumakov, M. P., Gaidamovich, S. Ya, Hannoun, C., Holmes, I. H., Horzinek, M. C., Mussgay, M., and Russel, P. K.,** Bunyaviruses and Bunyaviridae, *Intervirology,* 2, 270, 1973/74.

15. **Rosicky, B.,** *Ecology of arboviruses transmitted by ticks (excluding group B) with special respect to the localization of viruses in nature,* Int. Symp. Tick-borne Arboviruses (Excluding Group B), Gresikova, M., Ed., Publishing House of the Slovak Academy of Sciences, Bratislava, 1971, 95.

16. **Saidi, S., Casals, J., and Faghih, M. A.,** Crimean hemorrhagic fever — Congo (CHF-C) virus antibodies in man and in domestic and small mammals in Iran, *Am. J. Trop. Med. Hyg.,* 24, 353, 1975.

17. **Simpson, D. I. H., Williams, M. C., and Woodall, J. P.,** Four cases of human infection with the Congo agent, *E. Afr. Virus. Res. Inst.,* Rep. No. 14, 27, 1963/64.

18. **Simpson, D. J. H., Knight, E. M., Courtois, Gh., Williams, M. C., Weinbren, M. P., and Kibukamusoke, J. W.,** Congo virus: a hitherto undescribed virus occurring in Africa. Part 1. Human isolations — clinical notes, *E. Afr. Med. J.,* 44, 87, 1967.

19. **Varma, M. G. R.,** *Theoretical considerations of some factors determining the natural locality of tick-borne viruses,* Int. Symp. Tick-borne Arvoviruses (Excluding Group B), Gresikova, M., Ed., Publishing House of the Slovak Akademy of Sciences, Bratislava, 1971, 119.

20. **Woodall, J. P., Williams, M. C., Santos, D. F., and Ellice, J. M.,** Virology: laboratory studies. The 3010 group, *E. Afr. Virus. Res. Inst.,* Rep. No. 12, 21, 1961/62.

21. **Woodall, J. P., Williams, M. C., and Simpson, D. I. H.,** Congo virus: a hitherto undescribed virus occurring in Africa. Part 2. Identification studies, *E. Afr. Med. J.,* 44, 93, 1967.

22. **Woodall, J. P., Williams, M. C., Simpson, D. I. H., Ardoin, P., Lule, M., and West, R.,** The Congo group of agents, *E. Afr. Virus. Res. Inst.,* Rep. No. 14, 34, 1963/64.

23. **Zavodova, T. I., Butenko, A. M., Tkachenko, E. A., and Chumakov, M. P.,** in *Viral Hemorrhagic Fevers, Vol. 19.* Chumakov, M. P., Ed., p. 61, Works of the Institute of Poliomyelitis and virus Encephalitides, Academy of Medical Sciences of the U.S.S.R., Moscow, 1971.

TICK-BORNE CRIMEAN-CONGO HEMORRHAGIC FEVER*

H. Hoogstraal

NAME AND SYNONYMS

The tick-borne Crimean-Congo Hemorrhagic Fever (CCHF) complex is frequently called Crimean hemorrhagic fever (CHF), Central Asian hemorrhagic fever, Uzbekistan hemorrhagic fever, or other regional names in Eurasia and Congo (CON) fever in Africa. Since 1969, more uniformity in nomenclature has been appearing and CCHF is used throughout this chapter.

HISTORY

Significance of the Newborn Mouse Virus Isolation System.

The use of newborn (suckling) mice for arbovirus isolation has been the technological innovation most responsible for the great strides in the development of arbovirology since the 1940s.[582] Newborn mouse susceptibility to yellow fever virus has been known for decades.[521] Since Dalldorf and Sickles[126] demonstrated the sensitivity of these small animals to viral agents of paralysis in children, newborn mice have been used routinely for arbovirus isolation. These rodents, along with cell cultures, are now regarded as a basic tool for thorough investigation of any specimen likely to contain an arbovirus. Most arboviruses cause infection and disease when intracerebrally inoculated into the newborn mouse; therefore, white mice have long been mass-produced by American and European virological laboratories and by commercial entrepreneurs.[582]

Impact of This System on Knowledge of Hemorrhagic Fevers

In the U.S.S.R., results of the first use of newborn white mice (NWM) in 1967 for Crimean hemorrhagic fever research cleanly divide the long history of this disease into two periods. Numerous Soviet authors have stressed the significant advances in knowledge of Crimean-Congo hemorrhagic fever epidemiology following the 1967 technological "breakthrough." This single act provided the basis for a coordinated international study centered at the Yale Arbovirus Research Unit (YARU), which serves as a World Health Organization Arbovirus Reference Center.

* Reprinted with permission from the Journal of Medical Entomology, 15, 307-417, 1979 in which it was published with the title, "The Epidemiology of Tick-Borne Crimean-Congo Hemorrhagic Fever in Asia, Europe and Africa".

Publication of this article was supported in part by Grant No. 1-RO1-LM01954 from the National Library of Medicine, for support of a series of Review Articles appearing in the Journal of Medical Entomology. This is the 16th article to appear in the series.

This article is dedicated to my colleagues on the 1965 and 1969 U.S. Delegations on Hemorrhagic Fevers to the U.S.S.R., Drs. Jordi Casals, Brian E. Henderson, Karl M. Johnson, Alexis Shelokov, Ned H. Wiebenga, and Telford H. Work, and also to our chief Soviet hosts, Academician Mickhail P. Chumakov and Dra Elena V. Leshchinskaya, all of whom contributed to my knowledge of this disease. These delegations were organized by the National Institute of Allergy and Infectious Diseases (NIAID) of the National Institutes of Health.

From Research Project MR041.09.01-0152, Naval Medical Research and Development Command, National Naval Medical Center, Bethesda, Md. The opinions and assertions contained herein are the private ones of the author and are not to be construed as official or as reflecting the views of the Department of the Navy or of the naval service at large. This study was assisted by Agreements 03-036-N between the NIAID and NAMRU-3 and 03-063-N between the NIAID and Cairo University, Faculty of Science, Entomology Department.

From the 12th century to 1967, Central Asian and, later, Soviet and Bulgarian scholars, physicians, and scientists had recognized an association between ticks and various local manifestations of human hemorrhagic diseases. However, they were uncertain whether local syndromes were conspecific or differed and how the etiologic agent(s) survived in nature. During the 1944 to 1945 Crimean hemorrhagic fever epidemic following World War II, Chumakov[89,95,98] suggested the viral nature of the agent by reproducing the disease in humans inoculated with patients' blood and identified as the vector the only tick species commonly biting persons in the Crimea. The next two decades saw outbreaks of the same or "related" diseases, some with fearful mortality rates, in Central Asia and elsewhere in the U.S.S.R. and in Bulgaria. In the absence of a characterized agent and known antigens and antibodies for serological, diagnostic, experimental, and epidemiological survey purposes, the natural history and critical transmission factors of the disease(s) remained an enigma, and measures for prevention and control could be based only on guesswork.

In 1967, when blood from human hemorrhagic fever patients and corpses yielded the etiologic agent after intracerebral (i.c.) inoculation into NWM, an actual virus could be used for structural characterization by electron microscopy, and for physicochemical and serological classification. Identifiable antibodies and antigens could be produced for numerous experimental needs and for serological surveys. A new era in hemorrhagic fever history began.

The agents of the tick-borne hemorrhagic fevers in the major foci, from Kazakhstan and Uzbekistan to Bulgaria and across Africa from the Atlantic to the Rift Valley, were found to be indistinguishable from each other, thus giving rise to a new name for the disease — Crimean-Congo hemorrhagic fever (CCHF).

After 1970, results of studies using new serological and virological tools showed that India and Pakistan could be included in the known geographic range of CCHF virus circulation, as well as Iran, Afghanistan, all southern Republics of the Soviet Union, and numerous areas near or some distance from earlier recognized foci in republics where the disease was long known. Similarly, the presence of the virus was detected in other "new" areas of Africa. The approximate locations of known CCHF virus foci and disease outbreaks are shown in Figures 1 and 2.

Results of seroepidemiological surveys of human beings especially in remote areas, showed the incidence of unreported or misdiagnosed CCHF infections in various populations. Results of seroepidemiological surveys and of attempts to isolate the virus from wild and domestic vertebrates suggested the role of different vertebrates as active virus reservoirs, as nonreservoirs but significant contributors to the tick vector population density, or as epidemiologically unimportant members of the biocenose. Virus isolation rates from various tick species showed the role of individual species as a virus vector and/or reservoir and revealed the degree of risk to human health presented by these species in different foci. Demonstration of transstadial survival and transovarial transmission of the virus in ticks provided evidence of the biological properties permitting CCHF virus survival from season to season in dramatically differing ecological and zoogeographical zones and in 1-host, 2-host, and 3-host ticks feeding on very different groups of vertebrate hosts.

The post-1967 findings in Asia, Europe, and Africa have greatly expanded the knowledge of CCHF natural history, and certain earlier unanswered questions and perplexities can now be explained with some confidence. Nevertheless, numerous other significant epidemiological factors remain to be investigated. Within historic times, CCHF epidemics have been associated with environmental changes caused by war or by new agricultural practices such as collectivization, flood control, irrigation, virgin land exploitation, or increasing size and numbers of dairy herds. Recent studies are showing the presence of the virus and of sporadic human cases in an ever increasing

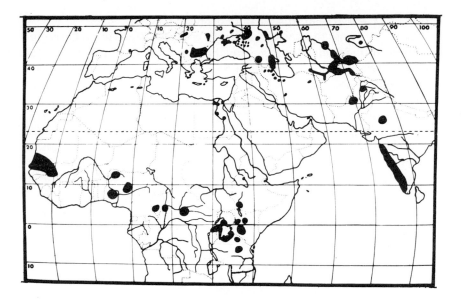

FIGURE 1. Distribution of Crimean-Congo hemorrhagic fever virus (outlines are approximate) based on virus isolations and results of seroepidemiological surveys. (From Royal Society of Tropical Medicine and Hygiene, London, Symposium Proceedings, November 23—25, 1977, 48. With permission.)

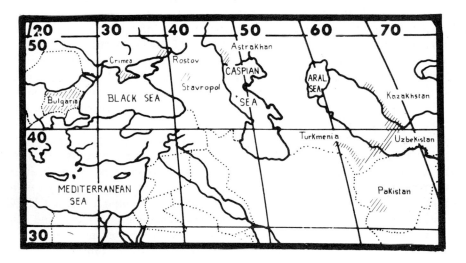

FIGURE 2. Locations (approximate) of some Crimean-Congo hemorrhagic fever epidemics and major outbreaks. (From Royal Society of Tropical Medicine and Hygiene, London, Symposium Proceedings, November 23—25, 1977, 48. With permission.)

number of more or less "silent foci" in numerous biotopes of Eurasia and Africa. We now know that a surprising number and variety of tick species maintain CCHF virus in nature. However, we have only a few rudimentary facts to answer the multifaceted question of how, when, and where new CCHF epidemics may appear. The most important of these facts have been gained within the past decade, especially during the latter half of this period. Thus, it is timely to consolidate the earlier and more recent information on CCHF epidemiology in order to inquire more intelligently — what needs to be done in CCHF research?

Early History of CCHF in Central Asia and European U.S.S.R.

In the Thesaurus of the Shān of Khwarazm[161] writtcn in Persian (in Soviet literature stated as written in the Tadzhik language), the physician Zayn ad-Dīn abū Ibrahim Ismacil ibn Muhamad al-Husayini al-Jurjām (died in 1136 at Merv) described a hemorrhagic disease, now considered to have been CCHF, from the area that is presently Tadzhikistan. The signs were presence of blood in the urine, rectum, gums, vomitus, sputum, and abdominal cavity. The arthropod causing the disease was said to be tough, small, related to a louse or tick, and normally parasitizing a black bird. Treatment, which was sometimes ineffectual, was application of *bodzkhar* and essence of red sandalwood at the site of the bite and the feeding the patient fresh goat milk together with butter, *khot'ma* flowers, and leaves or essence of *khovre* and essence of flax seed, chicory, and gourd.

CCHF was also recognized for centuries under at least three names by indigenous peoples of southern Uzbekistan. The first conclusive clinical accounts pertained to the World War II epidemic in the Crimea (1944-1945) and at about the same period to outbreaks in the present Asian Republics of the U.S.S.R.

ETIOLOGY

CCHF Virus Characterization (1967-1968) and Sequelae
Virus Characterization

In 1967, Chumakov and his colleagues at the Institute of Poliomyelitis and Viral Encephalitides, Moscow, first used newborn white mice (NWM) and rats (NWR) for CCHF virus isolation and the complement-fixation (CF) test with sera of convalescent CCHF patients to check the specificity of experimental infection and death of NWM and NWR.[64,95,98,101,105,112,115] The Drozdov strain of CCHF virus, isolated by this method from a patient (Drozdov) in Astrakhan, became the now-famous prototype CCHF strain for much experimental work in the U.S.S.R. and abroad (though for reasons discussed under Virus Taxonomy, the Drozdov strain is not the taxonomic prototype strain of the agent causing CCHF). After a 4- to 7-day incubation period, practically all the inoculated NWM and NWR died. The virus was passaged in these animals 27 times but was nonpathogenic for adult white mice, rats, guinea pigs, hamsters, rabbits, and monkeys. It had little or no cytopathogenic effect (CPE) in seven primary and passaged cell cultures but did reproduce in some of them. In infected cultures, virus multiplication was easily detected by the interference reaction with cytopathogenic viruses and by the fluorescent antibody (FA) technique. The CCHF virus contained RNA and was highly sensitive to sodium desoxycholate, ether, and chloroform. It passed through 220-nm Millipore® filter pores, resisted prolonged freezing on dry ice, and lyophilized well, but became inactivated when exposed to 60°C temperature for 15 min or to 37°C for 7 hr. Electron microscopy (EM) showed the virion to be spherical and to measure 100 to 130 nm. (More recent physicochemical and EM findings were reported by Donets,[140] Chumakov and Donets,[107] Jelinkova et al.,[235] Krasil'nikov and Donets,[294] Korolev et al.,[289] Popov and Zavodova,[412] and Donets et al.[142] Popov et al.[413] briefly mentioned certain properties observed by EM that appeared to be atypical of the family Bunyaviridae. Donets and Chumakov,[141] Korolev et al.,[288] and Donets et al.,[142] stressed that the single-stranded RNA in CCHF virions and other characteristics of these particles, and the morphogenesis of the virus, are typical of the family Bunyaviridae.)

Notably, attempts to obtain a hemagglutinating antigen from the brains of infected animals and from culture fluids of infected tissue cultures were unsuccessful. CF test results with serum of the Drozdov strain from Astrakhan, compared with other sera from CCHF patients from Rostov Oblast (both in European U.S.S.R.) and from Tadzhik S.S.R. and Bulgaria, showed the conspecificity of virus strains from each source. Of 96 CCHF patient sera from these areas that had been stored between 1954 and 1967, 72% showed CF test reactions specific for CCHF. The antigen did not react in the CF test with sera from healthy persons or from patients with hemorrhagic nephro-sonephritis, West Nile fever, tick typhus, Russian spring-summer encephalitis, Omsk hemorrhagic fever, etc.

In 1968, the Drozdov strain was sent for further characterization studies to YARU, where at the same time Casals was also investigating strains of "Congo virus" from human patients from Zaire and Uganda (Simpson et al.,[479] Woodall et al.,[580] and from *Hyalomma* ticks from Pakistan[30] The Drozdov strain, which had been transported from Moscow to New Haven in its 28th mouse passage in a mouse carcass frozen on dry ice, was easily reestablished in 1- or 2-day-old mice and immune sera and antigens were prepared for CF testing.[70] In summarizing his studies of these strains in the CF, agar gel precipitation, and neutralization (N) tests, Casals stated: "A viral strain isolated in the U.S.S.R. from a patient suffering from Crimean hemorrhagic fever and reported to be etiologically related to the illness, has been shown to be antigenically indistinguishable from Congo virus." Also included in the Casals paper is the statement that seven virus strains sent to YARU by Causey from ticks, cattle, *Culicoides,* and a hedgehog in Nigeria[82,261,262,577] were indistinguishable from Congo virus in the CF test.*

Thus less than 2 years after Chumakov and his colleagues first used NWM and NWR for virus isolation and characterization, it could be demonstrated that the CCHF agent occurs in nature from Pakistan to Bulgaria and in several regions of Africa. The remainder of this review will show the increase in depth and breadth of knowledge of CCHF epidemiology since the 1967-1968 "breakthrough," and will also ask where we go from here in CCHF research.

Virus Registry

By common agreement among arbovirologists throughout the world, an arbovirus name becomes "official," or is validated, when it is registered in the Catalogue of Arthropod-borne Viruses of the World.[39,507,514,515] Specialists from many countries, including the U.S.S.R., have warmly collaborated in providing arbovirus data for this unique international catalogue. However, Chumakov and his colleagues have not registered the Drozdov strain or any other related strain, despite having first discovered the virus properties in 1967-1968.

The taxonomic priority for the etiologic agent of this disease was established on June 10, 1969, when B. G. Kirya and G. W. Kafuko of the East African Virus Research Institute, Entebbe, Uganda, registered Congo virus strain V 3011. This strain had been isolated on March, 6, 1956 by C. Courtois at the Province Medical Laboratory, Kasangani (Stanleyville), Zaire (Belgian Congo), by venipuncture of a 13-year-old male patient presenting with fever, headache, nausea, vomiting, backache, general joint pains, and photophobia. The Casals paper[70] was quoted in the Registry, which was updated

---

*   In a comparative study of ten "CHF" virus strains from the U.S.S.R. and four "Congo" virus strains from Africa,[485] all results were identical for the dynamics of viremia in various mammals, sensitivity to standard chemicals, effect of temperature, optimum pH, virion size, immunogenic properties, etc. Nevertheless, because of the dearth of clinical and epidemiological data from Africa, these authors considered it premature to state that the infections caused by the Eurasian and African agents were identical. This attitude contrasts with that of the same and other authorities who immediately abandoned the names "Central Asian hemorrhagic fever" and "Uzbekistan hemorrhagic fever" for CCHF in 1967-1968 on the basis of similar comparative experimental results and of a similar disparity, at that time, in epidemiological data from European and Asian areas. Later, Donets et al.[142] studied the physicochemical characteristics, morphology, and morphogenesis of virions from three Soviet and two African ("Congo") strains and concluded that these agents are identical in every respect.

on May 20, 1973 with an official Subcommittee rating of Recognized Arbovirus, and again by Berge[39] with additional literature references.

Common Name

Following the official registry of Congo virus in 1969, some taxonomic purists have argued that the common name of this virus should also be Congo virus, but Soviet authorities have insisted that the long recognized name Crimean hemorrhagic fever (CHF) virus should be retained. As a compromise between "unofficial" historical antecedents and "official" Registry criteria, Casals et al.[75] suggested CHF-Congo virus as an acceptable common name. Some Soviet writers have adopted this term, others have continued to use only CHF, and others dealing with African strains refer to them as Congo virus. I find "CHF-Congo" to be awkward and have employed Crimean-Congo hemorrhagic fever (CCHF) virus in recent papers and throughout this review.

Before the conspecificity of CCHF strains from different Eurasian areas was determined, claims for different dissemination routes, degrees of disease severity, and mortality rates in the ecologically and zoogeographically diverse European and Central Asian foci led many writers to differentiate between Crimean hemorrhagic fever, "Uzbekistan hemorrhagic fever," "Central Asian hemorrhagic fever," etc. Since 1969, these discussions have dropped from the literature.

Virus Taxonomy and Systematics

The earliest attempt to place this virus in a taxonomic and systematic hierarchy was that of Ryzhkov,[443,444] who proposed the genus and species *Pantropus tchumakovi* in the Pantropiaceae. Order Pantropiales, Class Arthropodophilaceae. Zhdanov[604,605] recommended a different system: genus and species *Haemorrhagogenes tchumakovi,* family Acarophilaceae, and Order Arthropodophiliales. Zhdanov[606] briefly "characterized" H. *tchumakovi.* This 1950-1953 terminology has not appeared in subsequent literature.

Contemporary specialists consider the physical properties of CCHF virus to be characteristic of the family Bunyaviridae. However, generic relationships in this family remain unsettled and Fenner[169,170] recorded CCHF and Hazara (HAZ) viruses as "possible members of the family Bunyaviridae." The family Bunyaviridae, as proposed and characterized by Murphy et al.,[359] included more than 130 arboviruses with morphological and morphogenetic similarities of the Bunyamwera supergroup, originally defined serologically by Casals,[69] and of several other arboviruses. The genus *Bunyavirus* of these authors contained at least 88 viruses in 12 serogroups, and unassigned groups. Fifty-four other viruses, in 18 serogroups, including CCHF, were assigned to an "unnamed presumptive genus." The Arbovirus Study Group of the International Committee on the Nomenclature of Viruses (ICNV)[414] recognized the family Bunyaviridae and genus *Bunyavirus,* specified *bunyamwera* virus as the type-species, and suggested that the viruses in the "unnamed presumptive genus" be regarded as "other possible members" until their relationship(s) were clarified from results of further research. This family and genus were not mentioned in the list of names approved in June 1974 by the ICNV Executive Committee.[171] As already stated, Fenner[169,170] considers these viruses to be "possible members" of the family Bunyaviridae. Further ramifications of this question are mentioned under "Other possibly related agents".

All of the 12 serogroups included in the genus *Bunyavirus* were thought to be insect-rather than tick-associated when the Murphy et al.[359] paper was published. However, Converse et al.[124] isolated Bahig virus (Tete serogroup, genus *Bunyavirus*) from larvae of *Hyalomma marginatum rufipes* parasitizing a northward-migrating Common Wheatear, *Oenanthe o. oenanthe,* in Egypt, and from transovarially infected F_1 larvae and nymphs reared from an engorged female H. m. *marginatum* taken from a racehorse near Naples, Italy. Matruh virus, another member of the Tete serogroup, was also isolated from ticks in Egypt.[356]

Among the "possible members" of Bunyaviridae are a number of insect-associated viruses: 4 tick-associated serogroups (the number of viruses presently known in each serogroup is stated in parentheses), Uukuniemi (5), CCHF (2), Nairobi sheep disease (2 or 3), Kaisodi (3); and 4 ungrouped viruses, Lone Star, Sunday Canyon, Thogoto, and Bhanja.

Hazara Virus: a CCHF-Related Agent

The CCHF serogroup currently consists of two serologically related viruses, CCHF and Hazara (HAZ). HAZ virus was registered in the *International Catalogue of Arboviruses* as serologically ungrouped on July 25, 1967, reregistered in the "Congo" serogroup by the Subcommittee on Information Exchange American Committee. Arthropod-borne Viruses,[507] and given an official subcommittee rating of Possible Arbovirus in the Berge[39] revision of the Catalogue. The HAZ virus characterization was published by Begum et al.[29] This virus was isolated from one of two pools of *Ixodes (I.) redikorzevi* from a high mountain vole, *Alticola roylei,* trapped in alpine ("subartic") terrain at Gitidas, 3330 m altitude, Kaghan Valley, Hazara District, Pakistan. No HAZ virus was isolated from *Dermacentor* or *Haemaphysalis* ticks from Hazara District, but 4 of 150 human sera reacted positively in the CF and hemagglutination inhibition (HI) tests for infection by this virus. Nothing else is known of the natural history of HAZ virus. Notably, the HAZ isolate was from a rodent-infesting tick in an alpine zone; CCHF isolates from Pakistan are from cattle-infesting ticks (*Hyalomma a. anatolicum* and *Boophilus microplus*) in a lowland semiarid zone (Lahore) and from human patients from the Muree Hills and the Quetta area.

None of 1289 sera from humans and domestic animals in India showed CF antibodies to HAZ virus.

Biological and antigenic differences between HAZ and CCHF viruses are distinct. HAZ virus[492] and CCHF virus (Eurasian and "Congo" strains[164,495]) inoculated intracerebrally into NWM produced similar, diffusely distributed focal lesions in the brains. However, the HAZ antigen accumulations detectable by the FAT occurred in fewer cells and were less marked in individual cells of the brains, livers, and salivary glands. The CF titers of HAZ antigen in the brains and viscera were lower but the titers of infectious HAZ virus in the blood and viscera were considerably higher than those produced by the CCHF strains. The markedly edematous brain tissues of all HAZ virus-infected NWM appeared to be significant in determining the fulminating nature of the disease and in accounting for the absence of proliferative reactions usually present in brains of CCHF virus-infected NWM.[613]

Chumakov and Smirnova[110] reported results of a comparative study of pathogenicity, antigenic relationships, and reactions in tissue cultures of HAZ virus and of CCHF strains from Eurasia and Africa. Stefanov and Smirnova[504] briefly and ambiguously discussed morphometric differences between HAZ virus and CCHF strains from Eurasia and Africa.

The helical nucleocapsid found in an EM study of HAZ virus in the mouse brain[473] may explain certain discrepancies in observations of thin sections of members of the family Bunyaviridae.[142]

Buckley[59] used cloned HAZ and CCHF viruses to develop a cross-plaque neutralization test. Casals and Tignor[77] modified serological tests to overcome a nonspecifc antiviral factor in mouse serum that had complicated tests of the CCHF serogroup. Yunker and Cory[589] included HAZ among 123 other viruses tested for arbovirus plaque production in Singh's *Aedes albopictus* mosquito cell cultures.

Other Possibly Related Agents

In a lecture on the history and present status of international arbovirus research, Casals[73] briefly stated that distant serologic relationships seem to exist between CCHF virus (Congo strains) and Nairobi sheep disease (NSD) virus. Casals stated that "one begins to suspect that a second supergroup (may be involved) among the *Bunyavirus-like agents*." This supergroup, also containing Uukuniemi (UUK) virus, might eventually form a second genus based on UUK virus, in the family Bunyaviridae. The NSD serogroup consists of NSD virus in eastern Africa, the possibly identical Ganjam (GAN) virus in India, and Dugbe (DUG) virus in eastern and western Africa. It is still too early to evaluate the significance of these findings.

During the morphogenesis of both CCHF and UUK viruses, ringlike structures develop in infected cells.[290] This phenomenon, atypical of the genus *Bunyavirus,* lends support to the Casals suggestion that the CCHF, UUK, and NSD serogroups may constitute a separate genus within the family Bunyaviridae. The ringlike structures forming crystalline patterns in cells infected by CCHF virus may be virus-specific protein accumulations corresponding to fluorescent cytoplasmic masses characterizing later stages of infection.

DEFINITION

Probably described as early as the twelfth century in Central Asian U.S.S.R., CCHF has been extensively studied since the 1944-1945 epidemic in Ukranian S.S.R. It is recognized from Central Europe through the Middle East, U.S.S.R., Pakistan, and India, and in Africa in Egypt, Senegal, Nigeria, Central African Republic, Zaire, Uganda, Kenya, Ethiopia, and Tanzania. Inapparent to severe disease, from influenza-like to severe diphasic febrile disease with widespread hemorrhagic characterize the human infections. A variety of wild and domestic mammals are subclinically involved in the transmission cycles. A wide variety of ticks serve as lifelong carriers and transmitters of the virus.

ANIMAL INFECTION

Introduction

Like most arthropod-borne agents causing human disease, CCHF virus is generally a zoonosis circulating unnoticed in nature in an enzootic tick-nonhuman vertebrate-tick cycle. Humans become infected in caves, homes, or other buildings, in areas surrounding their homes, or when wandering (1) some or (2) a great distance away from their usual environment. Both the clinical and epidemiological differences between (1) and (2) are noteworthy. Zoonotic agents generally cause little or no damage to their usual hosts, but exceptions to this generalization do occur. What we wish to know, ideally, is the qualitative and quantitative role of each vertebrate species in maintaining the virus cycle in each of the ecologically and zoogeographically differing types of CCHF foci in Asia, Europe, and Africa. Before 1968, ignorance of the role of nonhuman vertebrates in the CCHF epidemiological process was total. Now we can present a broad outline of this subject and some significant data, but many specific questions remain to be answered.

Proof of Infection in Vertebrates

Details of methodology of arbovirus investigation are found in reports by Hammon & Work[199] Work,[582] and Hammon and Sather[198]. In brief, there are three major tools for obtaining proof of arbovirus infection in vertebrates. (Methods for obtaining proof of arbovirus infection in ticks are virtually identical.)

The first tool is intracerebral inoculation of tissues or body fluids from the suspect vertebrate into NWM, and reinoculation into other NWM of material (usually brain) from the mice becoming sick or dying after this procedure. (Blind passage of healthy-appearing mice may also yield virus.) Material from second-passage mice becoming ill or dying is passed through a Seitz or Millipore® filter, which retains bacteria but permits virus passage, and is then reinoculated into third-passage mice. If these mice become ill or die, and their brains are demonstrated to be free of bacterial infection, the agent is presumed to be a virus, which is then identified serologically.

A second tool is the use of cell cultures for virus detection and experimental studies. This method has been found to be particularly useful for primary isolation of viruses in the Kemerovo and Hughes serogroups in North America and for a few other ungrouped arboviruses and the Phlebotomus fever serogroup. Early cell culture techniques did not prove useful for primary isolation of CCHF virus but newer methods hold some promise that tissue culture may be applied for this purpose.

With both suckling mice and cell cultures, reisolation of the agent from the originally inoculated material assures that the agent was not an exogenous infection.

The third tool, the serological test, is used to identify the virus strain from animals or cell cultures. The chief serological tools for CCHF virus have been the agar gel diffusion and precipitation (AGDP), complement-fixation (CF), and neutralization (N) tests. During final stages of preparing this manuscript, reports of results using a recently developed indirect hemagglutination inhibition (IHI)-test began to appear and necessitated revision of several pages.

The fluorescent antibody (FA) test is also recommended for detecting CCHF virus in smears and sections of infected vertebrates and ticks.

Infections in Reptiles

In Tadzhikistan, a Horsfield tortoise, *Testudo horsfieldi,* 1 of 209 examined in the AGDP test was positive for CCHF antibodies.[373,386] I know of no other reports relating reptiles to CCHF virus, a subject that might well be investigated. Immature *Hyalomma a. anatolicum,* a common CCHF virus vector from Central Asia to northern Africa, sometimes feeds as larvae and nymphs on lizards.

Noninfection of Birds

Grobov[188] took immature *Hyalomma m. marginatum* from wild birds and domestic fowl in the original Crimean CCHF focus and postulated that birds may be reservoirs of the agent causing this disease. Following the 1953 appearance of clinical CCHF in the Volga River floodplains and delta (Astrakhan and Rostov Oblasts), birds became important factors for epidemiological consideration. In both areas, the rook, *Corvus f. frugilegus,* nesting in dense colonies in trees near rich cattle pastures, was the chief host of immature *H. m. marginatum,* and several other ground-feeding bird species were also infested. During this period, numerous immature specimens of the Eurasian *H. m. marginatum* and of the African *H. marginatum rufipes* were also being taken from southward- and northward-migrating birds in Egypt and Cyprus. However, the role of birds as virus reservoirs was unknown until after CCHF virus could be characterized.

Berezin et al.[33,35] experimentally inoculated the rook and the rock dove, *Columbia livia,* with CCHF virus. They observed no clinical signs in the inoculated birds, were unable to reisolate the virus, and obtained no serological evidence of viremia in the birds. In parallel tests with CCHF-inoculated hares and hedgehogs, antibodies to the virus could be demonstrated. The two brief reviews of Berezin's experimental results (also mentioned by Chunikhin[118]) were based on data which have never been published.

In the Astrakhan focus, Berezin et al.[34] and Chumakov et al.[103,104,106,112] isolated

CCHF virus from nymphal *Hyalomma m. marginatum* taken from birds which were serologically negative for antibody to CCHF virus. They investigated sera of 660 birds, mostly rooks, from the focus by the CF and AGDP tests. The results were uniformly negative, as were attempts to isolate the virus from blood and organs of 360 birds (35 species).

In the Rostov focus, Rabinovich et al.[421] isolated four CCHF strains from engorged nymphal *H. m. marginatum* taken from rooks, but none from 40 rooks and about 170 other birds. Kasymov et al.[257] also obtained negative CF and AGDP test results with numerous bird sera from Tadzhikistan. Three of the first five CCHF isolates from Kirgizia were from immature *H. m. marginatum* from birds.[244,328,329,538]

In summary, birds appear to be refractory to CCHF viremia even though some species support large numbers of CCHF-infected ticks. However, this conclusion is based on limited, poorly documented experimental results.

During the final stage of preparing this review, I received the following three papers that raise the question of birds anew. Using the conventional AGDP test, Semashko et al.[460] detected antibodies to CCHF virus in 1 of 428 sera from fowl (chickens and ducks) from Chimkent Oblast, Kazakhastan. Using the convential AGDP test, as well as the indirect HI test developed by Gaidamovich et al.[176] for samples from the Rostov Oblast CCHF focus, Zarubinsky et al.[591] detected antibodies in serum of a magpie, *Pica pica,* in the latter test, but five serum pools from other magpies and five pools from other birds were negative in both tests. The reported isolation of CCHF virus from a fowl-infesting tick, *Argas persicus,* from Samarkand Oblast, Uzbekistan[117] is discussed later.

Clearly more precise data on action of CCHF virus in birds and in bird-parasitizing ticks are required for epidemiological evaluation.

Infections in Wild Mammals

Large mammals

The larger wild mammals that once inhabited presently recognized Eurasian CCHF foci are now mostly or entirely replaced by humans and domestic animals. The first implication of a wild mammal larger than the hare followed use of the indirect HI (IHI) test in a seroepidemiological survey in Rostov Oblast in 1974.[591] Two of five sera from the common red fox, *Vulpes vulpes,* reacted positively in this test, but not in the AGDP test. Experimental studies of CCHF virus activity in the larger mammals that were the common hosts of tick vectors before the advent of domestic mammals should contribute to understanding basic epidemiological factors in CCHF circulation.

About 2% of 162 sera from baboons and gazelles from Kenya were positive for CCHF virus in the AGDP test.[98] The African tick species associated with CCHF virus all feed as adults on both larger wild mammals and on domestic mammals. The role of large African mammals in CCHF epidemiology has not been investigated.

Medium-Sized and Small Mammals

There are numerous more or less detailed accounts of negative results from attempts to demonstrate antibodies in sera or to isolate CCHF virus from mammals of this size range. Owing to the likelihood that technical problems may have influenced these results, negative data are not reviewed here. An example of a recent productive seroepidemiological survey is that of Saidi et al.,[447] who detected AGDP antibodies to CCHF virus in 3% of 274 small mammals from northern Iran. Medium-sized and small mammals are important hosts of many tick species; thus the success of these mammals, their ticks, and CCHF virus survival is interrelated. However, much remains to be learned about such interrelationships in nature. Reliable data are recent and limited.

Insectivora

Hedgehogs commonly inhabit Eurasian and African gardens, cultivated and irrigated lands, and savannas, steppes, and semideserts. They are infested by immatures of one or several tick species and genera, and also by adults of some species. The first CCHF virus isolates from hedgehogs were in Nigeria from the four-toed hedgehog, *Erinaceus (Atelerix) albiventris,* taken in the savanna and on the Jos Plateau.[78,80,262]

In Eurasia, there may be a significant difference in the epidemiological role of the hedgehog species present in certain CCHF foci. The European hedgehog, *Erinaceus europaeus,* and the long-eared hedgehog, *Hemiechinus auritus,* are both common in Rostov Oblast, and serve as hosts of immature *Hyalomma m. marginatum* and immature and adult *Rhipicephalus rossicus* and *Dermacentor marginatus.* Seven *E. europaeus* and two *H. auritus* were subcutaneously inoculated (1.0 and 0.5 mℓ, respectively) with a 10% NWM brain suspension containing CCHF virus in passages 56 to 58.[48] No clinical signs were observed in the animals during the 1-month observation period. No virus was detected in the *E. europaeus* blood 5 to 13 days postinoculation but titers in the blood of the two *H. auritus* were 10^{-4} on days 4 to 6. No immunological shifts were shown by CF and AGDP tests of both mammal species during the 1-month observation period. The virus was isolated from fed nymphal *H. m. marginatum* (on day 16 postfeeding) that had fed as larvae on an infected *H. auritus,* but *R. rossicus* and *D. marginatus* that fed on this hedgehog did not yield the virus. It was concluded that the susceptible *H. auritus* may be a reservoir in nature and a source of CCHF virus for ticks, but *E. europaeus* is not susceptible to infection.

Experimentally infected *Hemiechinus auritus* (and hares) were used as hosts of *Hyalomma m. marginatum* to demonstrate transstadial survival, transovarial transmission, and interseason survival of CCHF virus in this tick.[598] The hedgehogs and hares were inoculated with a 5% infected-NWM brain suspension intravenously (1 mℓ) and intramuscularly (3 mℓ). Both kinds of mammals proved to be susceptible to infection. The experimental results of Berezin[32] confirmed these conclusions.

During the original CCHF outbreak in the Crimea, no ticks were found on *Erinaceus europaeus.*[188] However, in Rostov Oblast, infected *Rhipicephalus rossicus* were taken from this hedgehog,[66,283,421] but the virus was not isolated from 17 hedgehogs.[421]

Hemiechinus auritus occurs in the entire steppe zone of southern U.S.S.R. and from Iran to northern Egypt and northeastern Libya. This hedgehog is numerous in the Volga floodplain and delta of Astrakhan Oblast.[418] Berezin et al.[36] found up to 40 larval and nymphal *Hyalomma m. marginatum* on hedgehog hosts during the peak season of immature tick activity. However, many more ticks infested groundfeeding birds and hares. *Hemiechinus auritus* frequently inhabits colonies of the Libyan redtailed jird, *Meriones libycus,* in the CCHF focus of Osh Oblast, Kirgizia. Both mammals in his focus are infested by immature *Hyalomma a. asiaticum, Rhipicephalus turanicus,* and *Haemaphysalis erinacei* subsp.[522] CCHF virus has been isolated elsewhere from the first two of these three tick species. Antibodies to the virus were detected in AGDP tests of sera from long-eared hedgehogs inhabiting two different biotopes of Turkmenia.[121,494] Ten percent of the hedgehogs in tugai vegetation were infested by immature *H. a. asiaticum.*

Chiroptera

AGDP antibodies to CCHF virus were detected in sera of the large mouse-eared bat, *Myotis blythi omari,* and the common noctule, *Nyctalus n. noctula,* in northern Iran[447] and in sera of 2 of 19 bats (species not stated) from southern France.[528] The possibility that bats, with their great mobility and specialized tick parasites, may have a role in the natural history of CCHF virus adds an intriguing dimension to the challenges facing biomedical researchers.

Lagomorpha

The European hare, *Lepus europaeus,* and the Cape or Tolai hare, *L. capensis,* occur in Soviet CCHF foci. The exact species is unstated in a good deal of epidemiological literature in which hares are mentioned. For purposes of the present review, it seems safe to assume that hares west of the Caspian Sea are *L. europaeus* and those east of the Caspian Sea are *L. capensis.* Some Soviet mammalogists prefer the name *L. tolai* for the common hares of Central Asia.

Hares are important hosts of ticks in many CCHF foci and probably serve as amplifying hosts of the virus. The broad generalization that hares are the vertebrates chiefly involved in epizootic CCHF virus circulation in Eurasia[45] is possibly true but should be treated with caution. More intensive and quantitative epidemiological research is needed to prove or disapprove this assumption. Birulya[45] stressed that CCHF foci are not found in biotopes where *L. europaeus* is abundant in the absence of extensive pastures, where adult ticks often find cattle and horses to serve as hosts.

The recent isolation of CCHF virus from the blood and livers of three tick-infested *L. europaeus* taken in the Crimea was hailed as the "first direct evidence of the important role of hares in the ecology of the causative agent of CCHF".[99] Zgurskaya et al.[598] and Perelatov et al.[400] had earlier found that viremia and antibodies to the virus develop in experimentally infected *L. europaeus,* and the former authors isolated the virus from *Hyalomma m. marginatum* which they fed on viremic hares. The virus persisted in hare blood for 15 days, with the highest titer (3.6 log $LD_{50}/0.02$ mℓ) on day 4.

The *Lepus europaeus* population explosion during the original CCHF outbreak in the Crimea, heavy infestation by *H. m. marginatum,* and daily and seasonal movements in relation to tick localizaion in the ecosystem are reviewed in a later section. In the subsequent Astrakhan Oblast CCHF outbreak, this hare, next to rooks, was the most common host of *H. m. marginatum.*[33,611] Serological data, especially from young hares, were useful indicators of the seasonal dynamics of the virus and of the risk of human infection in Astrakhan Oblast.[35] Antibodies to CCHF virus were also detected in sera of *L. europaeus* from Bulgarian foci[564,565] where this animal and two species of birds were the chief hosts of *H. m. marginatum.*[324] Numerous hares are bred and released for hunting in Bulgaria and elsewhere in eastern Europe.

L. europaeus yielded CCHF virus-infected adult *Rhipicephalus rossicus* in Rostov Oblast,[22,283,421] and antibodies to the virus were detected in AGDP tests of sera from hares as well as in the body contents of nymphal *Hyalomma m. marginatum* that had fed on hares.[421] In indirect HI tests, 4 of 20 hare sera from Rostov Oblast were positive for CCHF infection but in AGDP tests all were negative.[591]

Antibodies to CCHF virus were also detected in CF and AGDP tests of *Lepus capensis* sera from Turkmenia.[494] Hares are common in the Syr-Darya River floodplain of Kzyl-Orda Oblast of Kazakhstan, where CCHF virus circulates, but not nearby in the desert.[183] However, hares are said to be absent in the known CCHF foci of Tadzhikistan[383,522] did not list hares among the common wild vertebrates in CCHF foci of southeastern Osh Oblast, Kirgizia. Arata[15] indicated (in a table only) that antibodies to CCHF virus had been detected in sera of hares from Iran.

A recent report on the number and variety of ticks infesting *Lepus capensis* in Kenya[123] provides an example of how important these animals can be as hosts of immature stages of tick species known to participate in CCHF virus circulation in Africa. Seroepidemiological surveys of African hares may furnish rewarding clues to the natural history of CCHF virus and its geographical and ecological distribution on this continent.

Rodentia

Investigations into the role of rodents in CCHF foci where *Hyalomma m. margina-*

tum was the predominant tick revealed that immatures seldom if ever parasitize burrowing rodents.[188,324,338,417,418,611] For instance, Povalishina et al.,[418] who searched for ticks on 46,000 rodents and shrews in Astrakhan Oblast, found only three larval *H. m. marginatum* on a vole. Petrova-Piontkovskaya[406] did not mention rodents in her detailed pioneer study of *H. m. marginatum* biology and ecology during the original Crimean outbreak. However, immatures of *Dermacentor marginatus, Rhipicephalus rossicus,* and other tick species do parasitize rodents in the geographical and ecological areas occupied by *H. m. marginatum* and in nearby areas. Rodent hosts of these tick species might be virus-infected, as suggested by Butenko et al.[66] who reported a common field mouse, *Apodemus sylvaticus,* from Rostov Oblast to be serologically positive for CCHF virus (the test method was not stated). In another *A. sylvaticus* from Rostov Oblast, antibodies to the virus were detected in the IHI test but not in the AGDP test.[591] The epidemiological role of each rodent species inhabiting CCHF foci should be determined.

The role of the little suslik (ground squirrel), *Citellus pygmaeus,* in maintaining CCHF virus circulation in Rostov Oblast appears to be equivocal. Kondratenko[282] experimentally inoculated these rodents and used them as hosts for immature *Hyalomma m. marginatum, Rhipicephalus rossicus,* and *Dermacentor marginatus* in important studies on transstadial transfer and transovarial transmission of the virus. Blagoveshchenskaya et al.[50] concluded that *C. pygmaeus* has little epidemiological importance in Rostov Oblast. These authors inoculated CCHF virus into 50 young (4- to 6-week-old) little susliks, which showed no signs of illness afterward. Immunomorphological changes in the lymph nodes and spleens were most pronounced 5 to 7 days following inoculation; a month later the organs were normal. Virus was isolated from the blood and parenchymal organs 2 to 7 days after inoculation but not later.

Some very recent serological data show rodent involvement in CCHF virus circulation in Asia, where immatures of several infected tick species commonly parasitize these mammals. In the Murgab River Valley of Turkmenia, all long-clawed ground squirrels, *Spermophilopsis l. leptodactylus,* were infested by immature *Hyalomma a. asiaticum,* and antibodies to the virus were detected in the *S. l. leptodactylus* sera,[121] as well as in sera of this ground squirrel from the sandy Ashkhabad area[494] Smirnova et al.[491] also isolated the virus from adult *H. a. asiaticum* in Turkmenia, especially from adults parasitizing camels. The large-toothed suslik (or fulvous ground squirrel), *Citellus fulvus,* a common host of immature *H. a. asiaticum,* was numerous where the first human mortality from CCHF was recognized in the Kara-Tai foothills of Kzyl-Orda Oblast, Kazakhstan,[122] but was replaced by the great gerbil, *Rhombomys o. opimus,* in the Dzhalagash focus.[183] This gerbil is also a favorite host of immature *H. a. asiaticum.*

Starkov et al.[503] state that the prevalence of tick infestation of rodents is insignificant in Tadzhik CCHF foci but that high population densities of certain rodent species may lead to dense tick populations. As recorded for Tadzhikistan[383] and elsewhere, immatures of the important CCHF virus vectors *Hyalomma anatolicum antolicum* and *H. marginatum marginatum* rarely feed on rodents.

Results of experimental studies to determine the susceptibility of the African grass rat, *Arvicanthis abyssinicus,* to CCHF virus (Congo strain) infection[476,477,480] appear to be equivocal. Antibodies to the virus were detected in the serum of a multimammate rat, *Praomys (Mastomys) natalensis,* from Senegal.[120] The immature stages of several African tick species from which CCHF virus has been isolated (from adult ticks infesting domestic animals) commonly feed on rodents.

In Iran, Arata et al.[16] obtained evidence of CCHF virus infection in "small mammals" but, except for a brief remark,[15] they have not published their data. However, Saidi et al.[447] detected antibodies to CCHF virus in sera of the Williams' jerboa, *Al-*

lactaga euphrata williamsi; house mouse, *Mus musculus bactrianus;* and Swinhoe's jird, *Meriones crassus swinhoei,* from northern Iran. My unpublished data show numerous *Haemaphysalis, Hyalomma,* and *Rhipicephalus* and other ticks parasitizing Iranian rodents.

Arata[14] classified CCHF as a "representative rodent-born (sic) disease." However spelled, this statement is not based on proven fact. In the Crimean and in the Rostov Oblast CCHF epidemics, the virus was recorded only from *Hyalomma m. marginatum* that fed as immatures on birds or hares and as adults on domestic animals or humans. The fact is that the basic role of rodents in CCHF epidemiology remains to be determined. This role may differ significantly in foci of different ecological and zoogeographic zones depending on the intimacy, numbers, and species of ticks parasitizing immature rodents in their nests. Tick parasitism of adult rodents is possibly a less important factor in CCHF epidemiology than parasitism of immature rodents, but this suggestion also remains to be investigated.

Carnivora

Medium-sized and small carnivores are mentioned in passing in several faunal descriptions of CCHF foci. During seasons of local tick activity in Eurasia and Africa, these mammals are frequently infested, sometimes by a surprising number of ticks. CCHF virus antibodies were detected in sera of the common red fox, *Vulpes vulpes,* and the Pallas' (or steppe) cat, *Felis manul,* from the Ashkhabad area of Turkmenia,[494] and of the genet. *Genetta g. senegalensis,* from Senegal.[120]

Infections in Domestic Animals

Seroepidemiological survey results reviewed throughout the section on epidemiology indicate different percentages of positive reactions for CCHF antigens in sera of domestic cattle, horses, donkeys, sheep, goats and pigs in Eurasia and Africa. Some of the comparative data may be questionable owing to the influence of technical problems on the results.

Nevertheless, as stressed by Chumakov,[95] Smirnova et al.,[489] Vasilenko et al.,[564] and others, surveys of domestic animal sera can be useful to reveal the presence of otherwise unrecognized CCHF foci, as well as the prevalence of infection and thus the risk of human exposure to infected tick bites. Indeed, the results of such surveys did alert Armenian public health authorities to this risk, and almost immediately afterward laboratory-confirmed human cases were diagnosed in this Republic.[242,339,340,456] The first indication of CCHF virus in Iran was the finding that 45 of 100 sheep sera that were sent to Moscow from the Tehran abattoir reacted positively for CCHF virus infection.[108] The subsequent Saidi[446] and Saidi et al.[447] seroepidemiological surveys showed the presence of antibodies to the virus in several areas of northern and central Iran.

As in hares, antibody reaction rates in domestic animals decrease within 6 months after the season of peak tick parasitism. The most meaningful seroepidemiological data from Eurasia have been obtained in late summer.[248,489]

In a recent survey in the Crimea, 1.5% of sera from newly weaned calves being driven to pasture for the first time were positive for CCHF antigens in the AGDP test, as against 10.4% of the adult cattle from the same farms.[8] The same study showed no positive reactions in domestic animal sera from Crimean areas where no human cases had occurred during the 1944-1945 epidemic. These data illustrate the usefulness of domestic animal seroepidemiology in determining the localization of CCHF foci. Results of domestic animal surveys in Tadzhikistan were used to map the degree of risk to humans in different ecological and geographical zones.[372,377,383] Other productive surveys were made in Kirgizia,[523] Bulgaria,[560] Turkmenia,[491] and Hungary.[229]

Evidence for CCHF virus presence in India is based solely on results from testing a few human and domestic animal sera. African seroepidemiological survey data are limited to brief reports from Kenya and Egypt. African CCHF isolates from cattle and goats and from ticks infesting domestic animals were not accompanied by seroepidemilogical investigations.

Results of experimental CCHF infections in horses suggest that these animals are not virus reservoirs in nature but that they are useful in the laboratory to obtain serum for diagnostic and possibly for therapeutic purposes.[47,346] After a long inoculation series, the virus neutralizing activity of horse serum reached a quite high and stable level, which remained for 3 months (observation period) after the cycle ended.[46] Experimentally infected donkeys develop a low-level CCHF viremia.[422]

Causey et al.[80] inoculated two calves with different quantities of CCHF virus ("Congo" strain from a Nigerian goat) and observed mild illness characterized by dullness, lassitude, and decreased appetite. Blood samples from both calves were fatal for NWM on days 2 and 5 (from the calf with low-level viremia) postinoculation and on days 1 through 5 (from the calf with higher-level viremia). In the CF test, the agents in the NWM proved to be CCHF virus. A single female *Hyalomma marginatum rufipes* fed on an inoculated calf dropped on day 11 after virus injection, began ovipositing 4 days later, and was positive for CCHF virus when tested 18 days after dropping (24 days after viremia was last detected in the calf). The virus was not detected in F_1 larvae tested 27 days after deposit of eggs. Lee and Kemp[309] observed viremia in a calf on days 2 and 7 after infected *H. marginatum rufipes* fed on it. The question of CCHF virus causing bovine abortions remains unsettled.

In Rostov Oblast, Zarubinsky et al.[592] inoculated the Sudarkina CCHF strain into four calves; two were 2 months old and two were 4 months old. The day before virus inoculation, adult *Hyalomma m. marginatum, Rhipicephalus rossicus,* and *Dermacentor marginatus* were placed on the two younger calves for feeding. The four inoculated calves showed no clinical signs. Virus was recovered from the blood of a 2-month-old calf on days 3 and 7 after inoclation, but no strains were isolated from the ticks after feeding. The CF, N, AGDP, and indirect HI tests of sera from the calves gave greatly differing results between days 5 and 35 postinoculation. The authors concluded that the experiments showed an infectious process with relatively long-term viremia in the 2-month-old calves and that calves of this age may participate in circulating the virus in nature. However, 6-month-old calves showed no viremia and "developed high immunity in response to inoculating CCHF virus."

Calves can probably contribute to the quantity of CCHF virus flowing in a focus when previously uninfected ticks parasitize them during the viremic period. However, the nature of this contribution remains to be better qualified and quantified. Pak[374] considered cattle to have an important role as CCHF virus reservoirs in Tadzhikistan foci, where the numbers of infected *Hyalomma a. anatolicum* from cattle were much greater than from clay fences (duvals). Support is given to this thesis by the Chmakov et al.[116] report of three humans who became infected and died of CCHF after butchering a sick cow in Uzbekistan. Another human case which occurred in an abattoir in Chimkent, Kazakhstan, is reviewed in a later section.

Domestic buffalo (*Bubalus bubalis*) sera were among those tested in a preliminary seroepidemiological survey for CCHF virus in Egypt. CF antibodies were detected in 1 of 32 buffalo sera from the Port Said abattoir but in none from the abattoirs in Cairo (48), Alexandria (35), and Qena (16).[131]

Five lambs, 2 to 2½ months old, were inoculated by Zarubinsky et al.[592] in the Rostov Oblast studies with calves mentioned above. The virus was isolated from sera of each of the lambs on several days, up to day 8, of the 10-day postinoculation testing period. In the AGDP test, precipitating antibodies to CCHF virus were detected in four of the lambs on day 21 and in the fifth lamb on day 35 (observation period 5 to 35 days postinoculation). The authors concluded that lambs may also participate in circulating CCHF virus in nature during a relatively long viremic period. Other aspects of the role of sheep in CCHF epidemiology are reviewed in the sheep shearing section.

Camels are especially interesting to consider in CCHF epidemiology, owing to the large number and variety of ticks they acquire during their long treks in cargo caravans or in search of grazing and water.[576] Even when using the most sophisticated seroepidemilogical survey tools, Saidi et al.[447] found that none of 157 camel sera from southern Iran reacted positively for antibodies to CCHF virus. Chumakov and Smirnova[111] detected precipitating antibodies (AGDP test) to the virus in 19% of their camel sera from Iran but did not state the number tested or the collection area(s). Smirnova et al.[491] isolated 35 CCHF strains from 161 pools containing 1730 *Hyalomma a. asiaticum* from camels in the sandy zone of the Ashkhabad area, Turkmenia. These authors and Kurbanov et al.[302,303] appraised the camel as an important faunal element in CCHF epidemiology. *H. a. asiaticum* infested almost all camels inspected in a CCHF focus in Kzyl-Orda Oblast, Kazakhstan. However, the only report of seroepidemiological surveys including camel sera from the Soviet Union is from Astrakhan Oblast, where Berezin et al.[35] detected antibodies to CCHF virus in 1.4% of those examined in the AGDP test.

Infections in Laboratory Animals

The history of using suckling rodents to isolate and study CCHF and other arboviruses is reviewed elsewhere. Butenko et al.[64] first reported the Soviet experience with NWM and NWR; these and similar details have been repeated in scores of publications. CCHF virus in blood taken during the peak period of disease causes paralysis and death in most 1- to 2-day-old NWM or NWR after intracerebral inoculation. The incubation period is generally stated to be 4 to 7 (usually 7) days in initial passage and 3 to 5 days in subsequent passages. The virus is nonpathogenic for adult laboratory white mice and rats, guinea pigs, and hamsters. Using the FA test, Karmysheva et al.[250] detected maximum accumulation of virus antigen in the brains of NWM and NWR, chiefly in the cytoplasm of cortical neurons, and irregular accumulation in neuroglia cells and other cortical regions. Insignificant amounts were detected in spleen, liver, kidney, and lung macrophages, single reticular cells, and blood monocytes. By the CF test, antigen was detected only in the brains of infected animals.

The FA test and light microscopy were used by Tsypkin et al.[540] to study the interactions of CCHF virus in mouse embryo brain cell cultures, in which the virus reproduced in fibroblasts and different types of glial elements. The antigen was localized in fibroblast type cells, where it accumulated in the cytoplasm, and was visualized by light microscopy as peculiar basophilic inclusions reacting positively for RNA. Fibroblast elements in brain cell cultures originate chiefly from endothelium. Thus the selective involvement of fibroblast cells explains the genesis of the important hemorrhage syndrome in CCHF.

Using gel chromatography, Donets et al.[144] found that a soluble CF antigen present in the brains of experimentally infected NWM localizes in low molecular weight fractions, and that infections with large virus doses cause higher soluble antigen accumulations than do infections with small doses.

CCHF virus distribution and accumulation were studied in NWM by virological, serological, and histological methods and by the FA tests.[495] Virus found in the blood 2 to 3 hr after intracerebral, intraperitoneal, or subcutaneous inoculation of the maximal dose was considered to result from resorptive viremia with virus dissemination into the viscera. Subsequent viremic increase was apparently due to virus multiplication in the brain, liver, and (partially) salivary glands. Morphological lesions were observed only in the central nervous system. The highest titers of infectious virus and viral antigens and the presence of marked morphological lesions corresponded to the period of clinical infection before death. The CCHF strain used in this experiment (from a fatal human case in Uzbekistan) was highly virulent in NWM by each inoculation route.

Differences in reactions of NWM to infected blood samples from various sources, periods of illness, and after different times of storage were recorded by Butenko et al.[65]

Causey et al.[80] described the behavior of a Nigerian "Congo strain" of CCHF virus in NWM after inoculating material containing different virus levels, different numbers of passages, and different inoculation routes. They stated: "Virus has also been demonstrated in the liver, spleen, and urine of infected mice, but titers in these materials are low compared with the titers in the brain." (To the best of my knowledge, nothing has been published on CCHF virus dissemination in urine of infected vertebrates. The question of the spread of zoonotic infections in vertebrate urine is one of considerable epidemiological interest.[211])

Levi and Vasilenko[325] studied transmission of CCHF virus between *H. m. marginatum* and giant Belgian laboratory rabbits in Bulgaria. The virus was isolated from nymphal and adult ticks reared from larvae that had fed on viremic rabbits and also from F_1 larvae reared from infected adults. All virus strains isolated from the ticks were said to have low pathogenicity for NWM. There was a relationship between the antibody titer developing in rabbit hosts and the number of infected nymphs feeding on the host. When numerous infected larvae fed on a rabbit that was already immune to the virus (titer 1:128), the titer did not increase (possibly indicating that virus neutralization had occurred), but antibodies in the rabbit persisted for 6 months rather than for the usual 4 months (suggesting reinfection and reimmunization of the host). Virus neutralization in infected ticks that had fed on host blood containing antibodies to the virus is stressed as an epidemiologically important factor in "eliminating the infection in its natural source." The limited but fascinating Levi and Vasilenko study raises a number of questions regarding the epidemiological role of CCHF virus-infected vertebrates that should be investigated more intensively using vertebrate hosts of ticks normally occurring in CHF foci.

Results from investigating the susceptibility of young rabbits (kind unstated) to CCHF virus were briefly reviewed by Blagoveshchenskaya et al.[49] Threshold levels of CCHF virus concentrations in rabbits and hares needed to infect feeding *Hyalomma m. marginatum* were reported by Zgurskaya et al.[597]

Experimental infections of African primates have produced few or no signs of physical illness. Butenko et al.[65] inoculated an Astrakhan strain of the virus into five green monkeys, *Cercopithecus aethiops*, and observed them for about a month. CF and N tests were made of sera from the monkeys and/or from NWM inoculated with monkey blood. The temperature of one monkey rose to 40.3°C on day 4 postinoculation (PI). Antibodies to the virus were detected on day 30 PI in this monkey and on days 5 and 6 in two other monkeys. Fagbami et al.[165] inoculated a Nigerian ("Congo") strain into 2 Patas monkeys, *Cercopithecus (Erythrocebus) patas*, and one guinea baboon, *Papio papio*. Each animal experienced a low viremia 1 to 5 days PI and the baboon developed pruritus and a rash persisting on the extremities for 10 days. Biopsies from these areas showed a patchy infiltration of inflammatory cells in the dermis and vasculitis accompanied by hemorrhages. On day 137 PI, CF antibodies to the virus were detected only in the baboon serum. These authors employed the CF, N, and AGDP tests in their studies of monkey sera and discussed nonspecific neutralization of the virus with reference to difficulties in making seroepidemiological surveys for CCHF virus.

The early experiments of Chumakov and colleagues, using mice, guinea pigs, rabbits, monkeys, and cats as experimental animals, were widely discussed in pre-1967 Soviet literature. However, an outbreak of intestinal viral ectromelia was later recognized by Chumakov[98] to have confused the results of the experiments associated with the Crimean CCHF outbreak.

Hyalomma m. marginatum, which had been held for 7 to 9 months at 4°C, were able to transmit (CCHF) virus when biting guinea pigs and the hosts developed viremia on days 11 to 12 following tick attachment. The infection course was severe . . . and frequently fatal. CF antibodies were detected in surviving guinea pigs on day 21 following tickbites." This experience, quoted directly from Berezin,[32] appears to be unique.

HUMAN INFECTION

Historical

The 12th century account of CCHF in Tadzhikistan by Dzhurzhoni[161] is reviewed in an earlier section.

CCHF has been known for centuries among the populations of Termez and other districts of southern Uzbekistan as *khungribta* (blood taking), *khunymuny* (nose bleeding), or *karak halak* (black death).[462,467,468] (The appellation "black death," now frequently used for plague (*Yersinia pestis*), did not appear in Oriental literature on plague; it became common in European languages only in the 16th and 17th centuries.[137])

Some of the clinical descriptions of epidemics in the Crimea during the Crimean War[159] have been attributed to CCHF. After carefully studying the 1856 paper, I am convinced that CCHF is not involved and Academician Chumakov (personal correspondence) agrees with this conclusion. Gal'perin[180] stated that CCHF has long been known in the Crimea, but the first reliably described cases known to be from the Crimea[152] occurred there in April-June 1942, 2 years before the Crimean epidemic was recognized.

Gajdusek,[178] Shapiro and Levinzon,[469] Pak and Mikhailova,[383] and others have discussed the early clinical literature on CCHF. For instance, Fedulov et al.[166] described a pre-World War II outbreak in Uzbekistan. Sipovsky,[482] a pathologist, reported on the clinical signs and autopsy findings of 18 patients with gastrointestinal hemorrhages (now considered as CCHF) seen between 1927 to 1943 in Stalinabad (now Dushanbe, Tadzhikistan), as well as on nosocomial transmission and unsuccessful efforts to determine the disease etiology. Clinical aspects and autopsy findings of seven CCHF cases (five nosocomial) seen in a hospital (locality unstated) in Turkmenia during World War II were described by Mikhailov.[345] The 1944-1945 Crimean epidemic of CCHF, originally named acute infectious capillary toxicosis, resulted in two clinical-epidemiological books.[498] Grashchenkov,[185] and good clinical reviews by Kolachev,[280] Chumakov,[89] and others.

Differential characteristics of CCHF, hemorrhagic nephroso-nephritis, sandfly (Phlebotomus) fever, malaria, typhus, leptospirosis, Omsk hemorrhagic fever, Q fever, yellow fever, Colorado tick fever, etc., caused considerable concern during the earlier period of CCHF investigation,[43,89-92,179,280,341,342,439] and were later carefully defined by Leshchinskaya,[311,314-316] Gusarev,[194] and others.

Laboratory hosts in early (1944 to 1945) CCHF experimentation provided inconclusive results because adult animals were used and intestinal viral ectromelia in the animals caused symptoms similar to those of CCHF. Therefore, Chumakov and colleagues inoculated materials from Crimean CCHF patients into psychiatric patients needing pyrogenic therapy[91] as reviewed by Chumakov.[94] The subsequent disease courses in these experimental patients closely paralleled those observed in the Crimean patients and helped to establish the basic pattern of human illness caused by this virus. Suspensions of nymphal *Hyalomma m. marginatum* inoculated subcutaneously with antibiotics into healthy human volunteers caused a mild but characteristic clinical course of CCHF with recovery after 2 weeks.

Many clinical and epidemiological papers during the 1946 to 1968 period stated the individual author's view that the disease does, does not, or may possibly, differ in European and in Asian environments. This controversy ended after 1968, but similar clinical and epidemiological discussions for Eurasian and African environments until today.

The Disease in Eurasia
Introduction

Physicians in Bulgaria and in each Soviet republic, oblast, or region where CCHF epidemics or outbreaks occurred have published numerous clinical reports; these are listed in Volume 6 of the *Bibliography of Ticks and Tickborne Diseases (Annotated Bibliography of Tick-associated Viruses)*. The present paper is intended as only an epidemiological-biological review; thus only a few of the most salient characteristics of clinical CCHF are included. In the medical area, the widely experienced, perspicacious clinician Elena V. Leshchinskaya has served as mentor, consultant, and mother-confessor to all physicians dealing with hemorrhagic fevers.

Recent authoritative clinical papers from which I have drawn the following review of non-nosocomial CCHF are Leshchinskaya,[310,312-315,317] Yarovoy and Yarovaya,[587] Lazarev et al.,[308] Leshchinskaya and Butenko,[318] Pak and Mikhailova,[383] and Lazarev,[306] Other specialized clinical papers are mentioned in the text hereinunder. Important recent papers on autopsy findings (not reviewed here) are by Brumshtein and Leshchinskaya,[57] Gusarev,[191-195] and Karmysheva et al.[264] Increased chromosomal disorders in leukocytes during CCHF and their persistence during convalescence were reported by Timoshek and Kantorovich,[524]

CCHF is a disease of the nervous system. Neurological symptoms precede the dramatic hemorrhagic syndrome produced by vascular disorders.[315] The virus multiples in cells (especially Kupffer's cells and hematocytes) of the reticulo-endothelial system, in which specific antigens can be detected.[252-255] When death occurs, usually 6 to 8 days after disease onset, it is caused by profuse diapedetic hemorrhages, profound circulatory disturbances, general malaise, and brain edema, leading to cardiac arrest.

Leshchinskaya[315] categorized 174 CCHF cases (including only two nosocomial incidents) from Astrakhan and Rostov Oblasts as follows:

With hemorrhagic syndrome (161)	
Severe (77)	
Internal hemorrhages	
Absent	6
Present	71
Moderately severe (69)	
Internal hemorrhages	
Absent	12
Present	57
Mild	15
Without hemorrhagic syndrome (13)	
Moderately severe	5
Mild	8
Total	174

Diagnosis
Clinical

Persons presenting with an illness that *might* be CCHF must be hospitalized and studied as promptly as possible for correct diagnosis and proper care. Diagnosis is difficult during the prehemorrhagic period (1 to 7 days) and in mild cases. (Transporting hemorrhaging patients is contraindicated.) Average and severe disease courses are easily diagnosed, but only during the climax (hemorrhagic) period. Epigastric and lumbar pains and repeated vomiting on days 3 to 4 (but not on days 1 to 2) after disease onset are precursors of the hemorrhagic syndrome and important signs in early diagnosis. Early in the prehemorrhagic period, many patients have pronounced leukopenia and severe thrombocytopenia; leukocyte counts may decrease to 3000 to 2000 (or even to 800) per mm³ and thrombocyte counts to 50,000. More than one half of the patients have slight or pronounced albuminuria together with urinary sediment (1 to 2 erythrocytes and hyaline casts per microscope field) caused by increasing vascular permeability at this time.

Serological and Virological

Serological techniques for diagnosing CCHF are reviewed in another section. Virological-serological procedures are too time-consuming (5 to 6 days before results are obtained) to be useful for establishing diagnosis during the first few critical days of disease, but are important for confirming the diagnosis, especially of mild or uncertain cases. (In Krasnodar Region, 13 of 450 sera from convalescents from an "indistinct febrile disease" reacted against CCHF virus.[158])

Patients' blood taken during the febrile period and inoculated immediately afterward into NWM usually results in infecting the experimental animal.[65] Viremia generally continues to day 7 to 8, but sometimes to day 12, after onset of illness. Infected blood preserved at 4°C remains infective for NWM for 10 days, but afterward usually (but not always) produces negative results.[65] Blood, blood clots, and cerebrospinal fluid from patients, and autopsy materials (especially lung, liver, spleen, and bone marrow; also kidney and brain) may be used for CCHF virus isolation. Postmortem materials should be taken within 11 hr after death.

During 1968 to 1972 studies of 184 CCHF-suspect patients in Bulgaria, 121 were diagnosed clinically as CCHF; 114 patients or corpses were investigated for virus — 103 CCHF strains were isolated.[562] During 1968 to 1975 studies in Tadzhikistan, 22 CCHF strains were isolated from patients and corpses (and 41 strains were isolated from ticks).[129] Soviet and Bulgarian literature does not contain a scientifically satisfactory analysis of data on CCHF virus isolated from human beings, and of reasons for their failure to isolate the virus from certain patients who have been diagnosed by clinically astute physicians as suffering from CCHF.

Typical Disease Course

The typical progress of non-nosocomial CCHF cases consists of four periods: incubation, prehemorrhagic, hemorrhagic, and convalescence. (Most Soviet authors omit incubation as a period in the disease course.)

Incubation Period

The virus incubation period, between tickbite and onset of illness, is generally considered to be short, 3 to 6 days, but precise data are often difficult to obtain. Tickbites may be unnoticed by persons in whom they cause no pain. In certain situations, the patient may have been exposed to so many tickbites or crushed so many ticks that the exact date of infection cannot be determined.

Prehemorrhagic Period.

Onset of this 1- to 7- (average 3) day period is sudden and acute. Fever (39 to 41°C) is constant, irregular, or diphasic. Brief apyrexia (12 to 48 hr) develops in about one half of the patients on days 2 to 6 (usually 4 to 5) of disease. [Fever lasts for 3 to 16 (average 8.3) days.] Chills, headache, rheumatic, lumbar, and epigastric pains, nausea, repeated vomiting not associated with eating, liquid stools, adynamia, and loss of appetite are characteristic of the prehemorrhagic period. Hyperemia of the face, neck, and chest, congested sclerae, conjunctivitis, a slightly hyperemic pharynx, and spotted enanthemas on the soft and hard palates are common. Cardiovascular changes are shown by bradycardia and low blood pressure. As already stated, diagnosis during the prehemorrhagic period, aided especially by the peripheral blood picture, is important for proper subsequent handling of the patient.

Hemorrhagic Period

This short, climactic, rapidly developing period usually begins on day 3 to 5 of illness, when the condition deteriorates rapidly, and lasts 1 to 10 (average 4) days, or results in death at the peak of the period. In patients with diphasic fever curves, there is no relationship between degree of temperature and onset of hemorrhages. Hemorrhages from the size of petechiae to large hematomas appear on the mucous membranes and skin, especially on the upper body, along posterior axillary lines, in antecubital fossae, under the breasts of women, and at injection and pressure (tourniquet, etc.) sites. The buccal mucosa, gums, and nose bleed. Intestinal hemorrhages and uterine hemorrhages appear, sometimes together with bloody sputum and bleeding from the conjunctivae and ears. Stools are normal or tarlike. In some (ca 15%) patients, only a hemorrhagic rash appears. Bradycardia, muffled heart sounds, and low blood pressure characterize the hemorrhagic period. When hemorrhages are profuse, bradycardia may give way to tachycardia and the hyperemic face becomes pale. Respiratory organ involvement is manifest as hemorrhagic pneumonia in a few patients (ca 10%). Palpation of the epigastric region is usually very painful. The liver and spleen are enlarged in about one third of the patients. Autopsy usually reveals numerous hemorrhages into all organs and tissues and copious quantities of blood in the stomach and intestines.

Convalescent Period

Convalescence usually begins rapidly, about day 15 to 20 after onset of illness. There are no relapses of the hemorrhagic syndrome. Most patients are discharged from hospital 3 to 6 weeks after onset of illness, when blood and urine indices return to normal. Convalescence is characterized by prolonged, pronounced asthenia, labile pulse, and sometimes complete loss of hair (which is replaced 4 to 5 months later) and pronounced mono- or polyneuritis. Common problems, in addition to general weakness and rapid fatigability, are sweating, headache, dizziness, nausea, poor appetite, xerostomia, labored breathing, tachycardia, poor vision and hearing (or complete loss of hearing), loss of memory, etc. These problems may disappear rapidly or persist for longer than a year. Most convalescents can return to work about a month after discharge but only to light labor.

Mild Disease Course

From results of seroepidemiological surveys in Bulgaria,[560,563,564] European U.S.S.R.,[319] Kazakhstan,[490] and Tadzhikistan,[256] it appears that CCHF infections in humans may sometimes be asymptomatic or so mild as to cause no clinical concern. However, there is no scientifically documented verification for this phenomenon.

Of the 174 CCHF cases reported by Leshchinskaya,[315] 23 were mild; the hemorrhagic syndrome was present in 15 and absent in 8 of the 23. Four of the 42 well-described cases from Tadzhikistan were mild.[383] The four mild episodes were characterized by a brief "subfebrile" temperature, slight malaise, asthenia, appetite loss, moderate bradycardia, sparse rash, and profuse epistaxis ending rapidly. There was slight blood loss and moderate thrombocytopenia. Leukopenia disappeared by day 14 to 17. Patients could resume normal work a month after discharge from hospital. Some of Leshchinskaya's[315,317] cases lacking pronounced hemorrhagic syndrome had a relatively short (2- to 5-day) febrile period but moderately severe general malaise. In short, vascular disturbances of various kinds occur in mild CCHF cases but do not reach the stage of diapedetic hemorrhages.

Moderately Severe Disease Course

The fever lasts 4 to 7 days (average). Malaise is severe, hemorrhages are usually distinct, and the hypotonic patient becomes depressed or agitated but not unconscious. Dull heart sounds, functional murmurs, and tachycardia replacing bradycardia are usually observed during the hemorrhagic period but, despite bleeding mucosa, blood crusts do not form on the lips and mouth. Skin hemorrhages disappear slowly and rash may occur repeatedly. Blood loss from several organs may be profuse. Leukopenia (3000 to 4000), anemia (erythrocytes to 3 million or lower, hemoglobin 50 to 60%) and thrombocytopenia (70,000 to 90,000) (sometimes only thrombocytopenia) characterize the blood picture, which becomes normal 3 to 4 weeks later. Improvement in the patient's condition begins about 2 weeks after onset of illness, but the convalescence period may extend to 2 to 4 months.

Severe Disease Course

All signs and symptoms are acute or violent. The prehemorrhagic period is usually short (1 to 2 days). High temperature, chills, and severe malaise develop rapidly, often together with delirium and unconsciousness, and sometimes meningismus. Tachycardia is pronounced on the first day in fatal cases. There is severe blood loss (1 to 2 ℓ) from profuse nasal, gastrointestinal, pulmonary, and uterine hemorrhages. Petechiae and spontaneous diffuse s.c. hemorrhages appear, sometimes together with i.m. hemorrhages. There are numerous bleeding enanthemas on the oral mucosa and blood crusts on the gums and tongue. Pneumonia is frequent. The extreme blood picture becomes normal only after 5 to 6 weeks. The fatality rate is high. The convalescence period is long (3 to 4 to 12 months). (In a few atypical fatal cases with severe malaise, skin hemorrhages were absent but circulation disorders were present and numerous blood effusions into organs and tissues were observed at autopsy.)

CCHF During Pregancy

Four of seven CCHF patients who were 8 to 38 weeks pregnant aborted when the hemorrhagic period developed; a fifth aborted during convalescence, a month after disease onset. Three of the seven died from profuse hemorrhages. Pregnancy and labor were normal only in the single case with a mild disease course.[315] Three abortions were recorded by Pak and Mikhailova[383] in CCHF patients who were 9 to 10 weeks pregnant; two of the three died. Other reports of premature labor and abortions are scattered through the CCHF clinical literatures.

CCHF in Children

Leshchinskaya[315] observed that CCHF in children differs from that in adults by absence of bradycardia, fewer complaints of lumbar pains, and less pronounced leukopenia.

Sixteen CCHF cases in 3- to 13-year-old children (13 boys, 3 girls) in Rostov Oblast were reported in detail by Lazarev et al.[307] The disease course was severe in four, average-severe in nine, and mild in three; two died. Convalescence was slow and some of the children were partially disabled for 1 or 2 years. Ticks were known to have fed on 9 of the 13 children before illness. One 12-year-old boy had nursed his father, who died of CCHF the day before the boy was hospitalized; despite heroic treatment for his severe disease, the youngster died of cardiac arrest 41 days later. Of the 16 children, 5 were misdiagnosed before CCHF was determined. These authors' summary characterization of CCHF in children (early appearance of leukopenia and thrombocytopenia and of hemoconcentration followed by anemia) does not appear to differ greatly from the criteria for CCHF in adults.

Treatment

Leshchinskaya,[317] in the most recent publication by an outstanding authority on treatment of CCHF, states the following: "One of the most important conditions for successful treatment is that patients must be immediately hospitalized and kept in bed. Special attention should be devoted to the oral cavity to prevent reinfection. It is necessary to remove blood crusts, to brush the teeth regularly, and any sores on the lips or tongue must be painted with Vaseline® oil. The patient's room must be regularly ventilated. Sheets and pillowcases should have no creases in order to prevent bedsores, since it is at these sites that hemorrhages occur. Clothes must be loose for the same reason. There are no specific medicines against CHF. Antibiotics and sulfonamides are ineffective and can be applied only in cases of purulent complications. One of the most effective treatments is serum prepared from antibody-containing blood of recovered CCHF patients. The serum is injected intramuscularly in doses of 80 to 200 cm³. A similar effect is provided by gammaglobulin, obtained by immunization of horses. Rutin, ascorbic acid, and calcium chloride are also recommended for treating the hemorrhagic syndrome. With great blood loss, transfusions and blood substitutes (polyglutin, plasma, and hemodes) are necessary. Intravenous injections of gelatin and aminocaproic acid are also indicated. In severe cases accompanied by profuse hemorrhages, hemorrhagic pneumonia, and disturbances in vitally important functions in cardiovascular activity, hormonal preparations (prednisolone and hydrocortisone) are used."

The question of convalescent serum for treating CCHF has produced much controversy.[315] From personal data for 98 patients, Lazarev[305] concluded that convalescent serum is useful *only* on days 1 to 3 after disease onset, when it reduces the febrile period length and prevents or reduces the severity of the hemorrhagic period. Later, Lazarev[306] considered the earlier data to be insufficient and recommended continued study of serotherapy in CCHF. The Leshchinskaya and Martinenko[321] statements on using convalescent serum confirm this conclusion (this paper and Pak and Mikhailova[383] include detailed contemporary accounts of treating CCHF).

Transmission By Ticks

Field observations quoted in another section indicate, beyond a doubt, that bites by infected ticks, and also crushing infected ticks in ungloved hands, are the most common routes of transmitting CCHF virus to human beings. The species mentioned in this literature are chiefly *Hyalomma m. marginatum* and *H. a. anatolicum,* less often *Ixodes ricinus, Dermacentor marginatus,* and *Rhipicephalus rossicus.* However, almost all tick species associated with CCHF virus may feed on humans under certain circumstances. For instance, we have a few well-documented records that even *Boophilus* species bite humans, apparently after having been dislodged from cattle.

There have been no extensive scientific studies of the biological characteristics of CCHF virus transmission to experimental animals by biting ticks or by crushed ticks on scarified skin. Investigations using human subjects are obviously out of the question.

At this stage, we can postulate only that the degree of risk of human infection by CCHF virus-infected ticks is in direct proportion to ratios in the population dynamics and densities of the tick species most likely to utilize humans as an occasional host or to be handled by persons tending tick-infested animals.

Transmission By Contagion

Homes and Hospitals

Before the 1967 to 1968 breakthrough in CCHF knowledge; the extreme clinical severity and high mortality rates of CCHF reported from Uzbekistan and Kazakhstan contributed to the belief that the hemorrhagic fever(s) in these republics differed from that in the European zone of the U.S.S.R. The great ecological differences between these areas and the absence of reports of *Hyalomma marginatum* from foci recognized in the eastern republics tended to support this assumption. The 1967 to 1968 findings that virus strains from these geographical sources were serologically identical, together with a comparative study of clinical data,[315] brought universal acceptance of the single disease concept.

In retrospect, the clinical severity and high mortality of CCHF in Asia resulted largely from the numerous cases caused by contagion. In remote, primitive hamlets, villages, aid stations, and hospitals, members of closely-knit family groups solicitously caring for severely ill relatives, as well as physicians and medical attendants who were unaware of the nature of the disease, took no measures to prevent contamination by infected bloody discharges. After wide publicity was given to the dramatic home and hospital (nosocomial) infections, these outbreaks became exceptional . . . but nosocomial tragedies have continued until as recently as January 1976.

No nosocomial incidents were mentioned in the reports on about 200 CCHF cases seen in military hospitals in the Crimea in 1944 to 1945, but one proven and two suspected nosocomial cases occurred in civilian hospitals afterward. Medical attention and facilities during the Astrakhan and Rostov epidemics were quite good; only 4 or 5 of the more than 450 cases in these oblasts were nosocomial and multiple cases in single families were rare.

Six of the 25 (24%) CCHF cases recorded in Stavropol Region in 1953 to 1968 were in physicians, hospital attendants, and family members who cared for patients. The severe to very severe disease course in most Stavropol CCHF patients was probably partially responsible for the relatively large proportion of patient-transmitted disease in this region.

During the tumultuous 1953 to 1965 years of agricultural collectivization in Bulgaria, 717 CCHF cases were recorded from "natural" causes and 42 other cases were nosocomial. The mortality rates were 17.02% in the former group and 40.48% in the latter.

CCHF morbidity is sporadic in Turkmenia, but the presence of the disease was first recognized there when six medical attendants and roommates of a patient became ill with CCHF and five of the six died. Similarly, the earliest CCHF reports from Uzbekistan were associated with homes and hospitals; the literature on these cases is lurid but lacking in precise data. In a special study of 100 Uzbek CCHF case histories, Meliev[343,344] found that 14 of the patients had been in contact with a primary case 3 to 6 days before becoming ill; "most" died after very severe disease courses. One episode involved seven persons helping a sick cattle herder; three were friends who brought the herder to the hospital, two were nurses, and two were other persons in the same ward; four of the seven died. Another nosocomial case was in a surgical ward nurse after attending patients who had butchered a sick cow.

Kazakhstan is most notorious among CCHF foci for household and nosocomial incidents, several of which are reviewed in another section.

In Tadzhikistan, 14 cases in 1943 to 1972 and 5 in 1973 were attributed to CCHF patient contact.[384] In the 1943 to 1972 period, the mortality rates were 25.2% for tick-transmitted CCHF and 50.0% for patient-transmitted CCHF.[383] Sipovsky[482] first observed the importance of person-to-person transmission of the CCHF agent and the high mortality rate in these cases. In the Dushanbe Hospital for Infectious Diseases in 1943, a nurse who cared for a CCHF patient and a pathologist who performed autopsies contracted the disease.[470] In Moskovsky District during the summer of 1951, a shepherd died after hemorrhaging for 5 days in a mountain pasture camp; a relative with him at the time returned to his settlement and died of CCHF after a 3-day illness. Three persons who nursed the relative, his sister, a neighbor, and the neighbor's 18-year-old daughter, also contracted the disease. Only the daughter survived. More recently, two nurses and a medical student recovered after experiencing nosocomial CCHF infection in the Pyandzk and Dushanbe hospitals. Sixteen medical workers cared for a farmer who died of CCHF in the Dushanbe hospital in 1967. The farmer was first seen in the Rugar Regional Hospital, where five of the seven attendants who labored heroically to stem the profuse bloody discharges themselves became severely ill. Two died. After the farmer was transferred to the Dushanbe hospital, nine persons cared for him, but with less close and shorter contact periods; none of the nine became ill.[383]

Serologically and virologically proven CCHF cases in five persons (wife, son, and friend in home, and surgeon and physician in hospital) who cared for a typically ill patient in July 1973 are especially interesting because the disease course in each of the five was mild or inapparent.[384] This incident occurred in an unstated region of Tadzhikistan where CCHF cases lacking hemorrhages but having a fleeting roseolus rash are seen, as well as typically severe cases. The surgeon and physician had observed strict personal protective measures. The authors attributed the mild or inapparent infections to contamination by only a minute quantity of virus through pinpoint-size damage of gloves or through mucous membranes. They did not expand on their brief, epidemiologically provocative statement that these five infections occurred in a region where other mild CCHF cases were also being seen.

A nosocomial incident in the Central Government Hospital at Rawalpindi, Pakistan, in January 1976 began when a shepherd with CCHF was brought in and died the same night. His father had cared for the shepherd at home and also died. Of the 12 hospital personnel attending the shepherd, 10 became ill with CCHF; 2 died and 8 recovered after more or less severe illness. This sad experience, only 2 years ago in a medically enlightened area of the world, should be remembered by anyone who tends to think "it can't happen here."

The profuse bleeding and wide splattering of bloody discharges during the acute and violent phases of CCHF are vividly described in much literature. Any break in the skin or mucous membranes of persons tending CCHF patients may be a portal for virus entry into the body. The possibility of airborne (inhalation) infection is frequently discussed in the literature but has not been proven or disproven.

The signs and symptoms in nosocomial CCHF are generally reported as severe, and the stages in the clinical course are often said to be more rapid than in the tick-transmitted disease. In fact, the disease courses are similar in severely ill patients infected by either route. The clinical severity is usually postulated to be caused by direct infection by blood (through broken skin) containing a large quantity of virus. (There have been no satisfactory studies showing differences in virulence of CCHF virus strains from different sources.) Data for the frequently repeated statement that the incubation period for patient-transmitted CCHF is shorter than that for tick-transmitted CCHF are statistically unreliable.[315]

Methods for preventing nosocomial infections and a vaccine for medical and laboratory personnel who may be exposed to CCHF virus are reviewed elsewhere.

Laboratories

A laboratory assistant working with infected materials in Rostov Oblast died after a severe case of CCHF, but two surgeons recovered from the disease to which they were exposed in giving a transfusion and operating on CCHF patients.[23] The highly experienced technician, who had suffered from hepato-cholecystitis for the past 6 years (? a complicating factor in this case), may have become infected when a vial of material containing CCHF virus broke in the centrifuge or while doing other work with the live virus.

Chumakov[95] suspected the droplet-respiratory route of infection in four CCHF cases in virus-laboratory personnel; two in Sofia in 1968 and two in Rostov in 1969 to 1970.

Abattoirs and Animal Slaughter

A woman who skinned animals in the Chimkent City meat combine and became ill with CCHF[518] provided evidence for suggesting that the virus may be transmitted by contagion directly from infected animals to humans. In 1973 in Kashkadar'ya Oblast of Uzbekistan, three persons died of CCHF after skinning and butchering a sick cow (diagnosed as having acute gastritis); a nurse who cared for the three patients also became ill but survived.[99] Pak and Mikhailova[383] noted two CCHF cases after slaughtering a sick cow in Dangara district, Tadzhikistan, in 1967.

Sheep Shearing (And Sheep as Virus Reservoirs)

The potential role of sheep shearing in CCHF virus transmission to humans should not be overlooked. In many endemic foci, sheep greatly outnumber cattle, especially in steppes and semideserts where levels of economic development are relatively low and governmental and biomedical scrutiny is less intense than in controlled agroeconomic projects. Close human-sheep contact during shearing may result in virus invasion through broken skin contaminated by infected squashed or macerated ticks, or dislodged feeding ticks may transfer to the shearer and feed on him. Notably, when ixodid ticks reach a certain physiological phase in the several-day feeding process, they are avid to reach full engorgement. Following forced dislodgement during this feeding phase, ticks often eagerly attach to the first available matter: any other vertebrate (regardless of the usual host preference), another tick or arthropod, snake eggs, etc. (some published data and much unpublished data).

A virologically confirmed, clinically typical case of severe CCHF in an Armenian laborer, who found a tick (species unstated) attached to his skin after shearing heavily tick-infested sheep on the Norvan State Farm, was carefully recorded by Karapetyan et al.[242]

In Astrakhan Oblast in 1962 to 1963, ten CCHF patients sheared sheep on collective farms prior to illness; four observed ticks attached to themselves, two squashed or extracted ticks cut by shears, and four denied contact with ticks. Povalishina et al.[417] stressed that these cases occurred only among persons shearing privately owned sheep. The Stolbov et al.[506] review of 115 CCHF cases in Astrakhan Oblast attributed the cause of 20 cases to shearing sheep. Of the 20 manually sheared privately owned sheep, 17 were twice as heavily tick-infested as government-supervised sheep on collective and state farms. Only three persons became ill after mechanical shearing of 500 to 600 government-owned sheep. It is implied that each of the 20 cases was caused by skin contamination or inhalation of infected tick particles. Hemorrhagic pneumonia developing in some CCHF patients after shearing sheep has been suggested as evidence for airborne transmission of the virus. However, this condition may occur in any CCHF case.[318]

From results of the single study of experimentally infected sheep (five lambs, 2 to 2½ months old), it appears that lambs develop a relatively long-term CCHF viremia and can serve as virus amplifiers in nature.[592]

In Astrakhan Oblast, antibodies to CCHF virus are less prevalent in sera of sheep grazing in arid zones than in those of domestic animals from cultivated zones.[35] On Rostov Oblast farms where human CCHF occurred, antibody prevalence reached 2% in sera from sheep (vs. 17% in sera from cattle) but was negative in sheep sera from areas where no CCHF patients were recorded.[295] In Stavropol Region, where a CCHF case was reported from a sheep shearer, antibodies to CCHF virus were detected in 13 of 2747 sheep sera (vs. 1 of 350 cow sera).

Seroepidemiological survey results from Bulgaria to Iran, Kazakhstan, and Egypt often show high antibody prevalence in sheep sera. A Bulgarian survey showed prevalence of 28%. In Azerbaijan, antibodies were detected in sera of 15 of 99 sheep from two farms. Surveys in Turkmenia produced prevalences of 6 to 32% in sheep sera. The close associations between CCHF and shepherds in sheep-rearing areas of Kazakhstan are reviewed in another section. Seroepidemiological survey results for sheep and cattle in Kirgizia, reported by Timofeev et al.,[523] and in Tadzhikistan by Pak and Mikhailova,[383] are especially interesting. The antibody prevalence in sheep and goat sera from Iran is among the highest recorded anywhere. In Egypt, 12 of 66 sheep sera reacted in CF tests for CCHF virus infection.

The immatures and/or adults of many tick species associated with CCHF virus feed on sheep; those most commonly reported are *Ixodes ricinus, Haemaphysalis punctata, Dermacentor marginatus, Rhipicephalus bursa, R. pumilio, R. rossicus, R. turanicus, R. pulchellus,* and *Hyalomma impeltatum.* Notably, these species are generally considered, on the basis of available evidence, to be involved in epizootic rather than in epidemic CCHF virus circulation.

Mortality Rates

The staggering mortality rates in certain CCHF epidemics and outbreaks reflect (1) the extreme severity of some cases, (2) lack of knowledge in remote households and hospitals of how to avoid contaminative transmission, and (3) lack of experience in caring for very ill patients. Despite the absence of specific drugs for treating CCHF, and the continuing uncertainties over some therapeutic procedures, the Leshchinskaya[317] regimen of hospital care and treatment has resulted in considerable reduction of CCHF mortality rates.

Moving severely ill CCHF patients long distances over rough roads to hospitals was found to cause higher rather than lower fatality rates,[344] as was also observed in early yellow fever epidemics in the U.S.

Of 92 military patients, (and 18 of 161 military and civilian patients) 9 died during the first year (1944) of the Crimean CCHF epidemic. In Astrakhan Oblast, as medical awareness developed from 1953 to 1963, the accuracy of diagnosis improved, and suspected CCHF cases were hospitalized earlier; the mortality rate gradually dropped from more than 30% to 13%. The average annual mortality rate during the 1963 to 1969 Rostov epidemic was 15%. Most of the 25 CCHF cases recognized in Stavropol Region were severe; 11 of the patients died.

Bulgarian mortality rates were reported as 17.02% (1953 to 1965) and about 15% (1968 to 1973) for non-nosocomial cases and 40.8% for nosocomial cases during the former period. The higher mortality rate among patients from urban areas was explained by partial immunization of rural peoples. Seasonally decreasing mortality rates (from 27.3% in May to 1.6% in September) were explained by high virulence of the virus in overwintered ticks (a scientifically unproven, but interesting, hypothesis). Mortality rates were lower in patients below the age of 30 than in the 31- to 40-year age group (37.5%) and somewhat lower (33 to 25%) in older patients. About 19% of the male and 28% of the female patients died. These rates varied from area to area in

Bulgaria; subclinical cases were obviously not included in the statistics and many mild cases were probably not brought to the attention of medical authorities.

In Soviet Middle Asia (including southern Kazakhstan), household and nosocomial cases, resulting directly or indirectly from contact with bloody discharges of patients bitten by infected ticks, have been notorious for high mortality rates. The first reported outbreak in Turkmenia involved six patients and attendants in a ward with a CCHF patient; five of the six died. Several mortality reports for Uzbekistan are mentioned in the foregoing text. Meliev,[344] who studied 100 Uzbek cases, stated that 32% were fatal and also[343] that "most" of 14 cases contracted from CCHF patients ended fatally. Incidents of high (and low) mortality in Kazakhstan are described in some detail in the foregoing text. Household and nosocomial disease accounted for the high mortality rates in Tadzhikistan, where cases following tickbite are sporadic.[383] The Tadzhik mortality rate (1943 to 1970) was 25% for tick-bitten patients and 50% for patients infected by contact with primary cases.

In Pakistan in 1976, a nosocomial incident with high mortality occurred in the Rawalpindi Central Hospital, and two of five soldiers admitted to the Quetta military hospital died of CCHF.

The rather numerous references to papers containing a variety of theories regarding differences in CCHF mortality rates are listed, with annotations, in Volume 6 of the *Bibliography of Ticks and Tickborne Diseases* (Hoogstraal, in prep.).

Morbidity Rates

Eurasian morbidity data, arrived at by various methods or stated merely as "sporadic", are cited throughout the text. Morbidity in nature (exclusive of household and nosocomial cases) has almost everywhere been regarded as sporadic. Even in epidemic (epizootic) situations, associated chiefly with high population densities of *Hyalomma* ticks, disease distribution and incidence in farms, hamlets, and villages of a certain region have generally been scattered both spatially and from year to year. (This phenomenon has increased the expense and difficulty of designing specific measures for preventing CCHF.)

Morbidity rates in the Bulgarian epidemic were higher than any in the Soviet Union, and a larger number of Bulgarian villages and hamlets over a wider area were continuously active disease foci. In both Bulgaria and Rostov Oblast, the rates in certain districts were distinctly higher than in others. Nevertheless, cases were always scattered within and among different villages and often did not occur for a year or two before reappearing in a village. The gradual spread away from originally infected foci, and the "wandering" nature of morbidity rates throughout Rostov Oblast, were stressed in reports by local epidemiologists.

A notable feature of the history of CCHF epidemics is the decline to few or no reported cases immediately or soon after the major epidemic period has waned.

In many Soviet areas where the virus has been shown to be enzootic (confirmed human disease, virus isolations from ticks, results of seroepidemiological surveys of domestic animals, etc.), the number of recent publications on CCHF morbidity rates and on CCHF research have declined dramatically or dropped to nil. A dearth of morbidity data in available post-1975 Soviet literature may reflect (1) changing biomedical interests, research programs, and personnel, (2) less human contact with infected ticks owing to greater awareness of the danger of disease, (3) a cyclic reduction of virus prevalence in ticks in nature, or (4) a cyclic reduction of tick densities in nature.

The "sudden" appearance in 1976 of human CCHF in two widely separated areas of Pakistan, where the only previous evidence of the virus was two isolates from ticks, is a striking and tragic example of the unreliability of available CCHF virus data for predicting morbidity rates in most parts of Eurasia.

Seroepidemiological surveys of human beings should be useful indicators of the prevalence of previous CCHF infections; surveys of domestic animal sera should provide invaluable evidence pointing to the epidemiological potential of an area. However, the degree of reliability of serological tests used in many surveys reported in the literature is open to question. It appears best to regard most earlier seroepidemiological results as suggestive of the magnitude of a local morbidity problem at a specific time but not to weigh these results as positive proof.

The Disease in Africa
Incidence and Seroepidemiological Surveys

As in much of the Eurasian area where the virus is endemic but CCHF disease incidence is sporadic, few human cases have been reported from Africa and others have undoubtedly been overlooked or misdiagnosed. However, public health authorities must consider the potential for CCHF outbreaks or epidemics to be an ever-existing hazard in Africa.

Serological survey results of human beings and domestic and wild animals in Africa have been recorded in the foregoing text. However, the data are mostly too limited to be epidemiologically more meaningful than demonstrating the presence of the virus in certain geographical regions (for instance, Kenya, Tanzania, and Egypt). Most evidence that the virus occurs in Senegal, Nigeria, Central African Republic, and Ethiopia is based on isolations from ticks from domestic animals or, less often, on isolations from domestic or wild animals.

Antibodies to CCHF virus were detected in 24 of 250 febrile human sera from Ibadan, Nigeria.[133] Eighteen of the 24 sera were from children 14 years old or younger. Those authors believe that, under favorable circumstances, the virus presents a threat to human health in the Ibadan area. Except for this single study, there have been no surveys of human sera in Africa south of the Sahara.

Two isolates in Zaire in 1956 from human beings, one a physician who had treated a febrile boy, provided the first evidence of CCHF in Africa. No subsequent investigations have been reported from Zaire. During the heyday (1958 to 1968) of the East African Virus Research Institute, 13 CCHF strains were isolated from human beings in and near the Entebbe area of Uganda; 5 of the 13 were from laboratory personnel. Another CCHF infection occurred in a virus laboratory worker in Bangui, Central African Republic.

Clinical Symptoms and Mortality

Of the 16 virologically proven CCHF cases in Africa, 15 survived after courses of illness ranging from mild to severe.[277,435,479] Each infected person experienced fever of 1- to 3-day or longer (5 to 16 days) duration; temperatures up to 103°F (39.4°C) were recorded. Some patients had only a transient illness, others complained of nausea, severe headache, backache, photophobia, anorexia, joint pains, insomnia, etc. An Entebbe laboratory animal attendant died after severe hematamensis.

Despite the paucity of serious case histories in Africa, there are no scientific data to indicate that the virus is less virulent in Africa than in Eurasia, or that more serious cases might not occur in the future. The very recent histories of Lassa, Marburg, and Ebola viruses in Africa are poignant signals of how much remains to be learned about zoonotic viruses in relation to human disease on this continent.

Laboratory Techniques, Serological Tests

Serological techniques for CCHF virus identification and diagnosis and for biomedical research could be applied with more or less confidence following the 1967 to 1968 events reviewed in another section, although earlier experimental results had been reported.[333] The complete literature on this subject is presented in the forthcoming *Annotated Bibliography of Tick-borne Viruses.*

Except for a few strains of CCHF and all strains of Colorado tick fever, all tick viruses causing significant disease in humans yield agglutinating antigens.[71] Thus the HI test has not been generally applied to CCHF virus. For these reasons, results of serodiagnosis and seroepidemiological surveys for both diseases are difficult to evaluate and present. (The HI and N tests are considered "almost indispensable" for conducting antigenic relationship tests of arboviruses.[72])

Casals[74] stated: "There is need for improvement in the tests used for seroepidemiological surveys with (CCHF) virus. Some of the N test results reported are open to question due to the known nonspecific neutralizing activity of normal sera from many animal species, including man, on the virus . . . (Most) surveys . . . have been done by CF and ADGP tests; even in persons who had an overt infection there is a marked loss of positives within 3 or 4 years from onset, particularly among those who had a mild disease.[249]

As mentioned at the end of the section on morbidity rates: "It appears best to regard most earlier seroepidemiological results as suggestive of the magnitude of a local morbidity problem at a specific time but not to weigh these results as positive proof."

Those who have studied CCHF virus, as for instance Zavodova et al.[593] have agreed that the seldom-used N test is difficult to interpret owing to nonspecific antiviral activity of the sera in mice. To eliminate these nonspecific factors and to enable reproducible N tests in laboratory mice, Casals and Tignor[77] developed an acetone ether extraction technique and an antigen for use in HI tests, and confirmed the cross-reactivity between CCHF and HAZ viruses in the HI test. In this study, nonspecific antiviral factors were not found in human sera. For the same purpose, Buckley[59] developed cross-plaque N tests with cloned CCHF and HAZ viruses in LLC-MK$_2$ cell lines (derived from rhesus monkey kidney). (This cell line is the choice in vitro host system for these viruses according to Buckley. Stim[505] reported plaque formation as well as the cytopathogenic effect (CPE) of CCHF virus (Semunya strain) in these cells. Stim's results were confirmed by Buckley.[58])

Saidi et al.[447] found good correlation between the AGDP, N, and HI tests in total numbers of positive and negative results in Iranian sheep sera, as well as for individual sera. The CF test revealed only one third as many positives as the other tests. [Antibodies detected by the CF test are generally considered to be shorter-lived than those observed by the N and HI tests. Sera positive in the CF test, particularly when showing high titers, may indicate recent infection. The literature on this subject is often contradictory. See Donets et al.[143] for the dynamics of a soluble complement-fixing CCHF virus antigen in experimentally infected NWM.] However, the Saidi et al.[447] results with human sera were inconclusive and differed from those in sheep sera: none of the human sera positive in the AGDP test was positive in the N and CF tests and only 5 of 31 were positive at low titers in the HI test. (The Casals and Tignor[77] N test extraction technique was not employed in the Saidi et al.[447] work.)

David-West et al.,[133] using N tests based on mouse intracerebral inoculation, found no evidence of nonspecific antiviral activity in about 250 Nigerian human sera; 24 of the sera had a log neutralization index of 1.5 or greater. "This seems to be a very high proportion of positives by this test, particularly in view of the fact that no reports are available of natural diseases."[74]

The Ivanovsky Institute school has come to place reliance on an indirect hemagglutination (IHI) test developed by Gaidamovich for detecting and identifying CCHF virus (and Colorado tick fever virus) and for identifying antibodies to these viruses.[176,177]

In a CCHF survey of Rostov Oblast,[591] the IHI test produced seven times as many positives in cattle sera as the AGDP test. Sera from four persons positive in the IHI test were negative in the AGDP test; the IHI test also showed antibodies to the virus in persons 6 to 9 years from CCHF infection. All examined wild mammal and bird sera were negative in the AGDP test but, in the IHI test, antibodies to CCHF virus were detected in sera of hares, foxes, a field mouse, and a magpie (for the troublesome implications of detecting antibodies to CCHF virus in bird sera, see the section on noninfection of birds). Obukhova et al.[369] reported higher percentages of positive human and domestic animal sera from India in the IHI test than in the CF test; in the IHI test, titers were higher than in the IHA test.

Klisenko[275] recommended polyvinylpyrrolidone and albumin in place of horse serum as a stabilizer in the IHI and IHA tests for CCHF and other arboviruses.

Chastel[84] recommended the AGDP test for studying arenaviruses and arboviruses (including CCHF) in the following words: "This is a simple, quick, inexpensive, and often very specific method but the qualities of reagents limits its field of application; antigens are not sufficiently purified and the collection of antibodies is not very standardized . . . The best applications are in the epidemiological field: quick identification of wild strains of viruses, intratypic differentation, (and) serological surveys in man and animals . . . in connection with other analytical methods and providing the use of very purified antigenic fractions, immunoprecipitation helps to approach some more fundamental problems as antigenic structure of these viruses at the molecular level." Nevertheless, Casals[74] considers that the AGDP test "is not without problems of specificity" for CCHF virus. The AGDP test has been widely employed for seroepidemiological surveys of domestic animals and also of human beings.

In summary, the current status of serological techniques for use in CCHF studies[74] (personal communication) is as follows: The CF test is useful mainly for diagnosing current cases and possibly for surveys. The AGDP test should be applied chiefly to determine strain differences of the virus. The HI test is chiefly for diagnosis and surveys, and for studying comparatively strains of CCHF and other arboviruses. The IHI test is presumed to have the same application as the HI test. The N test, whether in the form of mouse neutralization, plaque reduction, or reduction of foci of infection,[496] is applicable to all studies, relationships, diagnoses, surveys, and strain differences detection (if any exist). The direct and indirect FA tests are used to diagnose disease in humans and for surveys and detecting the virus in vectors.

Fluorescent Antibody (FA) Technique (FA)

The FA test is used to detect CCHF virus in ticks and in smears and sections of infected vertebrates and for a variety of other experimental studies of the virus.

FAT methodology to detect CCHF virus in naturally and experimentally infected *Hyalomma m. marginatum* salivary and reproductive glands and to discover natural foci of the virus (using infected ticks as indicators) was developed by Zgurskaya et al.[601,603] and Popov et al.[411] This technique was enthusiastically applied by Chumakov and his colleagues during their latter years of studying CCHF epidemiology to reveal many new foci and species of infected ticks.

Karmysheva et al.[251-254] used the FA test (and cytochemical techniques and the electron microscope) to study cell lines inoculated with CCHF virus, antigenic and structural properties of the virus, comparative interactions between strains pathogenic for rodents and strains from cell cultures, and virus localization in impression smears and sections of the brain and other mammalian organs and in the bodies of persons who died of CCHF. The FA test and electron microscope studies are frequently combined in investigations into the nature of the CCHF virion.

The indirect immunofluorescence (IFA) technique is considered by Casals[74] to be an important candidate for research in relation to CCHF antibody surveys (results of a preliminary IFA test study of human sera from Bulgaria are presented). This technique may also be useful to shorten the time required for CCHF diagnosis by 1 to 3 days. Zgurskaya et al.[600] developed a "comparatively simple" IFA test on slides for determining and titrating antibodies to CCHF virus (the virus was said to be rendered harmless by acetone fixation; some authorities may disagree with this conclusion); antibody titers detected by this IFA test were eight (average) times higher than by the CF test. Zgurskaya and Chumakov[599] also discussed this technique. Semashko et al.[461] had earlier described experiments showing more distinct reactions by the IFA test than by the direct FA test in CCHF virus studies.

Cell Culture

The failure of Soviet attempts to isolate CCHF virus in cell culture lines delayed the era of modern CCHF virus research until the 1967 to 1968 period when NWM were first used.[105] The present status of employing cell cultures for CCHF virus is summarized by Casals[74] as follows: "CCHF virus replicates poorly or not at all in most cell lines tried with one exception, CER cells, and in all instances with no visible CPE under fluid medium. Plaque formation by some but not all strains has been reported in LLC-MK$_2$, CV-1 monkey cell line and African green monkey kidney primary cultures; such plaques are usually very small, delayed in appearing, and require skilled technical handling. HA antigens are not easily prepared with most strains, require special conditions in carrying out the test, and the titers at best are in the order of 1:50 to 1:100. Replication of the virus in CER cells, a hamster kidney cell line of somewhat dubious parentage,[496] is excellent but again with no CPE or plaque formation; the use of foci of infection detected by immunofluorescence (IF) and their neutralization by immune sera may lend itself to quantitative serological comparisons, as may also be done by titration of sera by indirect IF; no results are yet available."

Pre-1968 uses of cell culture for CCHF virus were reported by Khodukin et al.,[267] Angelov et al.,[13] Chumakov et al.,[109] Semashko et al.,[461] Shalunova et al.,[464] and others.

The earliest CCHF strains isolated from human patients after inoculation into NWM were also tested, with varying results, in different cell cultures.[64,65,174,594] For more recent information on cell culture and CCHF virus interrelationships, consult David-West[132] (on chicken embryo fibroblast, human cancer cell, and two African green monkey kidney cell lines), Tsypkin et al.[539] (on white mouse embryo brain lines), Buckley[59] (on the LLC-MK$_2$ line, discussed in relation to the N test), Chumakov[97,98] (on historical aspects), Semashko et al.[457] (on pig embryo kidney lines), Semashko et al.[460] (on pig embryo kidney, green monkey kidney, human embryo diploid, murine fibroblast (L cells), human carcinoma (HeLa), and chicken embryo cell lines), Donets et al.[144] (on 2 pig embryo kidney lines), and Hronovsky et al.[231] (on 3 lines employed in a modified plaque method on plastic panels).

Recognizing a need to develop a primary culture for large-quantity CCHF virus reproduction, Tatarskaya et al.[513] investigated human leukocyte cell culture. No CPE was produced, but whole and diluted culture fluids of infected cells were positive in the CF test with specific immune serum for the entire 49-day observation period, and several NWM infected with the culture fluid developed a typical clinical picture of CCHF with serological proof of CCHF virus infection. These authors stated that further investigation of human leukocyte lines is important for producing diagnostic preparations.

Benda et al.,[31] who made a profound study of CCHF virus adaptation to a CV-1 monkey cell line, ended their report with the following statement: "In spite of the knowledge accumulated by Soviet authors and the present results, we think that a detailed characterization of the relationship of CHF virus to cultured cells is not yet possible. The results of an electron microscope study on CHF virus-infected cells[235] will not substantially affect this situation."

CCHF virus and HAZ virus (as a representative of the CCHF serogroup) do not reproduce in mosquito cell lines.[58,589]

I have seen no reports of studies on CCHF virus in tick cell lines.

EPIDEMIOLOGY

Occurrence
Introduction

An ideal overview of the past and present status of CCHF epidemiology would be based chiefly on biological-ecological-zoogeographical-morbidity interrelationships of the virus and its vectors and reservoirs. Ecological boundaries would be emphasized, political boundaries would be deemphasized. However, CCHF epidemics have occurred because of major military or socioeconomic events within strictly circumscribed political areas. Where CCHF virus is endemic epidemiological data are all very recent and have been developed regionally. In each epidemiological category — epidemic or enzootic — the quantity and quality of data have been largely influenced by the numbers, abilities, resources, and attitudes of regional scientists in formulating and executing investigations and in publishing results. (The chief cohesive factor throughout the Soviet zone has been the guidance and support of the Chumakov school centered at the Institute of Poliomyelitis and Viral Encephalitides, Moscow.) Especially where CCHF morbidity has been sporadic, the kind of published data on virus circulation in nature has depended on a highly variable ratio of biomedical curiosity and virological-serological-zoological resources and capabilities in each region, republic, or nation. Thus it appears unrealistic, at this early stage, to compare available biomedical data as a whole outside the framework of the separate political regions in which the virus is known to exist.

Much of the geographic area under review is unfamiliar to most readers. To provide a generalized impression of the environments of known CCHF foci, I have briefly discussed topography, climate, vegetation, etc. A book-length review would be required to present properly environmental information for epidemiological analysis. Ecological terms such as steppes, plains, semideserts, etc., often loosely used in reports on the human disease and seroepidemiological results, have caused some problems in preparing this review.

European Foci (Southwestern Palearctic Faunal Region)

There are now varying levels of evidence for CCHF virus circulation in Europe from France, Hungary, Bulgaria, Yugoslavia, and European U.S.S.R.(to the Caspian Sea). Epidemics resulted from environmental changes caused by World War II devastation (Crimea, 1944 to 1945) and from converting swampy deltalands (Astrakhan, 1953 to 1969 and virgin steppes (Rostov, 1963 to 1969; Bulgaria, 1953 to 1972) to large-scale, collectivized agricultural enterprises under the ambitious 5-year plans following World War II.

The 1944 to 1945 Crimean experience provided a generalized background of information on the natural history of CCHF. Field research during the 1953 to 1969 outbreaks broadened the scope of this knowledge. New serological and virological tools were quickly applied after the 1967 technological breakthrough employing NWM for virus isolation. Use of these techniques contributed much new qualitative and quantitative epidemiological data. However, epidemics in each area waned following the long, excessively cold winter of 1968 to 1969 and the consequent decline in population densities of *Hyalomma m. marginatum,* the tick chiefly involved in epizootics. Virological and epidemiological research continued for 2 or 3 years following 1969, but then was directed mostly to other geographic regions. After 1969, many previously unrecognized foci were discovered and a number of vertebrate and tick species were demonstrated for the first time to be links in the CCHF transmission chain. Sporadic human cases continue to be seen in newly discovered foci and in some earlier recognized foci. One wonders whether, when, and where environmental changes during a period of increasing tick numbers, either influenced by human activities or in the course of a natural population density cycle, may again result in epidemics of this disease.

The Palearctic steppe region in which CCHF is known to occur is dominated epidemiologically by *Hyalomma m. marginatum,* but other tick species also maintain the virus in this ecosystem. Lightly wooded regions in the steppe biotope influence the vertebrate and ectoparasite composition of the fauna and also the virus circulation intensity, but *H. m. marginatum* does not invade the true forest biotope.

The Balkan plains and mountains of Bulgaria and mountains of Yugoslavia are also habitats of *H. m. marginatum*, together with the three species mentioned below from Moldavia (Palearctic broadleaf forest). However, to this date, CCHF in the Balkans has been associated chiefly with *H. m. marginatum*.

The rugged Caucasus and Transcaucasia areas have very recently produced new information on CCHF morbidity and epidemiology. *H. m. marginatum* is common here, as are many other tick species. The broad outlines of the tick fauna in this ecologically complex area have been fairly well documented.

The Palearctic broadleaf (deciduous) forest biotope, which originally covered much of Europe west of the steppes, interests us as the source of recent data on CCHF virus isolates from *Ixodes ricinus, Haemaphysalis punctata,* and *Dermacentor marginatus* from Moldavia and earlier records of ''Bukovinian hemorrhagic fever'' from forests in this Republic. These three tick species survive in suitable European habitats but not in true steppes. Part of Moldavia is steppeland but *H. m. marginatum* is rare or absent there. The fragmentary data on CCHF in Hungary and France arouse our interest to learn more about CCHF virus circulation in Europe.

Forests (Ixodes, Dermacentor, Haemaphysalis)

Hyalomma m. marginatum is common in the Mediterranean area of Europe but absent in contemporary and former European deciduous and mixed forest biotopes, where it is replaced chiefly by *Ixodes ricinus, Dermacentor marginatus,* and in more localized areas by *Haemaphysalis spp.* Little is known about CCHF virus in the European forest zone. However, a generalized picture of enzootic CCHF is beginning to emerge from recent investigations in Moldavia.

France

Tkachenko et al.[528] detected antibodies to CCHF virus in AGDP tests of sera from 2 of 19 bats (species not stated) from Perpignan, near the French-Spanish border. The possibility that these bats may have been infected elsewhere must be considered.

Hungary

Antibodies to CCHF virus were present in 6 of 687 cattle sera and 15 of 48 sheep sera from 8 Hungarian counties.[229] In sera from 587 persons working with animals in four areas of Hungary, antibodies to the virus were present in 17 (12 animal attendants, 3 veterinarians, 1 gardener from Hajdú-Bihar county, and 1 abattoir worker from Budapest); the highest titer was 1:16.[230] Each of 169 animal sera from Hajdú-Bihar county was negative. The AGDP test was used in both studies.

Moldavian S.S.R.

This mild, rich agricultural republic, formed in 1940 from parts annexed from Romania and southwestern Ukraine, differs ecologically and epidemiologically from other regions now known to be infected by CCHF virus. During the summers of 1946 and 1947, more than 60 persons, among them children and adults picnicking and gathering mushrooms and, also, timber-cutters, suffered from "Bukovinian hemorrhagic fever" in Carpathian foothill forests where *Ixodes ricinus* often bites people.[178,281,453] In retrospect, the Bukovinian disease may have been CCHF. Sporadic cases attributed to CCHF in 1958 to 1959 were reported by Drobinsky; wintertime hemorrhagic fevers recorded after 1955 were probably hemorrhagic fever with renal syndrome. Leshchinskaya[313] considered that there was no evidence to confirm earlier reports of CCHF from Moldavia.

All of Moldavia has long been "reclaimed" by humankind. Special circumstances leading to the 1946 to 1947 disease outbreak have not been mentioned in the literature. The republic is divided ecologically and zoogeographically into a European forest transition zone and a Palearctic steppe zone. *Hyalomma m. marginatum* is rare among the 21 tick species recorded in some detail from Moldavia by Uspenskaya,[541-552] and Uspenskaya and Konovalov,[553-556] and Uspenskaya and Motornyy,[556] and this species is not even mentioned in a monograph on parasites of Moldavian rodents and corvid birds.[11]

Chumakov et al.[100] stated that *H. m. marginatum* population densities have "sharply decreased" in Moldavia during the last 15 years owing to transferring most cattle to a stable-camp system and that "this probably also resulted in cessation of CCHF infections in Moldavia." They isolated eight CCHF strains from Moldavia in 1973 to 1974 from *Ixodes ricinus* (two strains, 57 pools/2948 ticks), *Dermacentor marginatus* (four strains, 43/1644), and *Haemaphysalis punctata* (two strains, 2/7).

Tick population densities are said to be generally low throughout Moldavia, but numbers in some habitats vary from moderate to very dense in different years. CCHF epidemiology should be especially interesing to study in Moldavian environments owing to the presence of the widely distributed *Ixodes ricinus* and other "secondary vectors" of CCHF virus, the number of isolates already obtained from these species, and the virtual absence of *Hyalomma m. marginatum*.

Steppes (Chiefly Hyalomma m. marginatum)
Ukrainian S.S.R.

Crimean (Krym) Oblast — In 1854, D'yakonov first observed "Crimean endemic disease" (or "malignant Crimean fever") while treating Crimean War casualties. From November 1855 to May 1856 he studied this disease in the Sevastopol, Bakhchisaray, and Simferopol military hospitals. More than 80% of about 2000 patients overflowing the Sevastopol hospital at the time experienced this illness, which D'yakonov distinguished from classic epidemic typhus, the inevitable wartime calamity of the period. Physicians and hospital assistants often became severely sick and many died. The D'yakonov report has been considered by some authors to include cases of CCHF. However, hemorrhages are not mentioned among the clinical signs, which are discussed at some length. I believe that the Crimean War patients experienced a different disease and in recent personal correspondence Academician M. P. Chumakov agreed with this opinion.

During the World War II enemy occupation of the Crimea (1941 to 1944), normal agricultural activities were disrupted and the common sport of hunting European hares, *Lepus europaeus*, was abandoned. When Soviet troops reoccupied the hilly Crimean steppes in 1944, hares had become excessively abundant and neglected pastures were overgrown by weeds. The *Hyalomma m. marginatum* population density had also exploded. Hares were heavily infested by immature ticks and cattle were heavily infested by adult ticks. This environmental disturbance produced the epidemiological conditions leading to the 1944 to 1945 epidemic of "acute infectious capillarotoxicosis," later named Crimean hemorrhagic fever. Subsequent investigations have shown the presence of numerous endemic CCHF foci in the Palearctic steppes infested by *H. m. marginatum.* The theory that the virus may have been introduced into the Crimea by extensive movements of birds disturbed by military action elsewhere[9] is justifiably considered as "not very convincing" by Pak and Mikhailova.[383]

Crimean hemorrhagic fever was first recognized between June and September 1944; 92 military personnel were hospitalized and 9 of the 92 died.[280] Morbidity data differ in various reports, apparently depending on whether the authors were concerned only with military cases or with both military and civilian cases. For instance, Grashchenkov[185] recorded 115 CCHF cases in a single hospital in the summer of 1944 but did not mention whether the patients were military or civilian or if there were also cases in other hospitals. Other reports state that there were 168 cases in 1944 and that 18 (11%) of them were fatal. Estimates including remote rural areas lacking medical facilities, especially in parts of Kerch peninsula, run to 200 or more cases in 1944. According to Drobinsky,[152] a similar disease was observed in the Crimea from April to July 1942.

Specialized military physicians travelled from the Far East to the Crimea in 1944 to study the alarming new hemorrhagic disease, and the first of three epidemiological research expeditions headed by Chumakov was sent from Moscow. "Most cases were seen among signalmen, drivers, and surveyors . . . who by their profession had even closer contact with ticks than the soldiers who harvested grain . . . . All patients had daily contact with ticks and were bitten during their entire stay on the steppe".[280] The epidemic began in June, reached peak numbers about mid-July, decreased in late August, and fell to only three cases in September. One to five people became ill in 63 scattered rural localities, mostly in northwestern Crimea but also in the Kerch peninsula.[406] The northwestern landscape was one of small farmsteads, vineyards, and plots of corn, sunflowers, and melons, larger grainfields bordered by rows of tree windbreaks, weedy pastures, and some virgin grassland with wormwood.

About 100 CCHF cases were again recorded in the summer of 1945, when counts of adult *H. m. marginatum* attacking a person who visited eight haystacks for 30 min on 6 August were 43, 100, 21, 32, 21, 18, 28, and 78 for the respective stacks. Numerous ticks survived the heavy rains and sleet of late 1944 and early 1945, but the 1945 densities of hares and rodents were considerably reduced.[188] In 1946, fewer than 9 ticks attacked persons in the same haystack situations where 18 to 100 ticks had been recorded in 1945.[406]

In a 12,000-ha study area, Grobov[188] observed eight hares per km in 1944 but only three in 1945. Only hares and some birds were infested by larval and nymphal *H. m. marginatum,* none fed on rodents, carnivores, or domestic dogs. The 1945 hare population reduction was paralleled by reduced numbers of ground squirrels, voles, house mice, and other rodents, many of which were found dead in flooded burrows. The relatively few hares available to serve as hosts for *H. m. marginatum* in 1945 and afterward appear to have "normalized" the subsequent tick population density. Crimean agricultural practices were gradually modernized[204] and CCHF morbidity fell to a low level.[608] However, recent reports show that CCHF virus continues to circulate in nature in the Crimea.

During the 1944 to 1945 outbreak, essentially similar results were obtained by Grobov[188] and Petrova-Piontkovskaya[406] in independent investigations of CCHF epidemiology. Adult *H. m. marginatum* were numerous on cattle from spring to fall in 1944 and 1945 but less numerous in 1946. Adults also fed on sheep, horses, humans, and sometimes on the European hare, greater bustard, *Otis tarda*, and Tengmalm owl, *Aegolius funereus*. Adult tick densities were greatest in fields where cattle grazed, in cattle enclosures, and in situations frequented by resting or feeding hares.

Immature *H. m. marginatum* infested all hares examined after mid-July and fed chiefly on the head and neck. As many as 194 larvae and 369 nymphs were found on a single hare in late July. Feeding activity of immature stages continued from mid-June to October. Nymphs becoming satiated and detaching in early summer molted to adults during the same season and overwintered in this stage. Fed nymphs detaching in September or October overwintered in this stage and molted to adults the following spring. Overwintering ticks were especially common under shocks and stacks of hay.

Hares rested during daytime, especially during rains, in fallow fields where the hard soil did not become muddy and stick to their fluffy feet. These fields were often near windbreaks where hares and birds sheltered and fed. Hares foraged at hayshocks and haystacks. In these situations and in cattle enclosures, *H. m. marginatum* densities were greatest — a person sitting on the ground in a cattle enclosure found 120 adult ticks attempting to bite him in a 30-min period. In colder weather, hares ventured closer to farmsteads where, after the first snowfall, they sheltered in barns and were easily shot or clubbed. Hunting hares throughout the year was recommended as a tick control and disease prevention measure.

Fewer immature *H. m. marginatum* were taken from resident and migrant ground-feeding birds: the partridge, *Perdix perdix;* Calandra lark, *Melanocorypha calandra;* short-toed lark, *Calandrella cinerea;* sparrow, *Passer domesticus,* stone curlew, *Burhinus oedicnemus;* swallow, *Hirundo rustica;* little owl, *Athene noctua;* and also on the Tengmalm owl, great bustard, and domestic chickens, turkeys, and ducks. Grobov[188] also listed immature *H. m. marginatum* from young cranes, *Megalornis grus,* which migrate to India and Thailand.

A few other tick species found on Kerch peninsula during the Crimean epidemic were dismissed as unimportant to CCHF epidemiology owing to their rarity or seasonal dynamics, which did not correspond to the spring-summer period of human infections. Immature *Haemaphysalis punctata* were common on partridges and adults were taken on cattle in late fall and spring. Some adult *Hyalomma* sp. (as *H. savignyi*), *Dermacentor marginatus,* and *Rhipicephalus sanguineus* were also found.

Chumakov,[88-91] Grashchenkov,[185] Sokolov et al.,[498] and others reported the early experiments leading to the belief that the agent causing CCHF is a virus common to ticks and that it is transovarially transmitted by and overwinters in *Hyalomma m. marginatum.* However, the Korshunova and Petrova-Piontkovskava[291] summary of 1946 studies of infected ticks from hares, bustards, and cattle from Crimean steppes and forests, and also of immunological properties of one of Chumakov's virus strains from a human patient, reveals ambiguously stated methods, experimental design, and results, which leave considerable doubt regarding the viral and/or rickettsial nature of the alleged isolates. Petrova-Piontkovskava[407] in discussing the same work, implied that only *Rickettsia* were isolated from these ticks. Avakyan[20] reviewed the early studies and concluded that the results from the humans experimentally inoculated with CCHF virus were reliable, but results of all other virological investigations were "objectionable" because of improper methods and observations. Lately, Chumakov[98] confirmed this opinion and straightforwardly and unequivocally stated: "In 1944, our first attempts to determine the question of . . . etiology and to create the laboratory model for studying this disease, including tests in white mice, guinea pigs, rabbits, monkeys, and cats, proved to be unsuccessful, despite the fact that the hemorrhagic syndrome was observed in infected mice and cats. Particularly discouraging results were obtained at the beginning of very promising tests in white mice because an outbreak of intestinal viral ectromelia developed in mice with different hemorrhages resembling CCHF symptoms in humans. This fact caused distrust in further use of these animals . . . . Therefore in the summers of 1945 to 1946, when new cases appeared in the Crimea, we experimentally induced the fever in psychiatric patients needing pyrogenic therapy (with permission of the People's Commissariat for Public Health)." Chumakov and the Soviet school now credit the 1967 to 1968 accomplishments as those in which the viral nature and properties of the agent of CCHF were defined.

In 1968 to 1969, more than 20 years after the initial Crimean outbreak, AGDP test results of cattle and horse sera (numbers not stated) from Kerch peninsula breeding farms showed up to 14.8% (average 2.8%) to be positive for CCHF infection.[8] These included 1.5% of the newly weaned calves being driven to pasture for the first time; 10.4% of the adult cattle from these farms were positive. In nearby Kirov area, where few human CCHF cases had earlier been recorded, there were no positive AGDP reactions in domestic animal sera. Pastures of the southern and northern coasts of Kerch peninsula to this day (1968 to 1969) remain heavily infested by *Hyalomma m. marginatum* and favorable environments for CCHF virus circulation.

Chumakov et al.[99] confirmed that scattered or single CCHF cases have been recorded in the Crimea during the 25 years following the 1944 to 1945 outbreak in military personnel. For instance, Domrachev[138] reported the clinical details of 31 mild, severe, and fatal CCHF cases seen in civilians in Crimean hospitals in 1945 to 1947; the Domrachev report was verified as pertaining to CCHF by Leshchinskaya.[315] One of the fatal cases was in a female sanitarian after nursing a gardener who died of CCHF. Two suspected cases of hospital (nosocomial) transmission of CCHF occurred in the Crimea in 1947;[320] notably, there were no nosocomial incidents during the 1944 to 1945 outbreak. However, Chumakov et al.[99] stated that no CCHF cases had been seen in the Crimea for the past 5 years but natural foci continue to exist.

In 1972 to 1973, 33 CCHF strains were isolated from five tick species from cattle in 11 localities (in central and eastern Kerch, Sevastopol area, and southern coastal areas) representing most of the varied ecological-geographical areas of the Crimea.[99] The 33 isolates were from 1663 *Hyalomma m. marginatum* (57 pools/28 positive), 33 *Ixodes ricinus* (3/2), 46 *Haemaphysalis punctata* (4/1), 97 *Rhipicephalus bursa* (2/1), and 132 *R. sanguineus* (2/1). These high rates of virus recovery are noteworthy. Tick control measures, and consequent reduction in *H. m. marginatum* numbers, were stated to be responsible for the absence of human CCHF cases after 1969; the possibility that tick densities were reduced by the severe 1968 to 1969 winter weather as in Astrakhan Oblast and elsewhere in southwestern U.S.S.R., was not mentioned. As usual, *Hyalomma scupense,* which parasitizes cattle during fall, winter, and early spring, was not considered as a potential reservoir or vector of the virus. Four (1.3%) of 299 cattle sera in the AGDP test and two (1.4%) of 143 cattle sera in the CF test were positive for CCHF antibody reactions; these were taken in 1973 in Inkerman region. The virus was also isolated from livers and blood of four hares, thus "proving their role in CCHF epidemiology," and from larval *H. m. marginatum* and nymphal and adult *R. bursa* from these hares.

Using the FA technique to demonstrate CCHF infections in *Hyalomma m. marginatum* salivary gland preparations, Chumakov et al.[113] obtained the following results (number of preparation/number of positive) from three regions of the Crimea in 1972 to 1973: Alushti (20/4), Leninsky (114/17), Sevastopol (120/46).

Voroshilovgrad and Kherson Oblasts — Voroshilovgrad (formerly Lugansk) is in central Ukraine, north of Rostov Oblast. In July 1969, a patient who had slept on the steppe, where he may have been bitten by ticks, was admitted to the Antrasit Regional Hospital with a diagnosis of CCHF, which was confirmed by CF and AGDP tests at the Rostov laboratory (Primakov[419]). Sera from two of three patients from rural areas of Antrasit Region were positive for CCHF in the same serological tests in 1969.[247]

In 1948, I. R. Drobinsky saw CCHF cases in Kherson Oblast, near the Dnieper River outlet into the Black Sea (northwest of the Crimea).[385,396]

Odessa and Chernigov Oblasts — Hemorrhagic fevers reported as CCHF from Odessa (Is-mail') Oblast in 1948 by Drobinsky[396] were hemorrhagic nephrosonephritis, not CCHF, according to Sakhno et al.[450] and Leshchinskaya.[315]

Outbreaks of "Bukovinian hemorrhagic fever" in Chernigov Oblast were reported by Zeitlenok and Mart'yanova[595] and "recently recorded single cases of this disease indicate the presence of a natural focus in this territory".[189] Whether these cases were CCHF has not been confirmed.

Astrakhan Oblast (RSFSR)

Nine years after the Crimean outbreak began, the first CCHF patients were recognized in Astrakhan Oblast. They were a 15-year-old shepherd and a 13-year-old fisherman seen in May and July 1953. The shepherd recovered but the fisherman died.[596] In May and June of 1954 there were nine cases, one housewife (fatal), three shepherds (two fatal), one fisherman, and four agricultural workers (one fatal). The patients were 16 to 54 years old. All had recently been bitten by ticks or had crushed ticks with their hands — some while pulling the parasites from animals, others while shearing sheep. *Hyalomma m. marginatum* was the chief tick species in the area.

Retrospectively diagnosed cases numbered 3 in 1953, 9 in 1954, 11 in 1955, 1 annually in 1956 to 1961, 32 in 1962, and 44 in 1963.[102] During this period, 18 of the 104 cases (17.3%) were fatal. In 45 of 70 agricultural settlements there were only single patients, but in one to nine other settlements there were two to five patients in one, two, three, or four seasons. No cases were reported from unmodified steppe landscape areas.[506]

Most patients had recently taken up residence in Astrakhan Oblast, when state agricultural and industrial enterprises were expanded or newly introduced. They worked chiefly in collective farms and other agricultural and rural industries as milkmaids, office employees, railroad inspectors, students, housewives, and pensioners. The 46 male and 58 female patients were 2½ to 78 years old, mostly in the 47- to 54-year age group. Three patients in one household had sheared heavily tick-infested sheep a few days before illness began, but most others were single cases from scattered settlements. Patients were seen from late March to about August 20.[102]

CCHF morbidity in the decade following 1953 was probably much higher than reported owing to misdiagnosis by physicians who were unacquainted with the disease.[506] As medical awareness developed, the mortality rate dropped from over 30% to 13%, chiefly because of better diagnosis and earlier hospitalization.

The 1962 to 1963 upswing in CCHF morbidity produced a flurry of epidemiological and parasitological investigations.

Astrakhan Oblast lies in a desert-semidesert-steppe transitional zone in the western part of the Caspian lowland. This dry area is traversed from northwest to southeast by the wide floodplain valley and lush alluvial delta of the Volga River before it flows into the Caspian Sea.[417,418,611] The important spring rains typically begin in late April, are heaviest in late May or early June, and end in late June or early July. The climate is continental dry with 150 to 300 mm annual rainfall. Following spring thaws, almost all the lowland is inundated. The entire delta has numerous ponds and complicated water channels. Poplar, willow, and elm form tree belts along waterways. The land is used chiefly for pasturing numerous cattle; some sheep, goats, pigs, horses, camels, and ducks are also kept there. Other parts are used for hay, vegetable gardens, melon fields, and rice and cotton plantations. Rodents and shrews of several species are common, as are hares, wild hogs, and foxes, the introduced raccoon-dog, and a large variety of resident and migrating birds. Extensive stands of reeds and willow remain in undeveloped delta land. The surrounding desert, semidesert, and steppe receive little or no water and their flora and fauna differ greatly from those in the floodplain and delta. Mapping the localities in which CCHF had occurred from 1953 to 1963 showed that most cases originated in or beside agricultural delta and floodplain areas where domestic animals were pastured near colonies of the rook, *Corvus f. frugilegus.*[416]

Seven tick species were taken in the Zimina et al.[611] survey of Astrakhan Oblast, but these and all other authors have stressed that adult *Hyalomma m. marginatum* made up the great majority (often 90% or more) of the numerous ticks collected in spring and summer from domestic animals in the floodplain and delta. Cattle and horses were the chief hosts of adults. Sheep and goats were less often infested. Picking these easily visible adult ticks from the ground or from vegetation by hand was found to be more effective than flagging to determine adult *H. m. marginatum* numbers and localization in nature.[590] Most adults were taken in sparse willow growth, others in hayfields and weedy meadows where cattle usually grazed. Tick incidence was low in weedy railway borders where fewer cattle grazed. Higher meadows heavily trampled by cattle also produced few ticks.

The first adults appeared at 5 to 9°C average daily temperature — April 8 in 1963 and April 20 in 1964.[611] Tick numbers per cow in 1963 reached 17 in late April, then decreased to 12 in May, 6 in June, and less then 1 by mid-July. In another 1963 survey, Zalutskaya[590] found an average of 23 ticks per cow during the 50-day period of peak population density (April 20 to June 10). The 1964 tick numbers were less than one third of those in 1963, and the adult activity cycle began later in the season. The first human illness occurred on April 24 in 1963 but on May 6 in 1964. The 1964 reduction in CCHF morbidity (44 cases in 1963 to 11 in 1964) was about proportional to the 1964 drop in *H. m. marginatum* population density. Most patients admitted tickbite or crushing ticks shortly before illness. A hospital nurse became infected while tending three CCHF patients.

I have seen no post-1964 morbidity data for all of Astrakhan Oblast, but Berezin et al.[38] state that in the Volga delta the number of cases was 23 in 1963, 7 in 1964, 9 in 1965, and 2 in 1967. The number of cases "increased" in 1968, when tick density also increased, but fell to zero in 1969 (to June 1), when tick numbers decreased.

Two major factors appear to regulate *H. m. marginatum* population density from year to year in Astrakhan Oblast: the level and length of the May to June Volga floods and critical winter temperatures.[38]

The peak May to June flood period, when much of the Volga delta and floodplain is inundated for several days, coincides with the season of greatest adult and unfed larval *H. m. marginatum* activity. The ticks can survive submersion for 5 to 7 days and females can oviposit afterward. However, adults and larvae drown in years of prolonged or erratic flooding. In 1963, the maximum flood level was 296 cm and the infestation index of immature ticks on rooks was approximately 88%. In 1964 and 1965, with lower flood levels (215 cm in 1965), peak parasitism indices rose to approximately 198 and 498. Consequently, in early 1966 adult ticks were extremely numerous. However, the late spring of 1966 brought an exceptionally high flood level (320 cm). The mass destruction of adults and immatures during the serious 1966 inundation caused lower tick numbers in 1967, and only two CCHF cases were recorded that year.

Before the Volga River flow was regulated to develop new agricultural areas in the early 1950s, spring flood levels had always been much higher. In retrospect, Berezin et al.[38] believed that this lowered flood level may have been a significant factor leading to increased tick numbers and to the first appearance of CCHF in 1953.

Temperatures rarely drop to −20°C in the relatively mild winters of the Volga delta. However, in the winter of 1968 to 1969 there was early frost and the temperature dropped to −30°C and remained at −20°C or lower for more than 2 months. Much

Table 1

IMMATURE *HYALOMMA M. MARGINATUM* FROM
GROUND-FEEDING BIRDS IN THE VOLGA DELTA,
1963 to 1964[35]

Species	Birds		Ticks	
	No. exam.	No. infest.	No. coll.	Infestation index
Rook (*Corvus frugilegus*)	461	431	31,780	68.9
Carrion crow (*Corvus corone*)	90	73	3717	41.3
Magpie (*Pica pica*)	32	21	891	27.9
Starling (*Sturnus vulgaris*)	111	85	603	5.4
White wagtail (*Motacilla alba*)	3	3	170	56.9
Tree sparrow (*Passer montanus*)	19	14	64	3.3
Crested lark (*Galerida cristata*)	2	1	18	9.0
Hoopoe (*Upupa epops*)	37	27	1150	31.1
Total	755	655	38,393	

ground was frozen to a depth of more than 1 m. After the severe winter, the adult tick abundance index per cow, which in 1968 had been approximately 20 with maximum numbers reaching 200, dropped to less than 0.1 in May 1969. No CCHF cases were reported during the summer of 1969.

A mathematical model for forecasting CCHF morbidity in Astrakhan Oblast, developed by Berezin,[32] is based on abundance of adult *H. m. marginatum* in spring after immatures have survived spring floods, and overwintering adults have survived cold winter temperatures and frozen soil conditions.

The rook was the most important host of immature *H. m. marginatum* in the Volga delta and floodplain. The tick also survived in smaller numbers on other birds and on nonburrowing medium-sized mammals here and in nearby semidesert and steppe areas. An important secondary host was the European hare, *Lepus europaeus*. In 1964, 6059 immature *H. m. marginatum* were taken from 32 hares (average 189.3 ticks/hare). There were four or five hares in each km² and 18,000 to 22,000 hares were shot annually in Astrakhan Oblast.[611] Numerous burrowing rodents and shrews were examined but only three larvae were found on a field vole. The common long-eared hedgehog, *Hemiechinus a. auritus,* was parasitized by as many as 40 ticks during the season of peak tick activity.[36]

The 1963 to 1964 studies of *H. m. marginatum* on birds in the Volga delta[36] produced important comparative data for infestation of 8 common bird species feeding chiefly on the ground (see Table 1). Six other bird species (falcon, kestrels, kite, roller, doves) periodically feeding on the ground were less often and less heavily infested, and seven other arboreal species rarely touching the ground were only seldom or not infested. Aquatic birds were infested only when they flew to feed in flooded pastures.

In the 44-km² Travinsky study station of Astrakhan Oblast, there were ten rook colonies containing 2776 nests, each occupied by two immature and two adult birds, with a total of 11,104 birds (average about 252/km²), on which about 2 million immature *H. m. marginatum* were estimated to feed.[37] In the same station there were about 100 pairs of nesting crows and magpies.

Adult *H. m. marginatum* began feeding on domestic animals in April, reached peak numbers in May, and disappeared from these hosts in early August. Larvae appeared about 55 days after females dropped from the host, just when young rooks were leaving the nests to feed in pastures and willow stands. The percentage of tick-infested rooks increased from 3.7 in mid-June, to 51.8 in late June, to 100% from mid-July to

August 20. Early in the season, immature ticks were found only in the ears of the birds; afterward, these orifices were completely filled with ticks and many others attached elsewhere on the head. Larvae molted to nymphs on these hosts (two-host life cycle); nymphs completed feeding and dropped to the ground about 2 weeks after they had attached as larvae. As some nymphs dropped they were replaced by new larvae so that a variety of feeding states were found on each bird. Some rooks were hosts to as many as 1170 immature ticks. Nymphs on the ground molted to adults and overwintered in this stage.

The rooks fed on the ground in cultivated fields, gardens, orchards, and fishery areas but chiefly in cattle pastures and hayfields. Dense flocks roosted or rested for many hours of the day in trees along canal banks and in single ("beacon") trees in pastures. Numerous satiated nymphs detached from rooks in these resting areas and molted to adults afterward. A person sitting under a beacon tree for 15 min was attacked by 78 adult ticks.

As immature rooks developed flying capability, their flight range increased from 10 or 15 km to as much as 500 km. They visited more or less distant fields, forests, villages, and cities just at the period when nymphs were engorging and dropping. This potential for infected tick dispersal was considered to be an important factor in CCHF virus dissemination in Astrakhan Oblast.

In undeveloped deltaland where cattle were not pastured, no *H. m. marginatum* was found, even on the bird species usually infested near pastures. Aquatic birds were parasitized when they flew to feed in flooded pastures. Notably, the Astrakhan area is an important breeding locale for birds that migrate to Africa for the winter.

An interesting tangential finding of the Berezin et al.[36] study was that the ground-feeding hoopoe, *Upupa epops*, may support as many as 330 larval *H. m. marginatum* but that most of these larvae shrivel and die 2 or 3 days after attaching to the hoopoe. The reason for this phenomenon is unknown.

In dry areas of Astrakhan Oblast and in Kalmyk A.S.S.R., wheatears and three species of larks are the most important hosts of immature *H. m. marginatum*.[32]

Serological investigations and attempts to isolate CCHF virus from birds in Astrakhan Oblast all gave negative results, but the virus was isolated from nymphal *H. m. marginatum* from some of these birds[35] and also from unfed and partially fed female ticks from the ground and from cattle.[104]

Sera from 8474 domestic animals from different localities in Astrakhan Oblast were examined from 1968 to 1970 in the CF and AGDP tests.[35] Antibodies to CCHF virus were detected in sera from each area, but the conversion ratios for different areas differed greatly. Antibodies were less often detected in sera of camels and sheep pastured in arid zones and of pigs held indoors than in sera of other animals feeding in delta and floodplain pastures where ticks were more numerous. Positives were 0.2% to 7.1% (average 6.1%) for cattle, 3.1% for horses, 0.3% for sheep, 1.4% for camels, and 1.6% for pigs. Following the decreased tick numbers after the cold 1968 to 1969 winter, the number of positive calf sera decreased from 3.2% in 1968 to less than 1% in 1969. Serological data from hares, especially from immature animals, were considered to provide the most accurate evidence of CCHF virus activity in Astrakhan Oblast. In August 1968, 40% of the sera from hares in the Volga delta were positive; in December 10% were positive.[34] Throughout the Oblast in 1968, 20% of hare sera were positive as compared to less than 10% in 1969. Notably, no antibodies were detected in sera from young hares in 1969, suggesting the absence of virus transmission that year.[35] As already stated, there also were no human cases of CCHF in Astrakhan Oblast in 1969.

The possibility of infection by inhalation was considered when 17 persons became ill with CCHF after shearing heavily tick-infested sheep on a private farm in Astrakhan

Oblast. On collective and state farms, where fewer persons participated in machine shearing of about 600 less heavily infested sheep, only three shearers became ill. Only "a few" of these 20 CCHF cases were accompanied by pneumonia.[506]

Vashkov and Poleshchuk[558] concluded, as had earlier workers, that most available control measures against *H. m. marginatum* were too expensive to consider because all pasture areas in the Oblast were potential microfoci. Spraying cattle during the period of adult tick parasitism was considered to be most efficient. These authors also reviewed earlier studies on tick repellents.

Rostov Oblast (R.S.F.S.R.)

CCHF in Rostov Oblast was first observed in 1963, 19 years after the first record from the Crimea and 10 years after the first record from Astrakhan Oblast. Epidemiological factors in the Rostov steppe area, where the Don River flows to the Black Sea, appear to be more complex than those to the east in the Volga delta (Astrakhan Oblast). The number of human cases recorded in Rostov Oblast gradually increased from 11 in 1963 to 24 (1964), 27 (1965), 38 (1966), 61 (1967), and 131 (1968)[22] but dropped to 31 in 1969,[404] "a few" in 1970 and 1971, and none in 1972 and 1973.[306] Thus the waning of the more serious Rostov Oblast epidemic followed the 1968 to 1969 cycle seen in Astrakhan Oblast, but morbidity in Rostov persisted at a low ebb for 3 years longer.

During this period, the geographic range of CCHF cases expanded from northwestern to southeastern and southwestern areas of Rostov Oblast. Known foci increased from 2 in 1963 to 13 in 1968 (but 9 in 1969), and infected settlements increased from 9 in 1963 to 49 in 1968 (but 26 in 1969). This geographic expansion, at the rate of 10 to 60 km per year,[44] was considered to have been caused by infected ticks dropping from infested rooks and other birds during postbreeding dispersal flights away from already established CCHF foci.[22] In 1969, the disease was also first recognized in regions adjacent to Rostov Oblast.[247]

Reasons for the 1963 CCHF outbreak in Rostov Oblast were attributed to changes in the rural economy and in agricultural and animal husbandry practices.[583] Late in the 1950s, agricultural enterprises were intensified and increased; weedy fields and pastures were plowed for growing grain; and cattle pastures were moved to virgin forest-steppes infested by numerous *Hyalomma m. marginatum*. Preliminary epidemiological studies began in 1964 as a cooperative program between the Rostov Regional Sanitary Epidemiological Station (V. D. Perelatov and colleagues) and the Moscow Institute of Poliomyelitis and Viral Encephalitides (M. P. Chumakov and colleagues). A multifaceted investigation initiated in 1966 included ecological, geographical, epidemiological, clinical, pathological, virological, and serological features of the disease and preventive and control measures and involved more than 20 senior scientists from four institutes. "In 1969, detailed study (of the disease) and determination of preventive measures by regional physicians and scientific workers of the four institutes reached a degree of harmony of action resulting in efficiency in the work". There is little published evidence of continuing research and surveillance in Rostov Oblast foci following the 1969 to 1971 decrease in CCHF morbidity.

The 11 cases observed from May to July 1963 were scattered in 9 or 10 settlements over a 1200-km² forest-steppe region along the stony northeastern slopes of Donets Ridge, where cattle were pastured between ploughed watershed areas and in forested and thicketed ravine bottoms. Ploughed fields and pastures near Donets Ridge were more extensive than in the loess hills and sandy soils elsewhere in Rostov Oblast.[409] Most CCHF patients were milkmaids who had crushed ticks with their hands (each milkmaid milked 18 to 25 cows two or three times daily[395]); others were dairy and agricultural workers, a child, and a physician accidentally infected in a hospital.[395,396]

Acaricide (1.5% chlorophos solution) treatment of cattle after July 1, 1964 was considered effective in reducing CCHF cases among milkmaids. Nine of the eleven patients were milkmaids in 1963 but only four milkmaids became ill in 1964 — all in May or June.[396,402]

The 1963 to 1969 morbidity rate in Rostov Oblast was 13.5 per 100,000 persons. The illness was seen each year in three endemic areas (Belaya Kalitva, Krasnyy Sulin, and Kamensk) with high morbidity rates (16.6, 22.8, and 50.5, respectively).[404] Most cases originated along the Donets Ridge, but smaller foci also appeared in the meadows, forests, and second-growth scrub of the Don River floodplain (Semikarakorsky and Tsimlysky regions). Male patients numbered 175, females 148. About 48% of the illnesses were severe, 32% moderate, and 20% mild; the average mortality was 15%. Among the 323 patients, there were 68 milkmaids, 65 cattleyard workers and shepherds, 43 farm workers, 55 other workers and employees, 3 medical workers (accidental infections), 55 housewives, 20 schoolchildren, and 14 "other persons."

An average of 13 adult *Hyalomma m. marginatum* were taken in each collection from cattle in 1968; in 1967 the average had been only 6. In the spring and summer of 1968, adult *H. m. marginatum* activity continued for 60 days and the highest CCHF incidence of any year was recorded. Many children in the 3- to 9-year age group were among the patients.

The winter of 1968 to 1969 was marked by exceptionally cold weather, high winds, and dust storms. In 1969, spring weather and adult tick activity began 3 or 4 weeks later than usual. Ticks were active for only 30 days and their numbers were considerably reduced. With less human-tick contact, CCHF cases fell from 131 in 1968 to 31 in 1969, and the number of recorded microfoci fell from 49 to 26. There was few cases in 1970 and 1971 and none in 1972 and 1973.

The 1971 abundance index of CCHF vector ticks infesting hosts (cattle, hares, rooks, and magpies) in the Rostov Oblast steppe biotope was only a small fraction of that rcorded in 1967, and *Rhipicephalus rossicus* replaced *Hyalomma m. marginatum* as the most commonly collected tick species. During this cycle of changing tick population numbers, *R. rossicus* and *Dermacentor marginatus* were found to have a role as CCHF virus reservoirs-vectors in Rostov Oblast. The timing of the first recognition of this role probably reflects researchers' use of the most easily available ticks in the 1969 to 1971 period of low *H. m. marginatum* density.

Until 1969, adult *H. m. marginatum* had made up 80% or more of the ticks taken from cattle, and this species was considered to be the only CCHF virus vector in Rostov Oblast. Numerous studies were devoted to the epidemiological aspects of adult *H. m. marginatum* on cattle (incidence, seasonal dynamics, distribution), methods for collecting ticks and data, risk of tick contact by different labor classes and age groups, control, etc. (Peralatov,[395] Peralatov et al.,[397,402,403] Pokrovsky et al.,[409] Perelatov and Chumakova,[399] Badalov et al.,[21,22] Bolovina et al.,[55] Karinskava et al.,[248] Maslennikov and Sorochinsky,[336] and Perelatov and Vostokova[404]). Special attention was given to educating agricultural workers and visitors to rural areas about the danger of handling or being bitten by *H. m. marginatum* and to adult tick control (Perelatov and Lazarev)[401] and many papers cited above). Because these measures proved to be expensive and inefficient, vaccination of high-risk personnel was suggested as a more realistic preventive action.[21] However, Kondratenko et al.[286] continued to recommend aircraft spraying of pastures (2% chlorophos at a rate of 50 to 100ℓ/ha) during the season of activity of unfed larval and adult *H. m. marginatum.*

Near the end of the 1963 to 1969 epidemic, 24% of the CCHF patients recognized *Hyalomma m. marginatum* as the tick that had bitten them before illness and 12% recognized *Dermacentor marginatus.* (The population density of *D. marginatus,*which is widely distributed in Rostov Oblast, apparently varied greatly from year to year.)

The percentages of human-tick contacts (ticks biting humans or being collected from animals) in May and June of 1968 in a CCHF focus were stated to be 57 for *H. m. marginatum,* 22 for *R. rossicus,* and 13 for *D. marginatus.*[22] The incidence of human-tick contacts was considered by other workers to be two or three times higher in the steppe than in the floodplain area.[284]

Following the cold 1968 to 1969 winter, the *Rhipicephalus rossicus* population density increased threefold over that of 1968, and this species replaced *H. m. marginatum* as the most common tick parasitizing cattle.[22] During 1969, 1429 ticks in 111 pools were tested for virus: *H. m. marginatum* (862 ticks/56 pools), *R. rossicus* (531/47), and *D. marginatus* (38/8).[283] CCHF virus was isolated from four pools of *H. m. marginatum* (nymphs from a rook; two females and one egg mass from cattle), from nine pools of *R. rossicus* (three adults from the European hare, two females from cattle, four females from the European hedgehog), and from the egg mass of a female *D. marginatus* from a cow.

Butenko et al.[66] also isolated CCHF virus from female *R. rossicus* parasitizing a hedgehog and from female *D. marginatus* parasitizing cattle in Belokalitvensky district of Rostov Oblast in May and June of 1971 (when there were few human infections). These findings were important because the immature stages of these two tick species parasitize a variety of small mammals (rodents, hedgehog, foxes, etc.) which are thus brought into the picture as part of the CCHF epidemiological chain. Unpublished serological and virological data showed CCHF virus infections in a common field mouse, *Apodemus sylvaticus,* and in hares and hedgehogs. Rabinovich et al.[421] also reported CCHF isolates from adult *R. rossicus* from hares and hedgehogs in Rostov Oblast and positive sera from hares in the AGDP test.

Rooks are hosts of immature *H. m. marginatum* in Rostov Oblast, but no detailed data on this subject appear to have been reported. Rabinovich et al.[421] isolated no virus from sera of 40 rooks and 171 other birds (12 species) in Rostov Oblast but did isolate CCHF virus from pools of nymphal *H. m. marginatum* from rooks. The early conclusion that rooks are the chief hosts of immature *H. m. marginatum* in Rostov Oblast[396,402] was later abandoned, and the European hare came to be considered as the chief host of *H. m. marginatum* and of *Rhipicephalus rossicus* in this Oblast.[400]

Of cattle sera from different Rostov Oblast, 9 to 52% CCHF foci were positive in the AGDP test for CCHF infection during 1968.[21] Neutralization test results gave "much higher" percentages of infections. Antibodies to the virus were also detected in horse sera but not in human sera (N, CF, and AGDP tests). The absence of immunity and the potential risk of infection in humans residing in rural communities were cited as showing the need for vaccinating these people. A more detailed serological study[248] also demonstrated a high rate of antibody reactions among domestic animals in September 1968 (at the end of the period of adult activity of *H. m. marginatum, Dermacentor marginatus, Rhipicephalus rossicus,* and *Haemaphysalis punctata*). Antibody rates were low in January to February 1969, and there were no antibodies in the same animals in May 1969. (Only *Hyalomma scupense* parasitized cattle from October to May; this species was not considered to be a vector.) Data from summer testing of domestic animal sera in different CCHF foci paralleled those from observations on human CCHF morbidity and tick population densities in the same foci.

The latest reported seroepidemiological survey in Rostov Oblast was in 1974. Zarubinski et al.[591] compared results of the AGDP test and the recently developed IHI test as tools for this purpose. In the Krasnyy Sulin focus, 26 (7.7%) of 336 cattle sera were positive in the AGDP test and 178 (53%) were positive in the IHI test. IHI tests were also positive for 4/20 sera from the European hare, *Lepus europaeus,* 2/5 sera from the common red fox, *Vulpes vulpes,* 1 common field mouse, *Apodemus sylvaticus,* one magpie, *Pica pica,* and four human beings who had recovered from CCHF 6 to 9 years earlier. In the AGDP test, all of these wild animal and human sera were negative. The unusual reaction in serum from a bird is discussed elsewhere.

A statistical analysis of interrelationships between CCHF morbidity, immature and adult *H. m. marginatum* numbers, and climatic factors in Rostov Oblast between 1964 and 1974 by Kondratenko et al.[285] pointed to certain critical epidemiological factors. The depth of frozen soil in winter was stated to be significant in the epidemiological process but the number of days with temperatures below −20°C was not a significant factor. I am unable to understand this reasoning. The experimental design on which these conclusions were based was only briefly described.

Kalmyk A.S.S.R.

Owing to its position between Astrakhan and Rostov Oblasts, favorable climatic conditions, and numerous *Hyalomma m. marginatum* on cattle, Durov[157] investigated sera of cattle and humans from this steppe area in May 1970 (too early in the season for reliable seroepidemiological results). Of 861 cattle sera, 3 were positive for antibodies to CCHF virus in the AGDP test but 360 human sera were negative. Two of 1443 earlier disease histories were suggestive of CCHF. When the seroepidemiological survey was extended,[158] 31 of 7966 cattle sera reacted against CCHF antigens. The virus was isolated from *H. m. marginatum* in the republic.[98,158]

Krasnodar Region (R.S.F.S.R.)

Krasnodar Region borders the Sea of Azov south of Rostov Oblast and extends to the Black Sea. On Taman peninsula, which projects into the Black Sea and is separated by a narrow strait from the Crimean Kerch peninsula, a few CCHF cases were seen during the 1944 epidemic. In 1948, 18 persons harvesting grain became ill with a disease[293] which Karinskaya et al.[247] and others considered as typical of CCHF.

In a 1970 to 1971 seroepidemiological survey using the AGDP test, no sera from 1035 apparently healthy persons were positive, but 13 of 450 sera from persons who had recovered from an "indistinct febrile disease" reacted against CCHF virus.[158] Nine of 11 sera from CCHF convalescents from Tuapse area, also reacted against the virus, and antibodies were detected in 2 of 5 patients from the 1948 outbreak more than 2 decades earlier. Thirty of 2567 cattle sera from Krasnodar Region were also positive for CCHF virus infection.

CCHF virus was isolated from a pool of 19 male *Rhipicephalus rossicus* taken from cattle in Seversky area in May 1971.[66] Infections in 12 of 60 preparations of *H. m. marginatum* salivary glands were demonstrated by the FA technique in May 1972.[113] Thus CCHF virus continues to circulate in Krasnodar, but human infections since 1948 have been diagnosed only retrospectively from results of seroepidemiological surveys.

Stavropol Region (R.S.F.S.R.)

Stavropol Region, an inland steppe plateau east of Krasnodar, lies between the Black Sea and the Caspian Sea. CCHF was first seen in agricultural and animal husbandry workers in 1953.[585,586] Among the 25 cases recorded in 1953 to 1968, 6 were in physicians, attendants, and relatives who had cared for CCHF patients. Twenty were from nine rural areas, five from Stavropol city. Most cases were traced to *Hyalomma m. marginatum* bites in spring and summer. The patients were a drayman, haymowers, an ox-driver in a brigade distributing water to haymowers, shepherds, a sheep shearer, and urban visitors to the countryside. Ages were 19 to 48 yr. Most were misdiagnosed before CCHF was proven by clinical or autopsy findings or by virus isolation. The disease was severe to very severe in 22 of the 25 patients and 11 died.[60,389,584,587]

Antibodies to CCHF virus were detected in AGDP and CF tests of sera from each of four regional residents who had experienced CCHF 12 years earliers.[158] An illness in a milkmaid, diagnosed in 1970 as "ulcerous gastric disease (with) hemorrhaging," was also proven serologically to have been CCHF and her clinical history was typical of CCHF. Sera from 1 of 350 cattle and 13 of 2748 sheep reacted positively for CCHF virus in AGDP tests in 1970 to 1971.

The tick fauna of Stavropol Region was reviewed by Reznik.[430]

Daghestan A.S.S.R.

This Autonomous republic, immediately southeast of Stavropol Region and bordering the western shore of the Caspian Sea, forms the northern sector of the Caucasus Mountain region. Berezin[32] discovered a CCHF focus in the Terek River delta of Kizlyar area, where the prevalence of antibodies to CCHF virus (average) was 23.5% in horses, 19.4% in cattle, and 2.3% in buffaloes. The prevalence in cattle was 35.1% in May, when adult *Hyalomma m. marginatum* were active, but decreased to 13.8% in September after the adult tick activity season. (Use of the HI, CF, N, and AGDP tests is mentioned in the introduction, but not elsewhere.)

Balkan Mountains/Plains (H. m. marginatum and Other Ticks)
Bulgaria

It has been suggested[234] that CCHF cases occurred in Razgrad and Kolarovograd areas in 1944 and that the virus was introduced into these and other Bulgarian areas by tick-infested horses or fodder of the Soviet army during World War II. There is no way to prove or disprove this theory. *Hyalomma m. marginatum* is common and widely distributed and since 1951 human CCHF has occurred in all Bulgarian districts except Gabrovo. Most of Bulgaria is an ecologically favorable environment for CCHF virus circulation in nature. Increased chances for human-tick contact, and other ecological and climatic factors, during the 1950 to 1960 period of agricultural collectivization provided the opportunity for a serious CCHF epidemic to develop.[139,234] The voluminous Bulgarian literature on CCHF published before 1967 contains many discrepancies and uncertain data which cannot now be resolved.

In 1953, during a massive effort to collectivize agriculture and plough virgin lands infested by *Hyalomma m. marginatum,* the occurrence of 50 CCHF cases with 6 fatalities aroused Bulgarian authorities to investigate the disease and its epidemiology. The first CCHF diagnosis in 1951[349,362] led Mironov[347] to examine disease histories and to recognize retrospectively that at least 10 CCHF cases from three localities had been hospitalized in Burgas distict from 1946 to 1952. In 1954 and 1955, there were 184 (36 fatal) and 248 (29 fatal) cases, respectively. From 1956 to 1959, the annual incidence fell to 20 to 29 and from 1960 to 1962 to 6 to 12 cases. Paralleling the morbidity pattern in Astrakhan Oblast, the incidence rose to 40 in 1963, 36 in 1964, and 29 in 1965.[139] In the 1953 to 1965 period, 717 cases were recorded. The morbidity rate in the Bulgarian population was 0.71%; the mortality rate among these cases was 17.02%. An additional 42 cases (17 fatal) resulted from contamination in hospitals where the disease was treated. I have seen no morbidity data for 1966 to 1967. The new scientific techniques to prove CCHF virus infection were first applied in 1968. In the 5-year period of 1968 to 1973, CCHF incidence fell to 129 cases (20 fatal).[560] During 1968 to 1972 virological and serological investigations of 184 CCHF suspect patients, 121 (16 fatal) were found to be infected and 103 CCHF strains were isolated from 114 patients or corpses.[562]

In 1953, 1954, and 1955, CCHF had been diagnosed in 8, 18, and 17 districts, respectively. From 1953 to 1965, 395 settlements (6.7%) of all those in Bulgaria) experienced the disease. The sporadic distribution of the disease in Bulgaria, as in Rostov Oblast, is noteworthy. In 79% of the known foci, the disease occurred only once. Cases were seen annually in some settlements but only for 1 or 2 years in others; in some villages there were intervals of several years between cases. Virus circulation throughout this period was especially intense in the Pazardzhik focus, where 13 cases were recorded in 1968 to 1970,[564] when the incidence elsewhere was waning.

Patients' age range was 3 to more than 60 years, but most were in the 21- to 50-year age group of robust working men (64.7%) and women (35.3%). Most patients were employed in agriculture or some form of animal husbandry; 6% worked in forests.

The seasonal dynamics of CCHF, appearing in April, reaching peak numbers in June, and disappearing by October, followed by about a month the first appearance, peak numbers, and declining numbers of adult *Hyalomma m. marginatum.*

Soon after the 1967 demonstration of the usefulness of NWM for CCHF virus investigations, Vasilenko et al.[561] isolated the virus from a human patient in Bulgaria and detected antibodies to the virus in AGDP tests of sera from people, sheep (28% positive), cattle (47%), and horses (82%). When they extended this survey, they also detected antibodies in sera of the European hare and found that goats showed high rates of positive reaction to the virus.[564,565] Between 1968 and 1972, the virus was isolated from human patients (as reported above) and from *Hyalomma m. marginatum, Rhipicephalus sanguineus,* and *Boophilus annulatus.*[560] In another brief report, Vasilenko et al.[563] stated that results of virological investigations of ticks from domestic animals showed these three species to have a role as vectors in Bulgarian CCHF foci, as well as *Ixodes (I.) ricinus, Rhipicephalus bursa* and *Dermacentor marginatus.* Serological results proved the presence of asymptomatic CCHF in humans. Different degrees of intensity of virus circulation were found in different localities, but in some places antibodies were detected in all domestic animals and in 18% of humans tending cattle. In CCHF foci during this 5-year period, antibodies were detected in 29.3% of 13,607 domestic animal sera, in 9.1% of 580 humans bitten by ticks, in 7.5% of 5398 persons working with cattle, and in 0.5% of other labor groups residing in these foci. A vaccine against CCHF given to 583 volunteers in 1970 and 1971 was considered to be highly efficient.

Hyalomma m. marginatum represented at least 50% of the ticks collected by Todorov et al.[529] in flat, hilly, and low mountain biotopes of southeastern Bulgaria, where 64 human cases involving 50 settlements had occurred from 1951 to 1958. Cattle were the chief hosts of adult *H. m. marginatum,* which first appeared in February, became more numerous in April, reached peak numbers in May, and decreased to a single specimen in November. During 1967 to 1968, *H. m. marginatum* represented about 90% of the 6565 ticks taken by Levi[323] from cattle (4856 ticks), horses (1278), and sheep (431) in settlements on the plains and in the foothills of the Pazardjik CCHF focus. Peak adult tick densities differed by a few weeks in lowland and foothill collection sites and from one summer to the next, depending on the number of rainy days. The first adult *H. m. marginatum* were seen in late March; otherwise, the Todorov et al.[529] and Levi[323] dynamics data are quite similar. (Studies by Levi and Vasilenko[325] on antibody reactions in laboratory rabbits and in ticks and on transstadial survival and transovarial transmission of CCHF virus in *H. m. marginatum* are reviewed elsewhere.)

Levi[324] collected ticks, mostly larvae and nymphs, from 513 wild birds, mammals, and reptiles in the Pazardjik CCHF focus. Of the 2582 ticks taken, 1243 were immature *H. m. marginatum* (Table 2). The chief hosts were the European hare, *Lepus europaeus,* little owl, *Athene noctua,* and European blackbird, *Turdus merula* — quite a different range of important hosts from those reported in Soviet foci of CCHF. Dryenski,[156] who studied *H. m. marginatum* biology in 1955 to 1957, stated that hares were uncommon in Bulgaria, but he did recommend hare destruction to control the tick.

In Bulgaria, larval *H. m. marginatum* parasitize birds and mammals from July to September (mostly July and August) and nymphs from July to October. (Many Euro-

Table 2

IMMATURE TICKS FROM WILD ANIMALS IN THE PAZARDJIK CCHF FOCUS, BULGARIA[324]

Host species	No. exam.	No. ticks	*Hyalomma m. marginatum*		*Haemaphysalis punctata*		*Dermacentor marginatus*		Other species	
			No.	Incidence (%)	No.	Incidence (%)	No.	Incidence (%)	No.	Incidence (%)
Testudo graeca	2	70	0		0		0		70	
Crocidura suaveolens	14	2	0		0		0		2	
Lepus europaeus	92	1836	1138	(62.0) 12.4	316	(17.2) 3.4	365	(19.9) 3.9	17	(0.9) 0.2
Rodents	174	73	3	(4.1) 0.02	1	(1.4) 0.01	61	(83.6) 0.4	8	(10.9) 0.05
Vulpes vulpes	2	7	0		0		0		7	
Pica pica	5	16	2	(12.5) 0.4	14	(87.5) 2.8	0		0	
Garrulus glandarius	9	8	2	(25.0) 0.2	6	(75.0) 0.7	0		0	
Passer montanus	13	1	0		1		0		0	
Alauda arvensis	3	1	0		1		0		0	
Motacilla flava feldegg	1	1	0		0		0		1	
Turdus merula	18	83	49	(59.0) 2.7	34	(40.9) 1.9	0		0	
Upupa epops	8	10	1	(10.0) 0.1	1	(10.0) 0.1	1	(10.0) 0.1	7	(70.0) 0.9
Caprimulgus europaeus	4	2	2		0		0		0	
Athene noctua	5	31	25	(80.6) 5.0	0		6	(19.4) 1.2	0	
Streptopelia turtur	11	1	0		1	0.1	0		0	
Charadrius dubius	1	1	1		0		0		0	
Perdix perdix	60	439	20	(4.6) 0.3	418	(95.6) 6.9	1	(0.2) 0.01	0	
Other species	91	0	0		0		0		0	
Total	513	2582	1243	(48.1)	793	(30.7)	434	(16.8)	112	(4.3)

pean bird species infested by immature *H. m. marginatum* begin their fall migration
to the Mediterranean area and Africa from late August to October). Earlier-detaching
nymphs molt to adults in the hot Bulgarian fall and overwinter before feeding; later-
detaching nymphs overwinter in the fed state and molt the following spring. Immature
Dermacentor marginatus and *Haemaphysalis punctata* also feed during the summer
but adults are active chiefly in spring and fall.[324]

The Bulgarian tick fauna has been listed by Surbova,[155,508-510] Levi, and Beron.[41,42]
Thirty-four species parasitizing mammals are recorded in the 1974 list. Among these
was a male *Amblyomma variegatum*, which had undoubtedly been carried to Bulgaria
as a nymph on a bird migrating from Africa,[322] where this species has been found
infected by CCHF virus. A male *A. hebraeum* (a common parasite of domestic and
wild animals in southern Africa) was also taken from a cow in southern Bulgaria.[390]

CCHF virus has not been isolated from the common field mouse, *Apodemus sylva-
ticus,* or from the other rodents or insectivores which are numerous in Bulgarian
CCHF foci.[338] These small mammals interest us as hosts of *Dermacentor marginatus,
Haemaphysalis punctata,* and *Ixodes ricinus,* which maintain endemic circulation of
CCHF virus in some areas.

Yugoslavia

Eight CCHF cases were diagnosed clinically in 21- to 54-year-old rural inhabitants
of Kosovo and Metokhiya Autonomous Oblasts in the summers of 1954 to 1967.[201,202]
About one half of the ticks found on domestic animals in CCHF foci in 1967 were
Hyalomma m. marginatum. Large flocks of rooks assembled in the evenings on roofs
of village houses and fed by day in fields. The role of these birds in maintaining the
H. m. marginatum population and other aspects of CCHF epidemiology has not been
investigated in Yugoslavia. In a brief symposium paper Smirnova and Chumakov[486]
stated that they had serologically confirmed the presence of CCHF foci in Yugoslavia.
However, "about 15 sera presumably containing CF antibodies when tested (in Yugoslavia) were sent (to YARU), where they were found to be negative or nonspecific".[74]

Obradović and Gligić (personal communication) stated in 1978 (Symposium on Arboviruses in the Eastern Mediterranean Countries, Brač) that the first serologically
confirmed CCHF epidemic in Yugoslavia occurred in 1970 in Čiflik village near Te-
tovo, Macedonia. Thirteen members of a family became ill; two died. AGDP and CF
antibodies were detected in sera of the survivors 3 years later; the CF titers were 1:4
to 1:32.

Greece

CCHF virus was isolated from *Rhipicephalus bursa* taken from goats in Vergina,
Macedonia, in May 1975.[388] In AGDP tests of sera from northern Greece, 139 (32.9%)
of 422 from goats and 34 (11.6%) of 294 from sheep were positive for antibodies to
CCHF virus.

Turkey

Of 1100 human sera from Turkey, 26 were positive in HI tests at YARU.[14]

Transcaucasia (*H. m. marginatum* and other ticks)

The first of several brief studies on CCHF virus in Transcaucasia was published
in 1972. Much remains to be learned epidemiologically in these highlands and lowlands, separated from the rest of the Soviet Union by the rugged, 800-km-long range
of great Caucasus mountains extending from the northeastern shore of the Black
Sea to the Apsheron Peninsula jutting into the Caspian Sea. Paralleling the Great
Caucasus to the south is the Rioni-Kuru depression and further south the Lesser Cau-

casus range. The Great Caucasus shelter the republics of Georgia, Armenia, and Azerbaijan from the bitterly cold air movements that characterize winters north of the mountains. Transcaucasia interests us ecologically and geographically because it represents the southeastern limit of *Hyalomma m. marginatum* in the Soviet Union. (The geographic range of this tick continues around the southern shores of the Caspian Sea in northern Iran.) However, other tick species have yielded the virus, and the environmental diversity of the area suggests that in Transcaucasia the CCHF epidemiological network may be more complex than in the steppe foci to the north.

Georgian S.S.R.

I have seen no mention of CCHF or of seroepidemiological surveys in this republic (or in Abkhaz A.S.S.R. to the north). One wonders whether the virus circulates in the broadly triangular Kholkida Lowland, facing the Black Sea, with its humid subtropical climate and rich evergreen vegetation. The Georgian lowlands are bordered in the south by treeless mountains extending from Armenia and in the east by dry elevated steppes extending from Azerbaijan.

Armenian S.S.R.

Chubkova[87] stressed the need to study natural foci of diseases in Armenia because of the constant growth of cities and villages and the establishment of population centers in recently reclaimed areas of the republic. Armenia is a high, dry tableland surrounded by mountains that prevent entry of humid winds. The lowest altitude, in the Araks Valley, is 900 m; the highest is more than 2500 m. At 1500 m, winter temperatures are like those in Moscow. Lake Sevan and high mountain streams provide water for irrigated agriculture and hydroelectric power for industry. Much of the landscape is semidesert or steppe, stony, boulder-strewn, or lava-covered. Forests occur only in the higher mountains. The scanty alpine meadows are used for summer pastures and hayfields. Grain is grown in some localities. Cotton and sugar beet fields and orchards are common where irrigation is available.

Semashko et al.[458] reported nine CCHF isolations during 1972 to 1974 from *H. m. marginatum* (five), *H. anatolicum* (one), *B. annulatus* (one), *R. bursa* (one), and *R. rossicus* (one). Matevosyan et al.[339,340] warned of the CCHF risk in Armenia after having detected AGDP antibodies to the virus in cattle sera from five areas of the republic and isolating seven CCHF strains from *Hyalomma m. marginatum* (four strains), *H. anatolicum* (one), *Rhipicephalus bursa* (one), and *Boophilus annulatus* (one) from cattle. No isolates were obtained from *Hyalomma detritum, H. scupense, Ixodes ricinus,* or *Argas persicus.*

Human CCHF in Armenia was first serologically proven in 1974 but clinically similar cases had been observed earlier in this republic. CCHF virus infection was confirmed in the CF and AGDP tests after inoculating the patient's blood into NWM.[242,456,458] The severely ill patient had removed an attached tick from his leg while shearing sheep on a collective farm in the Sisian mountain steppe. This zone, characterized by a dry, temperate climate and 350 to 400 mm annual rainfall, borders the Gissar Mountains where CCHF is most common in Tadzhikistan. Most positive domestic animal sera reported by Matevosyan et al.[339,340] from Armenia were from this mountain steppe belt.

Azerbaijan S.S.R.

This republic, in the southeastern corner of Transcaucasia, bordered by Armenia and the Caspian Sea to the west and east and by the Great Caucasus (Daghestan A.S.S.R.) and Iran to the north and south, is mostly a hot lowland steppe with a dry continental climate. Higher steppes and mountain slopes are cooler. Mountain forests are sparse except on the southern slopes of the Caucasus and in the Talysh range, where abundant rainfall supports a rich, diverse vegetation. The Kura River flowing from the Great Caucasus into the extensive Kura-Araks lowland steppe provides irrigation water for cotton, lucerne, wheat, rice, sesame, melons, and vegetables. Herdsmen use unirrigated lowland steppes for winter camps (kishlaks) and in the hot summer drive their animals to cooler mountains, some as far as Armenia. Fruit orchards, sericulture, and tobacco fields replace native vegetation in southern foothills and in Great Caucasus valleys. The southern strip of the Caspian Sea coastal plain, the Lenkoran (Talysh) lowland, is tropical and humid.

Results of a seroepidemiological survey of domestic animals from 12 administrative areas in four physical-geographical zones of Azerbaijan (the Kura-Araks floodplain, Great Caucasus, Lesser Caucasus, and Lenkoran) in 1967 to 1972 indicated that CCHF virus is widely but irregularly distributed throughout the republic, except possibly in the Kura-Araks floodplain, where there were no positive reactions in cattle sera. Elsewhere, antibodies to the virus were detected in 2 to 26% of the cattle sera tested. Antibodies in donkey sera from 4 villages ranged from 0 to 100% (average 18%), but all horse sera were negative, presumably because these animals are kept in tick-free barns. Of 99 sheep sera from two farms, fifteen were positive for antibodies to CCHF virus.[233,339]

Nikiforov et al.[364] isolated CCHF virus from a pool of 56 male *Rhipicephalus bursa* from a cow in the Ismail region of the northern Caucasus foothills. The cow had been grazing in a steppe pasture between higher foothill forests and the wormwood-saltwort semidesert of the Kura-Araks lowland. The likelihood of endemic CCHF in the steppe pastures of the southern foothills of the Great Caucasus, where cattle and *R. bursa* are common, is suggested. Ten CCHF strains were also isolated from *Hyalomma m. marginatum* parasitizing cattle in Dzhalilabad, Massalin, and Sabirabad districts.[455,458,459]

Using the FA test to demonstrate CCHF infections in tick salivary glands, Chumakov et al.[113] obtained the following results (number of preparations per number of positive): *Boophilus annulatus* from Lenkoran in May 1970 (16/1) and from Soalty in September 1970 (62/4), *Hyalomma m. marginatum* from Sabirabad in April 1972 (60/14), and *H. detritum* from Sabirabad in May 1972 (50/13).

Asian Foci [Southeastern Palearctic Faunal Region; Semideserts, Steppes, Foothills (**Hyalomma** and Other Ticks)]

Semideserts, steppes, river floodplains, irrigated valleys, or grassy foothill environments characterize most known southeastern Palearctic CCHF foci, together with a dry continental climate and hot summers but relatively moderate or mild winters. There also appears to be some virus activity in the mountains of southeastern Kazakhstan, but the very recent information is poorly documented. Local CCHF outbreaks, but no large-scale epidemics, have been reported from Asia. For this reason, and the remoteness of many infested foci, surveillance and awareness of the dangers of CCHF were often nil or slight. Unexpected episodes of the tick-transmitted disease frequently took a fearful toll of family members, friends, and medical attendants who were contaminated by bloody discharges from patients in their care.

The ticks incriminated in CCHF virus epidemiology in the southeastern part of the Palearctic faunal region are *Hyalomma anatolicum anatolicum, H. asiaticum asiaticum, H. marginatum turanicum, H. detritum, Rhipicephalus bursa, R. pumilio, R. sanguineus, R. turanicus, Dermacentor marginatus, D. daghestanicus,* and *Boophilus annulatus* (family Ixodidae), and *Argas persicus* (family Argasidae).

Soviet Middle Asia
Turkmen S.S.R.*

Mikhailov[345] reported a hospital outbreak in Turkmenia (locality unstated, apparently for military security reasons) in which a fatal CCHF case was the source of illness in six patients and attendants in the same ward. Only one survived. Human CCHF has occurred sporadically in Turkmenia since 1946[491] and the presence of endemic foci has recently been demonstrated with the aid of the new serological and virus isolation tools that became available in 1967 to 1968.

Formerly part of Iran, more than 90% of Turkmenia is clay or sand desert or arid steppe. This is the hottest and driest of the middle Asian republics. In the south, mountains up to about 3000 m altitude border Iran. The valleys of the Murgab and Tedzhen Rivers, flowing from the mountains some distance into the desert, are dotted with fertile oases which have been cultivated for centuries. After World War II, construction of the 500-mile (800-km) Kara Kum irrigation canal through the black sands (*kara kum*), from Kelif on the Amu Darya River in the east to Ashkhabad in the west, brought more than a million acres (400,000 ha) of desert into cultivation and numerous immigrants to southern Turkmenia from other parts of the U.S.S.R.

Kurbanov et al.[302,303] who studied the ticks of the newly irrigated and desert areas near the Kara Kum canal, summarized the climate as follows: mean annual air temperature 16 to 17°C, absolute maximum 48 to 50°C, absolute minimum −26 to − 30°C, sum of effective temperatures above 10°C 5000 to 5500°C, frostless period 210 to 250 days, annual rainfall 125 to 288 mm. Ticks recorded from cattle, camels, and sheep were *Hyalomma marginatum turanicum, H. asiaticum asiaticum, H. anatolicum excavatum, H. anatolicum anatolicum, H. dromedarii, H. detritum, Rhipicephalus turanicus,* and *Boophilus annulatus.* Camels were most heavily infested. The infestation patterns differed distinctly in deserts and in oases (considerable data are listed). Other authors also mention *R. pumilio, R. bursa,* and *R. sanguineus, H. a. asiaticum* is most closely associated with desert and semidesert landscapes; the other species are most common in and near cultivated areas.

Kurbanov et al.[302,303] isolated CCHF virus from *H. a. asiaticum* and detected CF antibodies against the virus in 2.5% of 283 human sera from four of five localities. However, their work is chiefly important for elucidating the tick fauna in the regions of southern Turkmenia where other workers have demonstrated the presence of endemic CCHF virus.

In and near the Murgab River valley, Chunikhin et al.[121] detected antibodies to CCHF virus in sera of the long-clawed ground squirrel, *Spermophilopsis leptodactylus,* taken from the smooth sand and shrub (*Calligonum*) desert, and of the long-eared hedgehog, *Hemiechinus auritus,* taken from riverside tugai vegetation (poplar, tamarisk, and other trees). Immature *Hyalomma a. asiaticum* infested all ground squirrels and 10% of the hedgehogs. *Rhipicephalus* spp. were most common on the hedgehog.

---

* The following reference was received while this manuscript was in press: Smirnova, S. E., Mamaev, V. I., Nepesova, N. M., Filipenko, P. I., Kalyaeva V. Ya., and Chumakov, M. P., 1978. Study of circulation of Crimean hemorrhagic fever vius in Turkmen S.S.R. *Zh. Mikrobiol. Epidemiol. Immunobiol.,* 55: 92-97. (In Russian). (In English, NAMRU3-T1296).

In May, 1976, CCHF virus was isolated from 2 of 56 pools containing 654 *Hyalomma dromedarii* from camels from Krasnovodsk Oblast. This is the first record of CCHF virus from *H. dromedarii.* (Thus 26 tick species are now associated with this virus.) Three strains were also isolated from 98 pools containing 1284 *H. a. asiaticum* from sheep from Geok-Tepe. By the IFA test, CCHF virus infections in salivary glands were detected in 9 of 52 *H. dromedarii* and in 5 of 36 *H. asiaticum.* No human cases were reported in the 1968 to 1976 period but CF antibodies to the virus were detected in sera of two students, two medical workers, four animal husbandry workers, and one farmer from four oblasts. Antibodies were also detected in sera from sheep, goats, cattle, camels, and long-clawed ground squirrels from different biotopes and oblasts. The potential for CCHF outbreaks in Turkmenia is discussed.

Domestic and wild animal sera collected from four localities in 1966 to 1967 showed positive reactions to CCHF virus in the CF and AGDP tests in sheep (80%) from the sandy Ashkhabad area and in the hedgehog, hare, fox, Pallas (steppe) cat, great gerbil, and long-clawed ground squirrel; antibodies were most often detected in the ground squirrel sera.[494] All of 445 sera from healthy humans from eight rural areas were negative in these tests. Serological studies continued in the summer of 1969 with 1252 samples from 12 state and collective farms in the Ashkhabad. Bakhardan, Geok-Teppe, and Tedzhen regions.[489] On 8 of the 12 farms, 3.5% to 31.0% of cattle sera and 5.9% to 32.0% of goat and sheep sera were positive against CCHF antibodies. Cattle sera positives increased from 31.0% to 58.6% from early to late summer. No virus was isolated from 284 specimens of *Rhipicephalus bursa,* 60 *R. pumilio,* or 44 *R. sanguineus* taken in a cultivated locality in 1970. However, using the FAT, CCHF virus, infection was demonstrated in the salivary glands from these 3 *Rhipicephalus* species as well as in *Hyalomma a. asiaticum* from several regions.[113,603] Also with aid of the FAT, Aristova et al.[19] found one pool of 30 male *H. anatolicum* to be infected; these ticks were from cattle in the Murgab valley. Negative results were recorded for 423 other specimens of *H. anatolicum,* 725 *H. a. asiaticum* and 40 *H. dromedarii,* all from domestic animals in and near cultivation in southeastern Turkmenia in the spring of 1972. Later, Smirnova et al.[491] isolated 35 CCHF strains from 161 pools (21.7%) of *H. a. asiaticum* (1730 ticks) from camels in the sandy zone of Ashkhabad area; 29 strains were from male and 6 from female ticks. Seven pools of 84 *H. a. asiaticum* from cattle, sheep, and goats in foothills near Ashkhabad yielded no virus and 24 pools of *Rhipicephalus turanicus* from cattle, sheep, and goats in the sandy and foot-hill zones were also negative. CF and AGDP tests of 1266 sheep and goat sera showed 149 (11.8%) reacting against CCHF antibodies; 18.4% of the positive responses were from sand deserts where infected *H. a. asiaticum* had been collected from camels.

Smirnova et al.[491] made a special point of the successful isolation of CCHF virus from ticks infesting camels, of the lowland desert landscape in which CCHF foci have been demonstrated in Turkmenia, and of the proximity of these foci to areas recently populated by nonimmune persons. Kurbanov et al.[302,303] also stressed the number of ticks and variety of species taken from camels in southern Turkmenia and the risk of human exposure to infected ticks.

Uzbek S.S.R.

CCHF in Uzbekistan was earlier considered to be a CCHF-related disease — "Uzbekistan hemorrhagic fever" or "Central Asian hemorrhagic fever" — because of the severe disease course, the frequent infections acquired from patients in hospitals or in rural homes, and the high mortality rate in this republic (and also in Kazakhstan). Obviously, great differences in the environments and in the biology of the tick species frequently biting humans in European and Asian areas of the Soviet Union contributed additional circumstantial support for this assumption. However, after the CCHF agent was characterized and the Uzbek virus (notably the Khodzha strain) was tested serologically against other strains from the Soviet Union and Bulgaria, all proved to be identical.[101,112,114]

Nine cases of an "infectious hemorrhagic capillary toxicosis" seen in the Termez City Hospital (on the Uzbekistan-Afhganistan border) during the summer of 1944[462] were retrospectively considered to have been CCHF. The patients were adult grain harvesters, four of whom died after 4 to 5 days in the hospital. Local farmers knew the disease as *khungribta* or *khunymuny.* Other cases acquired in the field and from association with patients in the Tashkent hospital in 1937 and in 1947 to 1948 were described by Fedulov et al.[166,258,259,519] (See also Khodukin[266] and Gajdusek.[178])

Many clinical observations and epidemiological results of hemorrhagic fever research by physicians, pathologists, entomologists, microbiologists, and epidemiologists during a 3-year program under the aegis of the Uzbek Ministry of Public Health were published in a 159-page book edited by Khodukin.[265] However, attempts to obtain experimental proof of infection in humans, domestic animals, and ticks failed because of the primitive research methods. *Hyalomma anatolicum* was considered to be the chief vector and 22 CCHF strains were purported to have been isolated from *H. anatolicum* (17), *H. detritum* (2), *R. turanicus* (2), and *R. sanguineus* (1) (see also Shapiro and Levinzon[469]).

Pre-1964 CCHF morbidity data from Uzbekistan were summarized by Meliev.[343,344] Uzbek physicians first recognized CCHF in 1944, but it had long been known as *karak halak,* or "black death", among the indigenous population. Between 1948 and 1963, 525 cases were recorded in 361 foci. Many other cases probably went unseen or misdiagnosed by physicians unacquainted with the disease; homestead and nosocomial cases were common.

Uzbekistan covers a variety of desert, semidesert, steppe, river floodplain, foothill, and high mountain landscapes. CCHF was recorded only from oases in semideserts, foothills, the plains-steppe subzone, and floodplains (not deserts) of six oblasts (Samarkand, Surkhandar'ya, Tashkent, Andizhan, Fergana, and Bukhara), but not from Khorezm Oblast or from Karakalpak A.S.S.R. *H. a. anatolicum* is apparently an important vector of the virus and common in much of Uzbekistan. Thus Meliev[343,344] believed that human cases are probably more widely distributed than the data show. *H. a. anatolicum* is active throughout the year in warm areas and some human cases have occurred in winter. However, the seasonal dynamics of peak tick numbers and activity and of human morbidity are closely interrelated; most ticks and most human cases occur in June, July, and August. Almost all patients inhabited rural areas: 60% were collective farm workers, 9% were rural school children; the age range was 2 to 70 years, with 83% in the working age group (15 to 50 years old). The findings for *H. a. anatolicum* were much like those reported from Tadzhikistan, but it was also observed that many ticks are present in rural homes where cattle are kept at night and that ticks fed on humans from March to November. *H. anatolicum* composed 48 to 94% of all *Hyalomma* collected throughout the year from different parts of Uzbekistan.[40]

An early study in Uzbek CCHF foci[358] showed the most common ticks on domestic animals to be *H. anatolicum* (49%), *H. detritum* (10%), and *Boophilus annulatus* (37%). Other species, *H. marginatum (turanicum), Rhipicephalus pumilio, Ornithodoros (Alveonasus) lahorensis,* etc. were less common.

In the Surkhandar'ya River tugai landscape, Chunikhin et al.[121] detected antibodies to CCHF virus in sera of cattle, 34% of which were infested by adult *Rhipicephalus pumilio.* In sedge and meadow grass landscapes of nearby foothills and low mountains, antibodies were also detected in sera of cattle and sheep. Several tick species infested the cattle; adult *R. pumilio* were found on approximately 10% of the sheep.

The only post-1968 attempts to isolate CCHF virus from ticks in Uzbekistan were reported briefly by Chumakov[98] and in more detail by Chumakov et al.[117] Isolates from adult ixodids taken from cattle in Samarkand and Andizhan Oblasts in April and May of 1973 were one from *Hyalomma marginatum turanicum* (1 pool/20 ticks), one from *H. anatolicum* (1/5), four from *H. detritum* (6/115), one from *H. asiaticum* (1/1), one from *Dermacentor marginatus* (1/3), two from *Rhipicephalus pumilio* (5/59), and one from *Boophilus annulatus* (5/57).

Two CCHF isolates from eight pools containing 515 *Argas persicus* from chicken coops in Samarkand Oblast[117] constitute the only record of this virus from an argasid tick and from a tick parasitizing only birds. Because of the perplexing questions regarding circulation of the virus in a tick-host chain confined to birds, it would be desirable to attempt to repeat these results.

A single CCHF isolate from *Rhipicephalus turanicus* was reported by Chumakov et al.,[117] but *R. turanicus* was not listed in the table. The report was repeated by Chumakov.[98]

Sidorova[475] stated the need to investigate CCHF virus circulation in *Hyalomma a. asiaticum* and in the great gerbil, *Rhombomys opimus,* and other small mammals inhabiting the burrow systems of this gerbil in southern Uzbekistan.

Human CCHF caused by contact with an animal from an endemic area, where it had probably been the host of infected ticks, occurred in Guzar region, Kashkadar'ya Oblast, Uzbekistan.[116] Three CCHF cases were described in persons who skinned and butchered a sick cow with a disease diagnosed as acute gastritis. The patients became ill 3 days afterward and died with typical CCHF symptoms 7 and 8 days after killing the cow. Five days after these deaths, a surgical ward nurse who had cared for the patients fell ill but survived despite a very severe disease course with numerous hemorrhages. CCHF virus was isolated from two patients and the convalescent serum of the nurse showed antibodies to the virus. In the same region in 1973, two more CCHF isolates were obtained at autopsy from organs of humans who had been bitten by ticks.

In this connection, it is interesting to recall that in the Rift Valley of Kenya, Nevill[363] had reported numerous deaths of adult Africans due to a rapidly progressive hemorrhagic disease (?CCHF) clinically similar to one in cattle in nearby forest margins.

Kazakh S.S.R.

About 75 CCHF cases, more than half of them fatal, were recorded between 1948 and 1968 in Kazakhstan.[135,442,518] Published data on early disease incidence differ. For instance, Kereev[263] (quoted by Pak and Mikhailova[383]) reported 80 cases from 1948 to 1964. Known foci gradually increased in number, but until 1964 evidence existed only for localities in the arid western part of Chimkent Oblast near the Kazakh-Uzbek border. The illness and the dangers of contact infection were seldom realized until too late in rural homes and in hospitals. Numerous relatives, friends, and hospital attendants died after contracting the disease from patients who had been bitten by infected ticks or who had crushed infected ticks. Subsequently CCHF has been recognized in different biotopes of this vast republic, and the most recent information suggests active virus circulation in Alma Ata, Chimkent, Dzhambul, and Kzyl-Orda oblasts of southern Kazakhstan. However, data are scanty and much remains to be learned about CCHF epidemiology in this republic.

Kazakhstan, stretching from the lower Volga and the Caspian Sea eastward to China and from the Trans-Siberia railway line south to the Tien Shan Mountains, is larger than all other Soviet republics combined, excluding R.S.F.S.R. Except for high mountains in the southeast (the Altai, Tasbagati, and ridges of the Tien Shan system), most of the republic is a vast plain, broken in the central area by hills, with less than 300 mm annual rainfall, few permanent rivers, and only salty lakes. Average January temperature is −20°C in the north, −4°C in the south; in July these averages are 20°C and 29°C, respectively. The grassy northern steppes were long used as pastures for animals from the south; in 1954 some 8 million ha of virgin land were ploughed for growing grain (CCHF virus is not known to occur in northern Kazakhstan). Wormwood and saltwort semideserts characterize much of the southern plains. The Caspian lowland and part of Ust-Urt Plateau are important topographical-ecological features of the west. Forests occur only in high mountains, river valleys (tugai), and in some southern sands (saxaul). The Altai and Tien Shan foothills are agriculturally rich.

Early CCHF patients in Chimkent Oblast were cattle herders, a woman who had been weeding cotton on the Karl Marx Collective Farm, a melon-field watchman, the family of a plum orchard worker, a pregnant wife of a railway employee, and several family members and hospital attendants who had cared for the patients.[135,518]

On June 11, 1962, a housewife from the Dzhilga railway settlement was brought on a cargo train to the Tashkent first aid station, where she died of CCHF.[135,387] Three days after her death, seven members of her family (son, daughter, husband, daughter-in-law, etc., 6 to 76 years old) were observed to be febrile and hospitalized. An eighth person, a neighbor, became ill 2 days later. All the patients except a 6- and 8-year-old son and daughter suffered a severe disease course; of the eight only the two children and a 45-year-old man survived despite the early hospitalization and intensive care given them. Notably in this instance, none of the medical and hospital personnel who had attended these patients and performed autopsies became ill. Dzhilga settlement was in an uncultivated sandy plain where water was obtained only from a railway pipeline and salty wells. Railway workers and state sheep farm employees grazed cattle and sheep among mounds 2 to 5 km from Dzhilga. The animals, which were tied up at night beside the clay huts of the village, were heavily infested by *Hyalomma anatolicum* and *H. detritum.* These ticks were numerous in cracks of practically all homestead walls. *Ornithodoros (Alveonasus) lahorensis* was also found in the walls. The platform on which the fatally ill housewife slept sheltered many ticks, and she often placed her mattress to air outdoors beside a clay wall sheltering ticks. Large colonies of ground squirrels were seen in the pastures.

Another example of contact infections occurred in 1966 in the Abay State Farm of Kelessky region.[518] A 60-year-old pensioner went to cut scripus (a weed) for the household cow in the Kur-Keles River floodplain, where he was attacked by some of the numerous *Hyalomma anatolicum* in the vegetation. Shortly afterward he became ill. At the hospital he was diagnosed as having influenza but died after intestinal hemorrhages and epistaxis developed. He was nursed by his wife and 18-year-old son, a tractor driver. Eight and 9 days after the pensioner had first become sick, they became ill and died a few days later despite medical assistance.

In Chimkent Oblast, CCHF foci are known in four areas in foothills and steppes, three areas in plains, floodplains, and irrigation canal systems, and one area in a semidesert where nomadic cattle pass.[518] In addition to the usual patients from state farms, animal husbandry enterprises, and rural homes with privately owned cattle, one patient was a woman who skinned animals in the Chimkent City Meat Combine. The inference was that she became ill from handling an infected carcass. Two wintertime (January) infections occurred on the 21st Party Conference State Farm in Bugun region, where *Hyalomma* ticks remain active throughout the year. A 46-year-old milkmaid died but her 16-year-old son survived the illness. However, most cases are seen during the spring-summer season of greatest *Hyalomma* tick activity. Efforts to control *H. anatolicum* in Chimkent Oblast were described by Dobritsa et al.[136]

Results of a seroepidemiological (ADGP test) survey of 26 farms in 11 regions of Chimkent Oblast in the winter of 1973 and spring and fall of 1974 indicated a low intensity of CCHF virus circulation.[460] None of 115 sera from healthy persons was positive. Six of 842 cattle sera, 3 of 832 sheep and goat sera, and 1 of 428 fowl sera were positive.

A total of 72 CCHF cases, chiefly among rural inhabitants was recorded in Chimkent Oblast between 1948 and 1972,[263,427] but the disease is now relatively rare there. Rapoport et al.[423] suggested that under the conditions of recent agricultural development, Chimkent Oblast CCHF virus foci have been reduced in numbers and extent.

Contemporary foci are chiefly in cotton fields and irrigated grain fields, orchards, and gardens near semidesert zones. The population densities of small- and medium-sized mammals are low in most of these agriculturally modified foci. The predominant vector species are *Hyalomma a. anatolicum, H. detritum,* and *Boophilus annulatus,* which spend their entire life cycles on domestic animals; *H. marginatum turanicum,* whose immatures infest chiefly birds; and *H. a. asiaticum,* whose immatures feed on burrowing mammals in the semidesert zone. The tick abundance index on domestic animals during the warm season is 1.6 to 8.3.[423]

In Kzyl-Orda Oblast, north of Chimkent Oblast, a shepherd died of CCHF in the Chili Regional Hospital and his wife, a nurse, and a sanitarian who attended him contracted the disease.[122] The shepherd had fallen ill on May 2, 1964 after spending April at an animal breeding farm in the grassy northern Kara-Tai foothills, where many large-toothed susliks, *Citellus fulvus,* were seen (these ground squirrels are common hosts of immature *Hyalomma a. asiaticum*). In mid-May, a season of low tick activity, 10% to 15% of the sheep at this farm were infested by adult *H. a. asiaticum,* but in April ticks were reportedly more numerous.

The 1964 disease episode led to a seroepidemiological and virological survey of Kzyl-Orda Oblast,[183,493] which became effective only after the 1967 characterization of CCHF virus.

This large oblast in the northern desert zone of Soviet Central Asia is traversed by the Syr-Darya River flowing from the Tien Shan Mountains south of Tashkent. The broad floodplain with tugai and pasture vegetation and irrigated fields (especially rice) is bordered by foothills, saltwort desert with sand islands, salt marshes, and clay flats (*takyr*).[183] The 100 to 180 mm of annual rainfall is confined chiefly to winter and spring, but snow is rare. Small carnivores (the wolf, common fox, corsac fox, and marten) are found everywhere. Large-toothed susliks were numerous but great gerbils were absent in the Chili CCHF focus, where CCHF occurred in 1964. Great gerbils, *Rhombomys opimus,* were abundant and susliks absent in the Dzhalagash focus, where CCHF occurred in 1967. Hares were common in the floodplain but absent in the desert. No nesting rooks were observed in Kzyl-Orda Oblast. Almost all (96 to 99.6%) goats, sheep, camels, and horses inspected were infested by adult *Hyalomma a. asiaticum* but only 2.5% of the cattle; the average numbers taken from sheep were 10.8 in April, 4.3 in May, 5.4 in June, and 5.2 in July. Fewer specimens were collected of *H. marginatum* (subspecies *turanicum*), *H. anatolicum* (subspecies probably *anatolicum*), *H. detritum, H. scupense, Dermacentor daghestanicus,* and *Rhipicephalus pumilio.*

Eight cases of CCHF with two fatalities were recorded between 1964 and 1968 in shepherds and village students on collective farms where sheep were raised in the sandy zone and in the floodplain-foothill zones of Kzyl-Orda Oblast. Three of the eight cases were caused by contact with patients. The 1968 illness was confirmed as CCHF in the CF test. CF tests of sera of shepherds from five regions of the oblast showed 2.7 to 5.9% to be positive for CCHF reactions, but all AGDP tests were negative. On two collective farms, none of 6 sheep and goat sera and none of 62 cattle sera were positive for CCHF in the AGDP test. However, in 701 sheep and goat sera from five other collective farms, positive AGDP reactions ranged from 14 to 44%. Infected *Hyalomma a. asiaticum* bites were the source of the human cases, but *H. anatolicum* was considered to be a potential vector in the floodplain and foothill zones.

The clinical and laboratory findings of a severe case of CCHF seen in a rice-field laborer from the Chili area in June 1972 were described by Smirnova et al.[488] The patient had found a tick biting him 2 days before the illness began. Karimov et al.[246] also reported CCHF virus isolation from two shepherds from the desert zone (where *Hyalomma a. asiaticum* is common) who died in the Kzyl-Orda Regional Hospital in 1974. They also detected AGDP antibodies to the virus in domestic animal sera from this oblast (Syr-Darya and Kazalin regions) and from Dzhambul Oblast (Dzhambul region). CF antibodies to CCHF virus were detected in 5 of 254 human sera from Kzyl-Orda and Dzhambul oblasts.

In 1971, 1500 *Hyalomma a. asiaticum* taken in the spring from two areas (details unstated) of Kzyl-Orda Oblast were innoculated into NWM and guinea pigs.[493] Of 29 pathogenic agents recovered from the inoculated mice, 16 were identified as CCHF virus by serial passage in NWM and by CF, AGDP, and N tests and the FA test. The results suggest a good deal of CCHF virus activity in Kzyl-Orda Oblast and the importance of *H. a. asiaticum* as a vector. This study capped a 5-year investigation (reported in more detail by Genis et al.[183]) during which serological results from domestic animal sera had provided data that permitted the authors to pinpoint the most likely times and places for collecting the tick species (*H. a. asiaticum*) most likely to be infected by CCHF virus. Before 1971, when fewer ticks were tested and there was a question of proper conditions for bringing ticks to the virus laboratory, no virus had been isolated from *H. a. asiaticum, H. detritum,* or *H. scupense* in Kzyl-Orda Oblast.

Using the FAT to demonstrate CCHF infections in salivary gland preparations of ticks taken during the 1970 to 1972 spring seasons in Kzyl-Ora Oblast, Chumakov et al.[113] obtained the following results (number of preparations per number of positive): *Hyalomma a. asiaticum* (379/128), *H. detritum* (10/2), *Dermacentor daghestanicus* (1/1) (all from Teremozchsky region), and *D. daghestanicus* from Chili region (59/10).

In Gur'yev Oblast (Degizsk district), an "authentic" CCHF case was retrospectively diagnosed by Chumakov et al.[102] This far-western oblast of Kazakh S.S.R. faces the Caspian Sea near Astrakhan Oblast. In Alma Ata Oblast of southeastern Kazakhstan, two early CCHF cases were seen according to Temirbekov et al.[518] (quoting Bartoshevich 1954) and Pak and Mikhailova[383] (quoting Kereev[265]). However, Zhumatov and Dmitrienko[610] pointedly referred to the absence of records of the disease in Alma Ata Oblast. Nevertheless, Karimov et al.[246] established a case for active circulation of the virus in the Balkash region of Alma Ata Oblast after detecting AGDP antibodies to the virus in 1.9% of animal blood sera from this source (the number of sera tested was not stated).

Kirgiz S.S.R.

Clinical CCHF is unusual in Kirgizia, but the virus is endemic in the southwestern climatic region of Osh Oblast. Two cases were recorded in 12- and 15-year-old brothers who had tended cattle in a mountain pass where *Hyalomma anatolicum* was found.[420] Other human cases occurred in 1948 and in 1951.[383] The paucity of human infection is postulated[243] to be owing to the infrequency of bites by *H. marginatum turanicum,* which appears to be the chief vector of CCHF virus in this republic.

Eleven CCHF strains were isolated in Osh Oblast in 1970 to 1974. Ten were from *H. marginatum turanicum* and one was from a person.[117,128,244,538] The tick isolates were from spring-early summer collections (April to June); the isolate from a human was in midsummer (August). Collecting regions were Frunze, Batken, Lyailyak, and Aravan. The *H. marginatum turanicum* isolates were from immatures infesting two crested larks, *Galerida cristata,* and a tree sparrow, *Passer montanus,* and from adults infesting cattle (1), sheep (5), and goats (1). (Dandurov et al.[128] reported their isolate as from "*H. p. plumbeum*", probably in error for *H. marginatum turanicum*.)

In a later investigation in Osh Oblast, Karas' et al.[243] took 12,045 ticks from domestic and wild animals; the most numerous were *Rhipicephalus turanicus* (5372), *Hyalomma a. asiaticum* (1895), *H. marginatum turanicum* (1867), and *Haemaphysalis punctata* (423) (only 9 *H. anatolicum* were collected). Nineteen CCHF strains were isolated from ticks from sheep, goats, and cattle: *H. marginatum turanicum* (17), *H. a. asiaticum* (1), and *R. turanicus* (1).

In the spring and summer seasons of 1971 to 1972, all of 782 human sera from southwestern Osh Oblast were serologically negative but 8% to 53% of sheep and cattle sera were positive against CCHF antigens in the CF test; none was positive in the HI test.[523]

The most common wild mammal in Kirgizian CCHF foci, the red-tailed Libyan jird, *Meriones libycus erythrourus,* is an important host of immature *Hyalomma a. asiaticum, Haemaphysalis erinacei turanica,* and *Rhipicephalus turanicus,* and is also parasitized by each feeding stage of *Ornithodoros tartakovskyi.* The long-eared hedgehog, *Hemiechinus auritus,* a frequent co-inhabitant of jird colonies, is infested by the same tick species.[371,522] The ixodid fauna of Kirgizia was reviewed in a monograph by Grebenyuk.[186]

The Osh Oblast semidesert has a total annual rainfall of 200 mm, mostly in winter. The winters are relatively mild, with mean January temperatures of $-3°$ or $-4°C$; the summers are warm and dry (July mean 24° or 25°C). The maximum is 40°C; the annual sum of effective temperatures (above 10°C) is 4000°C. The ticks providing the earliest CCHF isolates were collected between 600 and 1300 m altitude, where herding sheep on xerophilic vegetation is the chief occupation.[522]

Karas' et al.,[244] who described the four climatic regions of Kirgizia, discovered CCHF foci only in the southwestern part of Osh Oblast. The most active foci are in foothills beside Ferguna Valley (Naukatsky and Frunze regions) and in Chatkal Range foothills.[243] Kirgizian mountains, some rising to more than 5000 m altitude, generally have more gentle slopes and higher annual rainfall than those of Tadzhikistan.

Tadzhik S.S.R.

In the 12th century, human CCHF was described and associated with arthropod bites in Tadzhikistan. More recently, Sipovsky[482] reported observations from 18 autopsies of patients with gastrointestinal hemorrhages. He also stated that a similar illness had been observed in the Dushanbe (Stalinabad) city hospital in 1927. Later, specialists classified these cases as CCHF. The Sipovsky report aroused much interest among public health authorities in Middle Asia. Between this time and 1968, when new serological and virological tools became available for scientifically verifying clinical diagnoses, the official Tadzhik disease records (64 cases from 1951 to 1970) are clouded by misdiagnosis and failure to recognize the symptoms of this illness. The actual morbidity rate was said to have been higher. The number of cases differed in almost every report.

From studying hospital case histories and official data, Pak and Mikhailova[383] recorded 97 cases from 1943 to 1970. In most years, there were 1 to 6 cases, but in 1956, 1967, and 1970 there were 14, 21, and 10, respectively. The illnesses originated in 19 southern regions of the republic. One to eight patients were reported from most regions but 10 to 16 patients were from Dangara, Pyandzh, and Moskovski. Pak[374,376] stated that 120 CCHF patients had been recorded between 1943 and 1974. The disease course and its hemorrhagic manifestations were considered to be especially severe in Tadzhikistan.[264,469] Observations from nine autopsies between 1947 and 1967 were identical to those reported from the Crimea, Bulgaria, and Uzbekistan.[184] Five mild CCHF infections occurred in 1973 among persons who tended a patient with typical symptoms.[384] Other household-nosocomial cases are reviewed elsewhere. Pak and Mikhailova[383] first isolated CCHF virus from six patients from four districts in 1969 to 1970 and also from *Hyalomma a. anatolicum* from Dangara district.

Seroepidemiological surveys in 1968 to 1969[257,386,487] produced varying results which are difficult to interpret. Most positive reactions were from southern areas where 0.8 to 2.8% of the sera from domestic sheep, goats, cattle, and horses were positive in the AGDP test. But 39.5% of the donkey sera were said to be positive as well as 1 of 35 sera of the steppe tortoise, *Testudo horsfieldi.*[386] All wild bird and mammalian sera were negative. In the CF test, 25 of 2355 healthy human sera reacted against CCHF antigens.[257]

Tadzhikistan is divided geographically and climatically into northern, central, and southern regions, and the Pamir Mountains (Gorno-Badakhshan A.O.). CCHF cases occur only in the southern sector. However, infected ticks may be introduced into the cooler central area and into the Pamirs with cattle and sheep driven from the south to summer pastures.[383]

Southern Tadzhikistan is a lowland desert and semidesert plain with foothills and low mountains. Few peaks reach 2300 m altitude. From 500 to 2000 m altitude, there is much nonirrigated grain cultivation. Tugai vegetation persists in undeveloped river valleys; oases are developed for orchards and long-fiber cotton fields. The sum of effective annual temperatures is 3000 to 5700°C, but in warm years may exceed 6000°C. Annual rainfall increases from 150 to 300 mm at 500 m to 900 mm at 1200 m altitude. Rain falls mostly in spring (March). The relative humidity (mean annual 50 to 65%) is maximum in December and January (60 to 80%) and minimum in summer (20 to 50%). A large variety of reptiles, birds, and small mammals inhabit the plains and foothills. Pak and Mikhailova[383] stated that there are no hares in Tadzhik CCHF foci, but Kuima[300] reported *Hyalomma anatolicum anatolicum* from *Lepus capensis* in these areas.

Domestic cattle, sheep, and goats are common in foothills and low mountains where CCHF virus is enzootic. State-owned herds, treated with acaricide to control ticks, are driven from plains to hills and mountains, depending on the seasonal availability of grass; they can transport infected ticks over wide areas. Privately owned cattle, which graze the entire year near homesteads, are not treated for ticks and are usually heavily infested. People and cattle often sleep together in the summer within yards surrounded by clay fences.[382] In river valley cotton plantations, domestic animals are kept in stables where ticks do not thrive. CCHF has not been recorded from these plantations.

Pak and Mikhailova[383] found serological evidence of CCHF virus circulation in northern Tadzhikistan but were unable to account for the absence of disease records. They consider the north to be a potentially dangerous zone and suggested that the disease may be present but uncommon and unrecognized by northern physicians.

Almost all CCHF patients seen in 1967 to 1968 (and afterward) were from scattered rural localities in the Gissar Mountain foothills near Dushanbe and in the low mountains to the south.[240] These foci are ecologically similar. Humidity is low in most of these grassy or sedge and shrub semidesert zones; streams flowing from melting snow in the mountains provide irrigation water but most streams dry up in summer. Animals pastured in the higher mountains are brought to lower altitudes in the winter, when the average temperature is about 1°C in the southern area and −1° or −2°C in the Gissars. Annual rainfall is 400 to 600 mm in the former and 650 to 750 mm in the latter area. CCHF patients had been harvesting hay, guarding haystacks on collective farms, and shepherding calves and sheep. They often slept outdoors. Two villagers probably became infected from ticks brought to their homes with hay.

Thirty-one CCHF strains were isolated by Pak et al.[379] from ticks from southern Tadzhikistan between 1968 and 1973. Seven were from adult *Hyalomma a. anatolicum* [2 from ticks from cracks in the clay walls (*duval*) of cattle pens, 5 from ticks from cattle], 9 from adult *H. detritum* from cattle, and 15 from pooled adults of both species. Two of the strains were from unfed adult *H. a. anatolicum* collected as fed nymphs from ears of cattle. Two other strains were from unfed adults of this species taken in spring from *duval* cracks where cattle had been kept the previous summer. These isolations show transstadial survival and overwinter survival of CCHF virus in *H. a. anatolicum*. Pak[374,375] later stated that there had been "several" isolations of the virus from *H. a. anatolicum* after overwintering. During these studies, a strain of

Wad Medani virus was also isolated from unfed adult *H. a. anatolicum* from clay walls.[381]

Using the FAT to demonstrate CCHF infections in *Hyalomma a. anatolicum* salivary gland preparations, Chumakov et al.[113] obtained the following results (number of preparations per number of positive) from four regions of Tadzhikistan in 1970 to 1972: Dangara (48/9), Gissar (50/17), Leninsky (110/23), Yavan (28/7).

The virus was also isolated from a pool of 50 unfed female *H. marginatum turanicum* from privately owned cattle, which were not subject to antitick treatment, pastured in a steppe-semidesert zone beside wheat and barley fields in Gissar foothills near Dushanbe in the summer of 1971.[537] Pak and his colleagues did not mention *H. marginatum turanicum* in their numerous papers, but Starkov and Kalmykov[502] found this tick to be commonly associated with human activities and widely distributed except in desert and high mountain landscapes of southern Tadzhikistan. Examination of 1332 birds in CCHF foci resulted in collections of 329 ticks from 17 host species; 279 (85%) of the ticks were immature *H. marginatum turanicum.*[301] The chief hosts were the magpie and common carrion crow (eight or nine immatures per bird); other hosts were the Egyptian vulture, eastern black carrion crow, rock partridge, and Montagu harrier (three to five per bird), and the falcon, buzzard, rook, jackdaw, and cornish chough (0.2 to 1 per bird). These birds inhabit open areas. A few birds inhabiting burrows and others frequenting farmsteads and villages were also infested.

Hyalomma a. anatolicum is the most common tick throughout the Dangara area,[296,297] where CCHF virus has been isolated from this tick[374,375,379] and from human beings.[383] In 1968, 375(62%) of 605 cattle were infested by 7074 adults (average 19 per host) and 178 (13%) of 1066 sheep and goats were infested by 599 adults (average 3 per host). There were also 9475 nymphs and larvae on the cattle (32 to 52 per host). A male was taken from an argali (or red sheep) and Kuima[300] took 19 immatures and 9 adults from another argali. (Certain data on hosts of immature *H. anatolicum* in papers by these authors appear to apply to the subspecies *excavatum.*) *H. anatolicum* was found in 186 of the 237 areas searched for ticks in southern Tadzhikistan and constituted 82.4% of all specimens collected.[299] *H. detritum,* found in 101 of the 237 areas, was confined to floodplains, cultivated fields, and humid foothills, and made up 10.5% of all specimens. *H. detritum* was not taken from wild mammals or birds and *H. anatolicum* was not taken from wild birds.[300,301]

Nonfeeding *H a. anatolicum* are numerous in cracks in clay *duvals* where cattle are confined in Tadzhikistan; some are also found under shrubs but few in stables. Adults parasitize cattle throughout the year but are most numerous in June and July. Most larvae and nymphs feed in July and August; a few nymphs also feed in winter. Most ticks overwinter as eggs or unfed adults. Larvae molting from overwintered eggs spend the following winter as adults; overwintering adults overwinter in the egg stage the following year. Kuima[299] observed one or two generations annually in southern Tadzhikistan.

Pak and Makhailova[383] stated that Kuima[299] found substantial ecological differences in the distribution of *H. anatolicum anatolicum* and *H. anatolicum excavatum* (as is to be expected), but I have been unable to obtain a copy of this reference. The Starkov and Kalmykov[502] review of the 26 tick species in the Tadzhik fauna lumps the data for these two subspecies under a single heading. Kuima[300] mentioned both subspecies but may have mixed some data for immature stages (as stated above). Pak[374,375] specified the CCHF vector in Tadzhikistan as *H. anatolicum anatolicum.*

Measures taken after 1967 to prevent CCHF in Tadzhikistan included strict isolation of patients and of persons having contact with them, increased medical and laboratory investigations, questioning residents of the focus in which the patient lived about contacts with ticks and patients, antitick treatment of cattle and of stables and other buildings and clay fences sheltering ticks, and rodent control.[86]

Middle East Nations
Iran

Chumakov et al.[108] first suggested the presence of CCHF virus in Iran when they detected AGDP test antibodies to the virus in sera of 45 of 100 sheep sent to them from the Tehran abattoir. In 1970 to 1971, Chumakov and Smirnova[111] studied 580 serum samples from cattle (100), sheep and goats (201), camels (99), "wild animals" (175), and persons with undiagnosed febrile illness (5), from unspecified localities in Iran. The human sera were negative against CCHF antigens in the CF and AGDP tests. AGDP antibodies were detected in sera of five (2.9%) mammal specimens (house mouse, broad-toothed field mouse, Afghan pika, and Persian jird). AGDP tests in 1970 were positive with sera from cattle (19%) and sheep and goats (45%) and, in 1971, with sera from sheep (49%) and camels (19%). Approximately 62% of sheep sera from northern areas and 28% from northeastern areas (average 54%) were positive for antibodies to CCHF virus. Arata et al.[16] briefly mentioned evidence of CCHF virus infection in small mammals from Iran but have not published the data.

HI antibodies to CCHF infection were detected in 4 of 100 sera from preschool children from the Caspian Sea area.[446] Using the most recent and most sophisticated serological techniques, Saidi et al.[447] detected antibodies to CCHF virus in 48 of 351 (13%) sera from healthy humans (3 to 70 years old) from localities near the Caspian Sea and in East Azerbaijan Province of northern Iran. None of 157 camel sera were positive; the camels had been driven to the Tehran abattoir from southern and southeastern Iran. Domestic animal sera were obtained from local herds and from the abattoirs at Tabriz, Sarab, Rasht, Gorgan, Mashad, Isfahan, and Tehran — all in northern and central Iran. Positive reactions were obtained in sera of 280 (38%) of 728 sheep (mostly from near the Caspian Sea), 48 (36%) of 135 goats, and 23 (18%) of 130 cattle. Positively reacting small mammals from northern Iran were the large mouse-eared bat, *Myotis blythi omari,* common noctule, *Nyctalus n. noctula,* Williams' jerboa, *Allactaga euphratica williamsi,* house mouse, *Mus musculus bactrianus,* and Swinhoe's jird, *Meriones crassus swinhoei. Hyalomma, Rhipicephalus, Haemaphysalis, Argas,* and *Ornithodoros* ticks commonly infest mammals in Iran. *Ixodes, Dermacentor,* and *Boophilus* occur locally.

During investigation of an endemic focus of hemorrhagic purpura in a rural population of northeastern Azerbaijan Province, Karimi et al.[245] isolated no CCHF or other arboviruses from the patients.

Afghanistan

AGDP tests were positive for CCHF antigens in 9.0% of 233 goat sera and in 5.6% of 230 cattle sera from Afghanistan.[98] Semyatkovskaya and Sudtdykova[462] reported severe and fatal cases of CCHF seen in the Termez City Hospital, situated on the Soviet side of the Uzbekistan-Afghanistan border.

Asian Foci (Western Oriental Faunal Region)

CCHF virus was first reported in the Oriental faunal region in 1970 after two strains were isolated from ticks in Pakistan. The 1970 report was followed in 1973 and 1975 by surprising serological results indicating virus circulation in several states of India and in 1976 by outbreaks of the disease in shepherds and hospital and military personnel from different areas of Pakistan. These rapid developments in an extensive geomedical-zoogeographical zone where CCHF virus had not been considered to threaten human health demonstrate how much we yet have to learn about the natural history and epidemiology of the virus. The presence of CCHF virus in the Indian subregion, with its rich and diverse tick fauna largely differing from those of the Palearctic and Ethiopian faunal regions, adds a broad new dimension to biological-epidemiological factors urgently needing investigation. In this respect, prime candidates for virus reservoir-vector research are *Hyalomma marginatum isaaci* and the other *Hyalomma* ticks of the Indian subregion.[237] Spatially, *Hyalomma* species are sequential or overlapping links joining the three faunal regions in the area between southern India and western Africa. They are also likely to be important epidemiological links in these continents.

Pakistan

Begum et al.[30] reported two CCHF strains from cattle-parasitizing ticks in the Changa Manga forest plantation in the hot, irrigated, semiarid plain near Lahore. One was from *Hyalomma a. anatolicum*, the other from a mixed pool of *H. a. anatolicum* and *Boophilus microplus*.

In 1976, Pakistan outbreaks were investigated by Brigadier M. I. Burney, Director of the National Health Laboratories in Islamabad. Virological confirmation of isolates from patients was provided by specialists of the Center for Disease Control (CDC) in Atlanta (P. A. Webb) and YARU (J. Casals, G. H. Tignor, and S. M. Buckley). The full data are presented by these authorities in publications now in press and in preparation.

In brief, a shepherd from the Muree Hills, about 17 km from Rawalpindi, entered the Central Government Hospital with typical CCHF symptoms on January 27, 1976 and died the same night. The shepherd's father, who cared for his sick son at home, was hospitalized on February 8 and died of CCHF 2 days later, despite intensive care and repeated blood transfusions. The shepherd was operated upon when hospitalized on January 27; 12 persons attended him at the time. The surgeon, who cut his finger while operating, died of CCHF on February 11. An assistant surgeon who pricked his finger during the operation became ill on February 2 and was hospitalized on February 5; he recovered and was discharged on February 14. A female physician who admitted the shepherd, when he vomited blood onto her face and hands, showed signs of CCHF infection and was hospitalized on February 5 but slowly recovered. A nursing attendant who assisted in the operation was hospitalized on February 7 and died of CCHF 3 days later. The anesthesiologist also became ill and experienced bleeding from the gums, but recovered. Five of the seven other persons in the theatre during the operation also became ill and were hospitalized; all recovered.

In May 1976, a soldier who had recently been on leave was admitted to the military hospital in Quetta and died of CCHF the following day. About 20 other military patients, one a nursing officer, from at least two stations near Quetta were admitted with hemorrhagic fevers during May. Two of the first five patients died. I have not seen the final data on the remaining cases.

India

Results of a seroepidemiological survey made in 1973 to determine the presence of antibodies to CCHF virus in humans and domestic animals showed the wide distribution of the virus in southern states of India;[465,466] results from investigating 1289 sera were reviewed in the 1976 paper. There were 43 (3.3%) positive reactions in the AGDP test and 1 (0.08%) in the CF test. The 43 were 9 (1.4%) from humans in Kerala and Pondicherry and 34 (5.2%) from domestic animals (30 goats, 3 horses, 1 sheep) in Maharashtra, Karnataka (Mysore), Tamil Nadu, Pondicherry, and Kerala. The single positive CF test was in serum from an 18 year-old girl in Sorab taluk, Shimoga District, Karnataka. None of the 266 human sera from the urban populations of New Delhi and Madras were positive in either test. No sera from cattle and buffaloes from Pondicherry and Karnataka reacted positively in these tests. No human or domestic animal sera showed CF antibodies to HAZ virus.

In another study in 1973, antibodies were detected, chiefly in indirect HI tests, in sera of human beings (4/152), cattle (9/58), and buffaloes (3/42) from in and near Bharatpur in eastern-central Rajasthan.[369] The indirect HI test was considered to provide a more sensitive serological reaction than the CF and AGDP tests.

African Foci (Ethiopian and Palearctic Faunal Regions)

CCHF virus is endemic in a wide area of Africa from Senegal and Nigeria eastward to Kenya, Tanzania and Ethiopa (Ethiopian faunal region), but the scanty available data permit few epidemiological generalizations. Evidence for the presence of CCHF virus in Egypt (Palearctic faunal region) is based on results of a very recent preliminary seroepidemiological survey.

The information from Senegal, Nigeria, Central African Empire, and Ethiopia point to foci in semideserts or in savanna zones with long dry seasons. Data from Zaire, Uganda, Kenya, and Tanzania are difficult to evaluate ecologically but appear to be associated with higher rainfall regions where domestic animals and people live in close proximity. Immature stages of some of the African tick species known to be infected by CCHF virus commonly feed on birds and are transported long distances by migrating birds. The refrain, frequently repeated in Soviet literature, that CCHF cases are frequently overlooked or misdiagnosed in enzootic areas of the Soviet Union, also applies in Africa, where diagnostic facilities for CCHF are very few and far between. I submit that surveillance for CCHF in Africa has been too limited to suggest that the virus in Africa is less pathogenic than that in Eurasia. Soviet writers who make this assumption overlook their own rich experience in the epidemiology of this disease.

Senegal

In May and June of 1969, soon after adequate research tools became available, a joint Soviet-French team conducted a CCHF seroepidemiological survey in Senegal.[120] Of the 1608 sera taken, 137 were from wild mammals (2 positive), 43 from wild birds (all negative), 159 from febrile humans (all negative), and 1269 from domestic animals. The 41 positive reactions detected in the AGDP test were confirmed in the CF test. Four ecological areas were investigated: (1) The semidesert of northern Senegal (*sahel*) with large cattle populations and numerous *Hyalomma* ticks (chiefly *H. impeltatum*); about 6% and 12% of 747 sheep and cattle sera, respectively, were positive. (2) The northern Sudan savanna of central Senegal; cattle are nomadic and *H. truncatum* and *Amblyomma variegatum* were the most common ticks; in 263 goat, sheep, and cattle sera, 1.4% (sheep) and 6.2% (cattle) were positive. (3) The southern Sudan savanna of southeastern Senegal; 4 (15.4%) of 26 cattle sera were positive. (4) The Casamance dry deciduous forest, where cattle are fed on fodder; positives were 8 (8.6%) of 93 cattle and 1 (1.4%) of 70 goat sera. In wild animals, positive sera were from the multimammate rat, *Praomys (Mastomys) natalensis,* and the genet, *Genetta genetta senegalensis.*

Between 1969 and 1974, adult ticks collected from cattle at the Dakar abattoir yielded 26 CCHF strains: *Hyalomma marginatum rufipes* (7), *H. truncatum* (8), *H. impressum* (2), *H. impeltatum* (1), *Amblyomma variegatum* (7), and *Boophilus decoloratus* (1).[431-434,436] (Compare these data with data from ticks in Nigeria.) The virus was also isolated from the blood of a sentinel goat placed in Bandia Forest for arbovirus surveillance in 1972.[432]

Nigeria

The Rockefeller Foundation supported a program, based at the University of Ibadan, for surveillance and study of arbovirus infections of Nigerian vertebrates from 1964 to 1970.[78,82] CCHF virus infections were demonstrated in ticks, domestic animals, wild mammals, and a stray *Culicoides* midge taken in a light trap in a cattle barn. There were no isolates from humans, and no seroepidemiological surveys for human infections with CCHF virus were attempted during this program.[351] However, in 1973 to 1974, David-West et al.[133] detected antibodies in 24 of 250 sera from febrile human beings (9/141 male, 15/109 female) at the Ibadan University College Hospital. In the 0- to 14-year age group, 18 sera were positive (4/84 male, 14/79 female). The authors considered these results to suggest that, under favorable conditions, CCHF virus is a threat to human health in Nigeria.

Nigerian virus strains sent to the Yale and Moscow laboratories (as Congo virus) in the early stages of the Nigerian program proved timely and significant in establishing the common identity of CCHF strains from Eurasia and Africa.[70,115]

The 1964 to 1965 data[577] and the 1964 to 1968 data[80] on 27 CCHF strains from Nigerian ticks provided valuable information. The 24 strains from ticks from cattle were *Amblyomma variegatum* (1), *Boophilus decoloratus* (19), *Hyalomma marginatum rufipes* (1), *H. impeltatum* (1), and *H. truncatum* (2). Three additional strains were from *B. decoloratus* from sheep (2) and from *Hyalomma a. anatolicum* (as *H. excavatum*) from a camel (1). The infected *H. a. anatolicum* was taken from a pack camel at Sokoto; the infected *A. variegatum* was from the Upper Ogun Ranch in Western State. All the others were from animals at the Dugbe abattoir at Ibadan; their origins were unknown. The animals had been driven through a variety of ecological zones (see Causey et al.[81]) and had mingled with resident animals while en route to the abattoir.

Five CCHF strains were isolated from animals at the abattoir: four from cattle and one from a goat.[80,260] [The identity of the strain from a goat (AN 7620) was reported by Henderson et al.[200] of the East African Virus Research Institute and by Chumakov.[94]]

Two CCHF isolates from the African hedgehog, *Erinaceus (Atelerix) albiventris,* were from the Sudan savanna ecological zone in June[80,262] and from the Jos Plateau in December.[262] The Jos isolate appears to have been made while Kemp was on a mission to investigate a Lassa fever outbreak there.[175]

During the tenure of the Ibadan program, experimental studies were undertaken on transovarial transmission of CCHF virus in *Hyalomma marginatum rufipes*[309] and on experimental infections of NWM and calves.[80] These are mentioned elsewhere in this review.

Central African Republic

A CCHF strain was isolated at the Institut Pasteur, Bangui, from one of three pools of male *Hyalomma nitidum* taken from cattle at the Berberati abattoir (west of Bangui, near the Cameroon border) in September 1973.[434,511,512] In 1976, two strains were obtained from ticks from cattle at the Bangui abattoir, one from *Amblyomma variegatum* and one from *Boophilus annulatus*. Another strain was isolated from a Bangui laboratory worker who suffered a 3-day malaria-like illness beginning 5 days after handling CCHF virus-infected material.[435]

Zaire (Congo)

CCHF strain V3011, isolated in March 1956 from blood taken at the peak of fever from a 13-year-old African boy at the Kisangani (Stanleyville) hospital, became the prototype strain of Congo virus.[479,574] The following month, Courtois, the physician at the hospital, became ill, presumably from handling strain V3011, and experienced a 3-day fever, nausea, and vomiting. CCHF strain 3010 was isolated from Courtois.

These "Congo" strains were the subject of earlier reports on virus identify[337,481,579,581] and of later comparisons with Eurasian CCHF strains,[70,115] but nothing else is known about the virus in Zaire.

Uganda

Blood from febrile persons seen at the East African Virus Research Laboratory (Entebbe) from 1958 to 1965 produced ten CCHF strains as recorded in the two final reports on Congo virus studies by Simpson et al.[479] and by Williams et al.,[574] and in earlier papers.[14,278,573,575,578,579,581] Later, Knight et al.[277] reported two new case histories and Munube et al.[357] isolated the virus from an outpatient at the Entebbe dispensary. All the patients were from the Entebbe area, except one from Sazi District and one from Kigezi District. Of the 13 cases from Uganda, six were in laboratory workers; one died (an animal attendant). Uganda strains were also compared by Casals and Chumakov with others from Eurasia, as already mentioned for strains from Zaire and Nigeria.

One CCHF strain was isolated from a female *Amblyomma variegatum* from a cow in Ankole District,[268,270,272] but other recent attempts to recover the virus from ticks have been unsuccessful.[270,273,334] In AGDP tests of 104 sera from cattle from Mbarara, 38 (36.5%) reacted against CCHF virus antigens.[274] Kirya[269] commented on the difficulties of seroepidemiological surveys for CCHF virus in Africa because of the lack of reliable techniques at that time.

While this manuscript was in press, Kalunda and Mukwaya[241] reported two CCHF isolates from *Rhipicephalus appendiculatus* from cattle grazing 20 km apart in Uganda. One infected pool was of male ticks, the other of female ticks. Two laboratory workers handling the inoculated mice became ill 1 to 2 months afterward and CCHF virus was isolated from both; the infection route(s) could not be determind.

Twenty-five species of ticks associated with CCHF virus are discussed in another section. An additional species, *Hyalomma dromedarii* from Turkmen S.S.R. is listed elsewhere. The Uganda report of infected *Rhipicephalus appendiculatus*, the well-known vector of *Theileria parva* which causes East Coast fever, increases the number of ticks associated with CCHF virus to 27 species.

Kenya

In a letter to the editor of the *East African Medical Journal*, Nevill[363] of the Rift Valley Province Hospital at Nakuru stated: "During the past 2 years (there have) been a number of deaths in adult Africans in the Rift Valley due to a rapidly progressive hemorrhagic syndrome which may be a disease entity." He described some laboratory and postmortem findings and mentioned that "a clinically similar condition in cattle (occurred) in marginal forest areas in the same region." Whether these human and bovine illnesses were caused by CCHF virus is uncertain, but it is noteworthy that Woodall et al.[581] identified Nakuru-Dempster 9503 strain as CCHF (Congo) virus. This strain had been isolated by D. A. Haig at the Veterinary Research Institute, Kabete, from a febrile cow in a herd at Nakuru, where a series of unexplained abortions were being seen.

A total of 347 cattle sera were collected in four districts of Kenya during December 1974 and examined in the AGDP test at the East African Virus Research Institute (Entebbe); the following positive reactions were found: Eldoret 55 examined, 4 positive (7.3%), Isiolo 96/8 (8.3%), Kajiado 92/1 (1.1%), West Pokot 100/3 (3.0%) (A. M. Butenko and T. Minja, personal communication.)

Chumakov and Smirnova,[111] who investigated blood sera from 136 humans, 93 cattle, and 162 "wild animals" from Kenya and Uganda by the AGDP test, detected antibodies to CCHF virus in sera of 77 cattle and 3 wild animals (2 gazelles and 1 baboon). Identical results were obtained with antigens prepared from the Asian strain Khodzha and the "Congo" strain Nakivogo. Kirya et al.[274] detected no antibodies to the virus in sera of 226 baboons trapped in Kenya.

The 1974 to 1975 annual report of the London School of Hygiene and Tropical Medicine[327] recorded three virus strains "distantly related but not identical to Congo virus" from *Amblyomma variegatum* from cattle near Kisumu and CF and AGDP test antibodies to the virus in sera of 73/123 (59%) goats, 16/59 (27%) cattle, and sheep (data unstated).

At the Kabete laboratory in February 1975, Dr. F. G. Davies informed me that he had very recently isolated CCHF virus from *Rhipicephalus pulchellus* from a dying sheep at this laboratory.

Ethiopia

A CCHF strain was isolated from a pool of 20 partially fed adult *Hyalomma impeltatum* taken from sheep at Omo Ratay in southwestern Ethiopia. This station on the Omo River, at about 500 m altitude and 35 km upstream from Lake Rudolph, is in a narrow riparian bush zone surrounded by semidesert. The ticks were collected in March 1975 at the end of the long dry season. CCHF has not been recognized in people in the immediate area, but a hemorrhagic disease was reported in 1972 among the nearby Turkana tribesmen of Kenya (O. L. Wood, V. H. Lee, and J. S. Ash, NAMRU-5, Addis Ababa; personal communication). Other tick species taken at or within 10 km of Omo Ratay were *H. a. anatolicum, H. marginatum rufipes, H. truncatum, A. variegatum, Rhipicephalus e. evertsi, R. pravus, R. sanguineus,* and *R. simus.*

Tanzania

AGDP tests at the East African Virus Research Institute (Entebbe) of cattle sera from Tanzania in 1974 to 1975 gave the following positive reactions to CCHF antigens: Central Province, Mpwapwa 166 examined, 1 positive (0.6%); Northern Province (Longido, Monduli, Tengeru) 256/19 (7.4%), Sukumaland 209/10 (4.8%), Lake Victoria coastal region 417/68 (16.3%), total 1048/98 (9.0%) (A. M. Butenko and T. Minja, personal communication). This is the only effort to determine the presence of CCHF virus in Tanzania. Mpwapwa is in a low rainfall zone; the Lake Victoria coastal region is in a high rainfall zone.

Egypt

A total of 1174 sera, 433 from human beings and 741 from domestic animals, were examined in the CF test.[131] No antibodies were detected in sera from donkeys, horses, mules, pigs, goats, or dogs. Antibodies were detected in the serum of a 35-year-old male human from Asyut and in sera of 3 of 34 (8.8%) camels from Cairo, 3 of 21 (14.3%) cattle from Wadi Natroun, 2 of 15 (13.3%) cattle from Qena, 1 of 32 (3.1%) buffaloes from Port Said, and 12 of 66 (18.2%) sheep from Cairo. These are the only data for the presence of CCHF virus foci in northern Africa (Palearctic faunal region). *Hyalomma a. anatolicum, H. marginatum rufipes, H. impeltatum, Rhipicephalus sanguineus, R. turanicum,* and *Boophilus annulatus* are common members of the Egyptian tick fauna,[203,219] and numerous specimens of known vector tick species have been taken from northward- and southward-migrating birds passing through Egypt.

The Role of Birds in CCHF Virus Dissemination
Introduction

Although supporting data are scanty and more reliable evidence is desirable, it appears that CCHF virus causes no viremia in birds. In the natural history of CCHF virus, birds (1) serve as hosts of infected ticks and contribute to the numbers and success of vector species, and (2) transport ticks, some of which may be infected, (a) relatively short distances during local postbreeding flights, or (b) long distances during spring and fall migration flights.

The list of 25 different ticks already incriminated in CCHF epidemiology includes five frequently parasitizing birds in Eurasia (*Argas persicus, Ixodes ricinus, Haemaphysalis punctata, Hyalomma m. marginatum,* and *H. marginatum turanicum*) and 4 or 5 in Africa (*Hyalomma marginatum rufipes, H. impeltatum, H. truncatum, Amblyomma variegatum,* and probably *H. nitidum*). All feeding stages of the multihost *A. persicus* parasitize birds, but only the larvae of this species feed long enough to be carried away from the nest or roost by the bird host. The other species are two- or three-host ticks; immatures may parasitize birds; adults parasitize medium-sized or large mammals or large birds (ostrich, bustard, etc.).

Intracontinental (Local) Movements

Studies in Slovakia (outside the known geographic range of CCHF virus) beautifully illustrate the influence of seasonal activities of birds on *Ixodes ricinus* infestation in forest foci of tick-borne encephalitis (TBE) virus.[26,438] Tick and bird interrelationship patterns more or less similar to those in Slovakia occur in many temperate and tropical zones where land birds breed. The Slovakian studies are even more relevant when considering factors in CCHF epidemiology in Moldavia and Bulgaria, where infected *I. ricinus* have already been found.

The Slovakian forest focus study showed heavy tick infestations beginning in early April, when numerous resident and recently arrived migrating birds began to visit tick-inhabited biotopes for food and for nest-building material. In May, this bird population was augmented by later-arriving migrant species. In June, small-sized birds busily sought food and became tick-infested near their nests. Larger birds, particularly predaceous species, flew much greater distances for food. The predators could be attacked by ticks as they tangled with their prey on the ground. In May, and especially in June, young birds began leaving the nest to practice flying; they spent interflight intervals on the ground where they were parasitized. In July, both young and adult birds moved to different biotopes and greater distances in search of food. In August, local dispersals widened and some species began the fall migration. September and October saw birds from the north visiting Slovakia on their southward flight and local-breeding species departing. In November, the local bird fauna was increased by some winter visitors but long-distance movements stopped.

Some Slovakian birds, such as the nuthatch, pheasant, mountain grouse, and certain wrens, do not move far from their nests at any season. These birds participate in maintaining but not in dispersing the TBE foci. Birds that wander for some weeks after the nesting season may either leave tick-infested biotopes or enter new ones. Even species that seldom come to the ground as adults may be infested in the early-flight stage of their lives.

The chief studies of *Hyalomma m. marginatum* infestation of the rook, *Corvus f. frugilegus,* and of other ground-feeding bird species in CCHF foci, by Berezin and colleagues in Astrakhan Oblast, are reviewed elsewhere. The Levi studies in Bulgaria are also important. As immature rooks in Astrakhan Oblast developed flying capability, their flight range increased from 10 to as much as 500 km. At the same time, many nymphal *H. m. marginatum* were completing feeding on these rooks and dropping in more or less distant fields, forests, villages, and cities. This seasonal coincidence of bird and tick activity was credited with disseminating CCHF virus-infested ticks throughout Astrakhan Oblast. Such dissemination may be "routine" during years of enzootic virus activity but enhanced during cycles of increased tick numbers and epizootic virus activity.

Černý and Balát,[83] who found three *Hyalomma* nymphs in the ears of two tree pip-its, *Anthus trivialis,* migrating from the Mediterranean area or Africa to Moravia, in Czechoslovakia, where *Hyalomma* ticks do not occur, reviewed earlier literature on ticks associated with migrating birds in Europe and in the Soviet Union. Many early records are open to questions of available data. To spell out these problems in detail is outside the scope of the present review.

On Signildskär, the outermost island in the southwestern archipelago of Finland, 39 (approximately 2%) of 1928 migrants examined between March 15 and June 30, 1962 were infested by 79 immature ticks, all *Ixodes ricinus* except for a single *Hyalomma m. marginatum.*[368] Saikku et al.[449] took 312 immature ticks from 152 spring migrants (22 species) in southern Finland between 1961 and 1969. Of the 259 specimens identi-fied, 252 were *I. ricinus,* 1 was *I. arboricola,* and 6 were *Hyalomma marginatum* (these nymphs were identified as "positively" or as "probably" subspecies *rufipes,* but in the absence of reared adults, I hesitate to accept these subspecies identifications). Birds examined in this study numbered 3070. Many immature *I. ricinus,* some *I. arboricola,* and a single nymphal *H. marginatum* sp. were recorded from spring migrants at the Ottenby Bird Station on Öland Island in the Baltic Sea, Sweden.[56]

The ticks acquired by birds during stops in Europe, while en route to Finland and Sweden, may have easily molted to adults, fed on domestic animals during the summer, and transmitted infectious agents to be inbibed by the local tick population. Some introduced *I. ricinus* might survive the Scandinavian winter, but the *H. m. marginatum* would obviously succumb to cold in October or November.

In Europe and elsewhere, immature *Hyalomma* ticks found on migrating birds should be reared to adults for positive species and subspecies identification. A simple method for this purpose was suggested by Kaiser and Hoogstraal.[238] Some of the above records of nymphal *H. marginatum* spp. may pertain to the extra-European subspecies *H. m. rufipes* or *H. m. turanicum,* but unfortunately we do not know their actual identity or origin.

On each continent, dozens of bird species serve as hosts of immature stages of the nine or ten Eurasian and African ticks associated with birds and with CCHF virus. The wide geographic distribution of each of these tick species may be attributed to (1) ecological adaptability, (2) dissemination of immatures during local movements of host birds, and (3) ability of adults to parasitize numerous domestic animals pastured near farmsteads and in many other environments.

Intercontinental Migratory Movements

The classic, easily available book on Palearctic-African bird migration systems by the late Moreau,[352] with its excellent review of knowledge and long list of references, is must reading for anyone concerned with the transportation of viruses and ticks by birds migrating between Eurasia and Africa. The popular belief that most bird species use a "Nile Valley flyway" is true for relatively few bird species. Many species fly north or south in a broad front. They stop to rest when and where they can, and fly nonstop over the Mediterranean and the Sahara. Others veer and turn at specific lo-calities. Some use different routes for spring and fall migrations; each year in Egypt we see certain species in spring that we do not see in fall, and some in fall that we do not see in spring. In Figure 5 of his book, Moreau shows flight patterns of 6000 to 10,000 km from Tomsk, Yakutsk, and Lake Baikal to Khartoum, Nairobi, and Fort Lamy. Moreau estimates that 5 billion passerine birds migrate each fall from the west-ern and central Palearctic to vacation in Africa. Nonpasserine migrants, among them several species that figure in our lists of tick-infested birds, are estimated to number at least 200 million. Other estimates are 40 million for raptors and 700,000 for the stork, *C. ciconia.* Probably one half of all these birds are lost during migrations. Thus the numbers returning in spring from the African vacation to work at nest building and brood-rearing in Eurasia are smaller than the autumn numbers.

The only studies of ticks carried by migrating birds between Eurasia and Africa and Africa and Eurasia are those made in Egypt and Cyprus by the NAMRU-3 Medical Zoology Department from 1955 to 1973 (from1966 to 1973 in cooperation with the Smithsonian Palearctic Migratory Bird Survey based in our laboratories). A report on results obtained during the last 7 years of this project is in preparation.

Eurasia to Africa

The findings of adult *Hyalomma m. marginatum,* the European form of this tick, on camels and cattle in Kassala and Kordofan Provinces of the Sudan[203] and in northern Somalia[394] and on swine in Harar Province of Ethiopia (unpublished data), most probably result from nymphs that detached in these places from southward-migrating birds. Unlike large, colorful adult *Amblyomma,* which are quickly recognized in Europe and western Asia, where ticks of this genus do not normally occur (see below), foreign *Hyalomma* are difficult to recognize, except by specialists, in the African fauna, where they superficially resemble one or more *Hyalomma* species common in the local landscape.

All tick species taken in Egypt from fall migrants are characteristic of the fauna of Europe and nearby Asian areas of the Palearctic faunal region[218,225,227] (and unpublished). None is typical of Asia east of the Caspian Sea. (We have examined very few migrants that might have flown here from areas east of the Caspian. Most, though not all, bird species coming from Siberia and Central Asia arrive in Africa via routes to the east and/or south of the Mediterranean coast of Egypt, where we studied fall migrants.)

During the fall migrations of 1959, 1960, and 1961, we examined 32,086 birds (72 species and subspecies) in Egypt;[225] 40 of these taxa, represented by 31,434 birds, were infested. The 1040 tick hosts (3.31% of the infested taxa examined) bore 1761 immature ticks (1.69 per host). Of these, 686 (38.96%) were *Hyalomma m. marginatum,* 116 (6.60%) were *H.* sp. (probably mostly *H. m. marginatum*), 485 (28.11%) were *Haemaphysalis punctata,* 183 (10.39%) were *Ixodes ricinus,* 150 (8.52%) were *Ixodes* sp. (probably mostly *I. ricinus*), and the remainder were a few other species not known to be associated with CCHF virus. (In these and the following studies, large numbers of immature ticks were reared to adults to establish the species and subspecies identity.) During the 1962 fall migration, 11,036 birds (62 species and subspecies) were examined;[227] 24 of these taxa, represented by 10,612 birds, were infested. The 881 tick hosts (8.30% of the infested taxa examined) bore 1442 immature ticks (1.63 per host). Tick-host relationships in 1962 were similar to those in the 1959 to 1961 study, and the average number of ticks per host was the same, but in 1962 the prevalence of infestation was almost invariably much higher than the previous averages (and 5 bird species were added to the previous list of 40 infested taxa).

The following data summarize the prevalence of tick infestation in these studies: birds examined, 31,434 (1959 to 1961), 10,612 (1962); birds infested, 1040 (1959 to 1961), 881 (1962); percentage infested, 3.31 (1959 to 1961), 8.30 (1962). It is exciting to consider that the increased prevalence of tick-infested migrating birds recorded in Egypt in 1962 may be correlated with European climatic and other factors leading to greater population densities of *Hyalomma m. marginatum* and increased CCHF morbidity in 1962 to 1963 in Astrakhan Oblast and to the beginning of the CCHF epidemic in Rostov Oblast in 1963.

Among the southward-migrating birds most commonly examined in Egypt and most heavily infested by immature *H. m. marginatum* were the European quail, *Coturnix c. coturnix;* golden oriole, *Oriolus o. oriolus;* whinchat, *Saxicola rubetra;* wheatear,

Oenanthe o. oenanthe; rock thrush, *Monticola saxatilis;* common redstart, *Phoenicurus p. phoenicurus;* thrush nightingale, *Luscinia luscinia;* nightingale, *Luscinia m. megarhynchos;* willow warbler, *Phylloscopus trochilus;* spotted flycatcher, *Muscicapa s. striata;* tawny pipit, *Anthus c. campestris;* tree pipit, *Anthus t. trivialis;* and red-backed shrike, *Lanius c. collurio.*

Many other bird species were infested by immature *H. m. marginatum* when they reached Egypt, as well as during their passage through Cyprus.[239] These data point to the great need for more intensive European investigations of birds as hosts of immature *H. m. marginatum* and as disseminators of CCHF virus-infected ticks. Recent data from the Caspian Sea area show that even terns and other marine birds should be studied for their role in supporting and disseminating the *H. m. marginatum* population in that area.

Statistical analysis of our data for ticks from fall migrants in 1966, 1968, 1969, 1971, 1972 has not yet been completed but a brief review of some salient results was recently presented.[213] These results should be compared with the reports of the gradual decline of CCHF morbidity in Astrakhan and Rostov Oblasts between 1964 and 1968, the increase in 1968 morbidity correlated with increased tick density that year, and the precipitous drop to very few or no cases in 1969 following the excessively severe winter of 1968 to 1969 and the dramatic decrease in tick numbers. Our data for prevalence of tick infestation of fall migrants in Egypt follow exactly the same pattern, with 1969 results representing the lowest prevalence of the 13-year study period. In 1971, the prevalence of infestation in Egypt increased moderately and in 1972 almost reached the 1959 to 1961 level. To our great regret, we were unable to continue these studies after 1972. One wonders whether post-1972 data might have furnished clues to increasing or decreasing tick population densities in eastern Europe and southwestern U.S.S.R. and to consequent increasing or decreasing risk of human exposure to CCHF virus in recent years.

The results of 1967 fall migration studies in Cyprus[239] cannot be compared with those from Egypt because the birds were not as carefully examined as those in Egypt and data on noninfested birds were not recorded. However, with these reservations in mind, the Cyprus data do not contradict the Egyptian data.

Africa to Eurasia

Before reviewing data for ticks from spring migrants in Egypt and Cyprus, it is interesting to mention reports of large, brightly colored adult Africa *Amblyomma* ticks discovered in Eurasia. Each of these species feeds in Africa, as larvae and nymphs, on resident and migrating birds and on mammals. *Amblyomma hebraeum,* a tick of considerable medical and veterinary importance in Rhodesia, Botswana, Mozambique, and South Africa, was found feeding on a cow in Bulgaria.[390] Adult *A. variegatum* were taken feeding on a dog in France[304] and on cattle in Italy,[7] Bulgaria,[322] and Israel;[535] this species (from which CCHF virus has been isolated) inhabits much of the Ethiopian faunal region north of the range of *A. hebraeum.* Male *A. lepidum,* another economically important tick of eastern Africa, were removed from a stone curlew, *Burhinus oedicnemus,* shot in Azerbaijan S.S.R.[415] and from a white stork, *C. ciconia,* shot in Kharga Oasis of Egypt (unpublished data), and other adults were found on cattle and/or sheep in Syria,[279] Iraq,[437] and Israel.[167,535] Adult *A. gemma,* another economically important species of eastern Africa, were collected from cattle in the Crimea[276] and in Israel.[536]

From my relatively numerous records of immature *A. nuttalli* infesting spring migrants, I would not be surprised to learn of the presence of adult *A. nuttalli* in Europe. Obviously, less colorful ticks of other genera introduced into Eurasia are easily overlooked.

Results from northward-migrating birds in Egypt were reported by Hoogstraal and Kaiser[219] and Hoogstraal et al.[224,227] Hoogstraal[213] briefly reviewed the salient facts from much otherwise unpublished 1963 to 1973 data. The 1958 and 1961 reports were based on birds obtained in grub-baited traps or mist nets in the Cairo area (Cairo, Giza, and Fayium Governorates). Kestrels were caught in mouse-baited nooses. Subsequent data derive chiefly from birds mist-netted in the Bahig area, near Alexandria, on the Mediterranean coastal desert. Most spring migrants pass through northern Egypt in smaller flocks than fall migrants and, as stated earlier, migrants are generally less numerous in spring than in fall owing to heavy losses during these strenuous intercontinental flights. Thus fewer birds were examined in the spring. However, the high prevalence of tick infestation among those examined provided valuable data on ticks being carried northward. Almost every tick taken from these birds was *Hyalomma marginatum rufipes,* a form from which eight CCHF strains have been isolated in Senegal and Nigeria. The records for dates when these ticks dropped or were removed from infested birds and molted to adults show that, if the host had not been detained in Cairo, the ticks would have been carried deep into Eurasia, dropped, and molted to adults in late April or in May.

The 1955 to 1957 Cairo area spring migration data were from 77 hosts (10 species) carrying 504 ticks; 216 were reared to adult *Hyalomma marginatum rufipes* and 2 to female *H. impeltatum.*[220] The other 288 immatures (probably mostly *H. marginatum rufipes*) died before molting. In 1960, 128 (13 host taxa represented by 786 birds) of 959 birds examined in the Cairo area were infested by 347 ticks (average 1.0 to 5.6 per bird) from which 78 adult *H. marginatum rufipes* were reared.[224] Most of the remaining 269 immature *Hyalomma* probably represented the same species. Many other miscellaneous data are presented and discussed in the 1961 paper, and the winter and summer ranges of the 22 host taxa for this period are mapped.

The bird hosts taken in the spring of 1962 on the Mediterranean coast numbered 13 taxa, 8 of which were not among the 22 host taxa recorded earlier in the Cairo area, only about 250 km away.[227] This difference in itself illustrates how methods and localities may influence migration data. At any rate, 56 (6.4%) of the 867 birds examined in 1962 were infested by 186 ticks as follows: 166 *H. marginatum rufipes* (89.25%), 19 *Ixodes* spp. (10.21%), 1 *Amblyomma variegatum* (0.54%). There were 1 to 18 ticks per host (average 3.32).

Endemic Distribution and Epidemics in Animals
Endemic Distribution
Geographical

CCHF virus is known to circulate in nature (1) in areas where either epidemics or localized outbreaks of the disease have been followed by field investigations, (2) in the vicinity of several biomedical research laboratories with virological facilities, and (3) from the results of short-term or one-time-only field trips by interested specialists. Knowledge of the geographical distribution of CCHF virus was first (1944 to 1945) confined to the war-devastated focus in the Crimea. The post-World War II outbreaks in Uzbekistan and Kazakhstan and the epidemics during the 1950s and 1960s in Astrakhan and Rostov Oblasts and Bulgaria, together with the 1967 to 1968 "breakthrough" development of serological and other research tools, extended the confirmed range of the virus to these areas and to Pakistan, Zaire, Uganda, and Nigeria. The new tools also made possible the investigations into the natural history of the virus in the Astrakhan focus, as well as in Rostov Oblast and Bulgaria; the results have contributed significantly to understanding CCHF virus epidemiology.

The urgency to utilize all available research resources for keeping abreast of European epidemics waned when these epidemics faded following the severe 1968 to 1969 winter and spring seasons. Armed with the new tools for seroepidemiological surveys, investigators obtained evidence of CCHF virus in France, southern regions and all the southern republics of the Soviet Union, and the francophone areas of West and Central Africa. Some surveys were accompanied by more or less intensive attempts to isolate the virus from human beings, ticks, and domestic animals, but practically the only serious epidemiological study during this period was that of Pak and his colleagues in Tadzhikistan. During the past 4 or 5 years, bits and pieces of information have contributed to extending knowledge of the presence of CCHF virus into new localities within the known range in the Soviet Union and into several states of India, Pakistan, Iran, Egypt, Kenya, and Ethiopia. The very recent (1976) outbreak of the disease in Pakistan has not yet been documented in literature.

In terms of faunal regions of the world[130] endemic CCHF virus has thus far been reported from much of the southeastern zone of the Palearctic, neighboring western zones of the Oriental, and neighboring northern zones of the Ethiopian to slightly beyond the equator. Geographically and zoogeographically, these data, incomplete as they are, add up to a remarkably extensive distribution range for an arthropod-borne virus.

Evidence for postulating that birds may disseminate virus-infected *Hyalomma* and other ticks intracontinentally and intercontinentally and, thus, possibly account to some extent for the wide distribution of endemic CCHF virus was reviewed. Chunikhin[119] went so far as to state that the absence of antigenic differences between CCHF strains from Europe, Asia, and Africa may be explained through constant exchange of strains following transport of virus-infected ticks by migrating birds.

Ecological

In the Palearctic, Oriental, and Ethiopian regions, the chief common faunal denominator responsible for the enzootic distribution of CCHF virus appears to be the *Hyalomma* tick commonly infesting domestic and wild vertebrates in all zones except the deciduous forests of Moldavia. Enzootic CCHF virus is characteristically reported from areas where adults of one or two *Hyalomma* species are the very common or predominant ticks parasitizing domestic or wild mammals. (Immatures of some *Hyalomma* species parasitize the same hosts as adults; those of other species infest smaller-sized mammals, birds, or reptiles.) Of the 25 tick species and subspecies associated with CCHF virus, 10 are in the genus *Hyalomma*. Immatures and/or adults of 13 of the 15 ticks in other genera may feed in the same habitats and on the same hosts as the 10 hyalommas. The first exception is *Argas persicus,* but the reservoir-vector role of this bird parasite is cloudy. The second, chief, exception is *Ixodes ricinus,* both in Moldavia and in much of its range elsewhere in Europe, the British Isles, and Ireland. However, from southeastern Europe to the Caspian area of Iran, some *I. ricinus* and *Hyalomma* habitats are contiguous or overlap, and individual hosts may serve both tick groups. The Moldavian exception to the rule may represent a virus spillover into non-*Hyalomma* species and habitats remaining from nearby *Hyalomma* populations that have been eradicated in historical times by ecological change or by conscious human effort. *Hyalomma* distribution is quite circumscribed in Hungary and France, where little is known about the presence of CCHF virus. The paucity of reports of the virus from the Ethiopian faunal region south of the equator may be an artifact, due to lack of virological and serological search, or real, due to a climatic-ecological barrier to CCHF virus survival despite the common presence of *Hyalomma* ticks otherwise capable of serving as reservoirs and vectors. In the Oriental region, *Hyalomma* ticks fade out of the fauna in Burma immediately east of India.

Wherever and whenever enzootic CCHF virus has become epidemic, *Hyalomma* species have been the ticks chiefly involved. Whether this phenomenon will continue into the future remains to be seen.

There have been no sustained studies of the natural history and ecology of endemic CCHF virus anywhere in Asia, Europe, or Africa. The closest approach has been the several-year epidemiological survey throughout Tadzhikistan by Pak and colleagues. Even here, no effort was made to assess by rigorous scientific methods the biological role of individual small mammal, bird, and tick species in relation to the virus and how each component of the fauna interacts to maintain enzootic CCHF virus circulation.

"Silent", or enzootic, CCHF foci, in which the virus flows harmlessly between ticks and wild or domestic vertebrates, present the risk of human infection, misdiagnosis by unaware physicians, and possibly death, as frequently recorded in the earlier history of the disease in Asia and Europe. There is presently no surveillance for CCHF virus in Africa and the momentum for surveillance programs elsewhere has been declining since 1974 to 1975, owing to socioeconomic and political pressures to redirect biomedical and scientific research efforts to other subjects.

Not considering, for the moment, the disarrangements of nature caused by human activities, CCHF virus is enzootic in lowlands, foothills, and low mountain belts with arid or semiarid climates or long dry seasons, warm temperatures during summer or the year around, and relatively mild winters (by continental European-Siberian standards). Infected environments are deserts, semideserts, steppes (Eurasia), and savannas (Africa). Where rivers bordered by floodplains with rich meadows (as in Astrakhan Oblast and Egypt) or with tugai shrub and tree vegetation (as in Uzbekistan) course through deserts or semideserts, or where sparse saxaul forests dot the desert sands (as in Kazakhstan), or forests and thickets persist in rough steppelands (as in Rostov Oblast), the variety and population densities of vertebrates and ticks are greater than in the surrounding areas; in these belts, the intensity of virus circulation may also be greater.

Birulya et al.[45] concluded that all CCHF foci from Bulgaria to Central Asia are characterized by common physicogeographical conditions within the limits of the 2800 to 5000 sum of effective temperatures above 10°C in the transitional atmospheric humidity zone between forest-steppe and desert. How well the outside limits of this conclusion will stand the test of time remains to be determined. In Eurasia, the infected forest environments of Moldavia are marginal or an exception to this conclusion; the slight amount of information from India is impossible to fit into an ecological framework of any kind.

The Birulya et al.[45] conclusions regarding ecology and natural focality of CCHF virus in various landscapes are predicated on Soviet-Bulgarian experiences with the disease in human communities before 1970. Pragmatic as these assertions may be to epidemiologists of this geographical area, they do not include earlier and more recent data showing *enzootic* distribution of CCHF virus in various landscapes. Epidemiologists cannot fully appreciate and efficiently deal with the causes of enzootic activity while lacking detailed information on enzootic activity.

Climatically, the seasonal averages and extremes of the 1950s and 1960s in southeastern Europe were generally favorable for *Hyalomma m. marginatum* and CCHF virus survival. On this background, and aided by human-induced environmental changes, the intensity of virus circulation became epizootic. But this epidemic declined abruptly when *H. m. marginatum* densities drastically decreased during and following the severe 1968 to 1969 winter and spring seasons. While considering the enzootic cycle, we should recall that the virus did survive this severe winter and did remain active (i.e., enzootic) afterward in at least two northern tick species, *Rhipicephalus rossicus* and

Dermacentor marginatus, which are better adapted than *H. m. marginatum* for surviving cold winters.

African data derive chiefly from virus isolations from ticks from domestic animals driven long distances to abattoirs at Dakar, Ibadan, or Bangui, or from the host animals, or from a few human cases from hospitals in Kisangani and Entebbe and lacking field follow-up. Serological studies of East African wild mammals have been very limited. The single survey of African human sera consisted of no more than 250 samples from Nigeria. Only the most generalized ecological (and biomedical) conclusions can result from such insufficient data.

Infected landscapes in West Africa and the single focus reported from Ethiopia range from semidesert to grassy savannas, some with scattered trees and all with a long, harsh dry season. The scanty data from Zaire, Uganda, and Kenya provide an ecological enigma crying for elucidation. Ecologically and geographically, the recent discovery of enzootic CCHF virus in Egypt is not surprising.

Biological

Enzootic CCHF virus circulation is maintained by association between ticks and mammals. Transstadial and long interseasonal survival of the virus in the tick is of primary biological and epidemiological importance. Transovarial transmission of CCHF virus to successive tick generations is equally important, at least in the species in which this phenomenon has been investigated (this aspect of the virus-tick interrelationship should be studied qualitatively and quantitatively in a greater variety of tick species). Many but not all kinds of mammals (hedgehogs, rodents, ungulates) bitten by infected ticks develop a viremia of about 7 to 10 days duration (possibly longer) demonstrable serologically by antibody reactions which gradually decline over about a 6-month period. Uninfected ticks can become infected when feeding on an infected mammal. However, numerous factors determining the role of an individual mammal species in contributing to CCHF virus flow remain to be determined. Birds develop little or no detectable viremia but birds are biologically important in supporting populations of 9 or 10 of the 25 tick taxa associated with CCHF virus and also in disseminating virus-infected ticks. Tickbite is the only transmission route known to be significant in infecting mammals. However, in nature, infection from droplets or exudates or from contact with cadavers of infected mammals, especially in confined nests and burrows, should be considered as potentially possible. Urine apparently does not function as a CCHF virus-transport medium.

Enzootic CCHF virus has occasionally been associated with mild illness (lassitude, elevated temperature) or abortion in domestic ungulates. From experimental evidence with laboratory rodents, it would appear that newborn wild rodents bitten by CCHF virus-infected ticks can succumb to fatal illness. The epidemiological importance of CCHF virus in causing rodent mortality has not been investigated.

The feeding on a viremic host of two or more tick species with different biological patterns adds variety to the enzootic scene. A cow may become infected when serving as the host of transovarially infected adult *Hyalomma marginatum,* which had fed as immatures on birds, or of adult *Dermacentor,* which acquired the infection as larvae or nymphs from rodent or hedgehog hosts. Large numbers of one-host *Boophilus* parasitizing this cow throughout the viremic period may increase the virus activity in the host body. *Amblyomma, Rhipicephalus,* or *Haemaphysalis* species feeding on this viremic cow may become infected and transmit the virus via eggs to their progeny, which infest a variety of small vertebrates in different habitats and at varying periods and which disperse differently into the environment. In biota infected by CCHF virus, smaller-sized mammals as well as ungulates are often also infested simultaneously or in close succession by ticks of at least two genera.

One-host *Boophilus* ticks are important in maintaining virus circulation in herds of ungulates, which are very frequently also parasitized by two-host or three-host ticks of other genera. *Boophilus* rarely feed on humans.

Two-host ticks with similar (ungulate) hosts for both immature and adult stages differ from *Boophilus* mainly in that they infest two rather than one host and may attack humans. Two-host ticks with dissimilar hosts in the immature and adult stages feed as immatures chiefly on birds or on hares, depending on the nature of the local fauna. Birds or hares, so far as is known, are more or less equally acceptable food sources for these immatures. The local virus flow may be intensified by viremic hares but not by birds. However, CCHF virus acquired transovarially does persist through the combined larval-nymphal stages of two-host ticks feeding on birds, and adults molting from these immatures can infect a mammalian host.

A few species of three-host ticks feed on ungulates in each postembryonic stage, but most require small-sized hosts for immature stages and larger-sized hosts for the adult stage. This biological property enhances the epidemiological complexity of CCHF virus flow. In each virus focus, the degree of availability of two very different kinds of hosts, and the behavior patterns and seasonal and population dynamics of each animal, have a profound influence on tick population dynamics and consequently on virus flow dynamics.

Epizootics in Animals

Their Rise and Decline

Epizootics of certain zoonoses (typhus, plague, Kyasanur Forest disease, babesiosis, East Coast fever, etc.) become evident when wild or domestic animals, and sometimes also humans, sicken and die in larger numbers than usual. However, CCHF virus causes clearly defined disease only in people and newborn rodents. Therefore, epidemics in human populations have provided the only clues to epizootic episodes of CCHF virus in nature.

There have been four distinct epizootics of CCHF virus: in the Crimea in 1944 to 1945, Astrakhan Oblast in 1953 to 1968, Bulgaria in 1953 to 1973, and Rostov Oblast in 1963 to 1971. The 1976 outbreak in Pakistan may have assumed epizootic proportions, but accurate details are not yet available. Some outbreaks in southern republics of the Soviet Union probably occurred in conditions of epizootic virus circulation that were unrecognized as such owing to the sparse human population in undeveloped areas, misdiagnosis, and/or lack of epidemiological-virological follow-up.

In the Crimea, wartime devastation of the rural countryside steppe resulted in population explosions of hares and *Hyalomma m. marginatum,* much illness among nonimmune military personnel, and a high mortality rate. Climatic data for the first (1944) spring-fall season of the epidemic have not yet been recorded in literature that I have seen, but heavy rains and sleet in late 1944 and early 1945 caused a great reduction in the 1945 hare and tick populations and in human morbidity. Thereafter, CCHF virus became enzootic in the Crimea and only occasional human cases were seen between 1945 and 1969 despite dense *H. m. marginatum* populations in certain areas. No human cases have been reported from the Crimea since 1969, but more recent rates of CCHF virus isolation from four tick species have been high. Each of these four tick species is in close contact with domestic animals and humans. Owing to the lack of controlled investigations of interactions between the virus, different tick species, and wild and domestic animals in the Crimea, the anomaly of a high reported virus isolation rate but absence of human disease is difficult to explain.

The Astrakhan Oblast episode was biomedically the best studied of the 3 CCHF epizootics. It progressed from a low level of index cases of disease between 1953 and 1961 to higher levels in 1962 to 1963, fewer in 1964 to 1967, an increase in 1968, none in 1969, and few or none afterward. A combination of climatological factors necessary for *H. m. marginatum* survival in large numbers characterized the 1953 to 1968 period, which ended with the severe 1968 to 1969 winter-spring weather and drastically reduced *H. m. marginatum* density. (A detailed survey of the climate in Astrakhan Oblast preceeding, during, and after this period would be useful for epidemiological evaluation.) Epizootic virus circulation was indicated by disease among nonimmune inhabitants who had recently come to work in newly developed collective farms, other agricultural enterprises, and light industries in Astrakhan Oblast. Regulation of Volga floodwaters, instituted to make previously unexploited floodplains and deltalands available for the new agricultural schemes and human habitation, saved many ticks from drowning during the critical spring weeks when immature and adult *H. m. marginatum* quest for hosts. Flood control was considered to have been the critical initial factor in tick population density increase, leading to epizootic virus activity and epizootic human disease. Annual variations in the Volga spring flood level, even after control measures began, caused increased or decreased tick population densities the following summer. Hares, which were the chief hosts of immature *H. m. marginatum* in the Crimean CCHF epizootic, had a secondary host role in the Astrakhan epizootic. Here, rooks breeding in large colonies were the predominant hosts and dropped engorged nymphs in rich pastures where they molted to adults. The adults easily obtained from cattle the blood meals which provided energy for egg production.

From the results of limited seroepidemiological surveys of domestic animals in Astrakhan Oblast, it appears that CCHF virus was probably enzootic in the desert-semi-desert-steppe transitional zones on both sides of the Volga during the epidemic period in the riparian floodplains and deltalands. All cases of human illness — indicators of epidemic CCHF virus circulation — were traced to the floodplain-delta zone.

Thus the favorable climatological, faunal, and ecological nature of the Volga floodplain and delta areas of Astrakhan Oblast, together with the environmental changes wrought by a major socioeconomic drive, were interrelated in the development of epizootic CCHF virus. But only one factor — winter climate — reduced the virus flow from an epidemic to an endemic rate.

The tragic Bulgarian CCHF epidemic also became apparent in 1953, when 50 human cases with 6 fatalities were recognized. One Bulgarian case had been reported in 1951 and 10 occurring between 1946 and 1952 were diagnosed retrospectively from hospital records. Whether the pre-1953 data should be attributed to an epizootic (possibly involving other misdiagnosed or unrecorded cases) or to an enzootic period is moot. As in Astrakhan and Rostov Oblasts, the Bulgarian epizootic coincided with extreme environmental changes caused by countrywide collectivization of agricultural activities and frequent human contact with large numbers of *Hyalomma m. marginatum*. The pre-1969 Bulgarian morbidity rates, the highest recorded in any CCHF epidemic, show the same years of higher and lower disease incidence recorded in Astrakhan. However, the Bulgarian epizootic continued to 1973 (no later data are available to me), well beyond the 1969 "cutoff" date in Astrakhan, though at a lower ebb than in 1968 and earlier. This epizootic prolongation may have resulted from a milder Bulgarian winter climate, but precise evidence is lacking. Bulgarian CCHF foci were distributed through plains, hills, and low mountain biotopes, thus differing distinctly from the Volga floodplain-delta CCHF foci of Astrakhan but being similar, superficially at least, to certain environmental categories characterizing the Rostov epizootic.

The scattered studies of the natural history of CCHF virus during the Bulgarian epizootic listed hares and various ground-feeding bird species as hosts of immature *H. m. marginatum* and mentioned rooks only incidentally or not at all. As in Rostov Oblast, the 1968 breakthrough in CCHF research techniques provided the tools and impetus for isolating the virus in Bulgaria from other tick genera (*Ixodes, Dermacen-*

tor, Rhipicephalus, and *Boophilus*), as well as from *H. m. marginatum*. These other tick genera are undoubtedly involved, to a greater or lesser extent in enzootic CCHF but the data are too scanty for evaluating virus circulation dynamics in each.

Hopefully, Bulgarian authorities will analyze demographic, climatic, environmental-ecological, and morbidity data for the entire epizootic period and compare their results with data from Astrakhan and Rostov Oblasts to provide better understanding of factors responsible for CCHF epizootics and epizootics in human populations.

The severe Rostov Oblast CCHF epizootic began as a shock and surprise to all concerned in 1963, during the height of the Astrakhan and Bulgarian epizootics. It continued to 1969, with a few cases of human illness in 1970 and 1971. Again, the causes of greater *H. m. marginatum* numbers and of more frequent human contact with infected ticks were attributed to changes in the rural economy and in agricultural and animal husbandry practices under the impetus of an ambitious 5-year plan encompassing numerous environmental changes. The bitter winter-spring weather of 1968 to 1969 that reduced the tick population density in Astrakhan Oblast functioned with almost equal efficiency in Rostov Oblast. Although the natural history of tick-virus-vertebrate inter-relationships was not investigated as intensively as in Astrakhan Oblast, the gradual spread, sporadic incidence, and scattered source localities of CCHF cases throughout Rostov Oblast were well documented. This information nicely illustrates, in a generalized way, epizootic processes and temporal and spatial progress of CCHF virus flow. The climatological-acarological data for *H. m. marginatum* replacement by different reservoir-vector tick genera (*Rhipicephalus* and *Dermacentor*) in Rostov Oblast following the 1968 to 1969 winter provide valuable clues to epizootic/enzootic changeover and to the natural history of CCHF virus in the absence of large numbers of the usual epizootic-causing *Hyalomma* ticks.

The environments in which these four epizootics were localized differ ecologically but each was characterized by high population densities of *Hyalomma m. marginatum*. The brief Crimean episode occurred chiefly in primitively cultivated, partially abandoned steppeland. The Astrakhan epizootic (at the eastern margin of the European section of the Palearctic faunal region) was strictly confined to the lush Volga floodplain and delta, though there was some evidence of enzootic virus flow (with no human morbidity) in the desert-semidesert-steppe zones bordering this floodplain-delta zone. The Rostov epizootic was chiefly in rough, hilly, forest-steppe landscapes with nearby pastures and cultivated fields, but was less intense in the meadows, forests, and scrub areas of the relatively narrow Don floodplain. Bulgarian foci were scattered through newly and previously cultivated plains, hills, and low mountains. Riparian zones were not recorded as having an especially important epidemiological role in Bulgaria.

In each of the four epizootics, cattle were the chief hosts of adult *H. m. marginatum*. In the Crimea, a population explosion of hares and in Astrakhan huge numbers of rooks supported numerous immatures that molted to adult *H. m. marginatum* in pastures and field margins where cattle were easily available as hosts. Hares and rooks were both involved in the Rostov epizootic, but in Bulgaria hares and other species of ground-feeding birds were reported to be important hosts of immature *H. m. marginatum*.

In retrospect, we have a number of clues to how an enzootic CCHF focus may become epizootic, but little solid data of the scope desired by contemporary epidemiologists. Reasons for cessation of CCHF epizootics in a temperate area are well enough documented (except in Bulgaria) but different factors would operate in a CCHF focus in a tropical climate.

TRANSMISSION

Virus in Insects

More than 25,000 mosquitoes (six species) from the Astrakhan CCHF focus were tested for virus between 1967 and 1969. All results were negative and sentinel laboratory mammals on which mosquitoes fed in this focus showed no evidence of CCHF infection.[104]

Ardoin[17] inoculated a "Congo" strain intrathoracically into *Aedes aegypti* mosquitoes but was unable to recover the virus from the mosquitoes on the same day or later during the 15-day observation period. When Ardoin fed *Ae. aegypti* on blood containing the "Congo" strain, he recovered the virus immediately afterward but not later during the 22-day observation period. The failure of HAZ virus (CCHF serogroup) to plaque in Singh's *Aedes albopictus* cells[589] may suggest that neither member of this serogroup adapts to insects.

Causey et al.[80,81] isolated a CCHF strain from 1 of 377 pools of *Culicoides* spp. (Diptera: Ceratopogonidae) collected in light traps near a Nigerian cattle shed but mentioned that undigested vertebrate blood may have been present in this pool.

In summary, there is no evidence to suggest that insects have a role in the natural history of CCHF virus.

Virus in Ticks

To determine whether ticks (or insects) are infected by arboviruses, including CCHF, individual specimens or suitable specimen pools are triturated in physiological saline, usually containing 0.75% bovine albumin (pH 7.3), penicillin, and streptomycin sulfate. Following centrifugation at 2000 rpm for 20 min, supernatants are inoculated intracerebrally into NWM or cell cultures.

The FA technique has recently gained favor among Soviet researchers as a rapid, inexpensive, and efficient tool for demonstrating antibodies to CCHF virus in tick salivary glands and reproductive organs. FA test procedures developed by Popov[410] revealed CCHF-infected *Hyalomma m. marginatum* from Bulgarian cattle and horse[411] and in other *H. m. marginatum* from nature and following experimental infection.[601,602] Results of FA investigation of nine tick species from CCHF foci in six Soviet republics suggested to Zgurskaya et al.[603] and Chumakov et al.[113] that this technique is much more sensitive as an indicator of virus infection in ticks than inoculating NWM with tick suspensions.

There have been no detailed investigations of CCHF virus localization, multiplication, and dynamics in ticks on the order of those of Russian spring-summer encephalitis virus in *Haemaphysalis (H.) concinna* by Pavlovsky and Solovev.[391,392] Colorado tick fever virus in *Dermacentor andersoni* by Rozeboom and Burgdorfer,[440] and Quaranfil virus in *Argas (Persicargas) arboreus* by Kaiser.[236] The susceptibility of several tick species to experimental infection with CCHF virus is reviewed in the following section.

Virus Survival in Ticks

Introduction

The long survival of arboviruses in ticks is important epidemiologically. This is especially true where populations of the short-lived, small-sized bird or mammal hosts of long-lived ticks turn over rapidly in the ecosystem and also where these hosts rapidly develop antibodies to infections acquired in the nest during their first few days of life.[211] Results of experimental studies reviewed below suggest that in nature CCHF virus often survives throughout the life of the tick and may be transovarially (or vertically) transmitted from one tick generation to the next. However, better quantified and qualified data would be useful for epidemiological evaluation of these phenomena. The epidemiological importance of vertical transmission and the present state of knowledge of the subject in the plant and animal kingdoms were expertly reviewed by Fine.[173]

"Overwintering" of CCHF virus in unfed nymphal and female *Hyalomma m. marginatum* taken in spring in the Crimea and in Rostov and Astrakhan Oblasts was reported by Chumakov.[93,96] Pak et al.[380] isolated two CCHF strains from unfed adult *H. a. anatolicum* taken in the spring from cracks in clay walls in Tadzhikistan, and Pak[374,375] mentioned other isolations from unfed adults after overwintering.

Transstadial Survival and Transovarial Transmission

The transstadial survival of disease agents (from larva to nymph to adult) is frequent in argasid and ixodid ticks and is an important epidemiological property of these parasites.[74] This phcnomenon is rare in hematophagous insects. The reason for this biological difference lies in the tick's relatively insignificant structural changes during molting, when ectodermal derivatives and certain muscle groups are practically the only structures to undergo histolysis. Only the tick salivary gland alveoli are completely replaced while molting. The tick midgut, Malpighian tubules, and other organs that are intensely invaded by microorganisms are gradually replaced throughout the entire life cycle.

Transovarial transmission of pathogens is also more common in ticks than in insects; this complex, biologically important phenomenon requires more precise investigation for full epidemiological evaluation. Řeháček[428] and Burgdorfer and Varma[63] reviewed questions of transstadial survival and transovarial transmission of disease agents among arthropods, as did Balashov[24] [see pages 358, 359 in the Hoogstraal and Tatchell (Eds.)[226] translation of Balashov 1968].

During 1969 studies of CCHF epidemiology in Rostov Oblast, Kondratenko et al.[283] isolated the virus from eggs of *Dermacentor marginatus* and *Hyalomma m. marginatum*. They stated that this was the first demonstration of transovarial transmission of CCHF virus in *H. marginatum*. However, in describing "*Haemorrhagognes tchumakovi*," Zhdanov[606] had asserted, without citing evidence, that "*H. m. marginatum* is the vector transmitting the virus (causing CCHF) transovarially to the progeny."

The pioneer experimental study to determine the nature of transstadial survival and transovarial transmission of CCHF virus was made in Nigeria by Lee and Kemp,[309] who parenterally inoculated a local ("Congo") strain into fed nymphal *Hyalomma marginatum rufipes*. The inoculation processes caused trauma and only 99 of the 132 nymphs molted to adults. A variety of difficulties were encountered in feeding the adult ticks and keeping them alive and, apparently, also in obtaining a sufficiently high virus titer for meaningful experimental results. At any rate, on day 108 post-inoculation (PI) 11 adults that had molted from these nymphs were fed on a susceptible calf which experienced CCHF viremia 2 and 7 days later. The virus was recovered from two of the females removed from the calf and tested on day 135 PI, as well as from F₁ larvae tested on day 191 PI of the parents.

Zgurskaya et al.[598] fed clean, laboratory-reared larval *Hyalomma m. marginatum* on experimentally infected European hares, *Lepus europaeus,* and long-eared hedgehogs, *Hemiechinus auritus*. The larvae molted on the hosts to nymphs. Some nymphs were held at 4°C for 13 months (artificial overwintering and virus survival study) and checked monthly for presence of virus. After 6 months at 4°C, some nymphs were fed on uninfected guinea pigs to obtain engorged females and F₁ larvae and nymphs; thc guinea pig blood was tested afterward for evidence of CCHF virus infection by inoculation into NWM and by CF, AGDP, and N serological tests. Virus isolations from the fed nymphs and also from adults molting from fed nymphs provided evidence of transstadial survival. Adult ticks kept at 4°C for up to 7 months caused no clinical disease after being inoculated into NWM, but in the CF test the brain antigens of the mice reacted positively with immune serum against CCHF virus. The virus was also demonstrated in the ticks 8 to 10 months after dropping from the infected hosts. Two of 24 guinea pigs on which "overwintered" nymphs fed were viremic 11 and 12 days after the ticks attached, and CF test results showed evidence of infection up to day 35. Positive virus transmission results obtained in spring but not in winter were postulated to result from virus activation by increased environmental temperature, light, and solar radiation. Four CCHF strains were isolated from rabbit host blood 7 and 8 days after F_1 larvae began feeding, and 8 strains were isolated from unfed and partially fed F_1 nymphs from these rabbits. These data are not presented quantitatively but do demonstrate that CCHF virus survives in *Hyalomma m. marginatum* from season to season and in each developmental stage from the initially infected larva to the F_1 nymph (as far as tested). Each feeding stage can transmit the virus to a new vertebrate host. The presence of the virus in eggs could not be proven by inoculation into NWM owing to the extreme toxicity of tick eggs for the animals.

Kondratenko[282] investigated *Hyalomma m. marginatum, Rhipicephalus rossicus,* and *Dermacentor marginatus* from Rostov Oblast for infectibility with CCHF virus, virus survival in time and transstadially, and transovarial transmission. Larval *H. m. marginatum* and nymphal *R. rossicus* and *D. marginatus* were infected by feeding on the experimentally infected little suslik, *Citellus pygmaeus.* From 60 to 335 days after initial infection, suspensions of adults molting from these immatures were inoculated into NWM. One half of the 16 and 12 NWM inoculated with *H. m. marginatum* and *R. rossicus,* respectively, and about one third of the 23 NWM inoculated with *D. marginatus* were serologically positive for CCHF virus infection. Some of the adult ticks (exact numbers were not stated) had been held at 4°C to simulate overwintering. Nevertheless, the biological and epidemiological importance of transstadial survival and long (interseasonal) survival of the virus in these three species appears to be quite well established by these results.

For investigating transovarial transmission, Kondratenko[282] used the F_1 and F_2 progeny of 10 female *H. m. marginatum,* 10 female *R. rossicus,* and 12 female *D. marginatus,* each of which had oviposited normally after feeding on infected rabbits or susliks. Larvae were tested for infection 372 to 375 days (F_1) or 700 to 703 days (F_2) following initial infection of the mother generation, either by inoculation of suspensions into NWM or by feeding on infected susliks. The data for the 46 tests (28 positive to 18 negative) of these two generations (lumped in the text and in Table 1) were as follows: 8 of 14 tests with *H. m. marginatum* were positive (2700 larvae, 100 to 300 per test), 15 of 19 tests with *R. rossicus* were positive (4700 larvae, 100 to 400 per test), and 5 of 13 tests with *D. marginatus* were positive (2300 larvae, 100 to 200 per test). When about 800 F_1 nymphs and adults were tested 404 to 620 days after initial infection, 18 of 26 pools of *H. m. marginatum,* 22 of 34 pools of *R. rossicus,* and 18 of 27 pools of *D. marginatus* were positive for virus infection. When F_1 and F_2 larvae, nymphs, or adults of these three species were fed on susliks and laboratory rabbits 313 to 620 days following infection of the mother generation, virus was detected in 24 of the 38 host animals. These results show that in these three tick species transovarial transmission of CCHF virus is a significant biological phenomenon and an important process in the epidemiology of CCHF virus.

Levi and Vasilenko[325] reported transstadial survival and transovarial transmission of CCHF virus in *Hyalomma m. marginatum* which had fed on experimentally infected giant Belgian hares. They stated that all tests were positive for the virus. This is an unusually high rate of positive results for experiments on transovarial transmission of arboviruses in ticks.

Zgurskaya et al.[602] concluded from an interesting though limited experiment that *H. m. marginatum* is highly susceptible to CCHF virus by each of several infection methods tested. The small samples, low rates of positive results in some trials, and ambiguousness of certain statements leave many questions to be answered.

I have been unable to obtain the "preliminary report on experimental infections in *H. a. anatolicum*" by Pak et al.,[378] which Pak and Mikhailova[383] reviewed in a single sentence: "It was . . . established that larval *H. anatolicum* do not always become infected by feeding on NWM inoculated with CCHF virus." The Pak[375] conclusion that transovarial transmission of CCHF virus in *H. a. anatolicum* and in *H. detritum* is epidemiologically unimportant in Tadzhikistan was said to be based on negative results of virological testing of egg batches of these species. The data and methods were not stated. Numerous other workers have reported on the great toxicity of tick eggs for experimental animals.

Tick Species Associated with CCHF Virus

Introduction

Seventeen CCHF-associated tick species and subspecies from Eurasia are listed below. The virus has been isolated from 16. The 17th, *Dermacentor daghestanicus,* is included on the basis of FA demonstration of antigens to CCHF virus in salivary glands. All but 3 of the 17 species are fully representative of the Palearctic faunal region. *Boophilus microplus* (virus isolate from Pakistan), whose primary distribution is oriental, has been carried on cattle to Africa, Madagascar, the Americas, and Australia. *Hyalomma a. anatolicum* ranges from the Palearctic into nearby areas of the Ethiopian and oriental regions; CCHF virus has been isolated from this tick in all three regions. *Rhipicephalus sanguineus* has pushed northward from the Ethiopian region into the Palearctic with dogs and has also been widely transported elsewhere.

> Family Argasidae
> > *Argas (Persicargas) persicus* (Oken)
> Family Ixodidae
> > *Ixodes (Ixodes) ricinus* (Linnaeus)
> > *Haemaphysalis (Aboimisalis) punctata* Canestrini and Fanzago
> > *Hyalomma (Hyalomma) anatolicum anatolicum* Koch
> > *Hyalomma (Hyalomma) asiaticum asiaticum* Schulze
> > *Hyalomma (Hyalomma) detritum* Schulze
> > *Hyalomma (Hyalomma) marginatum marginatum* Koch [= *H. p. plumbeum* (Panzer)]
> > *Hyalomma (Hyalomma) marginatum turanicum* Pomerantsev
> > *Dermacentor (Dermacentor) daghestanicus* Olencv
> > *Dermacentor (Dermacentor) marginatus* (Sulzer)
> > *Rhipicephalus (Digineus) bursa* Canestrini and Fanzago
> > *Rhipicephalus (Rhipicephalus) pumilio* Schulze
> > *Rhipicephalus (Rhipicephalus) rossicus* Yakimov and Kohl-Yakimova
> > *Rhipicephalus (Rhipicephalus) sanguineus* Latreille
> > *Rhipicephalus (Rhipicephalus) turanicus* Pomerantsev and Matikashvili
> > *Boophilus annulatus* (Say) [= *B. calcaratus* Birula]
> > *Boophilus microplus* (Canestrini)

In Africa, CCHF virus has been isolated from the following 9 ixodid species. Each is typical of the Ethiopian Faunal Region, except *Hyalomma a. anatolicum,* which occurs south of the Sahara only near the borders with the Palearctic Region.

> *Hyalomma (Hyalomma) anatolicum anatolicum* Koch
> *Hyalomma (Hyalomma) impeltatum* Schulze and Schlottke
> *Hyalomma (Hyalomma) impressum* Koch
> *Hyalomma (Hyalomma) marginatum rufipes* Koch

> *Hyalomma (Hyalomma) nitidum* Schulze
> *Hyalomma (Hyalomma) truncatum* Koch
> *Amblyomma (Theileriella variegatum* (Fabricius)
> *Rhipicephalus (Lamellicauda) Pulchellus* Gerstäcker
> *Boophilus decoloratus* (Koch)

All verified CCHF strains from ticks were isolated after 1967. Of the more than 125 Soviet strains obtained between 1967 and 1970, about 30 were ticks.[95] After the 1944 to 1970 epidemics subsided in the U.S.S.R., epidemiological investigations turned to enzootic areas, and the number of virus strains and variety of tick sources increased greatly. Our previous list of CCHF-associated ticks[211] contained 10 species and subspecies; the present list contains 25. The Andrewes and Pereira[12] statement that CCHF virus has been isolated from *Ornithodoros* sp. appears to be mistaken.

Before the 1967 to 1968 use of NWM for CCHF virus isolation and the development of serological and other tools for strain identification and research, a few *Hyalomma* species with very different biological-ecological properties were circumstantially considered as vectors. These dissimilar properties were an important factor contributing to the nosological uncertainty over the poorly defined clinical and epidemiological types of hemorrhagic disease episodes described from Asian areas of the Soviet Union.

CCHF virus is remarkable among arthropod-borne viruses infecting humans for the number and variety of reservoir-vector species linked with it and the numerous ecological environments in which it circulates in three different faunal regions. The present list of 25 CCHF-associated tick species and subspecies will undoubtedly increase as epidemiological research extends to unexplored biotopes. The biological patterns among these 25 taxa include practically all of those recognized in ixodid ticks characteristic of temperate climates and many of those in tropical ixodids.

How best to condense the considerable quantity of biomedical information now available for these 25 taxa of ticks into a very few pages has caused me no little concern.* To present this information succinctly and meaningfully for the understanding of basic epidemiological processes, it appears most useful to arrange the tick species primarily by number of hosts parasitized by the larval, nymphal, and adult stages, and secondarily by geographical area (Eurasia and Africa).

The number of hosts parasitized by an individual tick during its lifetime, and the potential variety of hosts and degree of host specificity, are biological factors of utmost epidemiological importance. The equally important factors — virus survival in ticks in nature, and transstadial survival and transovarial transmission of the virus — have been mentioned elsewhere.

The general features of the three- , two- , or one-host types of ixodid life cycles were reviewed by Hoogstraal.[203,210,216] Balashov[24] stressed the physiological phases of development within the morphologically distinctive larva, nymph, and adult. A single argasid species, *Argas (P.) persicus,* is the only multihost tick reported to be a source of CCHF virus.

---

* (*The Bibliography of Ticks and Tickborne Diseases,* volumes 1 to 5 part II[206-209,212,217] lists all known literature on these subjects to December 31, 1976. Volume 6, now in an advanced stage of preparation, will be an annotated bibliography of CCHF virus and all other tick-associated viruses except those in the genus *Flavivirus* (B. serogroup). Volume 7, now partially completed, will be an annotated bibliography of tick-borne B serogroup viruses. The *Index-Catalogue of Medical and Veterinary Zoology,*[146-151,163,424,425,471,571] arranged by tick species and hosts, is a useful cross-reference. Persons using the *Index-Catalogue,* an excellent compilation, should be alerted to search for the taxa as originally cited, which will not necessarily be the currently accepted taxa used in the present review. For instance, much Soviet literature dealing with *Hyalomma marginatum* and *Boophilus annulatus* will be found in the *Index-Catalogue* under *Hyalomma plumberum* and *Boophilus calcaratus.* The most recent part of the *Index-Catalogue* devoted to ticks[145] is a checklist of families, genera, species, and subspecies.)

The three-host model is generally agreed to be the "original" ixodid host relationship pattern and remains so for at least 600 of the 650 contemporary ixodid species.[210,216] Three different vertebrates typically serve as hosts for the three parasitic stages of the tick. The three-host system thrice exposes the tick to possible environmental extremes or to the possibility of failing to reach an acceptable host before unfed larval, nymphal, or adult energy reserves are exhausted in questing for a host or merely in the process of survival. If more ixodids had been able to convert to a two- or one-host pattern, more tick species might have evolved and survived, and tick populations might be more ubiquitous than they are in the modern world.

A few ixodid species dwell solely in restricted microhabitats (burrows, caves, dens) for their entire life cycle but each feeds on three hosts. Pathogen circulation in this closed community is usually restricted to the one or few vertebrate species normally occupying these restricted habitats and to the one characteristic tick species in each situation. However, this ixodid species may share the restricted habitat and host(s) with 1 or more ixodid and/or argasid species, which may also participate in the pathogen circulation chain. The "additional" ixodid species remains in this microhabitat only during the larval and nymphal stages; the adults venture outside to the ground or to vegetation in search of larger-sized hosts and may transmit the agent from the closed community to the other vertebrate members of the biotope and, indirectly, to other tick species parasitizing these vertebrates. CCHF virus has not yet been reported from a tick species spending its entire life in restricted habitats, but has been isolated from *Hyalomma a. asiaticum* and other species whose immatures sometimes share burrows with various tick species.

Numerous ixodid species with a three-host pattern inhabit burrows or restricted shelters as larvae and nymphs but their adults search outside the shelter for larger-sized hosts. Nymphs of a few of these species typically leave the shelter; nymphs of other species may do so under conditions of stress or hunger. Hosts infested by immatures and adults of these three-host ixodids may differ vastly, as, for instance, mouse and buffalo, bird and goat, lizard and ibex, hedgehog and lion, or shrew and cow. The females of these species often oviposit along runways frequented by rodents or other small-sized vertebrates.

Some 30 ixodid species, involving representatives of all the large genera (i.e., 30 species or more), may feed as larvae, nymphs, and adults on larger-sized wandering vertebrates (deer, antelopes, buffalo, cattle, etc.), but this phenomenon is seldom *absolutely* established (see *Rhipicephalus pulchellus*).

Each active stage of other three-host species quests from the ground or from vegetation. Among these species, some such as *Ixodes (I.) ricinus,* a vector of CCHF virus and numerous other pathogenic agents, accept as a host almost any vertebrate coming within reach of the larvae, nymphs, and adults. Although this host catholicity characterizes less than 10% of all ixodid species, their exceptional adaptability and biological success place them among the world's most important and notorious tick vectors.

The two-host pattern is an occasional phenomenon in some *Hyalomma* species but a constant type in the *H. marginatum* complex, *H. detritum, Rhipicephalus bursa* and a few other species inhabiting steppe or savanna environments with low or moderate rainfall and long dry seasons. Adults, or both adults and immatures, of two-host ixodids infest wandering vertebrates, often in biotopes where the original host numbers (before the advent of domestic animals) were not dense. In this host pattern, the larva molts to the nymphal stage on the host and the nymph feeds on the same host before detaching and molting to an adult.

Reduction to the one-host pattern, the most extreme modification of the original three-host pattern, is confined to a few ixodid species parasitizing mobile, hoofed mammals with relatively extensive home ranges. The larvae, nymphs, and adults remain on the same host; only the mated, replete female detaches to oviposit on the ground. All *Boophilus* species are one-host ticks. *Hyalomma scupense* Schulze of the eastern Mediterranean and southwestern U.S.S.R. is a winter-feeding, generally one-host tick often mentioned in epidemiological studies of CCHF virus in this area. The virus has not yet been isolated from *H. scupense*.

It would be biologically proper to arrange the following discussion in the three-two-one-host order. However, the reverse sequence, from the epidemiologically most simple one-host to the more complex two- and three-host species, appears more practical for readers who are not intimately acquainted with tick biology.

One-Host Ticks

All *Boophilus* species (and presumably the three species of the closely related genus *Margaropus*) are one-host parasites of artiodactyl or perissodactyl mammals. There are very few one-host species in other genera (*Hyalomma, Rhipicephalus, Dermacentor, Aponomma*). If *Boophilus* ticks are accidently dislodged from the host before the final phase of female engorgement, they may reattach to a new host in the immediate vicinity of the dropping place. The feeding period of a *Boophilus* population usually extends over many weeks, during which the host parasite load is replenished by new larvae as replete females detach. Thus the *Boophilus* epidemiological role is in maintaining virus interaction betwen ticks and a single host over a relatively long period of the year. During this time, uninfected ticks of other genera parasitizing the same viremic host may easily become infected and subsequently transmit the virus to a different host. Or infected ticks of other genera may transmit a virus to a host; *Boophilus* feeding on this host at the same time or afterward may acquire and amplify the virus. Whether CCHF virus is transovarially transmitted in *Boophilus* species is unknown.

CCHF virus has been reported from three of the six recognized *Boophilus* species (see Hoogstraal[203] for identification criteria and illustrations). All hosts of the infected ticks were cattle, except that 2 of the 21 isolates from Nigeria were from *B. decoloratus* parasitizing sheep. In most *Boophilus*-infested biotopes, these ticks are numerous on cattle and horses and also parasitize all other available domestic and wild herbivores, but humans are seldom if ever attacked. The number of CCHF strains isolated from *Boophilus* in some surveys points to the usefulness of these ticks as indicators of the prevalence of CCHF infections in herds of domestic mammals.

Other viruses isolated from *Boophilus* are Dugbe (Bunyaviridae) and Jos (unclassified) from *B. annulatus* in Central African Republic; Dugbe, Bhanja, and Thogoto (Bunyaviridae) and Jos and Somone (unclassified) from *B. decoloratus* in Nigeria, Central African Republic, Cameroon, and Kenya; and Wad Medani and Seletar (Reoviridae) from *B. microplus* in Pakistan, Singapore, and Malaysia. *Boophilus* are notorious vectors of *Babesia* species and also transmit a variety of other infectious agents to domestic and wild herbivores.

Boophilus are biologically adapted to wandering hoofed mammals. They prospered when people pastured cattle and horses in or near their habitats and became very widely distributed when herds of infested domestic animals were driven great distances in search of food and water or transported to other continents.[210]

Boophilus annulatus

CCHF virus was isolated from *B. annulatus* in Bulgaria between 1968 and 1972, in Armenia about 1972, and in Uzbekistan in 1973. Infections were also demonstrated by the FA technique in *B. annulatus* from Azerbaijan in 1970.

B. annulatus is native to the southern part of the Palearctic faunal region, from Kazakhstan, Afghanistan, and Iran to the western Mediterranean area, where it probably originally fed chiefly on gazelles.[210] The Spanish probably transported *B. annu-*

latus to Mexico on horses or cattle; it became the famed "Texas fever tick" when cattlemen opened the American West. *B. annulatus* is also found in favorable biotopes of Africa north of the equator[203] but has not been well studied in this area. Some Soviet literature on *B. annulatus* (as the junior synonym *B. calcaratus*) is by Galuzo[182] for Kazakhstan (especially good), Dzhaparidze[160] for Georgia, and Grebenyuk[186] for Kirgizia.

The second Palearctic species, *B. kohlsi*,[222] is unique in this genus for parasitizing domestic sheep and goats rather than cattle. It occurs in Jordan, Iraq, Syria, Israel, and Yemen (outside of the presently known distribution area of CCHF virus).

Boophilus microplus

CCHF virus from *B. microplus* in Pakistan was reported in 1970. *B. microplus* originally infested forest-dwelling antelopes, deer, and wild cattle and buffalo in southern Asia (Oriental faunal region) but has been transported, chiefly on zebu cattle, to Australia, New Guinea, Madagascar, Taiwan, South and Central America (including southern U.S.), and southeastern Africa as far north as coastal Kenya. This highly adaptable tick is a serious economic problem almost everywhere it occurs. Within the known geographic range of CCHF virus, *B. microplus* is present only in India and Pakistan. A second oriental species of uncertain identity infests cattle in Sri Lanka.[572]

Boophilus decoloratus

One CCHF strain was isolated from *B. decoloratus* in Senegal between 1969 and 1974 but in Nigeria, between 1964 and 1968, 21 strains were isolated from this species, 19 from ticks from cattle and 2 from ticks from sheep. *B. decoloratus* is widely distributed in Africa south of the Sahara and is often numerous on cattle in present and former habitats of African antelopes and of the African, or cape, buffalo.[203] The available data point to *B. decoloratus* as a prime candidate for research in relation to the epidemiology of CCHF virus in Africa. Cattle are seldom exported from Africa; thus unlike *B. annulatus* and *B. microplus, B. decoloratus* has not become established on other continents.

Boophilus geigyi

The second Ethiopian species, *B. geigyi*,[3] is restricted to West Africa (Senegal, Nigeria, Ivory Coast, Benin, Chad, Central African Republic, Ghana, Togo, Liberia, Sierra Leone, Mali, etc.). Our files show that a certain number of *B. decoloratus* records in literature on Nigerian CCHF virus research are in fact based on *B. geigyi*. This species should be investigated for its role as a reservoir and vector of the virus.

Two-Host Ticks

These ticks can be considered in two subgroups reflecting distinct biological adaptations associated with the spatial movements and migrations of different kinds of preferred hosts.

In the first subgroup (3a), hosts of immature and of adult stages are generally similar (deer, wild pig, cow, horse, camel, goat, etc.). Birds are seldom involved with tick species of this category. In the second subgroup (3b), hosts of immature and adult stages are generally dissimilar; immature stages frequently feed on birds or hares, hedgehogs, or other small- or medium-sized mammals; adults feed on larger wild and domestic mammals, occasionally on large birds such as bustards, storks, or ostriches.

Similar-Host Subgroup

Tick-host-virus interelationships in the 3a *(B. annulatus)* subgroup are only slightly more complex epidemiologically than those of one-host ticks. In subgroup 3b *B. mi-*

croplus, these interrelationships can be as manifold as any found in heterogeneous three-host ticks. Among two-host ticks associated with CCHF virus, *Rhipicephalus bursa, Hyalomma detritum,* and *H. a. anatolicum* have a *B. annulatus* subgroup pattern. This pattern is characteristic of a few other Eurasian and African species in these genera but rarely of other ixodid ticks anywhere. Nomadic humans and their widely ranging camels, cattle, horses, sheep, and goats, and man-made structures serving as shelters, have undoubtedly contributed to extending the geographic range and to increasing the population densities of these three species.

Rhipicephalus bursa

Adults yielded CCHF virus in the Crimea, Bulgaria and Greece, Armenia and Azerbaijan, and Turkmenia. All strains were isolated between 1969 and 1975; all infected ticks were from cattle except those from Greece, which were from goats.

Other viruses isolated from *R. bursa* are West Nile (Togaviridae) in Azerbaijan,[499] and Bhanja in Azerbaijan[331] and Thogoto (both Bunyaviridae) in Sicily.[4-6] *R. bursa* is also a vector of *Babesia, Theileria,* and *Anaplasma* and causes paralysis in sheep.

The biologically and morphologically distinctive *R. bursa* ranges from the western Mediterranean (Portugal, Morocco, Algeria) eastward to Kazakhstan. It is especially common in suitable habitats in western Turkey, adjacent countries, and southwestern republics of the U.S.S.R. *R. bursa* also occurs in the Mediterranean climatic zone of Switzerland,[2] but records from tropical Africa are based on misidentifications.[203] Favorite habitats are grassy and lightly forested low and medium altitude mountain slopes. This tick has also adapted to certain modified steppe environments but less often to semidesert situations. All types of domestic mammals, and sometimes people and hares, are infested. The few records from bird,[196,197] lizard, or small mammal hosts require confirmation. Original hosts appear to be the roe deer, *Capreolus capreolus,* as reported from the Crimea and Italy,[441,501] the wild goat, *Capra hircus aegagrus,* and Asiatic mouflon (wild sheep), *Ovis orientalis,* as reported from Iraq and Iran,[223,228] and related artiodactyl mammals.

Hyalomma detritum

Infections with CCHF virus were demonstrated in this species after 1970 by the FA test or by virus isolations from specimens from Azerbaijan and from Uzbekistan, Kazakhstan, and Tadzhikistan. All hosts, where stated, were cattle.

Other viruses isolated from *H. detritum* are West Nile *(Togaviridae)* in Turkmenia, and Bhanja *(Bunyaviridae)* in Kazakhstan. *H. detritum* is important in veterinary medicine wherever it occurs, and dense populations often develop in areas grazed by livestock.

Geographically, the Asian *H. detritum* is discontinuously distributed through the area listed for *R. bursa,* but also occurs where *R. bursa* is not present, in the terai of Nepal, in northern India, Pakistan, and Afghanistan, and in Egypt. (Published records of *H. detritum* from China remain to be confirmed.) Domestic mammals and wild mammals related to those parasitized by *R. bursa* serve as hosts, but *H. detritum* is ecologically more adapted to desert, semidesert, and drier steppe biotopes, where its habitats are marshes, riparian floodplains (tugai), irrigated fields, and grassy slopes. *H. detritum* and *H. anatolicum* may be present in the same habitats, but *R. bursa* is seldom if ever associated with these species. Like *H. anatolicum, H. detritum* is often numerous in stables and houses where domestic animals rest. Adults generally feed from late spring to late summer, but in warmer areas during much of the year. Immature stages become active in late summer or fall. Satiated nymphs shelter under rocks or manure or in wall cracks, but some may remain on the host until spring. The seasonal dynamics vary in different biotopes.

Hyalomma anatolicum anatolicum

CCHF virus has been recorded from this tick from Armenia, Turkmenia, Uzbekistan, Tadzhikistan, Pakistan, and Nigeria. These isolates were mostly made in the 1969 to 1973 period; strains were isolated earlier in Nigeria but identified in 1968. *H. a. anatolicum* has also been circumstantially incriminated as a CCHF virus vector in Kazakhstan, but no isolations from this tick have been reported from this republic.

Other viruses recorded from *H. a. anatolicum* are Wad Medani (Reoviridae) in Pakistan and Tadzhikistan, and Thogoto and Tamdy (Bunyaviridae) in Egypt and Uzbekistan, respectively.

This tick, one of the most widely distributed in the world, is present in semidesert, steppe, and savanna biotopes from Bangladesh, India, and the terai of Nepal, through all the southern republics of the U.S.S.R., from Afghanistan to Arabia, in Mediterranean areas of southeastern Europe, and in Africa almost to the equator. The extensive dispersal of *H. a. anatolicum* from its original homeland, the steppe and semidesert lowlands east of the Caspian to Arabia and Africa north of the equator, has probably been through the agency of camel caravans and cattle movements rather than of migrating birds.

Structural and biological studies of *H. anatolicum* show the presence of two subspecies: the two-host *H. a. anatolicum* Koch throughout this vast geographical area and the three-host *H. a. excavatum* Koch in generally fewer numbers and usually in different habitats through much, but not all, of this area.[221] Our taxonomic-biological findings are in agreement with those of Soviet specialists. However, since the death of Serdyukova, the pioneer contemporary authority on the genus *Hyalomma* in the U.S.S.R., few writers have identified their materials to subspecies. From studying Soviet literature, it appears that most if not all records of CCHF virus infection in *H. anatolicum* pertain to the subspecies *H. a. anatolicum,* whose immature and adult stages are both often numerous on domestic mammals. (Most immatures are found on the ears of cattle.) Immatures occasonally infest smaller vertebrates but less consistently than matures of the subspecies *H. a. excavatum,* which typically infest rodents and other small burrowing mammals. Hares may be parasitized by large numbers of either subspecies. There is some intergradation between the two subspecies in cerain biotopes.

The question of transovarial transmission of CCHF virus in *H. a. anatolicum* remains unsettled but overwinter survival of the virus in nymphs or adults is apparenly common. Numerous *H. a. anatolicum* shelter in crevices of walls and clay fences near the sleeping places of people and domestic animals. Adults frequently bite people in these situations and in weedy pastures.[76] The bite causes little or no pain to some persons and may not be noticed until 3 days after attachment, when the tick enlarges with blood. In warm areas, *H. a. anatolicum* remains active throughout the year and causes wintertime cases of human CCHF.

Where irrigated agricultural fields replace the steppe-semidesert habitats of *H. a. anatolicum* in Asia, this tick is replaced by *H. detritum, Rhipicephalus turanicus,* and *Boophilus annulatus.*[76] However, *H. a. anatolicum* thrives in dry habitats within the richly cultivated Nile Valley of Egypt.

Fifty percent or often more of the ticks collected from domestic animals in certain Soviet studies of CCHF epidemiology have been *H. a. anatolium.* This tick was earlier considered to be the only CCHF vector in Soviet Asian foci. However, recent investigations have shown that several other *Hyalomma* and *Rhipicephalus* species, and also *Dermacentor* species, share a role in maintaining the virus on this continent. Chunikhin et al.[121] suggested that CCHF virus circulation caused by human activities ("anthropurgic foci") in Asia are maintained by the two-host ticks *H. a. anatolicum* and *H.*

detritum and natural foci are maintained by the three-host ticks *H. asiaticum, Rhipicephalus pumilio,* and *R. turanicus.*

H. a. anatolicum is undoubtedly a major vector CCHF virus and of other pathogens infecting humans and domestic animals in many relatively harsh biotopes now being extensively exploited for economic development projects. As such, the taxonomic, biological and biomedical interrelationships of the two *H. anatolicum* subspecies merit an intensive international research program for better understanding of their individual epidemiological roles and for devising practical control methods. A measure of this problem is that, owing to the taxonomic ambiguity of Soviet literature on this species, I am obliged to consider most or all CCHF virus records as pertaining to the subspecies *H. a. anatolicum,* which has a feeding pattern that utilizes similar hosts. The subspecies *H. a. excavatum,* with a dissimilar-host pattern would present quite a different epidemiological picture and control problem if it should prove to be involved in CCHF virus transmission.

Dissimilar-Host Subgroup

The immature and adult stages of very few two-host species feed on dissimilar animals. However, in this biological category, three of the four subspecies of the *Hyalomma marginatum* complex each have a prominent role in the natural history of CCHF virus in southern Europe, western and central Asia, and Africa. (The role of the fourth species in the Indian subregion remains to be investigated.) The taxon *H. marginatum* was used for this tick in the original Crimean CCHF reports. Subsequent Soviet authors have replaced this name with *H. plumbeum* (Panzer); most others consider *H. marginatum* to be correct.[76,203]

Ecologically, the *Hyalomma marginatum* complex is characteristic of steppe, savanna, and lightly wooded hill and valley biotopes with fairly low relative humidity, but not of deserts, semideserts, deep forests, or high mountains. The complex probably originated in the Caspian-Central Asian area, where the subspecies *H. m. turanicum* now occurs. It spread eastward to Pakistan, India, Nepal, and Sri Lanka (subspecies *H. m. isaaci*), westward to Spain and Morocco (subspecies *H. m. marginatum*), and southward to South Africa (subspecies *H. m. rufipes*).

The combined larval-nymphal stage of each *H. marginatum* subspecies characteristically feeds chiefly on ground-feeding birds or on the hare or hedgehog. Burrowing rodents seldom or never are parasitized. Infested birds are important in dispersing immature *H. marginatum* intracontinentally during postbreeding movements and intercontinentally during migratory flights. Adults feed on all domestic mammals, are especially common on cattle and horses, and eagerly attack human beings who present the opportunity. Wild hosts of adults are chiefly artiodactyl and perissodactyl mammals.

Hyalomma marginatum marginatum

CCHF virus has been isolated from the subspecies *H. m. marginatum* from Ukrainia and Kalmyk A.S.S.R., Astrakhan and Rostov Oblasts, and Krasnodar and Stavropol regions of the Russian Federation (R.F.S.F.R.), and Bulgaria and Armenia and Azerbaijan. This tick was also circumstantially associated with CCHF in Yugoslavia.

Other viruses reported from the subspecies *H. m. marginatum* are tick-borne encephalitis in Azerbaijan and West Nile (both Togaviridae) in Azerbaijan and the Russian Federation; Tete in Italy, Bhanja in Kirgizia, and Tamdy in Turkmenia (all Bunyaviridae); and Batken in Kirgizia and Dhori (both unclassified) in R.F.S.F.R., Armenia, Azerbaijan, and Portugal. This tick has also been incriminated as a vector of other infectious agents of human beings and lower animals.

The subspecies *H. m. marginatum* inhabits the Mediterranean climatic zone and steppe and foothill landscapes of southern Europe (southwestern Palearctic region) from the Caspian Sea to southern Ukrainia and Bulgaria, and westward to Spain, Portugal, and Morocco and Algeria.

The subspecies *H. m. marginatum* appears to be an efficient reservoir-vector of CCHF virus. Epidemiologically this property is enhanced by the adult's cursorial behavior and eagerness to bite people, and by the pasture habitats and cattle hosts provided by human beings, which contribute to the success of the tick wherever smaller wild vertebrates (especially hares, hedgehogs, and ground-feeding birds) are nearby to serve as hosts of immature stages. The virus survives in *H. m. marginatum* for at least a year and transstadially during the tick's postembryonic developmental stages and is also transovarially transmitted to the F_2 generation. Hare, hedgehog, and cattle hosts may serve as virus amplifiers, and birds serve to disseminate the ticks. When the tick population explodes due to a fortuitous combination of optimum weather during the critical winter-spring seasons and ecological-faunistic changes wrought by war, flood control, or land appropriation of new pastures or collectivized farming, zoonotic CCHF virus circulation in the *H. m. marginatum* population may also explode. Indeed, all the most important CCHF epidemics — those in the Crimea, Astrakhan and Rostov Oblasts, and Bulgaria — have been associated with increased *H. m. marginatum* densities. The epidemic lasted only 2 years in the Crimea but about 10 years elsewhere, then ended after tick numbers became reduced by exceptionally severe winter-spring weather. Even during the epidemic decade, disease distribution was sporadic and annual morbidity rates reflected the *H. m. marginatum* density due to climatic factors and the consequent rates of human-tick contacts. During nonepidemic periods, zoonotic CCHF virus circulation, with occasional human infections, is maintained in European steppes, plains, and low mountains by *H. m. marginatum* together with *Dermacentor marginatus, Rhipicephalus rossicus,* and other tick species. The *Dermacentor* and *Rhipicephalus* ticks also bite people, but less frequently than *Hyalomma* ticks.

A biologically and epidemiologically interesting variable in the natural history of *H. m. marginatum*-associated CCHF virus is the relative importance of various hosts of immature stages in different biotopes. The kinds and numbers of suitable birds and/or mammals available as hosts to questing larvae significantly influence both tick population numbers and localization of the unfed, questing adult *H. m. marginatum* in a specific area. A generalized picture of these biological variables is beginning to emerge from reviewing the literature. However, variations in research and reporting methods preclude precise comparative analysis of information on this subject. Notably, rodents are practically never hosts of immature *H. m. marginatum*.

In Astrakhan Oblast, where cattle grazed in the vicinity of large nesting colonies of rooks, engorged nymphs detached from rooks and molted to adults wherever the birds fed in pastures, cultivated fields, gardens, or orchards. Adult *H. m. marginatum* were most numerous under trees bordering canals and under lone trees in pastures, both favorite perches during rooks' long resting periods. Many rooks were heavily infested by immature *H. m. marginatum* (Table 1). Other ground-feeding birds, hares, and hedgehogs were also hosts; though common, they did not equal rooks in contributing to *H. m. marginatum* density in Astrakhan Oblast.

The published information on immature *H. m. marginatum* hosts in Rostov Oblast is generalized and contradictory. Hares, rooks, magpies, and larks are mentioned as hosts. Unfortunately, natural history studies of the caliber of those in Astrakhan were not undertaken in Rostov Oblast.

In the well-studied original Crimean CCHF episode, hares were dramatically involved as hosts of immature *H. m. marginatum,* a variety of ground-feeding birds including domestic chickens were less important hosts, and rooks were absent or rare.

Hares dropped satiated nymphal *H. m. marginatum* in pastures, fallow fields, windbreak tree rows, and near cattle enclosures, hay-shocks, and haystacks where they fed.

The hare was also the chief host of this tick in Bulgarian CCHF foci, where ground-feeding birds were secondary hosts, but rooks were rare or absent (Table 2).

Where hare populations are less dense and hares are more harried by hunters, their contributions of fed immature *H. m. marginatum* to human neighborhoods are likely to be fewer than they were in postwar Crimea. However, hares are tolerated for the hunting season and are commercially propagated in fields and lightly wooded areas of eastern Europe for shipping to hunting clubs elsewhere. These interests undoubtedly influence *Hyalomma m. marginatum* population densities. In view of Chumakov's recent suggestions that exposure to infected vertebrates may result in human CCHF, one wonders whether hunters may become ill from handling hare hosts of infected *H. m. marginatum.*

Hedgehogs were also secondary hosts of immature *H. m. marginatum* in the Astrakhan and Rostov CCHF foci. Hedgehog numbers and tick loads may be less than those of hares but hedgehogs do thrive in gardens, shrubby pastures, and field margins, where humans often regard them with amusement and children take them home as pets. This close association between humans and hedgehog hosts of immature *H. m. marginatum* might prove to be a village-farmstead localization factor in CCHF infections. Both the European and the long-eared hedgehog support the *H. m. marginatum* population where they occur, but only the latter species appears to be a CCHF virus amplifier.

The role of other small mammals as *H. m. marginatum* hosts is apparently insignificant. We have reared some typical adult *H. m. marginatum* from immatures infesting lizards.

The role of migrating birds in transporting immature *H. m. marginatum* from Europe and European Asia to Africa is reviewed later.

Hyalomma marginatum populations associated with migrating birds and marine birds near the Caspian Sea and on islands in the Caspian deserve special attention.

Zhemchuzhnyi Island, in the northern part of the Caspian Sea (Astrakhan Oblast), is a rest stop for thousands of migrating birds. During the fall (southward) migration, many of these resting birds drop engorged nymphs of the subspecies *H. m. marginatum,* which overwinter and molt to adults in spring. In the absence of mammals on Zhemchuzhnyi Island, adult *H. m. marginatum* have adapted to feeding on fledgling gulls (species unstated), and more than 40 adult ticks are sometimes found on a single fledgling.[32]

Nymphs of *H. marginatum rufipes,* the African representative of the *H. m. marginatum* complex, have been taken from redstarts during the spring (northward) migration in Astrakhan Oblast and adult *H. m. rufipes* are found on domestic animals in several regions of this Oblast.[32] Zimina and Ivanova[612] stated that in 1966 to 1969 tick collections, adult *H. "plumbeum impressum"* were found on cattle in eight steppe and floodplain localities of Astrakhan Oblast from April to August, and that these ticks had probably been carried here (as nymphs during the previous fall) on northward migrating birds from Africa. This report is probably based on misidentification of *H. marginatum rufipes. H. impressum* is less likely to be carried in appreciable numbers to Astrakhan Oblast than *H. marginatum rufipes.*

Another instance of adult *H. marginatum* (subspecies unspecified) biting marine birds on islands in Kara-Bogaz Bay, further south in the Caspian (Krasnovodsk Oblast, Turkmenia), was recorded by Andreev and Shcherbina.[10] (The only *H. marginatum* representative known in Turkmenia is the subspecies *H. m. turanicum,* but without voucher specimens one cannot be certain of the subspecies on these zoogeographically marginal islands.) These workers found 65% of the examined fledglings of the common tern, *Sterna hirundo,* to be each infested by 78 (average) adult *H. marginatum* subsp. on June 10 to 14, 1974. (Two strains of an unidentified B serogroup Togavirus were isolated from partially fed adult *Hyalomma* from these birds.) Several other marine bird species nesting on these islands may serve as tick hosts and persons collecting eggs are liable to tick attack. *Hyalomma* are said to be rare on the rabbits which have been introduced into these islands.[18] [Baku virus (Reoviridae, Kemerovo serogroup, Chenuda subgroup) commonly infects marine birds and *Ornithodoros* ticks on Caspian islands. West Nile virus infecting these *Ornithodoros*[1,190] may represent the "unidentified B serogroup Togavirus" from *H. marginatum* mentioned by Andreev and Shcherbina.[10] Another unidentified virus was isolated from adult *H. marginatum* taken from a dead Saiga antelope, *Saiga tatarica,* on Glinyany Island.[500]]

Hyalomma marginatum turanicum

CCHF virus has been isolated from 29 pools of the subspecies *H. m. turanicum* in Uzbekistan (1), Kirgizia (27), and Tadzhikistan (1). This tick is considered to be the chief CCHF virus vector in Kirgizia.

Bhanja virus (Bunyaviridae) was isolated in Kirgizia from this tick,[331] which is also a vector of *Coxiella burneti* (Q fever) and of *Babesia* and *Theileria* species infecting mammals.

H. m. turanicum inhabits chiefly wooded tugai (floodplain) meadows in semidesert and foothill and mountainside steppe biotopes in the southeastern part of the Palearctic faunal region, from the Caspian Sea eastward to Pakistan, and also south of the range of the subspecies *H. m. marginatum* through the Middle and Near East. Scattered populations occur in northeastern Africa. An extralimital population appearing to be *H. m. turanicum,* probably introduced with karakul sheep from Iran, occurs in the arid Karroo of South Africa.[203]

The only commonly reported hosts of immature *H. m. turanicum* are birds, usually those feeding on the ground. Kuima[301] recorded 17 bird host species in Tadzhikistan, and Shcherbinina[472] reviewed literature and data for 26 bird host species in Turkmenia. Hoogstraal[203] listed more than 30 bird host species from Soviet literature and reviewed information on *H. m. turanicum* biology.

Adult *H. m. turanicum* are usually recorded from domestic mammals, especially cattle, camels, and sheep. People are occasional or rare hosts. I have unpublished data for an adult *H. m. turanicum* from the burrow entrance of a jird, *Meriones rex buryi,* in Yemen and for an adult from a hare, *Lepus* sp., in Iraq. Hosts of adults in Iran are the Asiatic mouflon, *Ovis orientalis,* and wild goat, *Capra hircus aegagrus,*[228] and the wild boar, *Sus scrofa attila* (unpublished data). From other records, it appears that the subspecies *H. m. turanicum* is frequently carried to hospitable habitats by migrating birds.

Hyalomma marginatum rufipes

CCHF virus has been isolated from eight pools of the subspecies *H. m. rufipes* in Senegal (7) and Nigeria (1). Experimental studies of transovarial transmission of the virus in *H. m. rufipes* are reviewed elsewhere.

Other viruses of the family Bunyaviridae reported from *H. m. rufipes* are Bahig and Matruh in Egypt[215] and Dugbe in Nigeria.[79] This tick is also a vector of *Rickettsia conori* (boutonneuse fever)[61,205] and of other agents infecting herbivores.

The subspecies *H. m. rufipes* represents the *H. marginatum* complex in various savanna biotopes of much of the Ethiopian faunal region. Its range extends northward into the Nile Valley of Egypt and also into Yemen and scattered localities elsewhere in southern Arabia. Single specimens or small samples collected in nature in parts of northeastern Africa and Arabia can be difficult to differentiate from the subspecies *H. m. turanicum.* These samples may represent interbreeding between the local *H. m.*

rufipes population and individual *H. m. turanicum* introduced by birds migrating from southwestern Asia to Africa.

As usual in the *H. marginatum* complex, adult *H. m. rufipes* frequently parasitize domestic herbivores, especially cattle, and also horses, sheep, and goats. Wild antelopes, the cape buffalo, zebra, elephant, giraffe, rhinoceros, and warthog are common hosts, as are the ostrich, bustard, marabou stork, and other large birds. Adults occasonally attack people, dogs, and cats. Numerous species of ground-feeding birds, and hares and hedgehogs, are hosts of immature stages[203] (unpublished data).

Immature *H. m. rufipes* are carried each spring from Africa to the lower Volga basin of Astrakhan Oblast, where they molt to adults and infest domestic animals.[32] We have taken numerous immature *H. m. rufipes* from spring migrants in Egypt.

Hyalomma marginatum isaaci

The subspecies *isaaci* of the Oriental faunal region (northwestern Afghanistan, Pakistan, India, Sri Lanka, southern Nepal — mostly unpublished data) has not been studied in relation to CCHF epidemiology but is a likely candidate for investigation as a reservoir and vector linking Oriental to Palearctic and Ethiopian CCHF foci. Viruses reported from this tick in India are Wad Medani (Reoviridae) (V. H. Dhanda, personal communication) and Wanowrie (unclassified).[127]

Adult *H. m. isaaci* hosts in my collections are from cattle, buffaloes, sheep, goats, and camels, a dog, and the chital (axis deer), *Axis a. axis,* Asiatic mouflon, *Ovis orientalis punjabiensis,* Nilgai or blue bull, *Boselaphus tragocamelus,* Asian wild boar, *Sus scrofa cristatus,* and human beings. Immatures are from the blue rock thrush, *Monticola solitaria pandoo,* and Indian house sparrow, *Passer domesticus indicus.* Rebello and Reuben[426] recorded three immatures from 3 of 227 birds examined in southern India but none from 407 insectivores and rodents. An entirely different host picture was reported by Seneviratna[463] from Sri Lanka, where occasional immatures were found on the buffalo, mouse deer, hare, and mongoose; rodents were heavily invested. Adults were commonly taken from cattle and buffalo grazing near forests and jungles, but not on those in urban areas, where there were few or no small vertebrates to serve as hosts of immature stages.

Three-Host Ticks

Nine three-host species are associated with CCHF virus in Eurasia and six in Africa. Immatures of most of these species feed on small- or medium-sized hosts, but those of *Rhipicephalus pulchellus* feed either on small mammals or on the same large mammals as adults. Nymphal *Amblyomma variegatum* often infest cattle.

Eurasia

Ixodes ricinus

This common European tick was circumstantially associated with "Bukovinian hemorrhagic fever" in Carpathian foothill forests in 1946 to 1947 and two CCHF strains were isolated from adults from Moldavia in 1973 to 1974. Three other strains were isolated from *I. ricinus* in the Crimea (Ukraine) in 1972 to 1973, and this species is considered to have a role in CCHF epidemiology in Bulgaria.

I. ricinus is notorious as a vector of several viruses: tick-borne encephalitis,[51,497] louping ill,[557] Zimmern strain[52,53] (Togaviridae), Tribeč,[187] Kharagysh,[483] Eyach[429] (Reoviridae), and Uukuniemi[448] (Bunyaviridae). It is equally renowned as the vector of numerous other organisms among wild and domestic animals.

I. ricinus is often common in forests, weedy pastures, gardens, and shrubby margins of fields in Ireland, England, and Europe (see map in Smorodintsev[497]), southeastward to the Caspian forests and mountains of northern Iran.[172] I have numerous unpublished records of *I. ricinus* from this area of Iran from people, domestic animals, wild pigs, deer, goats, foxes, rodents, and ground-feeding birds. Wherever it occurs, *I. ricinus* is a prime candidate for investigation as a CCHF virus reservoir and vector.

I. persulcatus Schulze replaces *I. ricinus* in certain parts of eastern Europe and European U.S.S.R. and throughout Siberia,[287,288] in biotopes which appear to be ecologically unsuitable for CCHF virus survival. However, *I. gibbosus* Nuttall, which replaces *I. ricinus* in drier biotopes of Greece,[451] Italy,[452] Yugoslavia,[531-534] Turkey and Cyprus, (unpublished data), and Israel[168] should be investigated in relation to CCHF epidemiology.

I. ricinus has long been one of the most intensively studied tick species. Unlike several other species of importance in circulating CCHF virus, the vast literature on *I. ricinus* has been published chiefly in well-known journals easily available to most readers. Therefore, little space is devoted to *I. ricinus* in this review.

Each active stage feeds on practically any vertebrate coming within its reach. Larvae infest a wide variety of rodents, insectivores, birds, and lizards moving close to the ground. Nymphs quest from higher levels and often parasitize animals of somewhat larger size. Adults feed on domestic animals, deer and other wild herbivores, and carnivores. People are frequently attacked. Large numbers of immatures are taken from resident and migrating birds. The voluminous literature on tick-borne encephalitis includes many biological and ecological studies on *I. ricinus*.

Haemaphysalis punctata

CCHF virus was isolated from *H. punctata* in Moldavia and in the Crimea (Ukraine) during the 1972 to 1974 period. This species also occurs in Bulgarian CCHF foci.

H. punctata is a secondary vector of tick-borne encephalitis virus (Togaviridae),[367] and Tribeč virus (Reoviridae) has been isolated from it in Romania.[530] *H. punctata* appears to be a particularly important vector of Bhanja virus (Bunyaviridae) in Italy[445] and in Yugoslavia.[67,566] It is also a vector of *Babesia* and *Theileria* infecting domestic mammals.

H. punctata is locally distributed in much of Europe, from southern Scandinavia and northern Germany to Mediterranean islands, Morocco and Tunisia, and southeastward through all the Soviet republics, to Jordan and Iran. Earlier records of this species from Japan are incorrect.

Grebenyuk[186] summarized the extensive Soviet literature on *H. punctata* and included data from field observations and laboratory experiments in Kirgizia. Habitats are a wide variety of forest, shrub, and pasture zones, and also wooded areas of steppes and tugai vegetation along streams and rivers in deserts, to altitudes of 2000 or 2500 m. Adults parasitize all domestic mammals and practically all larger wild mammals, less often hares, ground squirrels, and larger-sized, ground-feeding birds. Nymphs and larvae frequently feed on birds; 80 bird species were listed as hosts by Ter-Vartanov et al.[520] and we have made almost 200 collections of immature *H. punctata* from 13 kinds of birds migrating through Egypt from Eurasia to Africa. Hares are also common hosts of immatures; occasional hosts of these stages are reptiles, certain rodents, wild carnivores, domestic sheep, and other domestic mammals. There are numerous records of *H. punctata* from human hosts.

Adult *H. punctata* feed mostly in March and April or in September and October, but in some areas are active into June or begin activity earlier in the fall. Nymphs and larvae are active chiefly in summer, but some may be found on hosts in spring and fall. The life cycle generally requires 2 years, but a 1-year cycle has been reported from the northern Caucasus. Adults, nymphs, or larvae may overwinter. Data for feeding periods vary widely, but are about 7 (7 to 18) days for females on sheep and cattle and 4 to 5 (3½ to 12) days for each immature stage.

Dermacentor marginatus

CCHF virus has been isolated from adult *D. marginatus* from Moldavia, Rostov Oblast, Bulgaria, and Uzbekistan. The earliest strain was obtained in 1969 in Rostov Oblast, when the population density of *Hyalomma m. marginatum* became greatly reduced following an exceptionally severe winter. A number of CCHF patients in this oblast recognized *D. marginatus* as a tick that had bitten them before the illness began. Transstadial survival and transovarial transmission of CCHF virus are common phenomena in *D. marginatus.*

D. marginatus has been incriminated in the epidemiology of tick-borne encephalitis virus (Togaviridae),[204] Dhori,[457] and Razdan viruses (Bunyaviridae).[331] *D. marginatus* is also a vector of *Rickettsia siberica* (Siberian tick typhus)[205] and *Francisella tularensis* (tularemia),[370] and is an important reservoir and vector of *Coxiella burneti* (Q fever) in Germany.[326] It transmits *Babesia* species to horses and dogs and has been more or less conclusively associated with the epidemiology of several other disease agents.

D. marginatus inhabits shrubby growth, forests, and marshes in lowlands, alpine steppes, and certain semidesert areas from Kazakhstan, Afghanistan, and Iran, through the Altai mountains to Central Europe and France.[454] In Central Europe, preferred *D. marginatus* biotopes are xerophilic plant communities.[365,366] Immatures feed chiefly on rodents and insectivores, also on hares and small carnivores. Most adults infest cattle, sheep, and horses and other domestic and wild herbivores. Adults are active throughout the year in southern parts of the range, with peak numbers in spring and late summer-fall; elsewhere they quest and feed during these seasons but not in summer. Immature stage activity is during summer months.

Dermacentor daghestanicus

The FA test was used recently to demonstrate CCHF infection in the salivary glands of the single *D. daghestanicus* examined from Kzyl-Orda Oblast in Kazakhstan. This species has frequently been associated with *Coxiella burneti, Francisella tularensis,* and piroplasms of domestic and wild mammals. Possibly the most xerophilic of all *Dermacentor* species, *D. daghestanicus* inhabits hot desert, semidesert, and foothill biotopes from the lower Volga area and Transcaucasia to Central Asia.[181,186,430] Adults are active chiefly in spring and in lesser numbers in fall; they parasitize all domestic mammals and also deer and people. Immature stages feed during summer on hedgehogs, rodents, and hares; their population densities are sometimes very high.

Hyalomma asiaticum asiaticum

CCHF virus has been isolated from 52 pools of adult *H. a. asiaticum* from Turkmenia (35) in 1974, Kazakhstan (16) in 1971, and, more recently, Kirgizia (1). In addition, 128 of 379 salivary gland preparations from Kzyl-Orda Oblast, Kazakhstan, during the spring seasons of 1970 to 1972 were positive for CCHF virus infections in the FA test.

Other viruses isolated from *H. a. asiaticum* are Tamdy (Bunyaviridae) from Uzbekistan[330] and Wad Medani (Reoviridae) from Turkmenia.[484] This tick also transmits *Coxiella burneti,*[24,25] *Rickettsia siberica* (Siberian tick typhus),[205,332] and *Theileria annulata, T. mutans,* and *Anaplasma marginale.*[24]

H. a. asiaticum is highly adapted to the various desert environments of southern republics of the U.S.S.R. Balashov[24] reviewed his numerous biological and behavioral studies of this subspecies and has continued to report subsequent investigations. Adults parasitize camels, other domestic herbivores, and also the mouflon, wild pig, gazelle, and human beings. Immatures infest burrowing mammals, especially rodents, and also hedgehogs, hares, and carnivores preying on rodents. The great gerbil, *Rhombomys opimus,* and two ground squirrels, *Spermophilopsis l. leptodactylus* and *Citellus ful-*

vus, are common hosts of immatures. After molting from the nymphal stage in burrows, adults await larger mammals on the soil, on low vegetation near burrow entrances, or under the shade of nearby trees or large leaves. The life cycle requires about a year. Adults are most numerous in spring, larvae in early summer, and nymphs in late summer, early winter, and spring. Adults molting from nymphs during summer or early fall may remain unfed in the burrow until spring and survive for at least a year. These exceptionally vigorous ticks can move as far as 500 m, but most remain within a radius of 25 to 100 m of the burrow. Unfed adults can lose up to 30% of their water content (about 20% of the tick weight) without harm. The quantities of blood ingested by immatures and adults are among the greatest of any ixodid species in the Palearctic fauna.

Rhipicephalus pumilio

CCHF infections in adult *R. pumilio* from Turkmenia were demonstrated by the FA technique in 1972, and two strains of the virus were isolated in 1973 from adults from Uzbekistan. *R. pumilio* is also infected by *Francisella tularensis*[405] and *Coxiella burneti.*[607]

This tick is found near lakes and rivers in desert and steppe biotopes from northern Astrakhan Oblast and Daghestan to Uzbekistan, Tadzhikistan, Turkmenia, Kazakhstan, and the Karakoram Mountains of Kashmir.[186] Adults feed chiefly on hares and hedgehogs, also on larger-sized rodents, domestic and wild mammals, and human beings. Immatures infest hares and hedgehogs as well as numerous rodents and some birds. Adults feed from spring through summer, nymphs through summer, and larvae in midsummer. There may be more than one generation a year and each developmental stage may overwinter.

Rhipicephalus rossicus

R. rossicus replaced *Hyalomma m. marginatum* as the most common tick species following the severe 1968 to 1969 winter in Rostov Oblast, where CCHF virus was isolated from adult *R. rossicus* from European hares and hedgehogs and from cattle. Other CCHF strains were isolated from adult *R. rossicus* from cattle in Krasnodar Region in 1971 and from Armenia in 1972 to 1974.

R. rossicus figures prominently in Soviet literature as a vector of *Francisella tularensis* and is also a vector of *Babesia bigemina* (Texas fever) and *Coxiella burneti.* West Nile (WN) virus (Togaviridae, B serogroup) is usually mosquito-borne in nature but survives in experimentally infected larval *R. rossicus* to the adult stage and is irregularly transmitted transovarially to the F_1 generation.[292]

R. rossicus occurs from Romania and Bulgaria to western Kazakhstan. Immature stages parasitize hedgehogs, rodents, and hares in lowland and mountain steppes. Adults feed on many kinds of wild and domestic mammals from the size of hares to camels. The European hare is an important host in Rostov Oblast, where this tick is also common on cattle and has close contact with people.

Rhipicephalus sanguineus

CCHF virus was isolated from the kennel tick in the Crimea (Ukraine) in 1972 to 1973, and in Bulgaria between 1968 to 1972. Infections in salivary glands of samples from Turkmenia were demonstrated by the FA technique in 1970.

Wad Medani virus (Reoviridae) was first isolated from *R. sanguineus* from goats in the Sudan.[516] This tick is reported to be a vector of *Rickettsia rickettsi* (Rocky Mountain spotted fever) (RMSF) in Canada, Mexico, Colombia, and Brazil and of *Rickettsia conori* (tick typhus or boutonneuse fever) in tropical and northern Africa and southern Europe (especially Bulgaria and Ukrainia).[205] A distinctly different member of the

RMSF rickettsial complex infects *R. sanguineus* in Mississippi.[62] *Coxiella burneti* has often been recovered from *R. sanguineus*. This tick is the chief vector of *Ehrlichia canis* (canine ehrlichiosis or tropical canine pancytopenia),[232,478] and of *Babesia canis*,[360,361] and numerous other agents infecting lower mammals.

In the Ethiopian faunal region, immature *R. sanguineus* parasitize chiefly insectivores and rodents; adults parasitize chiefly wild and domestic ungulates and carnivores.[203,354] This tick has been dispersed with domestic dogs to many parts of Europe, Asia, the Americas, and Australia. As is typical of an introduced tick species surviving away from its normal range in artificial conditions created by humans, immature and adult *R. sanguineus* almost always parasitize only one kind of vertebrate (the dog) outside of Africa. (However, cattle are infested in Mexico.) *R. sanguineus* is a notorious kennel tick, or "backyard parasite", in southeastern Europe and southwestern U.S.S.R. Notably, there is little or no evidence for the presence of *R. sanguineus* east of Iraq, except as a parasite of dogs. Taxonomic relationships in the *R. sanguineus* group were reviewed by Morel and Vassiliades[355] and Morel.[354]

Rhipicephalus turanicus

In Kirgizia, CCHF virus was isolated from *R. turanicus* from Osh Oblast, where this tick was the most numerous of several species collected from wild and domestic mammals in CCHF foci.[243] Chumakov[98] and Chumakov et al.[117] ambiguously referred to *R. turanicus* as a CCHF virus vector in Uzbekistan.

Tick-borne encephalitis and West Nile viruses (Togaviridae) were isolated from *R. turanicus* in Azerbaijan,[499] and Manawa virus (Bunyaviridae) was isolated from this species in Pakistan.[30] This tick has considerable importance in veterinary medicine.

R. turanicus is widely distributed through the southern Palearctic faunal region (southern Europe and northern Africa) to China[355] and India.[134,348] It has frequently been confused with *R. sanguineus,* but can be identified easily if carefully examined and differs distinctly in biological properties. The Soviet literature on hosts and biology was reviewed by Grebenyuk[186] together with his own observations in Kirgizia.

Africa

Hyalomma impeltatum

Two CCHF strains have been isolated from cattle-infesting *H. impeltatum,* one from Senegal and one from Nigeria. A third strain was from *H. impeltatum* from sheep in Ethiopia.

Wanowrie virus (unclassified, ungrouped) was isolated from *H. impeltatum* from camels in Egypt.[211,576] This virus was also isolated from the brain of a fatal human case in Sri Lanka.[393]

H. impeltatum is widely but erratically distributed in semidesert, steppe, and savanna biotopes from Iran and Arabia across northern Africa and southward to norther Tanzania in the east and Chad in the west.[203] Recently published data are from Tanzania,[588] Kenya,[570] northern Somalia,[394] and Ethiopia.[354] In Egypt, the greater Egyptian gerbil, *Gerbillus pyramidum,* a common resident of palm groves and sandy cultivated areas, is an important host of immature *H. impeltatum.*[220] Other hosts of immatures are different gerbils, jerboas, jirds, hedgehogs, hares, lizards, and ground-feeding birds. All domestic herbivores, gazelles, and antelopes are parasitized by adults, and also human beings, dogs, wild pigs, rhinoceros, etc. Infestations of camels and cattle are often heavy, and numerous adults may be taken from sheep.

Hyalomma impressum

Two CCHF strains were isolated from *H. impressum* from cattle in Senegal. *H. impressum* occurs in the Guinean and Sudanese savanna zones of West Africa, from the Atlantic to Darfur and Kordofan of western Sudan, but does not range south of the equator or into the northern desert zone.[203] Cattle are the chief hosts of adults, which also parasitize horses, camels, dogs, and sheep. Locality records from West Africa were published by Morel.[353] Camicas[68] reported two larvae from rat and a hedgehog in Senegal. Much remains to be learned about the biology of *H. impressum.*

Hyalomma nitidum

CCHF virus was isolated from male *H. nitidum* from cattle in Central African Republic. *H. nitidum,* long a "lost taxon" related to *H. truncatum,* is in the process of being redescribed. We have records from Cameroon, Central African Republic, Benin, Guinea, Ivory Coast, Mali, Senegal, and Upper Volta, where adults parasitize domestic cattle, horses, and goats, and the bush pig, cape buffalo, defassa waterbuck, and roan antelope (Hoogstraal collection, unpublished data). Our only records of immature *H. nitidum* are from hares. Ecologically and geographically, the relationship between *H. truncatum* and *H. nitidum* possibly parallels that between *Boophilus decoloratus* and *B. geigyi.*

Hyalomma truncatum

Ten CCHF strains have been isolated from cattle-parasitizing *H. truncatum,* eight in Senegal and two in Nigeria.

Different viruses reported from *H. truncatum* in Nigeria and Senegal are Dugbe and Bhanja (Bunyaviridae) and Jos (unclassified).[80,82,260,435,576] Other organisms infecting *H. truncatum* are *Rickettsia conori, Coxiella burneti, Wolbachia* sp., *Chlamydia* sp., *Theileria* spp., and *Babesia* spp. The bite of this tick causes paralysis in people and sheep, toxicosis (sweating sickness) in cattle, and lameness and deep wounds in domestic animals.

H. truncatum occurs between sea level and 2600 m altitude from the Cape to southeastern Egypt (see Hoogstraal[203], and more recent literature cited under *H. impeltatum*). *H. truncatum* habitats in this extensive area are reviewed by Morel.[354] The most common hosts of adults are domestic cattle, goats, and numerous wild antelopes; others are domestic sheep, horses, camels, pigs, and dogs and the rhinoceros, warthog, elephant, buffalo, giraffe, zebra, antbear, and porcupine. Carnivores, such as the lion, leopard, and jackal, are less often parasitized. Tortoises and birds as large as the ostrich and bustard are not infrequent hosts. Immatures have been recorded from birds, rodents, hares, and domestic animals but the biology of these stages remains poorly studied.

Amblyomma variegatum

CCHF virus was isolated from adult *A. variegatum* from cattle on seven occasions in Senegal and once each in Nigeria, Uganda, and Kenya.

Six other viruses recorded from *A. variegatum* (Hoogstraal, in preparation) are Nairobi sheep disease (Kenya, Somalia), Dugbe (Nigeria, Central African Republic, Cameroon, Chad, Uganda, Sudan), Bhanja (Nigeria, Senegal, Central African Republic), and Thogoto (Nigeria, Central African Republic, Cameroon, Uganda) (all Bunyaviridae); and (unclassified) Jos (Senegal, Nigeria, Central Africa Republic) and Somone (Senegal, Nigeria). *Rickettsia conori, Coxiella burneti, Cowdria ruminantum, Theileria parva, T. mutans, T. velifera,* etc. also infect *A. variegatum.*

The geographic range of *A. variegatum* is almost as extensive as that of *H. truncatum;* however, its southern limit is reached in Zambia and Angola. *A. variegatum* also occurs in the Yemen and Oman and has been introduced into Madagascar, Mauritius, Puerto Rico, and some islands of the West Indies, where it has become common.

This is possibly the most frequently seen tick in the African fauna. Hosts of adults, the same as mentioned for *H. truncatum,* and biological studies were reviewed by Hoogstraal[203] (see also literature mentioned under *H. impeltatum*). Habitats were reviewed by Morel.[354]

Immature *A. variegatum* feed on a large variety of ground-feeding birds and small mammals. Nymphs, and less often larvae, may also infest the same domestic animals as adults. Larvae sometimes cause severe irritation and inflammation in people. Immature *A. variegatum* have been taken in Egypt and Cyprus from several species of northward-migrating birds, and adults molting from bird-borne nymphs have been found parasitizing dogs and cattle in France, Italy, Bulgaria, and Israel.

Rhipicephalus Pulchellus

CCHF virus was isolated at the Veterinary Research Laboratory, Kabete, Kenya, from *R. pulchellus* from a dying sheep.

R. pulchellus is also a vector of Nairobi sheep disease virus (Bunyaviridae) and is infected by *Rickettsia conori, Babesia equi, Theileria* spp., *Trypanosoma theileri,* and *Wolbachia* sp.

In East Africa. *R. pulchellus* ranges from lowlands to 1800 m altitude, or higher, through open grassy plain and dry brush habitats with low rainfall and/or long dry seasons, from Ethiopia[354] and Somalia,[162,394] to Kenya[570] and northeastern Tanzania.[588] The adult and immature stages were defined and illustrated by Walker[567] and adults by Cunliffe[125] and Walker.[568,569] Adults and immatures generally parasitize the same kinds of mammalian hosts, all domestic and wild herbivores, and also carnivores. Immature stages, in the absence of adults, have been recorded from carnivores and hares and parasitize human beings more frequently and in greater numbers than adults. These "seed ticks" are especially pestiferous parasites of people, who complain afterward of inflamed, septic sores. Numerous adults often infest cattle and camels.

R. pulchellus is the only African three-host tick involved in CCHF epidemiology in which rodents and insectivores appear to have no role as hosts of immature stages. The single record from a bird is a male from an ostrich in Tanzania (Hoogstraal collection, unpublished data).

Multihost Ticks

Only members of the family Argasidae fall in the multihost category. Argasid ticks typically feed once as larvae, two to four times (or more often) as nymphs, and several times as adults. In a normal argasid lifetime, 5 to 20 hosts may furnish a blood meal for an individual tick. The family Argasidae is composed of the genera *Argas* (55 species), *Ornithodoros* (100 species), *Antricola* (5 species), *Otobius* (2 species), and *Nothoaspis* (1 specie). All inhabit dry niches in wood, stone, or soil where birds, mammals, or lizards nest or rest in tropical or warmer temperate climates.[210]

CCHF virus was reported from *Argas (Persicargas) persicus* in Uzbekistan.

A. persicus infests domestic chicken houses in the southern part of the Palearctic faunal region and has been widely transported elsewhere with domestic fowl. In southern U.S.S.R., Afghanistan, and Iran, *A. persicus* also parasitizes wild birds nesting in trees. However, almost everywhere else it survives only in the shelters constructed by people for chickens. The large majority of literature references to *A. persicus* published before 1966 pertain to other ticks misidentified as this species. The 1974 report of CCHF virus from *A. persicus* is especially interesting epidemiologically if for no other reason than that previously it was the only *Argas* species that had never yielded a virus of any kind in several laboratories where ticks of this genus were investigated for virus infections.[211]

Inasmuch as CCHF virus apparently causes no viremia in birds, the isolate from this bird-parasitizing tick, which often develops dense populations in or close to human habitations, points to the need for research in several critical areas. Can the virus survive in *A. persicus* populations only by transovarial (vertical) transmission? Are any of the numerous other *Argas* and *Ornithodoros* species common to CCHF virus-infected biotopes involved in virus maintenance and transmission? What is the epidemiological role of mammal-parasitizing argasids, some of which inhabit the same shelters and feed on the same hosts as ixodid tick species already incriminated as CCHF virus reservoirs and vectors? Can people who crush infected argasids become infected by contamination? The contagion route of infection, suggested by Chumakov and others for persons who handle infected domestic animals, would involve argasids in CCHF epidemiology even if the ticks do not bite persons or transmit the virus to birds.

Except for the single report of CCHF virus from *A. persicus* in Uzbekistan, and another report of failure to obtain the virus from this species in Armenia, there is no indication in literature of attempts to determine the role of multihost argasid ticks in CCHF epidemiology.

CONTROL

Introduction, Prevention

Efficient tick control, repelling and intercepting ticks attempting to feed on people, and avoiding contact between human skin and potentially infected ticks and their body fluids are basic measures for preventing CCHF virus infection in human beings. A vaccine is advantageous for persons in high-risk situations in nature, on farms, and in laboratories. Persons caring for and treating CCHF patients need to take strict precautions against contamination by bloody discharges and possibly by aerosols. At the first sign of an outbreak, a vigorous public awareness and education program should be initiated to prevent CCHF.

Multidisciplinary investigations of epidemiological factors were initiated during CCHF outbreaks in the Crimea, Bulgaria, Astrakhan, Rostov, Uzbekistan, and Kazakhstan to determine the most efficient course of actions for preventing human infections. Preventive measures applied during and after the fact have had mixed success. The need for preventive measures in both known and potential foci of CCHF virus is stressed by Chernovsky et al.[85] and many others.

The insight gained from studying these epidemiological experiences covering a 32-year period (1944 to 1976) (and from studying numerous other arthropod-borne disease episodes throughout the world) leads me to conclude that, despite the contemporary low ebb in reported CCHF morbidity, continued surveillance of potentially hazardous areas is necessary to save lives. Morbidity and mortality have been especially heavy where CCHF was unexpected. Recognizing the realities of financial restrictions and the need to show cost-effectiveness, one can design a reasonably inexpensive surveillance program based primarily on a twice, or thrice, annual spot check of (1) the population dynamics of the 1 to 3 tick species most commonly parasitizing domestic animals and (2) the parasitized animals' serological reactions to CCHF virus. More diversified biomedical investigations are, naturally, desirable and useful wherever circumstances and resources permit.

No continuing programs to determine the potential threat of CCHF infection have been mentioned in published literature or in reports from research institutions for the past 5 years or more.

Vaccine

The high prevalence of CCHF in Rostov Oblast during 1968 (1380 cases per 100,000 population, 16% fatal), the increasing number of foci, and the high cost and poor results in controlling *Hyalomma m. marginatum,* led Badalov et al.[21,22] and Tkachenko et al.[526] to consider it necessary to immunize the rural population of Rostov focal areas. Most other specialists have recommended vaccinating high-risk persons, such as milkmaids, cattleyard workers,[55] and others exposed to tick bites, and personnel in laboratories and infectious disease hospitals.

Tkachenko et al.[527] described the methods used at the Institute of Poliomyelitis and Viral Encephalitides, Moscow, for preparing an inactivated vaccine against CCHF virus in NWM brain tissue. These authors[52] gave the 3- or 4-dose vaccine to about 1500 persons in Rostov Oblast in 1970 and revaccinated them in 1971. Despite problems in interpreting serological results and low incidence of seroconversion in some tests, it was stated that "the first data show high frequency of detecting antibodies by the N test in revaccinated persons and confirm the conclusion of the high immunogenic effect of this preparation." Continuing the investigation, these authors[525] recommended a course of four subcutaneous 1.0-mℓ vaccine doses, the first three at 2-week intervals and the fourth 8 to 11 months later.

Martynenko and Badalov[335] reported changes in the peripheral blood of some persons after vaccination. Vasilenko[560] vaccinated 583 volunteers in Bulgaria and after revaccination detected antibodies to CCHF virus in 96.6% (CF test) and 82.1% (AGDP test).

Contagion

Soviet literature contains numerous more or less detailed accounts of measures to prevent CCHF virus transmission by contagion in households and hospitals. These procedures are nowadays universally recognized in developed and developing nations (though sometimes overlooked at critical times); description of their application to CCHF are chiefly of historical interest and outside the scope of this resume. Routes of contagious transmission are reviewed elsewhere.

All levels of medical, laboratory, and public health personnel should be alerted to protect themselves and others from infection by contagion when caring for CCHF patients. Complete isolation of CCHF patients and a 1-week observation period of persons tending hemorrhaging patients is routinely recommended. Transmission of CCHF virus by contamination (contagion) has consistently occurred in tragic numbers where medical personnel were uninformed or poorly informed about the dangers of this virus, especially in regions where the quality of medical attention and facilities were less than ideal.

I should stress that in Bulgaria and in European and Asian areas of the U.S.S.R. many CCHF cases have resulted from squashing infected ticks while pulling them from hosts (especially cattle) with bare hands — a practice to be strictly avoided in any danger zone. Sheep shearers in CCHF zones also need to protect themselves from contact with mutilated ticks.

Tickbite

The bionomics, seasonal dynamics, and behavior patterns of each tick species having a known or potential role as a chief or a secondary vector of CCHF virus should be well studied to provide clues to how persons may best avoid tickbite in hazardous zones. For instance, the information regarding *Hyalomma m. marginatum* in this respect is reasonably good but *H. marginatum turanicum* is virtually unstudied except for casual observations on avian and domestic animal hosts. Many questions relating to differences in behavior and dynamics (as well as to identification) of the subspecies *H. a. anatolicum* and *H. a. excavatum* of *Hyalomma anatolicum* remain unanswered. In the Eastern hemisphere, there have been casual observations on tick aggressiveness toward humans (on the order of that of Lamontellerie[304] in relation to *Rickettsia conori*-infected *Rhipicephalus sanguineus* and other species feeding on people in southwestern France), but surprisingly few serious studies of this subject. Chances for human contact with a single tick species depend on a variety of local factors, as studied for *H. m. marginatum* in Rostov Oblast by Perelatov et al.[397]

Warnings against tickbite in CCHF foci include admonishments to rest or sleep well away from tick-infested haystacks, cattle yards, hedgerows, clay fences, etc. (depending on terrain and habits and behavior of individual tick species), to examine hay bedding for ticks, to wear shoes, and to inspect one's clothing and body for crawling or attached ticks. Personal and/or mutual inspections should be at least three daily, or, in heavily infested habitats, at hourly intervals. During working hours, an alert should be maintained for crawling ticks. Examinations should include head hair, ears, neck, axillae, all hairy and/or moist skinfold areas, especially in the inguinal area and lower back, and legs. Folds of the clothes and pockets should also be inspected. A Rostov Oblast anti-CCHF propaganda poster (Figure 3) shows comrade farm workers inspecting each other for ticks.

In Eurasian CCHF foci, *Hyalomma* ticks are most aggressive in seeking human hosts. Hungry *H. m. marginatum,* often lurking in numbers in shaded spots where birds, hares, or cattle rest, and where people also prefer to rest, run quite rapidly for some distance to feed on a person.[205] *H. a. anatolicum* infestations are more likely in areas of low vegetation and near clay walls and fences where cattle rest.

The most simple practice to prevent tickbite is to tuck trouser cuffs into long socks, wear the shirttail under tightly belted trousers, and leave no opportunity for ticks to crawl under wristbands or neckbands of shirts. Wearing a tightly knotted kerchief around the neck to prevent ticks crawling from clothes to the body was often recommended in the U.S.S.R.

The latest of several Soviet designs in special clothing to protect humans from CCHF virus-infected ticks (*Hyalomma m. marginatum, Dermacentor marginatus, Rhipicephalus rossicus, Haemaphysalis punctata*) in Rostov Oblast is a two-piece knit fabric suit consisting of a fine net shirt with elastic cuffs and hood with elastic band borders, and wide trousers (*sharovar*) with elastic cuffs and a belt.[609] A more durable trouser fabric is recommended for hard-working shepherds, farmers, and forest guards. The suit is said to be comfortable, even on hot summer days, while stacking hay or cutting timber.

Commercially available repellents against ticks for application to exposed skin or for impregnating clothing may be more widely acceptable in warm climates than any closely confining hood-to-boots type of suit. Diethyl toluamide (Deet), which was developed by the U.S. Department of Agriculture to repel ticks and other bloodsucking arthropods, is widely used on the skin and for impregnating clothing. The Soviets have renamed this repellent Deta.

During the 1944 to 1945 CCHF outbreak in the Crimea, puttees, socks, and gauze leg wrappings were impregnated with "SK9", creolin, kerosene or carbolic acid to repel *H. m. marginatum.*[89,153,406] Perelatov and Lazarev[401] stated that no satisfactory repellent was available during the Rostov Oblast epidemic. In the Astrakhan Oblast CCHF epidemic, diethyl toluamide was recommended.[55] Various repellents commonly used in the U.S.S.R. and elsewhere were judged to be useless but diethylamide and dibutylamide of valerianic acid were said to give promising experimental results.[558] (For results of other studies, see Vashkov et al.[559] Deta, polychlorpinen (2% alcohol solution), "P-320", and terpenol were considered to be moderately useful against *Dermacentor marginatus* but less than satisfactory against *H. m. marginatum.*[474] In Uzbekistan, Bodanov[54] recommended impregnating clothing with "Pavlovsky repellent netting treatment" (3 to 5% emulsion of "K" preparation) and protecting the skin with a Vaseline® ointment containing 10 to 15% of the "K" preparation.

The tick species chiefly involved in transmitting CCHF virus to people on each con-

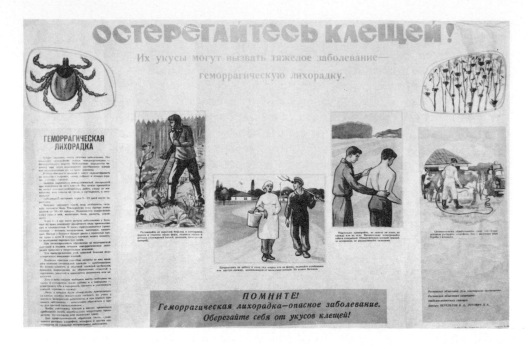

FIGURE 3.   CCHF propaganda poster. The title reads: "BEWARE OF TICKS. Tickbites may cause a severe disease: hemorrhagic fever." The illustration at the left, of a ♀ *Hyalomma m. marginatum (= p. plumbeum),* is followed by the text (freely translated): "HEMORRHAGIC FEVER. It is a severe, infectious disease. This disease is caused by the smallest living microorganisms (filterable viruses). The disease is transmitted to humans by an infected field tick or by crushing the tick on human skin. Ticks live in nature and may parasitize animals (cattle, sheep, hares) and birds (rooks, carrion crows, and magpies) Humans become infected with hemorrhagic fever after attack by ticks. This may occur while doing agricultural work, handling animals, or resting in grass or in shrubs and forests. The disease begins 3—12 days following infection. Patients suffer from chills, high temperature, exhaustion, and severe headache. The body temperature rapidly increases to 39-41°C. The skin of the face and neck becomes reddish, and muscular pains, asthenia, and somnolence appear. Three or 4 days followig disease onset, different types of hemorrhages and ecchymses appear on the skin. These are accompanied by nasal, gastric, uterine, and intestinal hemorrhages. Vomiting with traces of blood and blood in the urine are sometimes recorded. In severe cases, icteric discoloration of the skin may occur. Late hospitalization and late treatment of hemorrhagic fever lead to death. To protect ourselves against this severe disease, we should beware of tick attack. The most simple protective measure againt ticks is to wear special clothes, such as overalls. Usual clothes (shirts, trousers) may be substituted for overalls, but sleeves should fit as closely as possible, and trouser cuffs should be tucked into tight socks, but best tied with tape or elastic bands. Choose resting sites free of grass and shrubs. Personal and mutual inspection during rest periods and after work are obligatory; removed ticks should be destroyed. All persons on whom attached ticks are found must register with the local medical services and at the first signs of this disease must immediately appeal to a physician for urgent hospitalization. Places used for short visits should be treated with hexochlorane, or the glass should be burned. Chlorophos, metaphos, and other toxic chemicals should be used to treat cattle as recommended by veterinarians." The text below the illustration of the man spading a field reads: "Clear weeds and shrubs from all areas near roads, farms, field camps, and childrens' institutions (nurseries, pioneer camps, kindergartens)." The text below the illustration of a milkmaid and a farmer walking down a path reads: "Before going to work in fields, orchards, or farms, wear overalls or other clothes protecting against tick attack. Do not walk barefoot." The text below the illustration of one farmer inspecting another's body for ticks reads: "Carefully check to see if a tick is crawling on your clohes or on your body. Carefully inspect yourself and your comrades. Carefully remove ticks without squashing them with bare fingers." The illustration at the upper right is of nest of rooks (*Corvus f. frugilegus*) in a wooded area. Below it is an illustration of acaricide application to cattle followed by the text: "Regularly treat cattle with 1.5—2% chlorophos solution. This is a reliable measure against ticks." The lower central legend reads: "REMEMBER! Hemorrhagic fever is a very hazardous disease. Protect yourselves against tickbites!"

tinent are easily detached from one's body (if biting has not been prevented) with the aid of forceps or a bent or cleft twig or bent grass stem. Crushing ticks should be avoided; detached ticks should be burned or dropped into a lethal fluid (such as kerosene). Leaving tick mouthparts in the body has become a common fear in many nations but is seldom a problem with the tick species known to be chiefly involved in CCHF epidemiology. Early removal of attached ticks presumably reduces the possibility of virus transmission. Precisely how quickly the tick must be removed to prevent human infection is not known; the moment when effective agent inoculation into the host begins depends on a variety of biological and virological factors.

A 2-week observation period following tickbite is suggested where CCHF virus is known or suspected to infect ticks. (This observation period is usually stated as one week where contaminative transmission is a possibility; the incubation period of large virus doses under these circumstances is generally less than a week.)

Education and Propaganda

CCHF incidence is usually sporadic over an extensive, often thinly populated area. The warning directed toward at-risk populations in such regions, as said in Russian, "acquires a special character". Education and propaganda measures to prevent CCHF infection seen during two hemorrhagic fever delegations to the U.S.S.R. were, to us as visitors, quite impressive. One of the many propaganda posters distributed throughout Rostov Oblast is reproduced here in Figure 3. Despite their enthusiasm, Soviet authors have seldom claimed that educational efforts to prevent CCHF have produced the desired results. For instance, peasants who stubbornly refuse to control ticks on privately owned cattle, usually held close to or within their homestead plots (see several foregoing sections[76,383]), present a singular problem not easily overcome by education or propaganda.

The radio, television, and press were employed to disseminate information on preventing CCHF in each epidemic, as well as posters and lectures in schools and during the innumerable meetings held on State and collective farms and in village headquarters. Hospitals and rural health units and aid stations were centers for advising medical and paramedical personnel of the need for isolating suspected cases, preventing nosocomial and household infections by contamination, and hospitalizing all suspected cases as rapidly as possible. Persons who picked ticks from themselves or from animals were warned to report to hospitals or aid stations at the first signs of illness within the following week or two. Popular anti-CCHF literature (now termed "handouts" in the American vernacular) was distributed; an example is the 25-page booklet "What is Essential to Know about Hemorrhagic Fever" by Perelatov and Lazarev[401] published by the Rostov Oblast Sanitary Information House.

Environmental Control

During the Crimean CCHF epidemic, ditches were dug around camps in an effort to prevent *Hyalomma m. marginatum* from entering the grounds, rodent burrows were closed or tamped, and vegetation was cut or burned.[153] Various chemical solutions poured into the ditches and dusting the ground with pyrethrins had *no* noticeable effect on tick activity; "special antitick covers could not be used as a mass remedy." (Soldiers were also forbidden to rest or sleep near rodent burrows, in untreated vegetation, and in destroyed or abandoned houses.) In retrospect, early attempts at enviromental control and those of Petrova-Piontkovskaya,[408] who suggested that forest shelter belts tend to reduce *H. m. marginatum* numbers, reflect laudable attempts to overcome an emergency situation frustrated by lack of sufficient knowledge of vector-species bionomics.

Clearing areas around Young Pioneer camps, resorts, woodlots, and pathsides of shelters where ticks may survive (haystacks, brush piles, leaf litter, etc.) has been consistently stressed as a measure to reduce *H. m. marginatum* population density and the chances of human contact with ticks during CCHF epidemics.

Aerial spraying of acaricides (insecticides), a more or less common practice to control the forest-dwelling *Ixodes persulcatus* vectors of Russian spring-summer encephalitis virus, was seldom used where CCHF virus was a problem. However, helicopter and orchard sprayer-type spraying of chlorophos over 2600 ha of Krasnyy-Sulin pastureland (Rostov Oblast), together with controlling ticks on cattle, was said to reduce the tickload to low levels.[517] Aircraft spraying of 500 ha of Belaya Kaliteva pastureland with 10% DDT dust in 1966 was ineffective in controlling *H. m. marginatum*[286] The same authors considered springtime spraying of 2% chlorophos (100 liters/hactare) from KA-15 helicopters (at altitudes not exceeding 5 m and speed of 35 to 40 km/hr.) together with controlling ticks on cattle, to produce desirable results against *H. m. marginatum, Dermacentor marginatus,* and *Rhipicephalus rossicus.* On the other hand, Perelatov and Vostokova[404] concluded that none of the measures applied in Rostov Oblast had proved to be sufficiently effective for reventing CCHF.

Acaricides are recommended for use in the quite specific habitats where vector species density justify this action: usually in relation to domestic animal numbers, animal husbandry practices, and environmental changes.

To control *Hyalomma a. anatolicum* breeding away from cattle yards in Chimkent Oblast (Kazakhstan), Dobritsa et al.[136] suggested cutting dense grasses, especially on northern hill slopes, as well as reeds and rich vegetation in floodplain meadows and neglected alfalfa fields. Exposing larvae to sunlight, and in winter to cold, causes mortality. Irrigation and plowing also tend to reduce *H. a. anatolicum* numbers. Pasturing animals on infested fields during the first half of the year should be avoided. Tick control methods employed by veterinarians to prevent bovine theileriosis were considered to be equally effective in preventing CCHF infections in human beings.

In many environments of the world, the human populations and medical and veterinary authorities tolerate tick population densities that must be seen to be believed by persons habituated to a greater degree of tick control. Such environments are of primary concern in CCHF epidemiology.

Ticks On Wild Animals

Rodent control was recommended by a number of authors as a measure to reduce tick numbers in European CCHF foci. However, immature *Hyalomma m. marginatum* seldom if every parasitize rodents in these foci. Rodent destruction may help to decrease *Dermacentor marginatus* numbers in European foci and should be quite effective in controlling the important CCHF reservoir-vector *Hyalomma asiaticum* in Asian deserts and semideserts. Densities of other vector species whose immature stages feed on rodents may also be diminished by this method.

Hares are CCHF virus amplifiers and are often numerous and support large numbers of various tick species including *H. marginatum* subspp. and other known or potential CCHF reservoirs/vectors. Thus hare control was frequently recommended in Bulgaria and European U.S.S.R. Hedgehogs likewise are CCHF virus amplifiers and sometimes carry many ticks. Hedgehogs are seldom numerous but they commonly frequent gardens and pasture margins close to human habitations; their control might be considered in certain critical situations.

Except in some African areas, larger-sized wild mammals are usually too few in number to enter the picture of tick control to prevent CCHF.

Birds do not develop CCHF viremia but many species serve as hosts of ticks (especially of immatures) important in CCHF epidemiology and transport these parasites during intracontinental movements or intercontinental migrations. *Hyalomma m. marginatum* and other members of the *H. marginatum* complex feed chiefly on birds.

Large-scale control of rooks, *Corvus f. frugilegus,* might prove to be useful in reducing *H. m. marginatum* (and *Haemaphysalis punctata*) population densities in CCHF foci, but I have not seen this recommendation in Soviet literature. (Kondratenko et al.[286] briefly mentioned shooting birds to control these two tick species in Rostov Oblast.) All CCHF virus vector species associated in the immature stages with birds commonly feed as adults on domestic mammals, which are generally more economical targets for tick control than wild birds.

Ticks on Domestic Animals

Vashkov and Poleshchuk,[558] who reviewed various experiments to control *Hyalomma m. marginatum* in Astrakhan Oblast, concluded, as had earlier workers, that most available control measures were too expensive to consider because all pasture areas in the Oblast were potential microfoci. Spraying cattle during the period of adult tick parasitism was found to be most efficient. They recommended a mixture of 1% aqueous chlorophos solution with 0.3% polyvinyl alcohol (to hinder penetration of the insecticide through the skin into blood and milk), to be sprayed each 10 days, or a mixture of 1% aqueous Sevin® ["carbaryl" (International Standards Organization)] suspension with 0.5% polyvinyl alcohol to be sprayed each 13 days. Comparative tests with American and Soviet Sevin gave equally satisfactory results. Others[396] recommended spraying cattle at 7- to 8-day intervals. Chlorophos is the organophosphate "trichlorfon" (International Standards Organization), also known in the West as Dipterex®, Dylox®, Neguvon®, Tugon®, and trichlorophon. DDT had been used with poor results in Astrakhan Oblast[506] and elsewhere. Shevchenko et al.[474] considered DDT the most effective of several acaricides for *H. m. marginatum* control because of its long toxic effect but chlorophos more suitable for pasture control because of high toxicity, more rapid decomposition, and cheapness. Chlorophos is now the acaricide of choice in the U.S.S.R.

Barnett[27] reviewed methods for controlling ticks parasitizing livestock around the world. The subject is, of course, of primary concern in preventing CCHF. The reader is referred to more specialized literature for further information. The complete literature on tick control to prevent CCHF is included in the forthcoming *Annotated Bibliography of Tickborne Viruses* (Volume 6 of the *Bibliography of Ticks and Tickborne Diseases*).

EPILOGUE

The CCHF research programs that produced epic epidemiological and biomedical knowledge and history of CCHF during the 1968 to 1972 period in the U.S.S.R., and elsewhere in Europe, Asia, and Africa, have been discontinued or reduced to limited, opportunistic examinations of sera from domestic animals and occasionally from human beings. "Despite the contemporary low ebb in reported CCHF morbidity, continued surveillance of potentially hazardous areas is necessary to save lives".

Casals[74] stressed the high priority that should be given to research for rapid, early diagnosis of CCHF. The time required for specific diagnosis might be shortened by 1 to 3 days by IFA testing of brain tissue smears from mice inoculated with suspect material or of similarly inoculated CER cells in chamber-cells. The fastest way to diagnose CCHF would be by detecting the virus or its antigens in clinical specimens. Considering the high virus titer in blood between days 1 to 5 of illness (reportedly $10^{6.2}$ $LD_{50}/m\ell$), it may be possible to detect this virus by IFA tests or radioimmunoassay.

A highly sensitive test for detecting neutralizing antibodies also requires urgent development for seroepidemiological surveys and for determining possible antigenic differences among strains of CCHF virus. Studies of subvirionic particles may help to resolve the question of antigenic differences; however, the extent to which techniques for purification, fractionation, and polynucleotide analysis can be used may be curtailed by the risk involved in studies of this kind with this agent.[74]

In the interests of virological knowledge in general and of application for seroepidemiological surveys, especially in Africa and India, it is essential to learn more about the relationships and antigenic reactions between CCHF virus and the Nairobi sheep disease (NSD) serogroup (NSD, Ganjam, and Dugbe viruses).

I commenced work on this review some years ago after becoming enthused over the variety and quantity of information that was rapidly accumulating on the natural history of CCHF virus. I ended this review in the spring of 1978 distressed over our dearth of knowledge of *how CCHF virus survives as a zoonotic infection* in a large variety of zoogeographic regions, environments, ticks, and vertebrates. Fascinating information supported by more or less detailed data has derived from several CCHF epizootics (epidemics). Not a single substantial study has been made of interrelationships between the virus, large-sized and small-sized wild mammals, domestic mammals, and immature and adult ticks during the "silent" coursing of the virus in nature. Questions regarding CCHF viremia in birds also loom large. The role of reptiles as CCHF virus reservoirs has not been investigated.

It is disappointing to have to write, at this late stage, that there are still no detailed investigations of CCHF virus localization, multiplication, and dynamics in ticks. We should like to know if and/or how blood meals from different kinds of hosts affect virus dynamics in two-host and in three-host ticks. Also, do one-host species, such as *Boophilus,* have an independent reservoir-vector role or is their epidemiological importance related to and dependent on coexistance with other tick species?

I have postulated that epizootic CCHF appears to be closely associated with cyclic or human-caused peaks in *Hyalomma* population densities; this suggestion remains to be tested, modified, proven, or disproven. An authoritative Soviet-Bulgarian review of climatic factors prevailing before, during and after CCHF epidemics would be a scientifically valuable precursor for designing experimental protocols and models useful in predicting changes in tick population densities and CCHF outbreaks.

In Africa, CCHF is one of several hemorrhagic diseases caused by viruses; of these, the epidemiology of only Lassa virus is gradually being reasonably well elucidated.[350] Much of Africa is biomedically favorable testing ground for investigating the natural history of CCHF virus as a zoonoses, the incidence of inapparent and apparent infections in people and the questions of differences in virus strains and virulence.

For the biologist, virologist, and epidemiologist, the enormous enigma surrounding every aspect of the natural history of CCHF virus is its exceptional adaptability to such a large area of the earth's surface and to so many kinds of ticks and mammals. Explanations for this apparent adaptability await the results of future research.

ACKNOWLEDGMENTS

For furnishing critical comments on certain parts of this manuscript, I am grateful to Drs. Jordi Casals and R. E. Shope (Yale Arbovirus Research Unit), Donald Heyneman (University of California Medical Center, San Francisco), C. E. Yunker (Rocky Mountain Laboratory), M. W. Dols (California State University, Hayward), Gene Higashi (NAMRU-3, Cairo) and R. A. Bram (USDA, Hyattsville). Unpublished data were kindly furnished by Drs. P. A. Webb (Center for Disease Control, Atlanta), O. L. Wood, V. H. Lee, and J. S. Ash (NAMRU-5, Addis Ababa), and F. G. Davies (Veterinary Research Laboratory, Kabete).

Mrs. Olga Strekalovsky and Mrs. Sophie Korzelska (NAMRU-3 Medical Zoology

Department) expertly translated the Russian literature (under the auspices of NIH-NAMRU-3 Agreement 03-036-N), and Dr. Alexis Shelokov (University of Texas Medical School, San Antonio) helped with translating certain difficult Russian passages.

For making special efforts to provide otherwise unobtainable literature, I am grateful to Academician M. P. Chumakov and Drs. S. P. Chunikhin and E. V. Leshchinskaya (Institute of Viral Encephalitides and Poliomyelitis, Moscow), V. M. Neronov (Institute of Evolutionary Animal Morphology and Ecology, Moscow), D. K. L'vov (D. I. Ivanovsky Institute of Virology, Moscow), V. V. Kucheruk (Gamaleya Institute, Moscow), Brunhilde Rehse-Kupper (University Clinic for Nervous Diseases, Cologne), D. C. Gajdusek (National Institute of Neurological Diseases and Stroke, Bethesda), and J. Casals, R. E. Shope, and A. Shelokov.

Preparation of this review would have been impossible without the steadfast, expert assistance of Mrs. Alice Djigounian, Chief Bibliographer, and Mrs. Annie Massabki, Manuscript Specialist (NAMRU-3 Medical Zoology Department), and the support furnished by the National Institute of Allergy and Infectious Diseases (National Institutes of Health) Agreement 03-036-N with NAMRU-3.

ADDENDUM

On October 12, 1979, the World Health Organization Weekly Epidemiological Record contained a report of five cases, clinically resembling CCHF, seen in Baghdad, Iraq, where this disease had not previously been recognized. The index case, a pregnant woman from Ramadi, died in Yarmouk Hospital on September 9 and her hospital physician and nursing assistant died of the disease on September 19. The fourth case, a woman admitted to a different hospital in Baghdad on September 18, resided in the city and had no contact with the first three; she improved following transfusions of blood and platelets. The fifth patient, from a nearby town, was admitted to Yarmouk Hospital on September 21 and recovered following transfusions. The November 16 issue of the WHO Record contained the note that the CCHF diagnosis was now confirmed by isolation of "Congo" virus from the blood of "one of the patients". If this isolation was from one of the first three patients, it is reasonable to state that each was infected by this virus. However, in the absence of scientific proof, the similarity of clinical symptoms is insufficient evidence for positive diagnosis of CCHF in the other cases.

Several *Hyalomma* species thrive in Iraq and the presence of CCHF virus is not unexpected there. These three, and possibly five, cases point to the need for investigating the epizootiology of CCHF virus and its threat to human health throughout the Middle East and North Africa where *Hyalomma* are common.

REFERENCES

1. **Abushev, F. A., Sterkhova, N. N., and Akhundova, E. D.**, The role of herring gulls and common terns in forming the natural ornithosis focus on an island of Baku Archipelago, Azerbaijan S.S.R., *Mater. Simp. Itogi 6. Simp. Izuch. Virus. Ekol. Svyazan. Ptits.*, Omsk, December 1971, 124, 1972; in Russian. (In English, NAMRU3-T679.)

2. **Aeschlimann, A., Diehl, P. A., Eichenberger, R. Immler, and Weiss, N.**, Les tiques (Ixodoidea) des animaux domestiques au Tessin, *Rev. Suisse Zool.*, 75, 1039, 1968.

3. **Aeschlimann, A. and Morel, P. C.**, *Boophilus geigyi* n. sp. (Acarina: Ixodoidea) une nouvelle tique du betail de l'Ouest Africain, *Acta Trop.*, 22, 162, 1965.

4. **Albanese, M., Ajello, F., Tomasino, R. M., and Chiarini, A.,** Caratteristiche della infezione speri- mentale del topo e del criceto adulti con un arbovirus recentemente isolato in Sicilia, *Boll. Ist. Siero- ter. Milan.*, 52, 173, 1973.

5. **Albanese, M., Bruno-Smiraglia, C., di Cuonzo, G., Lavagnino, A., and Srihongse, S.,** Investigation on arboviruses in western Sicily: insect collection *Ann. Sclavo*, 13, 1, 1971.

6. **Albanese, M., Bruno-Smiraglia, C., di Cuonzo, G., Lavagnino, A., and Srihongse, S.,** Isolation of Thogoto virus from *Rhipicephalus bursa* ticks in western Sicily, *Acta Virol. (Engl. Ed.)*, 16, 267, 1972.

7. **Albanese, M., Bruno-Smiraglia, C., and Lavagnino, A.,** Notizie sulle zecche di Sicilia con Segnala- zione di *Hyalomma detritum* e *Amblyomma variegatum*, *Riv. Parassitol.*, 32, 273, 1971.

8. **Aleksandrov, Yu. V. and Kudryavtsev, M. G.,** Hemorrhagic fever in Crimea, *Tezisy Dokl. 2. Akarol. Soveshch. pt.* 1, 26, 1970; in Russian. (In English, NAMRU3-T858.)

9. **Aleksandrov, Yu. V. and Yagodinsky, V. N.,** Application of the comparative nosogeographical method for epidemiological analysis of Crimean type hemorrhagic fevers, *Mater. 2 Nauchn. So- veshch. Probl. Med. Geogr.*, No. 2, Leningrad, 1965; in Russian).

10. **Andreev, V. P. and Shcherbina,** New data on importance of polyspecies colonies of Kara-Bogaz as natural arbovirus foci, *Mater. 9 Simp. Ekol. Virus*, Dushanbe, October 1975, 88; in Russian. (In English, NAMRU3-T1140.)

11. **Andreiko, O. F. and Shumilo, R. P.,** *Parasites of birds and rodents in Moldavia*, Akad. Nauk Mold. S.S.R., Inst. Zool., Kishinev, 1970, 114; in Russian.

12. **Andrewes, C. (Sir) and Pereira, H. G.,** *Viruses of Vertebrates*, 3rd ed., Williams & Wilkins, Balti- more, 1972, 451.

13. **Angelov, St., Panaiotov, P., and Manolova, N.,** Essais de culture du virus de la fièvre hemorragique sur des cultures de tissus, *Dokl. Bolg. Akad. Nauk.*, 13, 211, 1960.

14. **Anon.,** Agents isolated, 1959-1960 (unnumbered table), *Rep. E. Afr. Virus Res. Inst.*, 10, 35, 1960.

15. **Arata, A. A.,** The importance of small mammals in public health, *Int. Biol. Programme*, 5, 349, 1975.

16. **Arata, A. A., Farhang-Azad, A., and Neronov, V. M.,** Study of the ecology of certain small-mam- mal-borne infections in Iran, *Trans. I. Int. Ther. Congr.*, 1,29, Moscow, June 1974.

17. **Ardoin, P.,** Congo group transmission experiments, *Rep. E. Afr. Virus Res. Inst.*, 14, 52, 1965.

18. **Aristova, V. A. and Gostinshchikova,** Clinyany Island of Baku Archipelago as a natural focus of arboviral infections, *Tezisy Dokl. Vop. Med. Virus. Inst. Virus. imeni Ivanovsky D. I. Akad. Med. Nauk SSR (October 1971) pt.* 2, 123, 1971; in Russian. (In English, NAMRU3-T507.)

19. **Aristova, V. A., Neronov, V. M., Veselovskaya, O. V., Lushchekina, A. A., and Kurbanov, M.,** Investigation of Crimean hemorrhagic fever natural foci in southeastern Turkmenia, *Sb. Tr. Ekol Virus*, 1, 115, 1973; in Russian. (In English, NAMRU3-T719.)

20. **Avakyan, A. A.,** Etiology of hemorrhagic fevers, Crimean and Crimean type, in *Clinical picture of infectious hemorrhagic diseases and fevers*, Gal'perin, E. A., Ed., Gos. Izd. Med. Lit. (Medgiz), Moscow, 1960, 122; in Russian. (In English, NAMRU3-T879.)

21. **Badalov, M. E., Butenko, A. M., Karinskaya, G. A., Leshchinskaya, E. V., Rubin, S. G., Tkach- enko, E. A., and Chumakov, M. P.,** Results from serological investigation of rural population and domestic animals in Rostov Oblast in connection with the problem of prophylaxis, *Mater. 16 Nauchn. Sess. Inst. Polio. Virus. Entsefalitov*, 2, 117, 1969; in Russian. (In English, NAMRU3-T834.)

22. **Badalov, M. E., Koimchidi, E. K., Semenov, M. Ya., and Karinskaya, G. A.,** Crimean hemorrhagic fever in Rostov Region, *Tr. Inst. Polio. Virusn. Entsefalitov Akad. Med. Nauk S.S.S.R.*, 19, 167, 1971; in Russian. (In English, NAMRU3-T923.)

23. **Badalov, M. E., Lazarev, V. N., Koimchidi, E. K., and Karinskaya, G. A.,** Contribution to the problem of Crimean hemorrhagic fever infections in hospitals and laboratories, *Mater. 3. Oblast. Nauchn. Prakt. Konf.*, 90 Rostov-on-Don, May 1970; in Russian. (In English, NAMRU3-T538.)

24. **Balashov, Yu. S.,** in *Bloodsucking ticks (Ixodoidea) — Vectors of Diseases of Man and Animals*, Nauka Publishers, Leningrad, 1968, 319; in English, *Misc. Publ. Entomol. Soc. Am.*, 8, 161, 1972.

25. **Balashov, Yu. S., Daiter, A. B., and Khavkin, T. N.,** Distribution of Burnet's rickettsiae in the tick *Hyalomma asiaticum*, *Parazitologiya*, 6, 22, 1972; in Russian, English summary.

26. **Balát, F. and Rosický, B.,** Die Bedeutung der Vögel in Naturherden der tularemie und encephalitis, *Česk. Parazitol.*, 1, 23, 1954; in Czech.

27. **Barnett, S. F.,** The control of ticks on livestock, *FAO Agric. Stud.*, 54, 115, 1961.

28. **Bartoshevich, E. N.,** Endemic cases of exanthematous typhus and tick relapsing fever in the Alma- Ata Province, *Tr. Konf. Prirod. Ochag. Zaraznykh. Bolez. Chelov. Sel. Khoz. Zhivot. Kazakh.*, 2, 127, 1954; in Russian. (In English, NAMRU3-T208.)

29. **Begum, F., Wisseman, C. L., Jr., and Casals, J.,** Tick-borne viruses of West Pakistan. II. Hazara virus, a new agent isolated from *Ixodes redikorzevi* ticks from the Kaghan Valley, W. Pakistan, *Am. J. Epidemiol.*, 92, 192, 1970.

30. **Begum, F., Wisseman, C. L., Jr., and Casals, J.,** Tick-borne viruses of West Pakistan. IV. Viruses similar to, or identical with, Crimean hemorrhagic fever (Congo-Semunya), Wad Medani and Pak *Argas* 461 isolated from ticks of the Changa Manga Forest, Lahore District, and Hunza, Gilgit Agency, W. Pakistan, *Am. J. Epidemiol.,* 92, 197, 1970.

31. **Benda, R., Plaisner, V., and Hronovsky, V.,** Experiences with the adaptation of Crimean hemorrhagic fever virus to the CV-1 monkey cell line, *Acta Virol. (Engl. Ed.),* 19, 340, 1975.

32. **Berezin, V. V.,** Investigation of the ecology of arboviruses in river deltas of the Caspian and Azov sea basins, (Avtoref. Diss. Soisk. Uchen. Step. Dokt. Biol. Nauk) *Inst. Polio. Virusn. Entsefalitov, Akad. Med. Nauk SSSR, Moscow,* 1971, 37; in Russian. (In English, NAMRU3-T1160.)

33. **Berezin, V. V., Chumakov, M. P., Reshetnikov, I. A., and Zgurskaya, G. N.,** Study of the role of birds in the ecology of Crimean hemorrhagic fever virus, *Mater. 6. Simp. Izuch. Virus. Ekol. Svyazan. Ptits.,* 94, Omsk, 1971; in Russian. (In English, NAMRU3-T721.)

34. **Berezin, V. V., Chumakov, M. P., Rubin, S. G., Stolbov, D. N., Butenko, A. M., and Bashkirtsev, V. A.,** Contribution to the ecology of Crimean hemorrhagic fever virus in the lower Volga River, *Mater. 16. Nauchn. Sess. Inst. Polio. Virus. Entsefalitov,* 2, 120, 1969; in Russian. (In English, NAMRU3-T836.)

35. **Berezin, V. V., Chumakov, M. P., Stolbov, D. N., and Butenko, A. M.,** On the problem of natural hosts of Crimean hemorrhagic fever virus in Astrakhan Region, *Tr. Inst. Polio. Virusn. Entsefalitov Akad. Med. Nauk. S.S.S.R.,* 19, 210, 1971; in Russian. (In English, NAMRU3-T912.)

36. **Berezin, V. V., Povalishina, T. P., Ermakova, R. M., and Stolbov, D. N.,** On the role of birds in feeding immature stages of *Hyalomma plumbeum* plumbeum ticks — vectors of hemorrhagic fever of the Crimean type in foci of the Volga Delta, *Tr. Inst. Polio. Virusn. Entsefalitov Akad. Med. Nauk S.S.S.R.,* 7, 296, 1965; in Russian. (In English, NAMRU3-T198.)

37. **Berezin, V. V., Stolbov, D. N., Povalishina, T. P., and Zimina, Yu. V.,** On the role of rooks in the epidemiology of Crimean hemorrhagic fever in Astrakhan Oblast, *Tr. Inst. Polio. Virusn. Entsefalitov Akad. Med. Nauk S.S.S.R.,* 7, 304, 1965; in Russian. (In English, NAMRU3-T376.)

38. **Berezin, V. V., Stolbov, D. N., and Zimina, Yu. V.,** Effect of natural factors on the rate of Crimean hemorrhagic infections, *Mater. 16. Nauchn. Sess. Inst. Polio. Virus. Entsefalitov.,* 2, 118, 1969; in Russian. (In English, NAMRU3-T835.)

39. **Berge, T. O., Ed.,** International Catalogue of Arboviruses Including Certain Other Viruses of Vertebrates, 2nd ed., Pub. (CDC) 75-8301, Public Health Service, U.S. Department of Health, Education and Welfare, Atlanta, 1975, 789.

40. **Bernadskaya, Z. M.,** Distribution of cattle ticks (Ixodidae) in Uzbek, S.S.R., *Byull. Uzbek Nauchno Issled Vet. Inst.,* 4, 29, 1935; in Russian, English summary.

41. **Beron, P.,** Catalogue des acariens parasites et commensaux des mammifères en Bulgarie. II, *Izv. Zool. Inst. Sofiya,* 38, 105, 1973.

42. **Beron, P.,** Catalogue des acariens parasites et commensaux des mammifères en Bulgarie, III, *Izv. Zool. Inst. Sofiya,* 39, 163, 1974.

43. **Bilibin, A. F.,** Omsk and Crimean hemorrhagic fevers, in *Symptomatology and diagnosis of infectious diseases,* Medgiz, Moscow, 1950, 200; in Russian. (In English, NAMRU3-T805.)

44. **Birulya, N. B., Badalov, M. E., Zalutskaya, L. I., and Koimchidi, E. K.,** Geography of Crimean hemorrhagic fever incidence in Rostov Oblast in 1963-1971, *Tezisy Konf. Vop. Med. Virus,* Moscow, October 1975, 268; in Russian. (In English, NAMRU3-T984.)

45. **Birulya, N. B., Zalutskaya, L. I., and Perelatov, V. D.,** Distribution area of natural foci of Crimean hemorrhagic fever, *Tr. Inst. Polio. Virusn. Entsefalitov Akad. Med. Nauk S.S.S.R.,* 19, 180, 1971; in Russian. (In English, NAMRU3-T962.)

46. **Blagoveshchenskaya, N. M., Butenko, A. M., Vyshnivetskaya, L. K., Zarubina, L. V., Kuchin, V. V., Milyutin, V. N., Novikova, E. M., and Chumakov, M. P.,** Dynamics of antibodies to Crimean hemorrhagic fever virus in hyperimmunized horses, *Mater. 3. Oblast. Nauchn. Prakt. Konf.,* 50, Rostov-on-Don, May 1970; in Russian. (In English, NAMRU3-T529.)

47. **Blagoveshchenskaya, N. M., Butenko, A. M., Vyshnivetskaya, L. K., Zavodova, T. I., Zarubina, L. V., Karinskaya, G. A., Kuchin, V. V., Milyutin, V. N., Novikova, E. M., Rubin, S. G., and Chumakov, M. P.,** Experimental infection of horses with Crimean hemorrhagic fever virus. II. Virological and serological observations, *Mater. 16. Nauchn. Sess. Inst. Polio. Virus. Entsefalitov,* 2, 126, 1969; in Russian. (In English, NAMRU3-T840.)

48. **Blagoveshchenskaya, N. M., Donets, M. A., Zarubina, L. V., Kondratenko, V. F., and Kuchin, V. V.,** Study of susceptibility to Crimean hemorrhagic fever (CHF) virus in European and long-eared hedgehogs, *Tezisy Konf. Vop. Med. Virus,* Moscow, October 1975, 269, in Russian. (In English, NAMRU3-T985.)

49. **Blagoveshchenskaya, N. M., Vyshnivetskaya, L. K., Gusarev, A. F., Zarubina, L. V., Kondratenko, V. F., Kuchin, V. V., Milyutin, V. N., Perelatov, V. D., Novikova, E. M., and Novikova, L. D.,** Investigation of susceptibility in rabbits to Crimean hemorrhagic fever virus, *Tezisy 17. Nauchn. Sess. Inst. Posvyashch. Aktual. Probl. Virus. Profilakt. Virus. Zabolev,* Moscow, October 1972, 353; in Russian. (In English, NAMRU3-T1062.)

50. **Blagoveshchenskaya, N. M., Vyshnivetskaya, L. K., Gusarev, A. F., Zarubina, L. V., Kondratenko, V. F., Kuchin, V. V., Perelatov, V. D., Novikova, E. M., and Novikova, L. D.,** Investigation of susceptibility in little susliks (*Citellus pygmaeus* Pall.) to CHF virus, *Tezisy 17. Nauchn. Sess. Inst. Posvyashch. Aktual. Probl. Virus. Profilakt. Virus. Zabolev,* Moscow, October 1972, 356; in Russian. (In English, NAMRU3-T1064.)

51. **Blaškovič, D. and Nošek, J.,** The ecological approach to the study of tickborne encephalitis, *Prog. Med. Virol.,* 14, 275, 1972.

52. **Blinzinger, K.,** Comparative electron microscopic studies of several experimental group B arbovirus infections of the murine CNS (CEE virus, Zimmern virus, yellow fever virus), *Ann. Inst. Pasteur Paris,* 123, 497, 1972.

53. **Blinzinger, K.,** Vergleichende elektronenmikroskopische Untersuchungen bei experimentellen Infektionen mit dem fränkischen Zimmern-Virus (Stamm ZIU VII-BM) und zwei bekannten Togaviren der Gruppe B, in *Arboviruserkrankungen des Nervensystems in Europa. Forschungsergebnisse, Klinische Beobachtungen und Diskussions-beträge auf dem Internationalen Symposion in Giessen,* Muller, W. and G. Schaltenbrand, Eds., Georg Thieme Verlag, Stuttgart, 1975, 124.

54. **Bodanov, M. I.,** Measures to be taken against ticks, *Vop. Kraev. Patol. Akad. Nauk Uzbek. S.S.R.,* 2, 155, 1952; in Russian. (In English, NAMRU3-T215.)

55. **Bolovina, V. N., Perelatov, V. D., Badalov, M. E., Koimchidi, E. K., Karinskaya, G. A., and Semenov, M. Ya.,** Study of Crimean hemorrhagic fever incidence and prophylactic measures in Rostov Oblast, *Mater. 3. Oblast. Nauchn. Prakt. Konf,* Rostov-on-Don, May 1970, 66.

56. **Brinck, P., Svedmyr, A., and Zeipel, G.,** Migrating birds at Ottenby Swenden as carriers of ticks and possible transmitters of tick-borne encephalitis virus, *Oikos,* 16, 88, 1965.

57. **Brumshtein, M. S. and Leshchinskaya, E. V.,** Clinical-anatomical characteristics of Crimean hemorrhagic fever, *Arkh. Patol.,* 30, 57, 1968; in Russian.

58. **Buckley, S. M.,** In vitro propagation of tick-borne viruses other than group B arboviruses, in (Intr. Lect. Proc. Symp.) *Int. Symp. Tick-borne Arboviruses (Excluding Group B) (Smolenice, September 1969),* 1971, 43.

59. **Buckley, S. M.,** Cross plaque neutralization tests with cloned Crimean hemorrhagic fever-Congo (CHF-C) and Hazara viruses, *Proc. Soc. Exp. Biol. Med.,* 146, 594, 1974.

60. **Bulynin, V. I. and Poshekhonov, S. A.,** The problem of the infectiousness of hemorrhagic fever in Stavropol, *Zh. Mikrobiol. Epidemiol. Immunobiol.,* 30, 147, 1959; in Russian.

61. **Burgdorfer, W., Ormsbee, R. A., Schmidt, M. L., and Hoogstraal, H.,** A search for the epidemic typhus agent in Ethiopian ticks, *Bull. WHO,* 48, 563, 1973.

62. **Burgdorfer, W., Sexton, D. J., Gerloff, R. K., Anacker, R. L., Philip, R. N., and Thomas, L. A.,** *Rhipicephalus sanguineus:* vector of a new spotted fever group *Rickettsia* in the United States, *Infect. Immun.,* 12, 205, 1975.

63. **Burgdorfer, W. and Varma, M. G. R.,** Trans-stadial and transovarial development of disease agents in arthropods, *Ann. Rev. Entomol.,* 12, 347, 1967.

64. **Butenko, A. M., Chumakov, M. P., Bashkirtsev, V. N., Zavodova, T. I., Tkachenko, E. A., Rubin, S. G., and Stolbov, D. N.,** Isolation and investigation of Astrakhan strain ("Drozdov") of Crimean hemorrhagic fever virus and data on serodiagnosis of this infection, *Mater. 15. Nauchn. Sess. Inst. Polio. Virus. Entsefalitov,* 3, 88, 1968; in Russian. (In English, NAMRU3-T866.)

65. **Butenko, A. M., Chumakov, M. P., Smirnova, S. E., Vasilenko, S. M., Zavodova, T. I., Tkachenko, E. A., Zarubina, L. V., Bashkirtsev, V. N., Zgurskaya, G. N., and Vyshnivetskaya, L. K.,** Isolation of Crimean hemorrhagic fever virus from blood of patients and corpse material (from 1968-1969 investigation data) in Rostov, Astrakhan Oblast, and Bulgaria, *Mater. 3. Oblast. Nauchn. Prakt. Konf.,* Rostov-on-Don, 1970, 6; in Russian. (In English, NAMRU3-T522.)

66. **Butenko, A. M., Donets, M. A., Durov, V. I., Tkachenko, V. A., Perelatov, V. D., and Chumakov, M. P.,** Isolation of Crimean hemorrhagic fever virus from *Rhipicephalus rossicus* and *Dermacentor marginatus* ticks in Rostov Oblast and Krasnodar Region, *Tr. Inst. Polio. Virusn. Entsefalitov Akad. Med. Nauk S.S.S.R.,* 19, 45, 1971; in Russian. (In English, NAMRU3-T828.)

67. **Calisher, C. H. and Goodpasture, H. C.,** Human infection with Bhanja virus, *Am. J. Trop. Med. Hyg.,* 24, 1040, 1975.

68. **Camicas, J. L.,** Contribution à l'etude des tiques de Sénégal (*Acarina,* Ixodoidea). I. Les larves d'Amblyomma Koch et de *Hyalomma* Koch, *Acarologia,* 12, 71, 1970.

69. **Casals, J.,** New developments in the classification of arthropod-borne animal viruses (Proc. 7th Int. Congr. Trop. Med. Malar., Rio de Janeiro, 1963), *An. Microbiol.,* 11, 13, 1963.

70. **Casals, J.,** Antigenic similarity between the virus causing Crimean hemorrhagic fever and Congo virus, *Proc. Soc. Exp. Biol. Med.,* 131, 233, 1969.

71. **Casals, J.,** Arbovirus infections, in *Serological Epidemiology,* Paul, J. R. and White, C., Eds., Academic Press, New York, 1973, 99.

72. **Casals, J.,** Serological techniques for Crimean hemorrhagic fever-Congo CHF-C) viruses, in *Trop. Med. Malar. Abstr. Inv. Pap. 9th Int. Congr. Trop. Med. Malar.,* 1, 35, 1973.

73. **Casals, J.,** International arbovirus research, (Int. Symp. Arbo., Helsinki and Lepolampi, June 1975) *Med. Biol.,* 53, 249, 1975.

74. **Casals, J.,** Crimean-Congo hemorrhagic fever, *Proc. Colloq. Ebola Virus and other Hemorrhagic Fevers, Antwerp, December 1977,* in press, 1979.

75. **Casals, J., Henderson, B. E., Hoogstraal, H., Johnson, K. M., and Shelokov, A.,** A review of Soviet viral hemorrhagic fevers, *J. Infect. Dis.,* 122, 437, 1970.

76. **Casals, J., Hoogstraal, H., Johnson, K. M., Shelokov, A., Wiebenga, N. H., and Work, T. H.,** A current appraisal of hemorrhagic fevers in the USSR, *Am. J. Trop. Med. Hyg.,* 15, 751, 1966.

77. **Casals, J. and Tignor, G. H.,** Neutralization and hemagglutination inhibition tests with Crimean hemorrhagic fever Congo virus, *Proc. Soc. Exp. Biol. Med.,* 145, 960, 1974.

78. **Causey, O. R. and Kemp, G. E.,** Surveillance and study of viral infections of vertebrates in Nigeria, *Niger. J. Sci.,* 2, 131, 1968.

79. **Causey, O. R., Kemp, G. E., Casals, J., Williams, R. W., and Madbouly, M. H.,** Dugbe virus, a new arbovirus from Nigeria, *Niger. J. Sci.,* 5, 41, 1971.

80. **Causey, O. R., Kemp, G. E., Madbouly, M. H., and David-West. T. S.,** Congo virus from domestic livestock, African hedgehog, and arthropods in Nigeria, *Am. J. Trop. Med. Hyg.,* 19, 846, 1970.

81. **Causey, O. R., Kemp, G. E., Madbouly, M. H., and Lee, V. H.,** Arbovirus surveillance in Nigeria, 1964-1967, *Bull. Soc. Pathol. Exot.,* 62, 249, 1969.

82. **Causey, O. R., Kemp, G. E., Williams, R. W., and Madbouly, M. H.,** West African tick-borne viruses, in *Abstr. Rev. 8th Int. Congr. Trop. Med.* Malar., Teheran, September 1968, 669.

83. **Černý, V. and Balát, F.,** Ein Fall der Einschleppung der Zecken *Hyalomma plumbeum* (Panz.) 1795 (Ixodidae) durch die Vögal auf das Gebiet der ČSR, *Zool. Listy,* 1, 81, 1957; in Czech. (In English, NAMRU3-T7).

84. **Chastel, C.,** Interet des techniques d'immunoprécipitation en gel (immunodiffusion double, immunoélectrophorèse) pour l'étude des arbovirus et des arenavirus, *Rev. Epidemiol. Med. Soc. Sante Publique,* 22, 231, 1974.

85. **Chernovsky, K. M., Kantorovich, R. A., Yasinsky, A. V., Kalmykov, E. S., Berdyev, Kh. B., Arsky, V. G., and Abdullokhodzhaev, Z. Ya.,** Hemorrhagic fever cases in Tadzhik SSR- *Zdravookhr. Tadzh.,* 2, 5, 1968; in Russian.

86. **Chernovsky, K. M., Yasinsky, A. V., Kalmykov, E. S., Berdyev, Kh. B., and Arsky, V. G.,** Liquidation measures of Crimean hemorrhagic fever outbreak in Tadzhik SSR, *Tr. Inst. Polio. Virusn. Entsefalitov Akad. Med. Nauk S.S.S.R.,* 19, 224, 1971; in Russian. (In English, NAMRU3-T979.)

87. **Chubkova, A. I.,** The landscape distribution of diseases with natural foci in the Armenian S.S.R. 10, *Sov. Parazitol. Probl.,* 1, 43, 1959; in Russian. (English translation, JPRS No. 10771, 1, 53, 1961.)

88. **Chumakov, M. P.,** A new tick-borne virus disease — Crimean hemorrhagic fever, in *Crimean Hemorrhagic Fever (Acute Infectious Capillary Toxicosis),* Sokolov, A. A., Chumakov, M. P., and Kolachev, A. A., Eds., Izd. Otd. Primorskoi Armii, Simferopol, 1945, 13; in Russian.

89. **Chumakov, M. P.,** *Crimean Hemorrhagic Fever (Acute Infectious Capillary Toxicosis). Short Reports,* Krymskiy Oblastnoi Otdel Zdravookhraneniya "Krymizdat", Simferopol, 1946, 27; in Russian. (In English, NAMRU3-T910.)

90. **Chumakov, M. P.,** A new virus disease — Crimean hemorrhagic fever, *Nov. Med.,* 4, 9, 1947; in Russian. (In English, NAMRU3-T900.)

91. **Chumakov, M. P.,** Crimean hemorrhagic fever, *Entsikl. Slovar Voenn. Med.,* 3, 268, 1948.

92. **Chumakov, M. P.,** Etiology, epidemiology and prevention of hemorrhagic fevers, *Tezisy Dokl. 4. Nauchn. Sess. Posvyashch. Probl. Kraev. Neiroinfekts. Patol.,* 1949, 40; in Russian. (In English, NAMRU3-T898.)

93. **Chumakov, M. P.,** A short story of the investigation of the virus of Crimean hemorrhagic fever, *Tr. Inst. Polio. Virusn. Entsefalitov Akad. Med. Nauk S.S.S.R.,* 7, 193, 1965; in Russian. (In English, NAMRU3-T189.)

94. **Chumakov, M. P.,** Crimean hemorrhagic fever, *Mater. 3 Oblast. Nauchn. Prakt. Konf.,* Rostov-on-Don, May 1970, 183; in Russian. (In English, *Misc. Publ. Entomol. Soc. Am.,* 9, 123, 1974.)

95. **Chumakov, M. P.,** Some results of investigation of the etiology and immunology of Crimean hemorrhagic fever, *Tr. Inst. Polio. Virusn. Entsefalitov Akad. Med. Nauk S.S.S.R.,* 19, 7, 1971; in Russian. (In English, NAMRU3-T953.)

96. **Chumakov, M. P.,** Investigations of arboviruses in the USSR and the question of possible association through migratory birds between natural arbovirus infection foci in the USSR and warm-climate countries, *Mater. 5. Simp. Izuch. Roli Pereletn. Ptits. Rasp. Arbovirus,* Novosibirsk, July 1969, 133, 1972; in Russian. (In English, NAMRU3-T876.)

97. **Chumakov, M. P.,** On the results of investigations of the etiology and epidemiology of Crimean hemorrhagic fever in the USSR, *Abstr. Inv. Pap. 9th Int. Congr. Trop. Med. Malar.,* 1, 33, 1973.

98. **Chumakov, M. P.,** On 30 years of investigation of Crimean hemorrhagic fever, *Tr. Inst. Polio. Virusn. Entsefalitov Akad. Med. Nauk SSSR,* 22, 5, 1974.

99. **Chumakov, M. P., Andreeva, S. K., Zavodova, T. I., Zgurskaya, G. N., Kostetsky, N. V., Mart'yanova, L. I., Nikitin, A. M., Sinyak, K. M., Smirnova, S. E., Turta, L. I., Ustinova, E. D., and Chunikhin, S. P.,** Problems of Crimean hemorrhagic fever virus ecology in natural foci of this infection in the Crimea, *Tr. Inst. Polio. Virusn. Entsefalitov Akad. Med. Nauk SSSR,* 22, 19, 1974; in Russian. (In English, NAMRU3-T1110.)

100. **Chumakov, M. P., Bashkirtsev, V. N., Golger, E. I., Dzagurova, T. K., Zavodova, T. I., Konovalov, Yu. N., Mart'yanova, L. I., Uspenskaya, I. G., and Filippsky, A. N.,** Isolation and identification of Crimean hemorrhagic fever and West Nile fever viruses from ticks collected in Moldavia, *Tr. Inst. Polio. Virusn. Entsefalitov Akad. Med. Nauk SSSR,* 22, 45, 1974; in Russian. (In English, NAMRU3-T1113.)

101. **Chumakov, M. P., Belyaeva, A. P., Voroshilova, M. K., Butenko, A. M., Shalunova, N. V., Semashko, I. V., Mart'yanova, L. I., Smirnova, S. E., Bashkirtsev, V. N., Zavodova, T. I., Rubin, S. G., Tkachenko, E. A., Karmysheva, V. Ya., Reingol'd, V. N., Popov, G. V., Kirov, I., Stolbov, D. N., and Perelatov, V. D.,** Progress in studying the etiology, immunology, and laboratory diagnosis of Crimean hemorrhagic fever in the USSR and Bulgaria, *Mater. 15. Nauchn. Sess. Inst. Polio. Virus. Entsefalitov,* 3, 100, 1968.

102. **Chumakov, M. P., Birulya, N. B., Butenko, A. M., Vasyuta, Yu. S., Egorova, P. S., Zalutskaya, L. I., Zimina, Yu. V., Leshchinskaya, E. V., Povalishina, T. P., and Stolbov, D. N.,** On the question of epidemiology of diseases of Crimean hemorrhagic fever in Astrakhan Oblast, *Mater. 11. Nauchn. Sess. Inst. Polio. Virus. Entsefalitov,* 263, 1964; in Russian. (In English, NAMRU3-T165.)

103. **Chumakov, M. P., Butenko, A. M., Rubin, S. G., Berezin, V. V., Bashkirtsev, V. N., Zavodova, T. I., Smirnova, S. E., Vasilenko, V. M., Stolbov, D. N., Karinskaya, G. A., and Birulya, N. B.,** Aspects of ecology of Crimean hemorrhagic fever (CHF) virus, *Tezisy Dokl. 5. Simp. Izuch. Rol' Pereletn. Ptitsepererab. Rasprostr. Arbovirus,* 89, 1969; in Russian.

104. **Chumakov, M. P., Butenko, A. M., Rubin, S. G., Berezin, V. V., Karinskaya, G. A., Vasilenko, S. M., Smirnova, S. E., Bashkirtsev, V. V., Derbedeneva, M. P., Badalov, M. E., and Stolbov, D. N.,** Question on the ecology of Crimean hemorrhagic fever virus, *Mater. 5. Simp. Izuch. Roli Pereletn. Ptitspererab. Rasprostr. Arbovirus,* Novosibirsk, July 1969, 222, 1972; in Russian. (In English, NAMRU3-T877.)

105. **Chumakov, M. P., Butenko, A. M., Shalunova, N. V., Mart'yanova, L. I., Smirnova, S. E., Bashkirtsev, Yu. N., Zavodova, T. I., Rubin, S. G., Tkachenko, E. A., Karmysheva, V. Ya., Reingol'd, V. N., Popov, G. V., and Savinov, A. P.,** New data on the virus causing Crimean hemorrhagic fever, *Vopr. Virusol.,* 13, 377, 1968; in Russian. (In English, NAMRU3-T596.)

106. **Chumakov, M. P., Butenko, A. M., Smirnova, S. E., Belyaeva, A. P., Voroshilova, M. K., Shalunova, N. V., Mart'yanova, L. I., Karmysheva, V. Ya., Tkachenko, E. A., Rubin, S. G., Bashkirtsev, V. N., Zavodova, T. I., Karinskaya, G. A., Vasilenko, S. M., and Popov, G. V.,** Some results of investigation of Crimean hemorrhagic fever, in *(Intr. Lect. Proc. Symp.) Int. Symp. Tick-borne Arboviruses (Excluding Group B),* Smolenice, September 1969, 167, 1971.

107. **Chumakov, M. P. and Donets, M. A.,** Virion and subvirion constituents of Crimean hemorrhagic fever virus, *Int. Virol. Abstr. 3. Int. Congr. Virol,* 3, 193, 1975.

108. **Chumakov, M. P., Ismailova, S. T., Rubin, S. G., Smirnova, S. E., Zgurskaya, G. N., Khankishiev, A. Sh., Berezin, V. V., and Solovei, E. A.,** Detection of Crimean hemorrhagic fever foci in Azerbaijan SSR from results from serological investigations of domestic animals, *Tr. Inst. Polio. Virusn. Entsefalitov Akad. Med. Nauk SSSR,* 18, 120, 1970; in Russian. (In English, NAMRU3-T941.)

109. **Chumakov, M. P., Shalunova, N. V., Semashko, I. V., and Belyaeva, A. P.,** Use of interference phenomenon in tissue culture for detecting Crimean hemorrhagic fever virus (CHF), *Tr. Inst. Polio. Virusn. Entsefalitov Akad. Med. Nauk SSSR.,* 7, 202, 1965; in Russian. (In English, NAMRU3-T832.)

110. **Chumakov, M. P. and Smirnova, S. E.,** Investigation of interrelationships between Pakistan Hazara virus (ShS JT 280) and CHF-Congo group viruses, *Tezisy 17. Nauchn. Sess. Inst. Posvyashch. Aktual. Probl. Virus. Profilakt. Virus. Zabolev.,* Moscow, October 1972; in Russian. (In English, NAMRU3-T1051.)

111. **Chumakov, M. P. and Smirnova, S. E.,** Detection of antibodies to CHF virus in wild and domestic animal blood sera from Iran and Africa, *Tezisy 17. Nauchn. Sess. Inst. Posvyashch. Aktual. Probl. Virus. Profilakt. Virus. Zabolev.,* Moscow, October 1972, 367; in Russian. (In English, NAMRU3-T1072.)

112. **Chumakov, M. P., Smirnova, S. E., Shalunova, N. V., Mart'yanova, L. I., Fleer, G. P., Sadykova, V. D., and Maksumov, S. S.,** Isolation and study of the virus from a Crimean hemorrhagic fever patient in Samarkand Oblast, Uzbek SSR; strain Khodzha, *Tr. Inst. Polio. Virusn. Entsefalitov Akad. Med. Nauk SSSR,* 19, 21, 1971; in Russian. (In English, NAMRU3-T956.)

113. **Chumakov, M. P., Smirnova, S. E., Shalunova, N. Y., Mart'yanova, L. I., Fleer, G. P., Zgurskaya, G. N., Maksumov, S. S., Kasymov, K. T., and Pak, T. P.,** Proofs of etiological identity of Crimean hemorrhagic fever and Central Asian hemorrhagic fever, *Abstr. Inv. Pap. 9. Int. Congr. Trop. Med. Malar.,* 1, 33, 1973.

114. **Chumakov, M. P., Smirnova, S. E., and Tkachenko, E. A.,** Antigenic relationships between the Soviet strains of Crimean hemorrhagic fever virus and the Afro-Asian Congo virus strains, *Mater. 16. Nauchn. Sess. Inst. Polio. Virus. Entsefalitov,* 2, 152, 1969; in Russian.

115. **Chumakov, M. P., Smirnova, S. E., and Tkachenko, E. A.,** Relationship between strains of Crimean hemorrhagic fever and Congo viruses, *Acta Virol. (Engl. Ed.),* 14, 82, 1970.

116. **Chumakov, M. P., Vafakulov, B. Kh., Zavodova, T. I., Karmysheva, V. Ya., Maksumov, S. S., Mart'yanova, L. I., Rodin, V. I., and Sukharenko, S. N.,** Cases of transmission of Crimean hemorrhagic fever virus in Uzbekistan by contacts with the blood of a sick cow and a human patient as well as by tick bites, *Tr. Inst. Polio. Virusn. Entsefalitov Akad. Med. Nauk SSSR,* 22, 29, 1974; in Russian. (In English, NAMRU3-T1111.)

117. **Chumakov, M. P., Zavodova, T. I., Mart'yanova, L. I., Mukhitdinov, A. G., Povalishina, T. P., Rodin, V. I., Rozina, V. F., Safarova, R. O., Sukharenko, S. I., Tatarov, A. G., Khachaturova, S. S., and Chunikhin, S. P.,** Detection of Crimean hemorrhagic fever virus in some species of blood-sucking ticks collected in 1973 in the Kirgiz and Uzbek SSR, *Tr. Inst. Polio. Virusn. Entsefalitov Akad. Med. Nauk SSSR,* 22, 35, 1974; in Russian. (In English, NAMRU3-T1112.)

118. **Chunikhin, S. P.,** Study of ecology of arboviruses in arid regions of Central Asia and some countries of Africa, (Avtoref. Diss. Soisk. Uchen. Step. Dokt. Biol. Nauk), *Inst. Polio. Virusn. Entsefalitov Akad. Med. Nauk SSSR,* Moscow, 1972, 41.

119. **Chunikhin, S. P.,** Investigation of the ecology of arboviruses in arid regions o Central Asia and Africa, *Tezisy 17. Nauchn. Sess. Inst. Posvyashch. Aktual. Probl. Virus. Profilakt. Virus. Zabolev.,* Moscow, October 1972, 272; in Russian. (In English NAMRU3-T1098.)

120. **Chunikhin, S. P., Chumakov, M. P., Butenko, A. M., Smirnova, S. E., Taufflieb, R., Camicas, J. L., Robin, Y., Cornet, M., and Shabon, Zh.,** Results from investigating human and domestic and wild animal blood sera in the Senegal Republic (western Africa) for antibodies to Crimean hemorrhagic fever virus, *Mater. 16. Nauchn. Sess. Inst. Polio. Virus. Entsefalitov,* 2, 158, 1969; in Russian. (In English, NAMRU3-T810.)

121. **Chunikhin, S. P., Chumakov, M. P., Smirnova, S. E., Pak, T. P., Pavlovich, A. N., and Kuima, A. U.,** Division into biocenotic groups of mammals and ixodid ticks in Crimean hemorrhagic foci of southern Central Asia, *Mater. 16. Nauchn. Sess. Inst. Polio. Virus. Entsefalitov,* 2, 156, 1969; in Russian. (In English, NAMRU3-T821.)

122. **Chun-Sun, F. and Genis, D. E.,** A natural focus of tick-borne hemorrhagic fever in the semi-desert zone of southern Kazakhstan, *Tr. Inst. Polio. Virusn. Entsefalitov Akad. Med. Nauk SSSR,* 7, 312, 1965; in Russian. (In English, NAMRU3-T199.)

123. **Clifford, C. M., Flux, J. E. C., and Hoogstraal, H.,** Seasonal and regional abundance of ticks (Ixodidae) on hares (Leporidae) in Kenya, *J. Med. Entomol.,* 13, 40, 1976.

124. **Converse, J. D., Hoogstraal, H., Moussa, M. I., Stek, M., Jr., and Kaiser, M. N.,** Bahig virus (Tete group) in naturally- and transovarially-infected *Hyalomma marginatum* ticks from Egypt and Italy, *Arch. Gesamte Virusforsch.,* 46, 29, 1974.

125. **Cunliffe, N.,** The variability of *Rhipicephalus pulchellus* (Gerstäcker, 1873), together with its geographical distribution, *Parasitology,* 6, 204, 1913.

126. **Dalldorf, G. and Sickles, G. M.,** An unidentified, filterable agent isolated from the feces of children with paralysis, *Science,* 108, 61, 1948.

127. **Dandawate, C. N., Shah, K. V., and D'Lima, L. V.,** Wanowrie virus: a new arbovirus isolated from *Hyalomma marginatum isaaci, Indian J. Med.,* 58, 985, 1970.

128. **Dandurov, Yu. V., Panteleev, V. A., Borisov, V. M., Smeshko, O. V., Arkhipov, P. N., Rybin, S. N., Risaliev, D. R., and Aleksandrov, A. K.,** Isolation of Crimean hemorrhagic fever virus from *Hyalomma plumbeum plumbeum* Panz. ticks in Osh Oblast, Kirgiz SSR, *Mater. 9. Simp. Ekol. Virus.,* Dushanbe, October 1975, 48; in Russian.

129. **Daniyarov, O. A., Pak, T. P., Kostyukov, M. A., Bulychev, V. P., and Gordeeva, Z. E.,** Results from virological investigations of Crimean hemorrhagic fever in Tadzhikistan, *Mater. 9. Simp. Ekol. Virus.,* Dushanbe, October 1975, 29, 1975; in Russian. (In English, NAMRU3-T1120.)

130. **Darlington, P. J., Jr.,** *Zoogeography: The Geographical Distribution of Animals,* John Wiley & Sons, New York, 1957, 675.

131. **Darwish, M. A., Imam, I. Z. E., Omar, F. M., and Hoogstraal, H.,** A seroepidemiological survey for Crimean-Congo hemorrhagic fever virus in humans and domestic animals in Egypt, *J. Egypt. Public Health Assoc.,* 52, 156, 1977.

132. **David-West, T. S.,** Tissue culture studies of common Nigerian arboviruses. Propagation in different tissue culture systems, *West Afr. Med. J.,* 21, 3, 1972.

133. **David-West, T. S., Cooke, A. R., and David-West, A. S.,** Seroepidemiology of Congo virus (related to the virus of Crimean haemorrhagic fever) in Nigeria. Brief communications, *Bull. WHO,* 51, 543, 1974.

134. **Dhanda, V. and Rao, T. R.,** The status of *Rhipicephalus sanguineus* (Latreille, 1806) and *R. turanicus* Pomerantzev, 1940 (Acarina: Ixodidae) in India, *J. Bombay Nat. Hist. Soc.,* 66, 211, 1969.

135. **Dobritsa, P. G.,** Epidemiology and prophylaxis of hemorrhagic fever in Chimkent Region of the southern Kazakhstan, *Tr. Inst. Polio. Virusn. Entsefalitov Akad. Med. Nauk SSSR,* 7, 262, 1965; in Russian. (In English, NAMRU3-T196.)

136. **Dobritsa, P. G., Abdulimov, M. A., Bakirova, M. N., and Mamontov, S. I.,** Investigation of Crimean hemorrhagic fever (CHF) in Chimkent Oblast. Kazakh SSR. II. Prevention of CHF in Kazakhstan conditions, *Tr. Inst. Polio. Virus. Entsefalitov Akad. Med. Nauk SSSR,* 19, 231, 1971; in Russian. (In English, NAMRU3-T977.)

137. **Dols, M. W.,** *The Black Death in the Middle East,* Princeton University Press, N.J., 1977, 390.

138. **Domrachev, V. M.,** Data on the problem of Crimean hemorrhagic fever, *Zh. Mikrobiol. Epidemiol. Immunobiol.,* 20, 69, 1949.

139. **Donchev, D., Kebedzhiev, G., and Rusakiev, M.,** Hemorrhagic fever in Bulgaria, Bulg. Akad. Nauk Mikrobiol., Inst. 1st Kongr. Mikrobiol., 1967, 777; in Bulgarian. (In English, NAMRU3-T465.)

140. **Donets, M. A.,** The effect of some physical and chemical treatments on the CHF-Congo group viruses, *Tr. Inst. Polio. Virusn. Entsefalitov Akad. Med. Nauk SSSR,* 22, 50, 1974; in Russian. (In English, NAMRU3-T1114.)

141. **Donets, M. A. and Chumakov, M. P.,** Certain characteristics of CHF and Congo virus virions, *Tezisy Konf. Vop. Med. Virus.,* Moscow, October 1975, 287; in Russian. (In English, NAMRU3-T993.)

142. **Donets, M. A., Chumakov, M. P., Korolev, M. B., and Rubin, S. G.,** Physicochemical characteristics, morphology and morphogenesis of virions of the causative agent of Crimean hemorrhagic fever, *Intervirology,* 8, 294, 1977.

143. **Donets, M. A., Rubin, S. G., and Chumakov, M. P.,** A soluble complement fixing antigen of Crimean hemorrhagic fever virus in experimental infection in newborne white mice, *Tezisy Konf. Vop. Med. Virus.,* Moscow, October 1975, 289; in Russian. (In English, NAMRU3-T994.)

144. **Donets, M. A., Rubin, S. G., Chumakov, M. P., Gavrilovskaya, I. N., and Dzagurova, T. K.,** Adaptation of CHF virus to SPEV and PEK cell cultures, *Tezisy Konf. Vop. Med. Virus.,* Moscow, October 1975, 290; in Russian. (In English, NAMRU3-T995.)

145. **Doss, M. A. and Anastos, G.,** *Index-Catalogue of Medical and Veterinary Zoology, Ticks and Tickborne Diseases. III. Checklist of Families, Genera, Species and Subspecies of Ticks,* Spec. Publ. No. 3, U.S. Department of Agriculture, Washington, D.C., 1977, 97.

146. **Doss, M. A., Farr, M. M., Roach, K. F., and Anastos, G.,** Index-Catalogue of Medical and Veterinary Zoology, Ticks and Tickborne Diseases. I. General and Species of Ticks. Part 1. Genera A-G, Spec. Publ. No. 3, U.S. Department of Agriculture, Washington, D.C., 1974, 429.

147. **Doss, M. A., Farr, M. M., Roach, K. F., and Anastos, G.,** Index-Catalogue of Medical and Veterinary Zoology, Ticks and Tickborne Diseases. I. Genera and Species of Ticks. Part 2. Genera H-N, Spec. Publ. No. 3, U.S. Department of Agriculture, Washington, D.C., 1974, 593.

148. **Doss, M. A., Farr, M. M., Roach, K. F., and Anastos, G.,** Index-Catalogue of Medical and Veterinary Zoology, Ticks and Tickborne Diseases. I. Genera and Species of Ticks. Part 3. Genera O-X, Spec. Publ. No. 3, U.S. Department of Agriculture, Washington, D.C., 1974, 329.

149. **Doss, M. A., Farr, M. M., Roach, K. F., and Anastos, G.,** Index-Catalogue of Medical Veterinary Zoology, Ticks and Tickborne Diseases. II. Hosts. Part 1. A-F, Spec. Publ. No. 3, U.S. Department of Agriculture, Washington, D.C., 1974, 1.

150. **Doss, M. A., Farr, M. M., Roach, K. F., and Anastos, G.,** Index-Catalogue of Medical and Veterinary Zoology, Ticks and Tickborne Diseases. II. Hosts. Part 2. G-P, Spec. Publ. No. 3, U.S. Department of Agriculture, Washington, D.C., 1974, 490.

151. **Doss, M. A., Farr, M. M., Roach, K. F., and Anastos, G.,** Index-Catalogue of Medical and Veterinary Zoology, No. 3, Ticks and Tickborne Diseases. II. Hosts. Part 3. Q-Z, Spec. Publ. No. 3, U.S. Department of Agriculture, Washington, D.C., 1974, 977.

152. **Drobinsky, I. R.,** Epidemiology and diagnosis of Crimean hemorrhagic fever, in *Crimean Hemorrhagic Fever (Acute Infectious Capillary Toxicosis),* Sokolov, A. A., Chumakov, M. P., and Kolachev, A. A., Eds., Izd. Otd. Primorskoi Armii, Simferopol., 1945, 49; in Russian.

153. **Drobinsky, I. R.**, Epidemiology and prevention of Crimean hemorrhagic fever (acute infectious capillary toxicosis), Report II, *Zh. Mikrobiol. Epidemiol. Immunobiol.*, 19, 36, 1948; in Russian. (In English, NAMRU-T934.)

154. **Drobinsky, I. R.**, Tickborne hemorrhagic fever in Moldavia, *Tezisy Dokl. 17. Ocheredn. Nauchn. Sess. Kishinev. Med. Itog. Nauchno Issled. Rabot.*, Kishinev, 1959, 126.

155. **Dryenski, P. St.**, Artbestand und verbreitung der Zecken (Ixodoidea) in Bulgarian, *Izv. Zool. Inst. Bulg. Akad. Nauk. Otd. Biol. Med. Nauk*, (4-5), 109, 1955; in Bulgarian.

156. **Dryenski, P. St.**, On the question of the study of dynamics of the principal species of ticks (Ixodidae) in the period 1955-1957 in relation to the spread of haemorrhagic fever in Bulgaria, *Izv. Mikrobiol. Inst. Sofiya*, 12, 199, 1960; in Bulgarian.

157. **Durov, V. I.**, Preliminary data on examination of blood sera from domestic animals and humans for antibodies to Crimean hemorrhagic fever in Kalmyk ASSR, *Mater. 3. Oblast. Nauchn. Prakt. Konf.*, Rostov-on-Don, May 1970, 64; in Russian. (In English, NAMRU3-T532.)

158. **Durov, V. I., Donets, M. A., Perelatov, V. D., Butenko, A. M., Tkachenko, E. A., and Chumakov, M. P.**, Survey of Crimean hemorrhagic fever foci in the southeastern part of the European RSFSR, *Tezisy 17. Nauchn. Sess. Inst. Posvyashch. Aktual. Probl. Virus. Profilakt. Virus. Zabolev.*, Moscow, October 1972, 358; in Russian. (In English, NAMRU3-T1066.)

159. **D'yakonov, P.**, Brief outline of characteristics of epidemics prevailing in Crimea during the Crimean campaign, *Voen. Med. Zh.*, 68, 1, 1856; in Russian. (In English, NAMRU3-T959.)

160. **Dzhaparidze, N. I.**, *Ixodid Ticks of Georgia SSR*, Akad. Nauk Gruz. SSR, Inst. Zool. Tbilisi., 1960, 259; in Russian.

161. **Dzhurzhoni, Z. A.**, *Compendium of the Sheikh of Khorezm*, 1110; in Tadzhik.

162. **Edelsten, R. M.**, The distribution and prevalence of Nairobi Sheep disease and other tickborne infections of sheep and goats in northern Somalia, *Trop. Anim. Health Prod.*, 7, 29, 1975.

163. **Edwards, S. J., Kirby, M. D., Crawley, L. R., Rayburn, J. D., Shaw, J. H., and Walker, M. L.**, Index-Catalogue of Medical and Veterinary Zoology, Parasite-Subject Catalogue: Hosts, Suppl. 18, Part 7, U.S. Department of Agriculture, Washington, D.C., 672, 1974.

164. **Fabiyi, A.**, Congo virus in Nigeria: isolation and pathogenetic studies, *Abstr. Inv. Pap. 9. Int. Congr. Trop. Med. Malar.*, 1, 35, 1973.

165. **Fagbami, A. H., Tomori, O., Fabiyi, A., and Isoun, T. T.**, Experimental Congo virus (IB-AN 7620) infection in primates, *Rev. Roum. Med. Virol.*, 26, 33, 1975.

166. **Fedulov, A. V., Grekov, A. D., and Terekhov, G. N.**, 1938; mentioned by Khodukin, N. I., 1952.

167. **Feldman-Muhsam, B.**, On two rare genera of ticks of domestic stock in Israel, *Bull. Res. Counc. Isr. Sect. B. Biol.*, 5, 193, 1955.

168. **Feldman-Muhsam, B. and Saturen, I. M.**, Notes on the ecology of ixodid ticks of domestic stock in Israel, *Bull. Res. Counc. Isr.*, 10, 53, 1961.

169. **Fenner, F.**, The classification and nomenclature of viruses. Summary of results of meetings of the International Committee on Taxonomy of Viruses in Madrid, September 1975, *J. Gen. Virol.*, 31, 463, 1976.

170. **Fenner, F.**, The classification and nomenclature of viruses. Summary of results of meetings of the International Committee on Taxonomy of Viruses in Madrid, September 1975, *Acta Virol. (Engl. Ed.)*, 20, 170, 1976.

171. **Fenner, F., Pereira, H. G., Porterfield, J. S., Joklik, W. K., and Downie, A. W.**, Family and generic names for viruses approved by the International Committee on Taxonomy of Viruses, June 1974, *Intervirology*, 3, 193, 1974.

172. **Filippova, N. A., Neronov, V. M., and Farhang-Azad, A.**, Data on ixodid tick fauna (*Acarina, Ixodidae*) of small mammals in Iran, *Entomol. Obozr.*, 55, 467, 1976; in Russian. (In English, NAMRU3-T1169.)

173. **Fine, P. E. M.**, Vectors and vertical transmission: an epidemiologic perspective, *Ann. N.Y. Acad. Sci.*, 266, 173, 1975.

174. **Fleer, G. P. and Smirnova, S. E.**, Detection of cytopathologic changes in tissue culture infected with Crimean hemorrhagic fever (CHF) virus. (Preliminary report), *Mater. 15. Nauchn. Sess. Inst. Polio. Virus. Entsefalitov*, 3, 99, 1968; in Russian. (In English, NAMRU3-T871.)

175. **Fuller, J. G.**, *Fever! The Hunt for a New Killer Virus*, Reader's Digest Press, New York, 1974, 297.

176. **Gaidamovich, S., Klisenko, G., Shanoyan, N., Obukhova, V., and Mel'nikova, E.**, Indirect hemagglutination for diagnosis of Crimean hemorrhagic fever, *Intervirology*, 2, 181, 1974.

177. **Gaidamovich, S., Klisenko, G., Shanoyan, N., Obukhova, V., and Mel'nikova, E.**, The indirect hemagglutination test with CHF-Congo group viruses, *Vopr. Virusol.*, 19, 705, 1974; in Russian.

178. **Gajdusek, D. C.**, Acute infectious hemorrhagic fevers and mycotoxicoses in the Union of Soviet Socialist Republics, *Med. Sci. Publ.*, 2, 140, 1953.

179. **Gajdusek, D. C.**, Hemorrhagic fevers in Asia: a problem in medical ecology, *Geogr. Rev.*, 46, 20, 1956.

180. **Gal'perin, E. A.,** *Clinical Features of Infectious Hemorrhagic Diseases and Fevers,* Gos. Izd. Med. Lit. (Medgiz), Moscow, 1960, 272; in Russian.

181. **Galuzo, I. G.,** *Bloodsucking ticks of Kazakhstan, Vol. 3, Genus* Dermacentor *Koch,* 1844; *Genus* Rhipicephalus *Koch,* 1844, Inst. Zool. Akad. Nauk Kaz.S.S.R., Alma-Ata, 1949, 372; in Russian.

182. **Galuzo, I. G.,** *Bloodsucking ticks of Kazakhstan, Vol. 4,* Genus Bophilus *Curtice,* 1891; Haemaphysalis *Koch,* 1844, *Genus* Ixodes *Latreille,* 1795, Inst. Zool. Akad. Nauk Kaz.S.S.R., Alma-Ata, 1950, 388; in Russian.

183. **Genis, D. E., Smirnova, S. E., Zgurskaya, G. N., and Chumakov, M. P.,** The results of investigation of Crimean hemorrhagic fever in Kzyl-Orda Region of the Kazakh SSR, *Tr. Inst. Polio. Virusn. Entsefalitov Akad. Med. Nauk SSSR,* 19, 92, 1971; in Russian. (In English, NAMRU3-T952.)

184. **Giller, A. S.,** Pathological anatomy of Crimean hemorrhagic fever in Tadzhikistan, *Tr. Inst. Polio. Vrusn. Entsefalitov Akad. Med. Nauk SSSR,* 19, 146, 1971; in Russian. (In English, NAMRU3-T978.)

185. **Grashchenkov, N. I. (Compiler),** *Reports on the 1944 Scientific-Investigations of the Institute of Neurology,* Akad. Med. Nauk S.S.S.R., Moscow, 1945, 123; in Russian.

186. **Grebenyuk, R. V.,** *Ixodid Ticks (Parasitiformes, Ixodidae) of Kirgizia,* Akad. Nauk Kirgiz. S.S.R., Inst. Biol., Frunze., 1966, 328; in Russian.

187. **Grešiková, M.,** Studies on tickborne arboviruses isolated in Central Europe, *Biol. Pr.,* 18, 1, 1972.

188. **Grobov, A. G.,** Carriers of Crimean haemorrhagic fever, *Med. Parazitol. Parazit. Bolezni,* 15, 59, 1946; in Russian. (In English, NAMRU3-T36.)

189. **Gromashevsky, L. V. and Vasil'eva, V. L.,** Arboviral infections in the Ukraine, *Mater. 11. Nauchn. Sess. Inst. Polio. Virus. Entsefalitov.,* 197, 1964; in Russian. (In English, NAMRU3-T1215.)

190. **Gromashevsky, V. L., L'vov, D. K., Tsirkin, Yu. M., Sidorova, G. A., Aristova, V. A., Gostinshchikova, G. V., and Andreev, V. P.,** New arboviral foci associated ecologically with birds in southeastern Azerbaijan, *Mater. Simp. Itogi 6. Simp. Izuch. Virus. Ekol. Svyazan. Ptits.,* (Omsk, December 1971), 118, 1972; in Russian. (In English, NAMRU3-T644.)

191. **Gusarev, A. F.,** Waterhouse-Friderichsen syndrome pathomorphology during certain hemorrhagic fever forms, *Mater. 16. Nauchn. Sess. Inst. Polio. Virus. Entsefalitov,* 2, 127, 1969; in Russian. (In English, NAMRU3-T841.)

192. **Gusarev, A. F.,** Pathomorphological changes in the liver during Crimean hemorrhagic fever, *Mater. 16. Nauchn. Sess. Inst. Polio. Virus. Entsefalitov,* October 1969, 130; in Russian. (In English, NAMRU3-T842.)

193. **Gusarev, A. F.,** Pathomorphological characteristics of Crimean hemorrhagic fever in Rostov Oblast, *Mater. 3. Oblast. Nauchn. Prakt. Konf.,* Rostov-on-Don, May 1970, 127; in Russian. (In English, NAMRU3-T544.)

194. **Gusarev, A. F.,** Dynamics of kidney changes and pathogenesis of the kidney-urinary syndrome in certain types of hemorrhagic fever, *Mater. 3. Oblast. Nauchn. Prakt. Konf.,* Rostov-on-Don, May 1970, 131; in Russian. (In English, NAMRU3-T545.)

195. **Gusarev, A. F.,** Data on characteristics of external examination of patients who died from hemorrhagic fever, *Tr. Inst. Polio. Virusn. Entsefalitov Akad. Med. Nauk S.S.S.R.,* 19, 149, 1971; in Russian. (In English, NAURU3-T945.)

196. **Gusev, V. M., Bednyy, S. N., Guseva, A. A., Labunets, N. F., and Bakeev, N. N.,** The ecological groups of birds on the Caucasus and their role in the life of ticks and fleas, *Tr. Nauchno Issled. Protivochumn. Inst. Kavk. Zakavk.,* 5, 217, 1961; in Russian.

197. **Gusev, V. M., Guseva, A. A., and Reznik, P. A.,** Role of birds in the distribution of fleas (Suctoria) and ticks (Ixodoidea) in Daghestan, *Med. Parazitol. Parazit. Bolezni,* 32, 738, 1963; in Russian. (In English, ABL No. 1414.)

198. **Hammon, W. McD. and Sather, G. E.,** Arboviruses, in *Diagnostic Procedures for Viral and Rickettsial Infections,* 4th ed., Lennette, E. H. and Schmidt, N. J., Eds., American Public Health Association, New York, 1969, 227.

199. **Hammon, W. McD. and Work, T. H.,** Arbovirus infection in man, in *Diagnostic Procedures for Viral and Rickettsial Disease,* Vol. 3, Lennette, E. H. and Schmidt, N. J., Eds., American Public Health Association, New York, 1964, 268.

200. **Henderson, B. E., Kirya, G. B., Mujomba, E., and Lule, M.,** Reference centre identification studies, *Rep. E. Afr. Virus Res. Inst.,* 18, 31, 1969.

201. **Heneberg, D., Heneberg, N., Celina, D., Filipović, Z., Marković, D., Žubi, D., Živcović, B., Simić, M., Zonjic, S., and Pantelic, M.,** Crimean hemorrhagic fever in Yugoslavia, *Vojnosanit. Pregl.,* 25, 181, 1968; in Croatian.

202. **Heneberg, N., Heneberg, D., Milošević, J., and Dimitrijević, V.,** Distribution of ticks in the autonomous provinces Kosovu and Metohiji. Regarding especially *Hyalomma plumbeum plumbeum* Panzer, reservoir and vector of Crimean haemorrhagic fever of man, *Zb. Vojnomed. Akad. Belgrad.,* 30, 1967; in Croatian. (In English, NAMRU3-T324.)

203. **Hoogstraal, H.,** African Ixodoidea. I. Ticks of the Sudan (with Special reference to Equatoria Province and with Preliminary Reviews of the Genera *Boophilus, Margaropus and Hyaloma*), Department of the Navy, Bureau of Medicine and Surgery, Washington, D.C., 1956, 1101.

204. **Hoogstraal, H.,** Ticks, in relation to human diseases caused by viruses, *Ann. Rev. Entomol.,* 11, 261, 1966.

205. **Hoogstraal, H.,** Ticks in relation to human diseases caused by *Rickettsia* species, *Ann. Rev. Entomol.,* 12, 377, 1967.

206. **Hoogstraal, H.,** *Bibliography of Ticks and Tickborne diseases from Homer (about 800 B.C.) to 31 December 1969, Intr. Remarks and Explanations, Authors A-E,* Vol. 1, NAMRU3, Cairo, 1970, 499.

207. **Hoogstraal, H.,** *Bibliography of Ticks and Tickborne Diseases from Homer (about 800 B.C.) to 31 December 1969, Authors F-M,* NAMRU3, Cairo, 1970, 495.

208. **Hoogstraal, H.,** *Bibliography of Ticks and Tickborne Diseases from Homer (about 800 B.C.) to 31 December 1969, Authors N-S,* Vol. 3., NAMRU3, 1971, 435.

209. **Hoogstraal, H.,** *Bibliography of Ticks and Tickborne Diseases from Homer (about 800 B.C.) to 31 December 1969, Authors T-Z,* Vol. 4, NAMRU3, Cairo, 1972, 355.

210. **Hoogstraal, H.,** *Acarina* (ticks), in *Viruses and Invertebrates,* Gibbs, A. J., Ed., North-Holland, Amsterdam, 1973, 89.

211. **Hoogstraal, H.,** Viruses and ticks, in *Viruses and Invertebrates,* Gibbs, A. J., Ed., North-Holland, Amsterdam, 1973, 349.

212. **Hoogstraal, H.,** *Bibliography of Ticks and Tickborne Diseases from Homer (about 800 B.C.) to 31 December 1973,* Vol. 5, Part 1, NAMRU3, Cairo, 1974, 492.

213. **Hoogstraal, H.,** Class Arachnida, in *Tropical Medicine,* 5th ed., Hunter, G. W., Swartzwelder, J. C., and Clyde, D. C., Eds., W. B. Saunders, Philadelphia, 1976, 712.

214. **Hoogstraal, H.,** Landscapes, epidemiology, tick species and some babesias and viruses transmitted to humans, Proc. 139th Ann. Meet. Br. Assoc. Adv. Sci., Birmingham, August to September 1977, 25; preprint.

215. **Hoogstraal, H.,** Viruses and ticks from migrating birds, *Int. ArbKolloq. Naturh. Infektionskr. ZentEurop.,* Graz, February 1976, 27, 1977.

216. **Hoogstraal, H.,** Biology of ticks, in *Tickborne Diseases and Their Vectors,* Proc. Int. Conf., Edinburgh, September to October 1976, Wilde, J. K. H., Ed., University of Edinburgh, Centre for Tropical Veterinary Medicine, Edinburgh, 1978, 3.

217. **Hoogstraal, H.,** *Bibliography of Ticks and Tickborne Diseases from Homer (about 800 B.C.) to 31 December 1976,* Vol. 5, Part 2, NAMRU3, Cairo, 1978, 456.

218. **Hoogstraal, H., Clifford, C. M., Keirans, J. E., Kaiser, M. N., and Evans, D. E.,** The *Ornithodoros (Alectorobius) capensis* group (Acarina: Ixodoidea: Argasidae) of the Palearctic and Oriental Faunal Regions. *O. (A.) maritimus:* identity, marine bird hosts, virus infections, and distribution in western Europe and northwestern Africa, *J. Parasitol.,* 62, 799, 1976.

219. **Hoogstraal, H. and Kaiser, M. N.,** Observations on Egyptian *Hyalomma* ticks (Ixodoidea, Ixodidae). II. Parasitism of migrating birds by immature *H. rufipes* Koch, *Ann. Entomol. Soc. Am.,* 51, 12, 1958.

220. **Hoogstraal, H. and Kaiser, M. N.,** Observations on Egyptian *Hyalomma* ticks (Ixodoidea, Ixodidae). III. Infestation of greater gerbils, especially by immature *H. impeltatum* S. & S., *Ann. Entomol. Soc. Am.,* 51, 17, 1958.

221. **Hoogstraal, H. and Kaiser, M. N.,** Observations on Egyptian *Hyalomma* ticks (Ixodoidea, Ixodidae). V. Biological notes and differences in identity of *H. anatolicum* and its subspecies *anatolicum* Koch and *excavatum* Koch among Russian and other workers. Identity of *H. lusitanicum* Koch, *Ann. Entomol. Soc. Am.,* 52, 243, 1959.

222. **Hoogstraal, H. and Kaiser, M. N.,** *Boophilus kohlsi* n. sp. (Acarina: Ixodidae) from sheep and goats in Jordan, *J. Parasitol.,* 46, 441, 1960.

223. **Hoogstraal, H. and Kaiser, M. N.,** Bat ticks of the genus *Argas* (Ixodoidea, Argasidae). VIII. *A. (Chiropterargas) ceylonensis,* new species, from Ceylon, *Ann. Entomol. Soc. Am.,* 61, 1049, 1968.

224. **Hoogstraal, H., Kaiser, M. N., Traylor, M. A., Gaber, S., and Guindy, E.,** Ticks (Ixodoidea) on birds migrating from Africa to Europe and Asia, *Bull. WHO,* 24, 197, 1961.

225. **Hoogstraal, H., Kaiser, M. N., Traylor, M. A., Guindy, E., and Gaber, S.,** Ticks (Ixodidae) on birds migrating from Europe and Asia to Africa, (1959-1961), *Bull. WHO,* 28, 235, 1963.

226. **Hoogstraal, H. and Tatchell, R. J.,** Eds., Bloodsucking ticks (Ixodoidea) vectors of diseases of man and animals, by Balashov, Yu. S., *Misc. Publ. Entomol. Soc. Am.,* 8, 161, 1972.

227. **Hoogstraal, H., Traylor, M. A., Gaber, S., Malakatis, G., Guindy, E., and Helmy, I.,** Ticks (Ixodidae) on migating birds in Egypt, spring and fall 1962, *Bull. WHO,* 30, 355, 1964.

228. **Hoogstraal, H. and Valdez, R.,** 1979. Ticks from wild sheep and goats in Iran and medical and veterinary implications, *Fieldiana Zool.,* in press.

229. **Horvath, L. B.,** Incidence of antibodies to Crimean haemorrhagic fever in animals, *Acta Microbiol. Hung.,* 22, 61, 1975; in Russian, English summary.

230. **Horvath, L. B.,** Precipitating antibodies to Crimean haemorrhagic fever virus in human sera collected in Hungary, *Acta Microbiol. Hung.,* 23, 331, 1976.

231. **Hronovsky, V., Benda, R., and Plaisner, V.,** A modified plaque method for arboviruses on plastic panels, *Acta Virol. (Engl. Ed.),* 19, 150, 1975.

232. **Huxsoll, D. L., Hildebrandt, P. K., Nims, R. M., and Walker, J. S.,** Tropical canine pancytopenia, *J. Am. Vet. Med. Assoc.,* 157, 1627, 1970.

233. **Ismailova, S. T., Rubin, S. G., Chumakov, M. P., Khankishiev, A. M., Manafov, I. N., Berezin, V. V., and Reshetnikov, I. A.,** Study of potential Crimean hemorrhagic fever foci in Azerbaijan after the data on serological investigation of domestic animals by the agar gel diffusion and precipitation (AGDP) test, *Tezisy 17. Nauchn. Sess. Inst. Posvyashch. Aktual. Probl. Virus. Profilakt. Virus. Zabolev,* Moscow, October 1972, 365; in Russian. (In English, NAMRU3-T1071.)

234. **Ivanov, N.,** Epidemiology of hemorrhagic fever in Bulgaria, *Izv. Mikrobiol. Inst. Sofiya,* 12, 151, 1960; in Bulgarian.

235. **Jelínkova, A., Benda, R., and Novak, M.,** Electron microscopic demonstration of Crimean hemorrhagic fever virus in CV-1 cells, *Acta Virol. (Engl. Ed.),* 19, 369, 1975.

236. **Kaiser, M. N.,** Viruses in ticks. II. Experimental transmission of Quaranfil virus by *Argas (Persicargas) arboreus* and *A. (P.) persicus, Am. J. Trop. Med. Hyg.,* 15, 976, 1966.

237. **Kaiser, M. N. and Hoogstraal, H.,** The *Hyalomma* ticks (Ixodidae) of Pakistan, India, and Ceylon, with keys to sub-genera and species, *Acarologia,* 6, 257, 1964.

238. **Kaiser, M. N. and Hoogstraal, H.,** Redescription of *Hyalomma (H.) erythraeums* Tonelli-Rondelli (resurrected), description of the female and immature stages, and hosts and distribution in Ethiopia and Somali Republic, *Ann. Entomol. Soc. Am.,* 61, 1228, 1968.

239. **Kaiser, M. N., Hoogstraal, H., and Watson, G. E.,** Ticks (Ixodoidea) on migrating birds in Cyprus, fall 1967 and spring 1968, and epidemiological considerations, *Bull. Entomol. Res.,* 64, 97, 1974.

240. **Kalmykov, E. S. and Yasinsky, A. V.,** Landscape associations of Crimean hemorrhagic fever foci in Tadzhik SSR, *Tr. Inst. Polio. Virusn. Entsefalitov Akad. Med. Nauk. SSSR,* 19, 186, 1971; in Russian. (In English, NAMRU3-T946.)

241. **Kalunda, M. and Mukwaya, L. G.,** Isolation of Congo virus from man and ticks in Uganda, *Abstr. 4. Int. Congr. Virol.,* Hague, August to September 1978, 1978, 290.

242. **Karapetyan, R. M., Vorobiev, A. G., Semashko, I. V., and Matevosyan, K. Sh.,** A case of Crimean hemorrhagic fever in the Armenian SSR, *Tr. Inst. Polio. Virusn. Entsefalitov Akad. Med. Nauk. SSSR,* 22, 260, 1974; in Russian. (In English, NAMRU3-T1115.)

243. **Karas', F. R., Risaliev, D. D., and Vargina, S. G.,** Crimean hemorrhagic fever foci in southwestern climatic region of Kirgizia, *Tezisy Dokl. Vses. Konf. Prirod. Ochag. Bolez. Chelov. Zhivot.,* Omsk, May 1976, 128; in Russian. (In English, NAMRU3-T1175.)

244. **Karas', F. R., Vargina, S. G., Osipova, N. Z., Grebenyuk, Yu. I., Steblyanko, S. N., Usmanov, R. K., Tsirkin, Yu. M., Timofeev, E. M., Gromashevsky, V. L., and L'vov, D. K.,** Investigation of arbovirus infection foci in Kirgizia, *Sb. Tr. Ekol. Virus.,* 1, 69, 1973; in Russian (In English, NAMRU3-T746.)

245. **Karimi,Y., Hannoun, C., Ardoin, P., Ameli, M., and Mohallati, H. B.,** Sur le purpura hemorrhagique observe dans l'Azarbaidjan-Est de l'Iran, *Med. Malad. Infect.,* 6, 399, 1976.

246. **Karimov, S. K., Kiryushchenko, T. V., Usebaeva, G. K. and Rogovaya, S. G.,** On investigations of Crimean hemorrhagic fever in southern Kazakhstan, *Tezisy Konf. Vop. Med. Virus.,* Moscow, October 1975, 297; in Russian. (In English, NAMRU3-T986.)

247. **Karinskaya, G. A., Badalov, M. E., and Primakov, S. V.,** Detection of new Crimean hemorrhagic fever foci (CHF) in Rostov and Luga Oblasts, *Mater 3. Oblast. Nauchn. Prakt. Konf.,* Rostov-on-Don, May 1970, 108; in Russian. (In English, NAMRU3-T540.)

248. **Karinskaya, G. A., Chumakov, M. P., Butenko, A. M., Badalov, M. E., and Rubin, S. G.,** Investigation of blood samples from animals in Rostov Oblast for antibodies to Crimean hemorrhagic fever virus, *Mater. 3. Oblast. Nauchn. Prakt. Konf.,* Rostov-on-Don, May 1970, 55; in Russian. (In English, NAMRU3-T530.)

249. **Karinskaya, G. A., Chumakov, M. P., Butenko, A. M., Badalov, M. E., and Rubin, S. G.,** Certain data on serological investigation of patients recovered from CHF in Rostov Oblast, *Mater 3. Oblast. Nauchn. Prakt. Konf.,* Rostov-on-Don, May 1970, 45; in Russian. (In English, NAMRU3-T528.)

250. **Karmysheva, V. Ya., Borisov, V. M., Tkachenko, E. A., Butenko, A. M., and Chumakov, M. P.,** Characteristics of certain cell cultures infected with rodent-pathogenic Crimean hemorrhagic fever (CHF) virus strain, *Mater. 15. Nauchn. Sess. Inst. Polio. Virus. Entsefalitov,* 3, 92, 1968; in Russian. (In English, NAMRU3-T867.)

251. **Karmysheva, V. Ya., Borisov, V. M., Zavodova, T. I., Tkachenko, E. A., Butenko, A. M., Smirnova, S. E., and Chumakov, M. P.,** Investigation of interaction between rodent-pathogenic Crimean hemorrhagic fever virus strains and cell cultures, *Tr. Inst. Polio. Virusn. Entsefalitov Akad. Med. Nauk SSSR,* 19, 48, 1971; in Russian. (In English, NAMRU3-T932.)

252. **Karmysheva, V. Ya., Butenko, A. M., Bashkirtsev, V. N., and Chumakov, M. P.,** Indication of Crimean hemorrhagic fever virus in smear impressions from the brain and certain other organs of animals using the fluorescent antibody method, *Mater. 15. Nauchn. Sess. Inst. Polio. Virus. Entsefalitov,* 3, 94, 1968; in Russian. (In English, NAMRU3-T827.)

253. **Karmysheva, V. Ya., Butenko, A. M., Bashkirtsev, V. N., and Chumakov, M. P.,** Use of the fluorescent antibody technique for detection of Crimean hemorrhagic fever virus in impression smears and sections of the brain and some other organs of animals, *Tr. Inst. Polio. Virusn. Entsefalitov Akad. Med. Nauk. SSSR,* 19, 56, 1971; in Russian. (In English, NAMRU3-T960.)

254. **Karmysheva, V. Ya., Leshchinskaya, E. V., Butenko, A. M., Savinov, A. P., and Gusarev, A. F.,** Results of some laboratory and clinical-morphological investigations of Crimean hemorrhagic fever, *Arkh. Patol.,* 35, 17, 1973; in Russian. (In English, NAMRU3-T763.)

255. **Karmysheva, V. Ya., Leshchinskaya, E. V., Savinov, A. P., Gusarov, A. F., and Mochalova, E. A.,** Results of clinical-morphological and immunofluorescent study of Crimean hemorrhagic fever latent infections, *Mater. 16. Nauchn. Sess. Inst. Polio. Virus. Entsefalitov,* 2, 139, 1969; in Russian. (In English, NAMRU3-T847.)

256. **Kasymov, K. T., Daniyarov, O. A., Pak, T. P., Pavlovich, A. N., Smirnova, S. E., and Chumakov, M. P.,** Isolation and study of Crimean hemorrhagic fever virus from *Hyalomma* ticks in Tadzhikistan, *Tr. Inst. Polio. Virusn. Entsefalitov Adad. Med. Nauk SSSR,* 19, 38, 1971; in Russian. (In English, NAMRU3-T815.)

257. **Kasymov, K. T., Pavlovich, A. N., and Daniyarov, O. A.,** Results of examination of normal human and animal sera in CF and AGDP tests with the antigen of Crimean hemorrhagic fever virus in Tadzhikistan, *Tr. Inst. Polio. Virusn. Entsefalitov Akad. Med. Nauk SSSR,* 19, 80, 1971; in Russian. (In English, NAMRU3-T928.)

258. **Katsenovich, A. L. and Itskovich, I. D.,** The clinical picture of hemorrhagic fevers, *Klin. Med. (Moscow),* 28, 51, 1950; in Russian.

259. **Katsenovich, A. L. and Itskovich, I. D.,** Clinical characteristics of the Uzbekistan hemorrhagic fever, in *Hemorrhagic Fever in Uzbekistan,* No. 2, Khodukin, N. I., Ed., Vop. Kraev. Patol. Akad. Nauk. Uzbek, SSR, 1952, 34.

260. **Kemp, G. E., Causey, O. R., and Causey, C. E.,** Virus isolations from trade cattle, sheep, goats and swine at Ibadan, Nigeria, 1964-1968, *Bull. Epizoot. Dis. Afr.,* 19, 131, 1971.

261. **Kemp, G. E., Causey, O. R., Moore, D. L., and O'Connor, E. H.,** Viral isolates from livestock in Northern Nigeria, 1966-1970, *Am. J. Vet. Res.,* 34, 707, 1973.

262. **Kemp, G. E., Causey, O. R., Setzer, H. W., and Moore, D. L.,** Isolation of viruses from wild mammals in West Africa, 1966-1970, *J. Wildl. Dis.,* 10, 279, 1974.

263. **Kereev, N. I.,** *Natural Focal Diseases in Kazakh SSR,* Izd. "Kazakhstan," Alma-Ata, 1965, 310; in Russian.

264. **Khashimov, D. M. and Mikhailova, L. I.,** Materials on the study of the clinical pattern of Crimean hemorrhagic fever in Tadzhikistan, *Tr. Inst. Polio. Virusn. Entsefalitov Akad. Med. Nauk SSSR,* 19, 134, 1971; in Russian. (In English, NAMRU3-T976.)

265. **Khodukin, N. I., Ed.,** *Hemorrhagic Fever in Uzbekistan,* No. 2, Vop. Kraev. Patol. Akad. Nauk Uzbek. S.S.R., 1952, 159; in Russian. (In English, NAMRU3-T215.)

266. **Khodukin, N. I., Ed.,** Introduction, in *Hemorrhagic Fever in Uzbekistan,* No. 2, Vop. Kraev. Patol. Akad. Nauk Uzbek. S.S.R., 1952; in Russian. (In English, NAMRU3-T215.)

267. **Khodukin, N. I., Lysunkina, V. A., and Kamenshteyn, I. S.,** The search for vectors of hemorrhagic fever in Central Asia, in *Hemorrhagic Fever in Uzbekistan,* No. 2, Khodukin, N. I., Ed., Vop. Kraev. Patol. Akad. Nauk Uzbek., S.S.R., 1952, 112; in Russian. (In English, NAMRU3-T215.)

268. **Kirya, B. G.,** New data on Congo virus in East Africa: isolation of Congo virus from *Amblyomma variegatum* ticks, *Tezisy 17. Nauchn. Sess. Inst. Posvyashch. Aktual. Probl. Virus. Profilakt. Virus. Zabolev.,* Moscow, October 1972, 348; in Russian. (In English, NAMRU3-T1057.)

269. **Kirya, B. G.,** The significance of Congo virus infection in Africa, *Abstr. Inv. Pap. 9th Int. Congr. Trop. Med. Malar.,* Athens, October 1973, 1, 34.

270. **Kirya, B. G. and Lule, M.,** Congo virus (AMP 10358), *Rep. E. Afr. Virus Res. Inst.,* 20, 18, 1971.

271. **Kirya, B. G. and Lule, M.,** Congo virus studies, *Rep. E. Afr. Virus Res. Inst.,* 22, 10, 1972.

272. **Kirya, B. G., Lule, M., and Mujomba, E.,** Isolation of Congo virus from the tick *Amblyomma variegatum* in East Africa, in *Proc. E. Afr. Med. Res. Council Sci. Conf.,* 1972, 267.

273. **Kirya, B. G., Lule, M., Sekyalo, E., Mukuye, A., and Mujomba, E.,** Arbovirus isolation and identification, *Rep. E. Afr. Virus Res. Inst.,* 22, 7, 1972.

274. **Kirya, B. G., Semenov, B. F., Tret'yakov, A. F., Gromashevsky, V. L., and Madzhomba, E.**, Preliminary report on investigation of animal sera from East Africa for antibodies to Congo virus by the agar gel diffusion and precipitation method, *Tezisy 17. Nauchn. Sess. Inst. Posvyashch. Aktual. Probl. Virus. Profilakt. Virus. Zabolev.*, Moscow, October 1972, 368; in Russian. (In English, NAMRU3-T1073.)

275. **Klisenko, G. A.**, Use of different stabilizers for the IHA test with arboviruses, *Sb. Tr. Inst. Virus. imeni D. I. Ivanovsky Akad. Med. Nauk. SSSR*, 1, 62, 1974; in Russian. (In English, NAMRU3-T1231.)

276. **Klyushkina, E. A.**, The occurrence of *Amblyomma gemma* Don. (Ixodidae) in the Crimea, *Parazitologiya*, 6, 306, 1972; in Russian. (In English, NAMRU3-T571.)

277. **Knight, E. M., Henderson, B. E., Tukei, P. M., Lule, M., and West, R.**, Case histories with arbovirus isolations, *Rep. E. Afr. Virus Res. Inst. (1967)*, 17, 14, 1968.

278. **Knight, E. M. and Santos, D. F.**, Clinical notes, *Rep. E. Afr. Virus Res. Inst. (1960-1961)*, 11, 21, 1961.

279. **Köhler, G., Hoffmann, G., Janitschke, K., and Wiesenhutter, E.**, Untersuchungen zur Kenntnis der Zeckenfauna Syriens, *Z. Tropenmed. Parasitol.*, 18, 375, 1967.

280. **Kolachev, A. A.**, Data on the clinical aspects and treatment of the so-called acute infectious capillary toxicosis, *Voen. Med. Zh.*, 6, 21, 1945.

281. **Kolachev, A. A. and Kosovsky, I. I.**, Clinical aspects of hemorrhagic fever in Bukovina, *Klin. Med. (Moscow)*, 27, 42, 1949; in Russian.

282. **Kondratenko, V. F.**, Importance of ixodid ticks in transmission and preservation of Crimean hemorrhagic fever agent in infection foci, *Parazitologiya*, 10, 297, 1976; in Russian. (In English, NAMRU3-T1116.)

283. **Kondratenko, V. F., Blagoveshchenskaya, N. M., Butenko, A. M., Vyshnivetskaya, L. K., Zarubina, L. V., Milyutin, V. N., Kuchin, V. V., Novikova, E. M., Rabinovich, V. D., Shevchenko, S. F., and Chumakov, M. P.**, Results of virological investigation of ixodid ticks in Crimean hemorrhagic fever focus in Rostov Oblast, *Mater. 3. Oblast. Nauchn. Prakt. Konf.*, Rostov-on-Don, May 1970; in Russian. (In English, NAMRU3-T524.)

284. **Kondratenko, V. F., Kuchin, V. V., and Vyshnivetskaya, L. K.**, Associations between human population and the vector of Crimean hemorrhagic fever agent in infection foci of Rostov Oblast, *Tezisy 17. Nauchn. Sess. Inst. Posvyashch. Aktual. Probl. Virus. Profilakt. Virus. Zabolev.*, 359, Moscow, October 1972; in Russian. (In English, NAMRU3-T1067.)

285. **Kondratenko, V. F., Myskin, A. A., and Zhuravel', L. A.**, Relationship between Crimean hemorrhagic fever (CHF) incidence rate and adult *H. plumbeum* Panz. tick numbers and meteorological conditions (from the data on Rostov Oblast), *Tezisy Konf. Vop. Med. Virus*, Moscow, October 1975; 540; in Russian. (In English, NAMRU3-T989.)

286. **Kondratenko, V. F., Shevchenko, S. F., Perelatov, V. D., Badalov, M. E., Ionov, S. S., Semenov, M. Ya., Romanova, V. A., Lobanov, V. V., and Tekut'ev, I. V.**, Two year experiment on application of chemical campaign method against ixodid ticks in Crimean hemorrhagic fever focus of Rostov Oblast, *Mater 3. Oblast. Nauchn. Prakt. Konf.*, Rostov-on-Don, May 1970, 157; in Russian. (In English, NAMRU3-T550.)

287. **Korenberg, E. I., Dzyuba, M. I., and Zhukov, V. I.**, Range of *Ixodes ricinus* in the USSR, *Zool. Zh.*, 50, 41, 1971; in Russian.

288. **Korenberg, E. I., Zhukov, V. I., Shatkauskas, A. V., and Bushueva, L. K.**, The distribution of *Ixodes persulcatus* in the USSR, *Zool. Zh.*, 48, 1003, 1969; in Russian. (In English, NAMRU3-T1088.)

289. **Korolev, M. B., Donets, M. A., and Chumakov, M. P.**, Electron microscope study of Crimean hemorrhagic fever virus in brains of infected mice and in pig kidney cell cultures, *Tezisy Konf. Vop. Med. Virus.*, Moscow, October 1975, 302; in Russian. (In English, NAMRU3-T1001.)

290. **Korolev, M. B., Donets, M. A., Rubin, S. G., and Chumakov, M. P.**, Morphology and morphogenesis of Crimean hemorrhagic fever virus, *Arch. Virol.*, 50, 169, 1976.

291. **Korshunova, O. S. and Petrova-Piontkovskaya, S. P.**, On the virus isolated from the ticks *Hyalomma marginatum marginatum* Koch, *Zool. Zh.*, 28, 186, 1949; in Russian. (In English, NAMRU3-T793.)

292. **Kotel'nikova, G. M. and Kondrashova, Z. N.**, Survival of West Nile virus in *Rhipicephalus rossicus* ticks, *Sb. Nauchn. Tr. Diagnost. Profilakt. Virus. Infekts.*, 160, 1974.

293. **Koval'sky, G. N. and Rybkina, L. G.**, Infections of the hemorrhagic fever group in the steppe region of Krasnodar Oblast, *Sb. Nauchn. Tr. Kuban. Med. Inst.*, 15, 1957; in Russian.

294. **Krasil'nikov, I. V. and Donets, M. A.**, Determination of the size and molecular weight of Crimean hemorrhagic fever virus virions, *Tezisy Konf. Vop. Med. Virus.*, Moscow, October 1975, 309; in Russian. (In English, NAMRU3-T987.)

295. **Kuchin, V. V., Yanovich, T. D., Butenko, A. M., and Kirsanova, K. S.,** Serological examination for antibodies to Crimean hemorrhagic fever virus in domestic animals of Rostov Oblast, *Mater. 3. Oblast, Nauchn. Prakt. Konf.,* Rostov-on-Don, May 1970, 61; in Russian. (In English, NAMRU3-T531.)

296. **Kuima, A. U.,** Species composition of ixodid ticks in hemorrhagic fever foci of Tadzhikistan, *Soveshch. Leish. Drug. Trans. Trop. Prirodnoochag. Bolez. Lyud. Sred. Azii Zakav.,* Ashkhabad, May 1969, 204; in Russian.

297. **Kuima, A. U.,** The host range and phenology of *Hyalomma anatolicum* Koch development in hemorrhagic fever foci of Dangara region, Tadzhikistan, *Tr. Inst. Polio. Virusn. Entsefalitov Akad. Med. Nauk. SSSR,* 19, 204, 1971; in Russian. (In English, NAMRU3-T831.)

298. **Kuima, A. U.,** Biological characteristics of tick subspecies, *Mater. Konf. Itog. Nauchno Issled. Rab. Dushan. Inst. Epidem. Gig.,* Dushanbe, 1970, 1971; in Russian.

299. **Kuima, A. U.,** Some characteristics of distribution and numbers of Crimean hemorrhagic fever vectors in southern Tadzhikistan, *Tezisy Konf. Vop. Med. Virus.,* Moscow, October 1975, 310; in Russian. (In English, NAMRU3-T1002.)

300. **Kuima, A. U.,** Ixodidae of wild mammals in Crimean hemorrhagic fever foci of southern Tadzhikistan, *Mater. 9. Simp. Ekol. Virus.,* Dushanbe, October 1975, 70; in Russian. (In English, NAMRU3-T1134.)

301. **Kuima, A. U.,** The role of birds as ixodid tick hosts in the zone of CHF foci of southern Tadzhikistan, *Mater. 9. Simp. Ekol. Virus.,* Dushanbe, October 1975, 73; in Russian. (In English, NAMRU3-T1135.)

302. **Kurbanov, M. M., Berezina, L. K., Zakaryan, V. A., Kiseleva, N. V., and Vatolin, V. P.,** Results of serological investigation of human and domestic animal blood sera with 13 arboviruses in the Karakum canal zone and southeastern Turkmen SSR, *Sb. Tr. Ekol. Virus,* 2, 113, 1974; in Russian. (In English, NAMRU3-T778.)

303. **Kurbanov, M. M., Gromashevsky, V. L., Berdyev, A., Skvortsova, T. M., Kiseleva, N. V., and Vatolin, V. P.,** Isolation of arboviruses from ticks in the Karakum canal zone, *Sb. Tr. Ekol. Virus,* 2, 109, 1974; in Russian. (In English, NAMRU3-T777.)

304. **Lamontellerie, M.,** *Les Ixodoides du Sud-Ouest de la France. Espèces Recontrées, Agressivite, Rôle Pathogène. Imprimerie E.,* Drouillard, Bordeaux, 1954, 145.

305. **Lazarev, V. N.,** Therapy of patients ill with Crimean hemorrhagic fever with the sera of convalescents, *Mater. 16. Nauchn. Sess. Inst. Polio. Virus. Entsefalitov,* 2, 142, 1969; in Russian. (In English, NAMRU3-T849.)

306. **Lazarev, V. N.,** Some features of the clinical picture of Crimean hemorrhagic fever in Rostov Region, *Tr. Inst. Polio. Virusn. Entsefalitov Akad. Med. Nauk SSSR,* 22, 155, 1974; in Russian. (In English, NAMRU3-T937.)

307. **Lazarev, V. N., Lazarev, A. N., and Badalov, M. E.,** Crimean hemorrhagic fever in children, *Mater. 3. Oblast. Nauchn. Prakt. Konf.,* Rostov-on-Don, May 1970, 121; in Russian. (In English, NAMRU3-T543.)

308. **Lazarev, V. N., Reunova, N. M., Manukyan, N. S., Badalov, M. E., and Koreneva, G. D.,** Certain clinical laboratory features of Crimean hemorrhagic fever in Rostov Oblast, *Mater. 3. Oblast, Nauchn. Prakt. Konf.,* Rostov-on-Don, May, 1970, 115; in Russian. (In English, NAMRU3-T542.)

309. **Lee, V. H. and Kemp, G. E.,** Congo virus: experimental infection of *Hyalomma rufipes* and transmission to a calf, *Bull. Entomol. Soc. Niger.,* 2, 133, 1970.

310. **Leshchinskaya, E. V.,** Clinical features of hemorrhagic fever of Crimean type in Astrakhan Oblast, *Mater. 11. Nauchn. Sess. Inst. Polio Virus. Entsefalitov,* 1964, 266; in Russian. (In English, NAMRU3-T166.)

311. **Leshchinskaya, E. V.,** Differential diagnosis of hemorrhagic fever of the Crimean type, *Mater. 11. Nauchn. Sess. Inst. Polio. Virus. Entsefalitov.,* 1964, 268; in Russian. (In English, NAMRU3-T168.)

312. **Leshchinskaya, E. V.,** Clinical picture of Crimean hemorrhagic fever (CCHF), *Tr. Inst. Polio. Virusn. Entsefalitov Akad. Med. Nauk SSSR,* 7, 226, 1965; in Russian. (In English, NAMRU3-T856.)

313. **Leshchinskaya, E. V.,** Crimean hemorrhagic fever, *Jpn. J. Med. Sci. Biol.,* 20, 143, 1967.

314. **Leshchinskaya, E. V.,** Clinical aspects of Crimean hemorrhagic fever, *Sov. Med.,* 30, 74, 1967; in Russian.

315. **Leshchinskaya, E. V.,** Clinical picture of Crimean hemorrhagic fever and its comparison with hemorrhagic fevers of other types, *Avtoref. Diss. Soisk. Uchen. Step. Dokt. Med. Nauk,* Akademiya Meditsinskikh Nauk S.S.S.R., Moscow, 1967; in Russian. (In English, NAMRU3-T1180.)

316. **Leshchinskaya, E. V.,** Comparative analysis of clinical symptoms of hemorrhagic fever accompanied by hepatic syndrome and Crimean hemorrhagic fever, *Abstr. Rev. 8th Int. Congr. Trop. Med. Malar.,* Teheran, September 1968, 846; in Russian. (In English, NAMRU3-T764.)

317. **Leshchinskaya, E. V.,** Clinical course and treatment of Crimean hemorrhagic fever (CCHF), *Med. Sestra,* 32, 6, 1973; in Russian. (In English, NAMRU3-T819.)

318. **Leshchinskaya, E. V. and Butenko, A. M.**, Comparison of clinical and laboratory data in Crimean hemorrhagic fever, *Tr. Inst. Polio. Virusn. Entsefalitov Akad. Med. Nauk SSSR,* 19, 140, 1971; in Russian. (In English, NAMRU3-T961.)
319. **Leshchinskaya, E. V., Butenko, A. M., Karinskaya, G. A., Martynenko, I. N., Rubin, S. G., Stolbov, D. N., Zimina, Yu. V., Derbedeneva, M. P., and Chumakov, M. P.**, Results of clinical-epidemiological and serological examination of healthy persons in foci of Crimean hemorrhagic fever, *Mater. 16. Nauchn. Sess. Inst. Polio. Virus. Entsefalitov,* 2, 143, 1969; in Russian. (In English, NAMRU3-T850.)
320. **Leshchinskaya, E. V. and Chumakov, M. P.**, Comparative study of Crimean hemorrhagic fever in different endemic foci and of similar diseases in Central Asia, *Sb. Tr. Inst. Polio. Virus. Entsefalitov Akad. Med. Nauk SSSR,* 7, 315, 1965; in Russian. (In English, NAMRU3-T372.)
321. **Leshchinskaya, E. V. and Martinenko, I. N.**, Certain questions of CHF therapy, *Mater. 3. Oblast. Nauchn. Prakt. Konf.,* Rostov-on-Don, May 1970, 111; in Russian. (In English, NAMRU3-T541.)
322. **Levi, V.**, Findings of African tick *Amblyomma variegatum* (Fabricius) in Bulgaria, *Letop. Chig. Epidem. Inst.,* 3, 201, 1969; in Bulgarian.
323. **Levi, V.**, Seasonal activity of the ticks of the family Ixodidae in focus of Crimean hemorrhagic fever in Pazarkjick Region, *Suvrem. Med.,* 23, 44, 1972; in Bulgarian. (In English, NAMRU3-T981.)
324. **Levi, V.**, Distribution and seasonal activity in the preimago phases of the ixodid ticks in a focus of haemorrhagic fever (Crimean type), *Proc. 3rd Int. Congr. Acarol.,* Prague, August 1971, 1973, 609.
325. **Levi, V. and Vasilenko, S.**, Study on the Crimean hemorrhagic fever (CHF) virus transmission mechanism in *Hyalomma pl. plumbeum* ticks, *Epidemiol. Mikrobiol. Infekts. Boles.,* 9, 182, 1972; in Bulgarian.
326. **Liebisch, A.**, Die Rolle einheimischer Zecken (Ixodidae) in der Epidemiologie des Q-Fiebers in Deutschland, *Dtsch. Tieraerztl. Wochenschr.,* 83, 274, 1976.
327. **London School of Hygiene and Tropical Medicine,** *Report on the Work of the School,* 1974-1975, 1976, 143.
328. **L'vov, D. K.**, Results of three-year-long field trials performed by the department of ecology of viruses, *Sb. Tr. Ekol. Virus,* 1, 5, 1973; in Russian. (In English, NAMRU3-T739.)
329. **L'vov, D. K.**, The role of birds in transportation and survival of arboviruses, *Med. Parazitol. Parazit. Bolezni,* 43, 473, 1974; in Russian. (In English, NAMRU3-T896.)
330. **L'vov, D. K., Sidorova, G. A., Gromashevsky, V. L., Kurbanov, M., Skvortsova, T. M., Gofman, Yu. P., Berezina, L. K., Klimenko, S. M., Zakharyan, V. A., Aristova, V. A., and Neronov, V. M.**, Virus "Tamdy" — a new arbovirus, isolated in the Uzbec, S.S.R. and Turkmen S.S.R. from ticks *Hyalomma asiaticum asiaticum* Schulce et Schlottke, 1929, and *Hyalomma plumbeum plumbeum* Panzer, 1796, *Arch. Virol.,* 51, 15, 1976.
331. **L'vov, D. K., Timofeeva, A. A., Gromashevsky, V. L., et al.**, New viruses isolated in the USSR in 1969-1974, *Tezisy Konf. Vop. Med. Virus,* Moscow, October 1975, 322; in Russian. (In English, NAMRU3-T1005.)
332. **Lyskovtsev, M. M.**, *Tickborne Rickettsiosis,* Medgiz, Moscow, 1963, 275; in Russian. (In English, *Misc. Publ. Entomol. Soc. Am.,* 6, 41, 1962.)
333. **Lysunkina, V. A. and Khozinsky, V. I.**, The reaction or complement fixation by brain antigen in hemorrhagic fever, in *Hemorrhagic Fever in Uzbekistan,* No. 2, Khodukin, N. I., Ed., Vop. Kraev. Patol. Akad. Nauk. Uzbek. S.S.R., 1952, 96.
334. **McCrae, A. W. R., Manuma, P., and Kitama, A.**, Tick collections from Entebbe, *Rep. E. Afr. Virus. Res. Inst. (1969),* 19, 22, 1970.
335. **Martynenko, I. N. and Badalov, M. E.**, Peripheral blood condition in persons vaccinated against Crimean hemorrhagic fever, *Mater. 3. Oblast. Nauchn. Prakt. Konf.,* Rostov-on-Don, May 1970, 146; in Russian. (In English, NAMRU3-T548.)
336. **Maslennikov, I. I. and Sorochinsky, V. V.**, Study of Crimean hemorrhagic fever in Belaya Kalitva Region of Rostov Oblast (1963-1969), *Mater. 3. Oblast. Nauchn. Prakt. Konf.,* Rostov-on-Don, 1970, 88; in Russian. (In English, NAMRU3-T537.)
337. **Mason, P. J.**, Agents sent from other laboratories for identification: agent 3010, *Rep. E. Afr. Virus Res. Inst. (1956-1957),* 7, 23, 1957.
338. **Mateva, M.**, Bulgaria's mammals as reservoirs of infection, *Trans. 1st Int. Ther. Congr.,* 1, 392, 1974.
339. **Matevosyan, K. Sh., Semashko, I. V., Marutyan, E. M., Rubin, S. G., and Chumakov, M. P.**, Discovery of Crimean hemorrhagic fever virus in *Hyalomma plumbeum plumbeum, Hyalomma anatolicum, Rhipicephalus bursa, Boophilus calcaratus* ticks in the Armenian SSR, *Tr. Inst. Polio. Virusn. Entsefalitov Akad. Med. Nauk SSSR,* 22, 169, 1974; in Russian. (In English, NAMRU3-T938.)
340. **Matevosyan, K. Sh., Semashko, I. V., Rubin, S. G., and Chumakov, M. P.**, Antibody for Crimean hemorrhagic fever virus in human and cattle blood sera in the Armenian SSR, *Tr. Inst. Polio. Virusn. Entsefalitov Akad. Med. Nauk SSSR,* 22, 173, 1974; in Russian. (In English, NAMRU3-T939.)

341. **Mayer, C. F.**, Epidemic hemorrhagic fever of the Far East (EHF) or endemic hemorrhagic nephrosonephritis; morphology and pathogenesis, *Lab. Invest.*, 1, 291, 1952.

342. **Mayer, C. F.**, Medical aspects of the Korean campaign, *Lancet*, 1, 974, 1952.

343. **Meliev, A.**, A contribution to epidemiology of hemorrhagic fever in Uzbekistan, *Zh. Mikrobiol. Epidemiol. Immunobiol.*, 44, 93, 1967; in Russian. (In English, NAMRU3-T413.)

344. **Meliev, A.**, Data on investigating hemorrhagic fever in Uzbek SSR, *Avtoref. Diss. Soisk. Uchen. Step. Kand. Med. Nauk*, Inst. Epidem. Mikrobiol., Gamaleya, N. F., Ed., Akad. Med. Nauk S.S.S.R., Moscow, 1967, 18; in Russian. (In English, NAMRU3-T1179.)

345. **Mikhailov, G. I.**, On the epidemiology of an acute infectious hemorrhagic disease, *Klin. Med. (Moscow)*, 24, 67, 1946; in Russian.

346. **Milyutin, V. N., Butenko, A. M., Artyushenko, A. A., Bliznichenko, A. G., Zavodova, T. I., Zarubina, L. V., Novikova, E. M., Rubin, S. G., Chernyshev, N. I., and Chumakov, M. P.**, Experimental infection of horses with Crimean hemorrhagic fever virus. I. Clinical observations, *Mater. 16. Nauchn. Sess. Inst. Polio. Virus. Entsefalitov*, 2, 145, 1969; in Russian. (In English, NAMRU3-T851.)

347. **Mironov, P.**, Hemorrhagic fever in Burgas District, *Suvrem. Med.*, 6, 62, 1953; in Bulgarian. (In English, NAMRU3-T1101.)

348. **Mitchell, C. J. and Spillett, J. J.**, Ecological notes on *Rhipicephalus turanicus* Pomerantzev in West Bengal, India (Acarina: Ixodidae), *J. Med. Entomol.*, 5, 5, 1968.

349. **Mitov, A. and Neklyudov**, First published record of CCHF in Bulgaria, 1952; in Bulgarian; as cited in **Donchev, D., Kebedzhiev, G., and Rusakiev, M.**, Bulg. Akad. Nauk Mikrobiol. Inst. 1st Kongr. Mikrobiol., 1967, 77.

350. **Monath, T. P.**, Lassa fever: past, present and possible future status, *Medicina (Buenos Aires)*, 37 (Suppl. 3), 167, 1977.

351. **Moore, D. L., Causey, O. R., Carey, D. E., Reddy, S., Cooke, A. R., Akinkugbe, F. M., David-West, T. S., and Kemp, G. E.**, Arthropod-borne viral infections of man in Nigeria, 1964-1970, *Ann. Trop. Med. Parasitol.*, 69, 49, 1975.

352. **Moreau, R. E.**, *The Palaearctic-African Bird Migration Systems*, Academic Press, London, 1972, 384.

353. **Morel, P. C.**, Les tiques des animaux domestiques de l'Afrique occidentale francaise, *Rev. Elev. Med. Vet. Pays Trop.*, 11, 153, 1958.

354. **Morel, P. C.**, *Etude sur les tiques d'Ethiopie (acariens, ixodides)*, Inst. d'Elev. Med. Vet. Pays Trop, Maisons-Alfort, France, 1976, 326.

355. **Morel, P. C. and Vassiliades, G.**, Les *Rhipicephalus* du groupe *sanguineus:* especes africaines, (Acariens, Ixodoidea), *Rev. Elev. Med. Vet. Pays Trop.*, 15, 343, 1963.

356. **Moussa, M. I., Imam, I. Z., Converse, J. D., and El-Karamany, R. M.**, Isolation of Matruh virus from *Hyalomma marginatum* ticks in Egypt, *J. Egypt. Public Health Assoc.*, 49, 341, 1974.

357. **Munube, G. M. R., Yazama, G. W., and Nsubuga, E.**, The out-patient dispensary, *Rep. E. Afr. Virus Res. Inst.*, 22, 6, 1972.

358. **Muratbekov, Ya. M.**, Ticks as transmitters of hemorrhagic fever in Uzbekistan, in *Hemorrhagic Fever in Uzbekistan*, No. 2., Khodukin, N. I., Ed., Vop. Kraev. Patol. Akad. Nauk Uzbek. S.S.R., 1952, 122; in Russian. (In English, NAMRU3-T215.)

359. **Murphy, F. A., Harrison, A. K., and Whitfield, S. G.**, Bunyaviridae: morphologic and morphogenetic similarities of Bunyamwera serologic supergroup viruses and several other arthropod-borne viruses, *Intervirology*, 1, 297, 1973.

360. **Neitz, W. O.**, A consolidation of our knowledge of the transmission of tickborne diseases, *Onderstepoort, J. Vet. Res.*, 27, 115, 1956.

361. **Neitz, W. O.**, Classification, transmission, and biology of piroplasms of domestic animals, *Ann. N.Y. Acad. Sci.*, 64, 56, 1956.

362. **Neklyudov, M.**, A case of hemorrhagic fever (Crimea), *Suvrem. Med.*, 5, 92, 1952; in Bulgarian.

363. **Nevill, L.**, Correspondence, *East Afr. Med. J.*, 38, 174, 1961.

364. **Nikiforov, L. P., Gromashevsky, V. L., and Veselovskaya, O. V.**, Isolation of Crimean hemorrhagic fever virus in Azerbaijan, *Sb. Tr. Ekol. Virus*, 1, 125, 1973; in Russian. (In English, NAMRU3-T742.)

365. **Nŏsek, J.**, The ecology and public health importance of *Dermacentor marginatus* and *D. reticulatus* ticks in Central Europe, *Folia Parasitol. (Prague)*, 19, 93, 1972.

366. **Nŏsek, J.**, The ecology, bionomics, behaviour and public health importance of *Dermacentor marginatus* and *D. reticulatus* ticks, *Wiad. Parazytol.*, 18, 721, 1973.

367. **Nŏsek, J. and Blaskovič, D.**, Ticks as vectors of tick-borne encephalitis virus in Europe, *Proc. 3rd Int. Congr. Acarol.*, Prague, 1971, 589, 1973.

368. **Nuorteva, P. and Hoogstraal, H.**, The incidence of ticks (Ixodoidea, Ixodidae) on migratory birds arriving in Finland during the spring of 1962, *Ann. Med. Exp. Biol. Fenn.*, 41, 457, 1963.

369. **Obukhova, V. R., Gupta, N. P., Klisenko, G. A., Gaidamovich, S. Ya., Gosh, S. N., and Myasnenko, M.,** Antibodies to viruses of the CHF-Congo group in sera collected in India, *Sb. Tr. Inst. Virus. imeni D. I. Ivanovsky Akad. Med. Nauk SSSR,* 2, 77, 1975; in Russian. (In English, NAMRU3-T1138.)

370. **Olsuf'ev, N. G. and Dunaeva, T. N.,** *Natural Focality, Epidemiology and Prophylactic Measures Against Tularemia,* Izd. "Meditsina", Moscow, 1970, 271.

371. **Osipova, N. Z., Karas', F. R., Vargina, S. G., and Grebenyuk, Yu. I.,** Ectoparasites of wild animals in Crimean hemorrhagic fever natural focus of southern Kirgizia, in *Entomological Investigations in Kirgizia,* Protsenko, A. I., Ed., Izd. "Ilim," Frunze, 1975, 124; in Russian. (In English, NAMRU3-T1164.)

372. **Pak, T. P.,** Epidemiological zonation of Crimean hemorrhagic fever in Tadzhik SSR, *Zh. Mikrobiol. Epidemiol. Immunobiol.,* 49, 112, 1972; in Russian. (In English, NAMRU3-T615.)

373. **Pak, T. P.,** Problems of ecology of Crimean hemorrhagic fever in the Tadzhik SSR, *Sb. Tr. Ekol. Virus,* 1, 91, 1973; in Russian. (In English, NAMRU3-T725.)

374. **Pak, T. P.,** Contribution to the question on development of Crimean hemorrhagic fever noso-distribution area, *Tezisy Konf. Vop. Med. Virus,* Moscow, October 1975, 336; in Russian. (In English, NAMRU3-T1007.)

375. **Pak, T. P.,** Seasonal circulation dynamics of Crimean hemorrhagic fever virus in Tadzhikistan, *Mater. 9. Simp. Ekol. Virus,* Dushanbe, October 1975, 35; in Russian. (In English, NAMRU3-T1126.)

376. **Pak, T. P.,** Structure of the distribution area of Crimean hemorrhagic fever in Tadzhikistan, *Mater. 9. Simp. Ekol. Virus.* Dushanbe, October 1975, 39; in Russian. (In English, NAMRU3-T1131.)

377. **Pak, T. P.,** Division of Tadzhik SSR into landscape-endemic regions with Crimean hemorrhagic fever, *Tezisy Dokl. 9. Vses. Konf. Prirod. Ochag. Bolez. Chelov. Zhivot,* Omsk, May 1966, 1976, 129; in Russian. (In English, NAMRU3-T1176.)

378. **Pak, T. P., Daniyarov, O. A., and Kasymov, K. T.,** Transovarial transmission of Crimean hemorrhagic fever virus in ticks. I. Contribution to the infection method of *Hyalomma antolicum* ticks with Crimean hemorrhagic fever virus, *Mater. Konf. Itog. Nauchno Issled. Rab. Dushan. Inst. Epidem. Gig.,* Dushanbe, 1970, 1971; in Russian.

379. **Pak, T. P., Daniyarov, O. A., Kostyukov, M. A., Bulychev, V. P., and Kuima, A. U.,** Biocenotic interrelationships between Crimean hemorrhagic fever, ixodid ticks and their hosts. I. Results from virological investigations of ixodid and argasid ticks in Tadzhik SSR, *Sb. Tr. Inst. Virus. imeni D. I. Ivanovsky Akad. Med. Nauk. SSSR,* 2, 135, 1974; in Russian. (In English, NAMRU3-T783.)

380. **Pak, T. P., Daniyarov, O. A., Kostyukov, M. A., Bulychev, V. P., and Kuima, A. U.,** Ecology of Crimean hemorrhagic fever in Tadzhikistan, *Mater. Resp. Simp. Kamenyuki "Belovezh. Puscha",* Minsk, September 1974, 93; in Russian. (In English, NAMRU3-T968.)

381. **Pak, T. P., Kostyukov, M. A., Daniyarov, O. A., and Bulychev, V. P.,** A combined focus of arbovirus infections in Tadzhikistan, *Mater. 9. Simp. Ekol. Virus.* Dushanbe, October 1975, 38; in Russian. (In English, NAMRU3-T1127.)

382. **Pak, T. P., Kuima, U. A., and Bratushchak, V. N.,** Contact of the population with ticks in a region endemic for Crimean hemorrhagic fever, *Tr. Inst. Polio. Virusn. Entsefalitov Akad. Med. Nauk. SSSR,* 19, 221, 1971; in Russian. (In English, NAMRU3-T948.)

383. **Pak, T. P. and Mikhailova, L. I.,** *Crimean Hemorrhagic Fever in Tadzhikistan,* Izd. "Irfon", Dushanbe, 1973, 154; in Russian. (In English, NAMRU3-T1000.)

384. **Pak, T. P., Mikhailova, L. I., and Zykov, M. F.,** Contact infections with Crimean hemorrhagic fever in Tadzhik SSR, *Sov. Med.,* 1, 153, 1975; in Russian. (In English, NAMRU3-T1020.)

385. **Pak, T. P. and Pashkov, V. A.,** Criteria for epidemiological assessment of a locality for Crimean hemorrhagic fever, *Sb. Tr. Ekol. Virus.* 2, 129, 1974; in Russian. (In English, NAMRU3-T782.)

386. **Pak, T. P., Smirnova, S. E., Zgurskaya, G. N., Yasinsky, A. V., Berdyev, Kh. B., Apostoli, L. A., Karovkin, V. P., Feldman, E. M., Derlyatko, K. I., Golovko, E. N., Makhmudov, R. Kh., and Chumakov, M. P.,** Results of a serological survey of Crimean hemorrhagic fever in Tadzhik SSR in 1969, *Tr. Inst. Polio. Virusn. Entsefalitov Akad. Med. Nauk. SSSR,* 19, 72, 1971; in Russian. (In English, NAMRU3-T936.)

387. **Pan'kina, M. V. and Kannegiser, N. N.,** An outbreak of contact infections of Central Asian fever in southern Kazakh SSR, *Tr. 5. Konf. Prirod. Ochag. Bolez. Vop. Parazit. Respub. Sred. Azii Kazakh,* Frunze, September 1962, 1964, 41; in Russian. (In English, NAMRU3-T860.)

388. **Papadopoulos, O. and Koptopoulos, G.,** Isolation of Crimean-Congo hemorrhagic fever (CCHF) virus from *Rhipicephalus bursa* ticks in Greece, *Acta Microbiol. Hell.,* 23, 20, 1978; in Greek, English summary.

389. **Pavlov, B. P., Sizyy, L. P., Taran, I. F., and Yarovoi, L. I.,** A case of hemorrhagic fever in Stavropol' resulting from contact, *Mater. Konf.,* Stavropol-on-Caucasus, October 1966; in Russian.

390. **Pavlov, P. and Popov, A.,** *Amblyomma hebraeum* (Koch 1844) in Bulgaria, *Izv. Inst. Eksp. Vet. Med. Sof.,* 1, 211, 1951; in Bulgarian.

391. **Pavlovsky, E. N. and Solovev, V. D.,** On circulation of the virus of spring-summer encephalitis in the organism of the tick-vector *Haemaphysalis concinna, Tr. Voen. Med. Akad. Krasnoi Armii,* 25, 9, 1941, in Russian.

392. **Pavlovsky, E. N. and Solovev, V. D.,** Circulation of the virus of spring-summer encephalitis in the organism of tick-vector *Haemaphysalis concinna, Rab. Eksp. Parazit. (Pavlovsky),* 1963, 197; in Russian. (In English, NAMRU3-T115.)

393. **Pavri, K. M., Anandarajah, M., Hermon, Y. E., Nayar, M., Wikramsinghe, M. R., and Dandawate, C. N.,** Isolation of Wanowrie virus from brain of a fatal human case from Sri Lanka, *Indian J. Med. Res.,* 64, 557, 1976.

394. **Pegram, R. G.,** Ticks (Acarina, Ixodoidea) of the northern regions of the Somali Democratic Republic, *Bull. Entomol. Res.,* 66, 345, 1976.

395. **Perelatov, V. D.,** Hemorrhagic fever in the Rostov Region, *Zh. Mikrobiol. Epidemiol. Immunobiol.,* 41, 117, 1964; in Russian. (In English, NAMRU3-T232.)

396. **Perelatov, V. D.,** *Hemorrhagic Fever in Rostov Oblast,* Rostov Oblast Sanit. Epidem. Sta., Rostov-on-Don, 1966, 40; in Russian. (In English, NAMRU3-T1186.)

397. **Perelatov, V. D., Birulya, N. B., and Zalutskaya, L. I.,** Interrelationships between the human population and vectors in the Rostov Oblast Crimean hemorrhagic fever focus, *Mater. 3. Oblast. Nauchn. Prakt. Konf.,* Rostov-on-Don, 92, 1970; in Russian. (In English, NAMRU3-T539.)

398. **Perelatov, V. D., Butenko, A. M., Vostokova, K. K., Donets, M. A., Kataitseva, T. V., Alekseev-Malakhov, A. G., and Durov, V. I.,** Ecological association between Crimean hemorrhagic fever virus and ixodid tick hosts in Rostov Oblast and Krasnodar Region, *Tezisy 17. Nauchn. Sess. Inst. Posvyashch. Aktual. Probl. Virus. Profilakt. Virus. Zabolev,* Moscow, October, 1972, 357; in Russian. (In English, NAMRU3-T1065.)

399. **Perelatov, V. D. and Chumakova, I. V.,** Contribution to the ecology of *Hyalomma plumbeum* ticks in the Donets Crimean hemorrhagic fever focus, *Med. Parazitol. Parazit. Bolezni,* 36, 356, 1967; in Russian. (In English, NAMRU3-T422.)

400. **Perelatov, V. D., Kuchin, V. V., Donets, M. A., Zarubina, L. V., Kondratenko, V. F., Blagoveshchenskaya, N. M., Vostokova, K. K., Novikova, L. D., and Novikova, E. M.,** Results of experimental infection of European hares with Crimean hemorrhagic fever virus, *Tezisy 17. Nauchn. Sess. Inst. Posvyashch. Aktual. Probl. Virus. Profilakt. Virus. Zabolev,* Moscow, October, 1972, 354; in Russian. (In English, NAMRU3-T1063.)

401. **Perelatov, V. D. and Lazarev, V. N.,** *What is Essential to Know About Hemorrhagic Fever,* Rostovskoe Knizhnoe Izd. Rostov-on-Don, 1965, 28; in Russian. (In English, NAMRU3-T182.)

402. **Perelatov, V. D., Leshchinskaya, E. V., Chumakov, M. P., Birulya, N. B., and Zalutskaya, L. I.,** On epidemiology of Crimean hemorrhagic fever in Rostov Region, *Tr. Inst. Polio. Virusn. Entsefalitov Akad. Med. Nauk SSSR,* 7, 279, 1965; in Russian. (In English, NAMRU3-T371.)

403. **Perelatov, V. D., Leshchinskaya, E. V., Vasyuta, Yu. S., Lang, N. N., Petrovsky, P. Ya., and Chumakov, M. P.,** Incidence of Crimean hemorrhagic fever (CHF) in Rostov Oblast, *Mater. 11. Nauchn. Sess. Inst. Polio. Virus. Entsefalitov,* 1964, 283; in Russian. (In English, NAMRU3-T174.)

404. **Perelatov, V. D. and Vostokova, K. K.,** Epidemiology of Crimean hemorrhagic fever in Rostov Region, *Tr. Inst. Polio. Virusn. Entsefalitov Akad. Med. Nauk S.S.S.R.,* 19, 174, 1971; in Russian. (In English, NAMRU3-T924.)

405. **Petrov, V. G.,** Ixodid ticks and gamasid mites as vectors of the agent of tularemia infection, *Tezisy Dokl. l. Akarol. Soveshch.,* 1966, 155; in Russian. (In English, NAMRU3-T424.)

406. **Petrova-Piontkovskaya, S. P.,** Materials on the biology and ecology of *Hyalomma marginatum marginatum* Koch in the northwest reservoir of the Crimean hemorrhagic fever, *Nov. Med.,* 5, 21, 1947; in Russian. (In English, NAMRU3-T864.)

407. **Petrova-Piontkovskaya, S. P.,** *Hyalomma marginatum marginatum* Koch as vector of rickettsia, *Zool. Zh.,* 28, 419, 1949; in Russian. (In English, NAMRU3-T40.)

408. **Petrova-Piontkovskaya, S. P.,** Influence of agriculture on the population of *Hyalomma marginatum marginatum* Koch in the areas of the field protection plantations, *Zool. Zh.,* 29, 297, 1950; in Russian.

409. **Pokrovsky, S. N., Perelatov, V. D., Popov, G. M., Birulya, N. B., and Zalutskaya, L. I.,** Hemorrhagic fever in Rostov Oblast, *Mater 11. Nauchn. Sess. Inst. Polio. Virus. Entsefalitov,* 1964, 282; in Russian. (In English, NAMRU3-T173.)

410. **Popov. G. V.,** Immunofluorescent and electron-microscopic investigations of Crimean hemorrhagic fever virus with application of comparative investigations of model viruses, *Avtoref. Dokt. Diss., Moscow,* 1971, 41; in Russian. (In English, NAMRU3-T1185.)

411. **Popov, G. V., Levi, V. D., Vasilenko, S. M., and Chumakov, M. P.,** Application of fluorescent antibody method (FAM) in the isolation of Crimean haemorrhagic fever virus from ticks, the vectors of the disease, *Proc. 3. Int. Congr. Acarol.,* Prague, August September 1971, 1973, 615.

412. **Popov, G. V. and Zavodova, T. I.**, Morphology of the virus of Crimean hemorrhagic fever (Congo virus), *Int. Virol. Abstr. 3. Int. Virol.*, 3, 257, 1975.
413. **Popov, G. V., Zavodova, T. I., and Semashko, I. V.**, Electron microscopy of tissue cultures and the brain of newborn white mice infected with Crimean hemorrhagic fever virus, *Tezisy Konf. Vop. Med. Virus.*, Moscow, October 1975, 345; in Russian. (In English, NAMRU3-T1008.)
414. **Porterfield, J. S., Casals, J., Chumakov, M. P., Gaidamovich, S. Ya., Hannoun, C., Holmes, I. H., Horzinek, M. C., Mussgay, M., and Russell, P. K.**, Bunyaviruses and Bunyaviridae, *Intervirology*, 2, 270, 1974.
415. **Pospelova-Shtrom, M. V. and Abusalimov, N. S.**, A case of collecting *Amblyomma lepidum* Dönitz, 1909, tick in Azerbaijan, *Med. Parazitol. Parazit. Bolezni*, 26, 56, 1957; in Russian. (In English, NAMRU3-T1.)
416. **Povalishina, T. P.**, Utilization of the cartographic method for study of a focus of hemorrhagic fever of Crimean type, *Mater. 11. Nauchn. Sess. Inst. Polio. Virus. Entsefalitov*, 1964, 285; in Russian. (In English, NAMRU3-T175.)
417. **Povalishina, T. P., Stolbov, D. N., Zimina, Yu, V., Egorova, P. S., Berezin, V. V., and Butenko, A. M.**, Parasitological information on foci of incidence of Crimean type hemorrhagic fever in Astrakhan Oblast, *Mater. 11. Nauchn. Sess. Inst. Polio. Virus. Entsefalitov*, 1964, 271; in Russian. (In English, NAMRU3-T169.)
418. **Povalishina, T. P., Zimina, Yu. V., Egorova, P. S., Berezin, V. V., Stolbov, D. N., and Ivanova, N. A.**, Landscape characteristics of foci of Crimean type hemorrhagic fever in Astrakhan Oblast, *Mater. 11. Nauchn. Sess. Inst. Polio. Virus. Entsefalitov*, 1964, 278; in Russian. (In English, NAMRU3-T172.)
419. **Primakov, S. V.**, A case of Crimean hemorrhagic fever in Voroshilovgrad Region, *Vrach. Delo*, 12, 130, 1971; in Russian. (In English, NAMRU3-T796.)
420. **Proreshnaya, T. L.**, Hemorrhagic fever, *Sov. Zdravookhr. Kirg.*, 1, 3, 1955; in Russian.
421. **Rabinovich, V. D., Blagoveshchenskaya, N. M., Butenko, A. M., Zarubina, L. V., Kondratenko, V. F., and Milyutin, V. N.**, Virological and serological examination of wild animals and birds in the Rostov Oblast Crimean hemorrhagic fever focus, *Mater. 3. Oblast. Nauchn. Prakt. Konf.*, Rostov-on-Don, May 1970, 35; in Russian. (In English, NAMRU3-T525.)
422. **Rabinovich, V. D., Milyutin, V. N., Artyushenko, A. A., Buryakov, B. G., and Chumakov, M. P.**, Possibility of extracting hyperimmune gammaglobulin against CHF from donkey blood sera, *Tezisy 17. Nauchn. Sess. Inst. Posvyashch. Aktual. Probl. Virus. Profilakt. Virus. Zabolev*, Moscow, October 1972, 1350; in Russian. (In English, NAMRU3-T1059.)
423. **Rapoport, L. P., Mamontov, S. I., and Dobritsa, P. G.**, Crimean hemorrhagic fever foci in Chimkent Oblast, *Tezisy Dokl. 9. Vses. Konf. Prirod. Ochag. Bolez. Chelov. Zhivot*, Omsk, May 1976, 129; in Russian. (In English, NAMRU3-T1177.)
424. **Rayburn, J. D., Hood, M. W., Edwards, S. J., and Shaw, J. H.**, Index-Catalogue of Medical and Veterinary Zoology. Parasite-Subject Catalogue: Subject Headings and Treatment, Suppl. 20, Part 6, U.S. Department of Agriculture, Washington, D. C., 1975, 483.
425. **Rayburn, J. D., Hood, M. W., Kirby, M. D., and Shaw, J. H.**, Index-Catalogue of Medical and Veterinary Zoology. Parasite-Subject Catalogue: Parasites: Arthropoda and Miscellaneous Phyla, Suppl. 19, Part 5, U.S. Department of Agriculture, Washington, D. C., 1975, 403.
426. **Rebello, M. J. and Reuben, R.**, A report on ticks collected from birds and small mammals in North Arcot and Chittoor Districts, South India, *J. Bombay Nat. Hist. Soc.*, 63, 283, 1967.
427. **Reformatskaya, A. D., Pan'kina, M. V., and Krinitsky, N. I.**, Hemorrhagic fever in Kazakh SSR, *Zdravookhr. Kaz.*, 1965, 5; in Russian.
428. **Řeháček, J.**, Development of animal viruses and rickettsiae in ticks and mites, *Annu. Rev. Entomol.*, 10, 1, 1965.
429. **Rehse-Kupper, B., Casals, J., Rehse, E., and Ackermann, R.**, Eyach — an arthropod-borne virus related to Colorado tick fever virus in the Federal Republic of Germany, *Acta Virol. (Engl. Ed.)*, 20, 339, 1976.
430. **Reznik, P. A.**, Peculiarities of distribution areas and formation routes of the ixodid tick fauna in the Soviet Union, *Fauna Stavropol.*, 1970, 3; in Russian.
431. **Robin, Y.**, Centre régional O.M.S. de référence pour les arbovirus en Afrique de l'Ouest, *Rapp. Inst. Pasteur, Dakar*, 1972, 15.
432. **Robin, Y.**, Centre régional O.M.S. de référence pour les arbovirus en Afrique de l'Ouest, *Rapp. Inst. Pasteur Dakar*, 1973, 17.
433. **Robin, Y.**, Centre régional O.M.S. de référence pour les arbovirus en Afrique de l'Ouest, *Rapp. Inst. Pasteur Dakar*, 1974, 20.
434. **Robin, Y.**, Centre collaborateur O.M.S. de référence et de recherche pour les arbovirus, *Rapp. Inst. Pasteur Dakar*, 1975, 22.

435. **Robin, Y.**, Centre collaborateur O.M.S. de référence et de recherche pour les arbovirus, *Rapp. Inst. Pasteur Dakar*, 1977, 16.

436. **Robin, Y. and le Gonidec, G.**, Activities du laboratoire des arbovirus. *Rapp. Fonct. Tech. Inst. Pasteur Dakar*, 1972, 37.

437. **Robson, J., Robb, J. M., Hawa, N. J., and Al-Wahayyib, T.**, Ticks (Ixodoidea) of domestic animals in Iraq. VI. Distribution, *J. Med. Entomol.*, 6, 125, 1969.

438. **Rosicky, B. and Balat, F.**, Die Zecke *Ixodes ricinus* L. als Parasit der Vogel, *Cesk. Parazitol.*, 1, 45, 1954; in Czech.

439. **Rowe, A. J.**, Epidemic haemorrhagic fever, *Lancet*, 2, 980, 1952.

440. **Rozeboom, L. E. and Burgdorfer, W.**, Development of Colorado tick fever virus in the Rocky Mountain wood tick, *Dermacentor andersoni*, *Am. J. Hyg.*, 69, 138, 1959.

441. **Rukhlyadev, D. P.**, Parasitic diseases and reason for wild mammals abandoning Crimean game reserve, *Nauchno Metod. Zap. Glav. Uprav. Zapov.*, 8, 78; in Russian.

442. **Rybalko, S. I., Pankina, M. V., Kannegiser, N. I., and Burlakova, T. S.**, Hemorrhagic fever in southern localities of Kazakhstan, *Med. Parazitol. Parazit. Bolezni*, 32, 619, 1963; in Russian. (In English, NAMRU3-T154.)

443. **Ryzhkov, V. L.**, Test on the systematic of viruses, *Vopr. Med. Virusol.*, 3, 9, 1950; in Russian.

444. **Ryzhkov, V. L.**, Systematics of viruses in the contemporary literature, *Mikrobiologiya*, 21, 458, 1952; in Russian.

445. **Sacca, G., Mastrilli, M. L., Balducci, M., Verani, P., and Lopes, M. C.**, Studies on the vectors of arthropod-borne viruses in central Italy: investigations on ticks, *Ann. 1st Super. Sanita.*, 5, 21, 1969.

446. **Saidi, S.**, Viral antibodies in preschool children from the Caspian area, Iran, *Iran. J. Public Health*, 3, 83, 1974.

447. **Saidi, S., Casals, J., and Faghih, M. A.**, Crimean hemorrhagic fever-Congo (CHF-C) virus antibodies in man, and in domestic and small mammals, in Iran, *Am. J. Trop. Med. Hyg.*, 24, 353, 1975.

448. **Saikku, P.**, Uukuniemi Virus, Academic Dissertation, Medical Faculty, University of Helsinki, 1974, 67.

449. **Saikku, P., Ulmanen, I., and Brummer-Korvenkonito, M.**, Ticks (Ixodidae) on migratory birds in Finland, *Acta Entomol. Fenn.*, 28, 46, 1971.

450. **Sakhno, I. M., Sidorkin, A. P., and Simonovich, E. H.**, The steppe nidus of hemorrhagic fever, *Sb. Rab. Posvyashch. 70. Let. Yubil. En N. Pavlovsky*, 216, 1955; in Russian.

451. **Saratsiotis, A.**, Etude morphologique et observations biologiques sur *Ixodes gibbosus* Nuttall, 1916, *Ann. Parasitol. Hum. Comp.*, 45, 661, 1970.

452. **Saratsiotis, A. and Battelli, C.**, Comparison morphologique d'une nouvelle espece de tique dans la faune d'Italie *Ixodes gibbosus* Nuttall, 1916 avec les especes voisines, *Parassitologia (Rome)*, 14, 183, 1972.

453. **Savenko, S. N. and Ruzinova, Yu. G.**, The clinical picture and symptomatology of a hemorrhagic fever type of disease in Bukovina, *Nevropatol. Psikhiatr.*, 20, 56, 1951; in Russian.

454. **Schulze, P.**, Die heutige Verbreitung einzelner Tierarten im Lichte der ergeschichtlichen Vergangenheit (besonders der Zecken *Dermacentor reticulatus* Auct. und *Hyalomma marginatum* Koch), *Z. Morphol. Oekol. Tiere*, 15, 735, 1929.

455. **Semashko, I. V., Chumakov, M. P., Bannova, G. G., Ismailova, S. T., Berezin, V. V., Bernshtein, A. D., Reshetnikov, I. A., and Khankishiev, A. M.**, Isolation and study of CCHF virus strain K-618 from *Hyalomma pl. plumbeum* ticks collected in Azerbaijan SSR, *Tezisy 17. Nauchn. Sess. Inst. Posvyashch. Aktual. Probl. Virus. Profilakt. Virus. Zabolev*, Moscow, October 1972, 373; in Russian. (In English, NAMRU3-T1077.)

456. **Semashko, I. V., Chumakov, M. P., Karapetyan, R. M., Vorob'ev, A. G., Zavodova, T. I., Matevosyan, K. Sh., Nersesyan, M. A.**, First isolation of the CHF virus in Armenia from the blood of the patient with Crimean hemorrhagic fever, *Tr. Inst. Polio. Virusn. Entsefalitov Akad. Med. Nauk SSSR*, 22, 25, 1974; in Russian. (In English, NAMRU3-T1029.)

457. **Semashko, I. V., Chumakov, M. P., and Matevosyan, K. Sh.**, Production of CHF-Congo virus group plaques (colonies) in piglet kidney tissue culture, *Tr. Inst. Polio. Virusn. Entsefalitov Akad. Med. Nauk SSSR*, 22, 165, 1974; in Russian. (In English, NAMRU3-T935.)

458. **Semashko, I. V., Chumakov, M. P., Matevosyan, K. Sh., Safarov, R. K., Marutyan, E. M., Postoyan, S. R., Karapetyan, R. M., Bashkirtsev, V. N., Tkachenko, E. A., and Chunikhin, S. P.**, Results from the 1972-1974 works on isolation and investigation of CHF-Congo, Dhori, and Bhanja viruses in Azerbaijan and Armenia, *Tezisy Konf. Vop. Med. Virus*, (Moscow, October 1975,) 354; in Russian. (In English, NAMRU3-T1010.)

459. **Semashko, I. V., Chumakov, M. P., Safarov, R. I., Tkachenko, E. A., Bashkirtsev, V. N., and Chunikhin, S. P.**, Isolation and identification of Crimean hemorrhagic fever and Dhori-Astra virus strains from *Hyalomma plumbeum plumbeum* ticks collected in the Azerbaijan SSSR, *Tr. Inst. Polio Virusn. Entsefalitov Akad. Med. Nauk SSSR*, 22, 57, 1974; in Russian. (In English, NAMRU3-T1031.)

460. **Semashko, I. V., Dobritsa, P. G., Bashkirtsev, V. N., and Chumakov, M. P.**, Results from investigating blood sera from healthy persons, animals, and birds collected in southern Kazakhstan for antibodies to CHF-Congo virus, *Mater. 9. Simp. Ekol. Virus.*, Dushanbe, October 1975, 43; in Russian. (In English, NAMRU3-T1128.)

461. **Semashko, I. V., Shalunova, N. V., Karmysheva, V. Ya., and Chumakov, M. P.**, Isolation and reproduction of a few Crimean hemorrhagic fever virus strains in tissue cultures using the fluorescent antibody technique for virus study, *Tr. Inst. Polio. Virusn. Entsefalitov Akad. Med. Nauk SSSR*, 7, 215, 1965; in Russian. (In English, NAMRU3-T814.)

462. **Semyatkovskaya, Z. V. and Sudtdykova, N. K.**, On the clinical aspects of infectious hemorrhagic fever, *Klin. Med. (Moscow)*, 28, 69, 1950; in Russian.

463. **Seneviratna, P.**, The Ixodoidea (ticks) of Ceylon. II and III, *Ceylon Vet. J.*, 13, 28, 1965.

464. **Shalunova, N. V., Semashko, I. V., and Chumakov, M. P.**, Plaque formation of CHF virus in tissue cultures, *Tr. Inst. Polio. Virusn. Entsefalitov Akad. Med. Nauk SSSR*, 7, 209, 1965; in Russian. (In English, NAMRU3-T813.)

465. **Shanmugam, Dzh., Smirnova, S. E., and Chumakov, M. P.**, Detection of antibodies to CHF-Congo viruses in human and domestic animal blood sera in India, *Tr. Inst. Polio. Virusn. Entsefalitov Akad. Med. Nauk SSSR*, 21, 149, 1973; in Russian. (In English, NAMRU3-T955.)

466. **Shanmugam, Dzh., Smirnova, S. E., and Chumakov, M. P.**, Presence of antibody to arboviruses of the Crimean haemorrhagic fever-Congo (CHF-Congo) group in human beings and domestic animals in India, *Indian J. Med. Res.*, 64, 1403, 1976.

467. **Shapiro, S. E. and Barkagan, Z. S.**, History of haemorrhagic fever in Central Asia, *Vopr. Virusol.*, 5, 245, 1960; in Russian.

468. **Shapiro, S. E. and Barkagan, Z. S.**, History of haemorrhagic fever in Central Asia, *Probl. Virol. (USSR)*, 5, 267, 1960.

469. **Shapiro, S. E. and Levinzon, E. N.**, Epidemiological and clinical peculiarities of Central Asiatic strains of haemorrhagic fever, *Voen. Med. Zh.*, 3, 55, 1955; in Russian.

470. **Shapiro, S. E. and Zhitomirsky, V. K.**, *Hemorrhagic Fever*, Stalinabad, 1953; in Russian.

471. **Shaw, J. H. and Hood, M. W.**, Index-Catalogue of Medical and Veterinary Zoology. Parasite-Subject Catalogue: Parasites: Arthropoda and Miscellaneous Phyla, Suppl. 20, Part. 5, U.S. Department of Agriculture, Washington, D.C., 1975, 223.

472. **Shcherbinina, O. Kh.**, Bird hosts of *Hyalomma plumbeum* (Panzer) ticks in Turkmenia, *Izv. Akad. Nauk Turkm. SSR, Biol. Nauk*, 5, 54, 1971; in Russian. (In English, NAMRU3-T588.)

473. **Shestopalova, N. M., Reingol'd V. N., Averina, S. M., and Smirnova, S. E.**, Electron microscope study of Hazara virus in white mouse brains, *Tezisy Konf. Vop. Med. Virus.*, Moscow, October 1975, 375; in Russian. (In English, NAMRU3-T1193.)

474. **Shevchenko, S. F., Bul'ba, N. P., and Turchinov, G. A.**, Contribution to the study of effect of acaricides on certain ixodid ticks species. II. Effect of acaricidal properties on unfed adult *Hyalomma plumbeum* Panzer in experimental conditions, *Mater. 3. Oblast. Nauchn. Prakt. Konf.*, Rostov-on-Don, May 1970, 162; in Russian. (In English, NAMRU3-T551.)

475. **Sidorova, G. A.**, Some problems concerned with the existence of arbovirus natural foci in arid regions of Uzbekistan, *Sb. Tr. Ekol. Virus.*, 2, 98, 1974; in Russian. (In English, NAMRU3-T774.)

476. **Simpson, D. I. H.**, The susceptibility of *Arvicanthis abyssinicus* (Rüppell) to infection with various arboviruses, *Trans. R. Soc. Trop. Med. Hyg.*, 60, 248, 1966.

477. **Simpson, D. I. H.**, Arboviruses and free-living wild animals, *Symp. Zool. Soc. London*, 24, 13, 1969.

478. **Simpson, D. I. H.**, Arbovirus diseases, *Br. Med. Bull.*, 28, 10, 1972.

479. **Simpson, D. I. H., Knight, E. M., Courtois, G., Williams, M. C., Weinbren, M. P., and Kibukamusoke, J. W.**, Congo virus: a hitherto undescribed virus occurring in Africa. I. Human isolations — clinical notes, *East Afr. Med. J.*, 44, 87, 1967.

480. **Simpson, D. I. H. and Lule, M.**, Further experimental infection in *Arvicanthis abyssinicus*, *Rep. E. Afr. Virus. Res. Inst. (1963—1964)*, 14, 48, 1965.

481. **Simpson, D. I. H., Williams, M. C., and Woodall, J. P.**, Four cases of human infection with the Congo agent, *Rep. E. Afr. Virus Res. Inst. (1963—1964)*, 14, 27, 1965.

482. **Sipovsky, P. V.**, Atypical cases of gastro-intestinal hemorrhage, *Klin. Med. (Moscow)*, 22, 64, 1944; in Russian.

483. **Skofertsa, P. G., Korchmar', N. D., Yarovoy, P. I., and Gaidamovich, S. Ya.**, Isolation of Kharagysh virus of the Kemerovo group from common starlings (*Sturnus vulgaris* L.) in Moldavian SSR, *Sb. Tr. Inst. imeni D. I. Ivanovsky, Akad. Med. Nauk SSSR*, 1, 100, 1974; in Russian. (In English, NAMRU3-T1154.)

484. **Skvortsova, T. M., Kurbanov, M. M., Gromashevsky, V. L., L'vov, D. K., Aristova, V. A. Neronov, V. M., and Berdiev, A.**, Identification of Wad Medani virus in Turkmen SSR, *Mater. 9. Simp. Ekol. Virus.*, Dushanbe, October 1975, 45; in Russian. (In English, NAMRU3-T1130.)

485. **Smirnova, S. E. and Chumakov, M. P.**, Comparative study of CHF and Congo virus strains, *Tezisy 17. Nauchn. Sess. Inst. Posvyashch. Aktual. Probl. Virus. Profilakt. Virus. Zabolev.* Moscow, October 1972, 340; in Russian. (In English, NAMRU3-T1052.)

486. **Smirnova, S. E. and Chumakov, M. P.**, Study of the distribution area of arboviruses of the CHF-Congo-Hazara group, *Tezisy Konf. Vop. Med. Virus.*, Moscow, October 1975, 356; in Russian. (In English, NAMRU3-T988.)

487. **Smirnova, S. E., Daniyarov, O. A., Zgurskaya, G. N., Kasymov, K. T., Pavlovich, A. N., Pak, T. P., Chumakov, M. P., and Yasinsky, A. V.**, Serological examination of people and animals for antibodies to Crimean hemorrhagic fever virus in the Tadzhik, SSR, 1968, *Tr. Inst. Polio Virusn. Entsefalitov Akad. Med. Nauk SSSR,* 19, 66, 1971; in Russian. (In English, NAMRU3-T964.)

488. **Smirnova, S. E., Genis, D. E., Zgurskaya, G. N., and Chumakov, M. P.**, Isolation of CHF virus from the blood of a patient in Kzyl-Orda Oblast, Kazakh SSR, *Tezisy 17. Nauchn. Sess. Inst. Posvyashch. Aktual. Probl. Virus. Profilakt. Virus. Zabolev,* Moscow, October 1972, 372; in Russian. (In English, NAMRU3-T1076.)

489. **Smirnova, S. E., Nepesova, N. M., Tachmuradov, G., Kir'yanova, A. M., and Chumakov, M. P.**, Materials on the study of Crimean hemorrhagic fever in the Turkmen SSR, *Tr. Inst. Polio. Virusn. Entsefalitov Akad. Med. Nauk SSSR,* 19, 86, 1971; in Russian. (In English, NAMRU3-T804.)

490. **Smirnova, S. E., Shalunova, N. V., and Mart'yanova, L. I.**, Study of Samarkand and Rostov viral strains of the Crimean hemorrhagic fever type, *Mater. 15. Nauchn. Sess. Inst. Polio. Virus. Entsefalitov,* October 1968, 96; in Russian. (In English, NAMRU3-T868.)

491. **Smirnova, S. E., Shanmugam, D., Nepesova, N. M., Filipenko, P. I., Mamaev, V. I., Chumakov, M. P.**, Isolation of Crimean hemorrhagic fever virus from *Hyalomma asiaticum* ticks collected in the Turkmenian SSR, *Tr. Inst. Polio. Virusn. Entsefalitov Akad. Med. Nauk SSSR,* 22, 176, 1974; in Russian. (In English, NAMRU3-T940.)

492. **Smirnova, S. E., Shestopalova, N. M., Reingol'd, V. N., Zubri, G. L., and Chumakov, M. P.**, Experimental Hazara virus infection in mice, *Acta Virol. (Engl. Ed.)* 21, 128, 1977.

493. **Smirnova, S. E., Zgurskaya, G. N., Genis, D. E., and Chumakov, M. P.**, Isolation of Crimean hemorrhagic fever virus from *Hyalomma asiaticum* ticks collected in Kzylorda Region of the Kazakh SSSR, *Tr. Inst. Polio. Virusn. Entsefalitov Akad. Med. Nauk SSSR,* 19, 41, 1971; in Russian. (In English, NAMRU3-T951.)

494. **Smirnova, S. E., Zgurskaya, G. N., Nepesova, N. M., Pak, T. P., Chumakov, M. P., and Chunikhin, S. P.**, Examination of animal blood samples in Central Asia for antibodies to Crimean hemorrhagic fever virus (CHF), *Mater. 16. Nauchn. Sess. Inst. Polio. Virus. Entsefalitov,* 2, 146, 1969; in Russian. (In English, NAMRU3-T820.)

495. **Smirnova, S. E., Zubri, G. L., Savinov, A. P., and Chumakov, M. P.**, Pathogenesis of experimental Crimean hemorrhagic fever infection in newborn white mice, *Acta Virol. (Engl. Ed.),* 17, 409, 1973.

496. **Smith, A. L., Tignor, G. H., Mifune, K., and Motohashi, T.**, Isolation and assay of rabies serogroup viruses in CER cells, *Intervirology,* 8, 92, 1977.

497. **Smorodintsev, A. A.**, Tickborne spring-summer encephalitis, *Prog. Med. Virol.,* 1, 210, 1958.

498. **Sokolov, A. A., Chumakov, M. P., and Kolachev, A. A., Eds.**, *Crimean Hemorrhagic Fever (Acute Infectious Capillary Toxicosis),* Otd. Primorskoi Armii, Simferopol, 1945; in Russian.

499. **Sokolova, E. I., Mirzoeva, M., and Kulieva, N. M.**, Isolation of arboviruses from ticks in Azerbaijan SSR, *Tezisy Dokl. 3. Vses. Soveshch. Akarol.,* Tashkent, October 1976, 218; in Russian. (In English, NAMRU3-T1161.)

500. **Sokolova, E. I., Mirzoeva, N. M., Kulieva, N. M., Sultanova, Z. D., Kanbai, I. G., Obukhova, V. R., and Gaidamovich, S. Ya.**, Islands of Baku Archipelago-natural arbovirus foci, *Sb. Tr. Ekol. Virus,* 1, 126, 1973; in Russian. (In English, NAMRU3-T715.)

501. **Starkoff, O.**, *Ixodoidea d'Italia. Studio monografico,* II Pensiero Scientifico Editore, Rome, 1958, 385.

502. **Starkov, O. A. and E. S. Kalmykov**, Ixodid ticks of Tadzhikistan and other landscape associations, *Tr. Inst. Polio. Virusn. Entsefalitov Akad. Med. Nauk SSSR,* 19, 195, 1971; in Russian. (In English, NAMRU3-T944.)

503. **Starkov, O. A., Kuima, A. U., Panova, V. V., and Kalymkov, E. S.**, The species composition of ixodid ticks and their hosts in foci of Crimean hemorrhagic fever in Tadzhikistan, *Tr. Inst. Polio. Virusn. Entsefalitov Akad. Med. Nauk SSSR,* 19, 190, 1971; in Russian. (In English, NAMRU3-T963.)

504. **Stefanov, S. B. and Smirnova, S. E.**, Morphometric differences in cell cultures infected with CHF, Congo and Hazara viruses, *Tezisy Konf. Vop. Med. Virus,* Moscow, October 1975, 359; in Russian. (In English, NAMRU3-T1196.)

505. **Stim, T. B.**, Arbovirus plaquing in two simian kidney cell lines, *J. Gen. Virol.,* 5, 329, 1969.

506. **Stolbov, D. N., Butenko, A. M., Egorova, P. S., Leshchinskaya, E. V., and Chumakov, M. P.**, Crimean hemorrhagic fever (CHF) in Astrakhan Oblast, *Tr. Inst. Polio. Virusn. Entsefalitov Akad. Med. Nauk SSSR,* 7, 271, 1965; in Russian. (In English, NAMRU3-604.)

507. Subcommittee on Information Exchange American Committee on Arthropod-borne Viruses, Catalogue of arthropod-borne viruses of the world, *Am. J. Trop. Med. Hyg.,* 19, 1082, 1970.

508. **Surbova, St.,** Distribution, biology and ecology of Ixodidae in the Balchish region with special considerations on epizootiologic and epidemiologic factors, *Suvrem. Med.,* 6, 13, 1955; in Bulgarian.

509. **Surbova, St.,** Species composition and seasonal dynamics of ticks of the family Ixodidae in Iskra Village, district of Pervomaisk., *Tr. Nauchno Issled. Inst. Epidemiol. Mikrobiol.,* 3, 209, 1956; in Bulgarian.

510. **Surbova, St.,** Verbreitung und epidemiologische Bedeutung der Zecken von der Famille Ixodidae in Bulgarien, *Izv. Zool. Inst. Sofiya,* 15, 135, 1964; in Bulgarian, Russian, and German summaries.

511. **Sureau, P., Ed.,** *Rapport sur le fonctionnement technique de l'Institut Pasteur de Bangui, 1974,* 1974, 162.

512. **Sureau, P., Cornet, J. P., Germain, M., Camicas, J. L., and Robin, Y.,** Enquête sur les arbovirus transmis par les tiques en Republique Centrafricaine (1973—1974). Isolement des virus Dugbe, CHF/Congo. Jos et Bhanja, *Bull. Soc. Pathol. Exot.,* 69, 28, 1976.

513. **Tatarskaya, G. A., Reznikova, O. Yu., Milyutin, V. N., and Kukharchuk, O. N.,** Investigation of Crimean hemorrhagic fever virus in human leukocyte cell culture, *Tezisy 17. Nauchn. Sess. Inst. Posvyashch. Aktual. Probl. Virus. Profilakt. Virus Zabolev,* Moscow, October 1972, 371; in Russian. (In English, NAMRU3-T1075.)

514. **Taylor, R. M.,** Purpose and progress in cataloguing and exchanging information on arthropod-borne viruses. The 26th Charles Franklin Craig Lecture, *Am. J. Trop. Med. Hyg.,* 11, 169, 1962.

515. **Taylor, R. M.,** Catalogue of Arthropod-Borne Viruses of the World, No. 1760, Public Health Service Publications, Washington, D.C., 1967, 898.

516. **Taylor, R. M., Hoogstraal, H., and Hurlbut, H. S.,** Isolation of a virus (Wad Medani) from *Rhipicephalus sanguineus* collected in Sudan, *Am. J. Trop. Med. Hyg.,* 15, 75, 1966.

517. **Tekut'ev, I. V., Lobanov, V. V., and Perelatov, V. D.,** Hemorrhagic fever in Krasnyy Sulin, *Mater. 3. Oblast Nauchn. Prakt. Konf.,* Rostov-on-Don, May 1970, 83; in Russian. (In English, NAMRU3-T536.)

518. **Temirbekov, Zh., Dobritsa, P. G., Kontaruk, V. M., Vainshtein, E. K., Marushchak, O. N., Dobritsa, and Shvets, M. Ya.,** Investigation of Crimean hemorrhagic fever in Chimkent Region of the Kazakh SSR, *Tr. Inst. Polio. Virusn. Entsefalitov Akad. Med. Nauk SSSR,* 19, 160, 1971; in Russian. (In English, NAMRU3-T949.)

519. **Terekhov, G. N.,** Pathological anatomy of Uzbekistan hemorrhagic fever, *Vopr. Kraev. Patol. Akad. Nauk Uzbek. SSR,* 2, 59, 1952; in Russian. (In English, NAMRU3-T215.)

520. **Ter-Vartanov, V. N., Gusev, V. M., Reznik, P. A., Guseva, A. A., Mirzoeva, M. N., Bocharnikov, O. N., and Bakeev, N. N.,** Contribution to the transmission of ticks and fleas by birds. Second communication, *Zool. Zh.,* 35, 173, 1956; in Russian.

521. **Theiler, A. (Sir),** Un nouveau medicament pour le traitement des piroplasmoses, *Bull. Soc. Pathol. Exot.,* 23, 506, 1930.

522. **Timofeev, E. M., Grebenyuk, Yu. I., Karas', F. R., Osipova, N. Z., and Tsirkin, Yu. M.,** Characteristics of CHF natural foci in southeastern Osh Oblast, Kirgiz SSR, *Mater. Simp. Itogi 6. Simp. Izuch. Virus. Ekol. Svyazan. Ptits.,* Omsk, December 1971, 103, 1972; in Russian. (In English, NAMRU3-T670.)

523. **Timofeev, E. M., Shakhgil'dyan, I. V., Rybin, S. N., Grebenyuk, Yu. I., and Karas', F. R.,** Results of serological examination of human blood sera and domestic animals with 15 arboviruses in southwestern districts of Osh Oblast in Kirgiz SSR, *Sb. Tr. Inst. Virus. imeni D. I. Ivanovsky Akad. Med. Nauk SSSR,* 1, 80, 1973; in Russian. (In English, NAMRU3-T694.)

524. **Timoshek, G. M. and Kantorovich, R. A.,** Test on clinical-cytogenic study of Crimean hemorrhagic fever, *Mater. 16. Nauchn. Sess. Inst. Polio. Virus. Entsefalitov,* 2, 149, 1969; in Russian. (In English, NAMRU3-T852.)

525. **Tkachenko, E. A., Butenko, A. M., Badalov, M. E., and Chumakov, M. P.,** Results of remote revaccination against Crimean hemorrhagic fever, *Tezisy 17. Nauch. Sess. Inst. Posvyashch. Aktual. Probl. Virus. Profilakt. Virus. Zabolev.,* Moscow, October 1972, 349; in Russian. (In English, NAMRU3-T1058.)

526. **Tkachenko, E. A., Butenko, A. M., Badalov, M. E., Zavodova, T. I., and Chumakov, M. P.,** Investigation of the immunogenic activity of killed brain vaccine against Crimean hemorrhagic fever, *Tr. Inst. Polio. Virusn. Entsefalitov Akad. Med. Nauk SSSR,* 19, 119, 1971; in Russian. (In English, NAMRU3-T931.)

527. **Tkachenko, E. A., Butenko, A. M., Butenko, S. A., Zavodova, T. I., and Chumakov, M. P.,** Characteristics of prophylactic vaccine against Crimean hemorrhagic fever, *Mater. 3. Oblast. Nauchn. Prakt. Konf.,* Rostov-on-Don, May 1970, 136; in Russian. (In English, NAMRU3-T546.)

528. **Tkachenko, E. A., Khanun, K., and Berezin, V. V.**, Serological investigation of human and animal sera in agar gel diffusion and precipitation (AGDP) test for the presence of antibodies of Crimean hemorrhagic fever and Grand Arbaud viruses,, *Mater. 16. Nauchn. Sess. Inst. Polio. Virus. Entsefalitov*, 2, 265, 1969; in Russian. (In English, NAMRU3-T620.)

529. **Todorov, T., Dzhankov, I., and Lekov, Zh.**, Epidemiological significance of the tick *Hyalomma plumbeum* (Panz.) in Bulgaria, *Vet. Med. Nauki*, 3, 961, 1966; in Bulgarian, Russian and English summaries.

530. **Topicu, V., Rosiu, N., Georgescu, L., Gherman, D., Arcan, P., and Csaky, N.**, Isolation of a cytopathic agent from the tick *Haemaphysalis punctata*, *Acta Virol. (Engl. Ed.)*, 12, 287, 1968.

531. **Tovornik, D.**, Tick fauna (Ixodidae) in foci of central European encephalitis, *Acta Parasitol. Iugosl.*, 1, 103, 1970; in Croatian, English summary.

532. **Tovornik, D.**, On natural foci of tickborne meningoencephalitis in Slovenia, *Celj. Zb.*, 159, 1974; in Slovenian.

533. **Tovornik, D. and Brelih, S.**, Angaben über einige Zeckenarten aus Jugoslawischen gebieten des Adriabereiches, *Wiad. Parazytol*, 18, 731, 1973.

534. **Tovornik, D. and Černy, V.**, The ecology of the tick *Ixodes gibbosus* Nuttall, 1916 on the Island of Brač (Yugoslavia), *Biol. Vestn.*, 20, 89, 1972.

535. **Tsafrir, N. and Rauchbach, K.**, *Amblyomma variegatum* (Ixodoidea: Ixodidae) in Israel, *Isr. J. Zool.*, 22, 197, 1973.

536. **Tsafrir, N., Rauchbach, K., and Cohen, R.**, On the finding of *Amblyomma gemma* Dönitz 1909 in Israel, *Refu. Vet.*, 31, 90, 1974.

537. **Tsilinsky, Ya. Ya., Lebedev, A. D., Pak, T. P., Gromashevsky, V. L., Timofeev, E. M., Ershov, F. I., Tsirkin, Yu. M., and L'vov, D. K.**, Isolation of Crimean haemorrhagic fever (CHF) virus from *Hyalomma plumbeum* ticks in Tadzhikistan, *Mater. Simp. Itogi 6. Simp. Izuch. Virus. Ekol. Svyazan. Ptits.*, Omsk, December 1971, (1972), 94; in Russian. (In English, NAMRU3-T665.)

538. **Tsirkin, Yu. M., Karas', F. R., Timofeev, E. M., L'vov, D. K., Gromashevsky, V. L., Veselovskaya, O. V., Osipova, N. Z., Grebenyuk, Yu. I., and Vargina, S. G.**, Isolation of Crimean hemorrhagic fever virus (CHF) from *Hyalomma plumbeum* ticks in Kirgizia, *Mater. Simp. Itogi 6. Simp. Izuch. Virus. Ekol. Svyazan. Ptits.*, Omsk, December 1971. (1972), 98; in Russian. (In English, NAMRU3-T661.)

539. **Tsypkin, L. B., Smirnova, S. E., and Fleer, G. P.**, Morphological investigation of white mouse embryo brain cell cultures infected with CHF virus, *Tezisy 17. Nauchn. Sess. Inst. Posvyashch. Aktual. Probl. Virus. Profilakt. Virus. Profilakt. Virus. Zabolev.*, Moscow, October 1972, 569; in Russian. (In English, NAMRU3-T1089.)

540. **Tsypkin, L. B., Smirnova, S. E., and Fleer, G. P.**, Morphological and immunofluorescence study of Crimean hemorrhagic fever virus interaction with white mouse embryo brain cell cultures, *Acta Virol. (Engl. Ed.)*, 18, 264, 1974.

541. **Uspenskaya, I. B.**, Fauna and ecology of ixodid ticks of Moldavia: genera *Haemaphysalis* Koch and *Dermacentor* Koch, *Izv. Akad. Nauk Mold. SSR Ser. Zool.*, 5, 28, 1963; in Russian.

542. **Uspenskaya, I. G.**, Zoogeographical characteristics of ixodid tick fauna of Moldavian SSR, *Tr. 4. Nauchn. Konf. Parazitol. UkSSR Kiev*, 1963, 407; in Russian.

543. **Uspenskaya, I. G.**, Zoogeographical characteristics of the fauna of ixodid ticks in Moldavian SSR, *Parazity Zhivotn. Rast. Mold.*, 1963, 91; in Russian.

544. **Uspenskaya, I. G.**, Data on the fauna and ecology of ixodid ticks of Moldavia. Genus *Ixodes* Latr., *Parazity Zhivotn. Mold. Vopr. Kraev. Parazitol.*, 1963, 73; in Russian.

545. **Uspenskaya, I. G.**, Variability of some characters in three species of ixodid ticks in Moldavia, *Zool. Zh.*, 43, 815, 1964; in Russian, English summary.

546. **Uspenskaya, I. G.**, Biology of *Ixodes ricinus* L. in Moldavia conditions, *Tezisy Dokl. I. Akarol. Soveshch.*, 1966, 213; in Russian.

547. **Uspenskaya, I. G.**, Biology of *Haemaphysalis (Alloceraea) inermis* in Moldavia, *Abstr. 3. Int. Congr. Acarol.*, Prague, August to September 1971, 192; in Russian.

548. **Uspenskaya, I. G.**, Influence of culturing areas on the ixodid tick fauna, *Parazity Zhivotn. Rast. Akad. Nauk. Mold. SSR*, 7, 115, 1971; in Russian. (In English, NAMRU3-T649.)

549. **Uspenskaya, I. G.**, Biologic peculiarities of ticks *Haemaphysalis inermis* and *H. punctata* in Moldavia, *Parazity Zhivotn. Rast. Akad. Nauk. Mold. SSR*, 8, 75, 1972; in Russian.

550. **Uspenskaya, I. G.**, Ixodid tick fauna of Moldavia and cultivation of the republic territory, *Tr. 13. Mezhdunar. Entomol. Kongr.*, 3, 266, 1972; in Russian.

551. **Uspenskaya, I. G.**, Biology of *Haemaphysalis (Alloceraea) inermis* in Moldavia, *Proc. 3. Int. Congr. Acarol.*, Prague, August to September 1971, 1973, 483.

552. **Uspenskaya, I. G.**, Ecology of *Ixodes vespertilionis* Koch in Moldavia, *Proc. 3. Int. Congr. Parasitol.*, 2, 958, 1974.

553. **Uspenskaya, I. G. and Konovalov, Yu. N.,** Seasonal interchange of population composition of *Ixodes ricinus* L. in Moldavian SSR, *Parazity Zhivotn. Rast. Akad. Nauk. Mold. SSR,* 2, 187, 1966.

554. **Uspenskaya, I. G. and Konovalov, Yu. N.,** Contributions to the biology of *Ixodes apronophorus* P. Sch. in conditions of Moldavia, *Tezisy Dokl. 2. Akarol. Soveshch.,* 2, 175, 1970; in Russian.

555. **Uspenskaya, I. G. and Konovalov, Yu. N.,** *Ixodes apronophorus* focus in the Prut River floodland, *Parazity Zhivotn. Rast. Akad. Nauk Mold. SSR,* 5, 88, 1970; in Russian.

556. **Uspenskaya, I. G. and Motornyy, I. A.,** Ixodid ticks of Moldavia and some peculiarities of their ecology (*Rhipicephalus* Koch and *Hyalomma* Koch), *Parazity Zhivotn. Rast. Mold.,* 1963, 100; in Russian.

557. **Varma, M. G. R. and Smith, C. E. G.,** The epidemiology of louping ill in Ayrshire, Scotland, II. Ectoparasites of small mammals (Ixodidae), *Folia Parasitol.,* 18, 63, 1971.

558. **Vashkov, V. I. and Poleshchuk, V. D.,** Measures for control of vectors of CHF - *Hyalomma plumbeum plumbeum* Panz. ticks, *Tr. Inst. Polio. Virusn. Entsefalitov Akad. Med. Nauk SSSR,* 19, 239, 1971; in Russian. (In English, NAMRU3-T983.)

559. **Vashkov, V. I., Poleshchuk, V. D., Latyshev, V. I., Gleiberman, S. E., Stolbov, D. N., Tsetlin, V. M., and Zhuk, E. B.,** Investigation of the effect of some acaricidal preparations and repellents on ticks *Hyalomma plumbeum plumbeum* Panzer, *Tezisy 17. Nauchn. Sess. Inst. Posvyashch. Aktual. Probl. Virus. Profilakt. Virus. Zabolev.,* Moscow, October 1972, 376; in Russian. (In English, NAMRU3-T1080.)

560. **Vasilenko, S. M.,** Results of the investigation on etiology, epidemiologic features and the specific prophylactic of Crimean hemorrhagic fever (CHF) in Bulgaria, *Abstr. Inv. Pap. 9. Int. Congr. Trop. Med. Malar.,* 1, 32, 1973.

561. **Vasilenko, S. M., Chumakov, M. P., Butenko, A. M., Smirnova, S. E., Teokharova, M., and Popov, V.,** Contribution to the question of Crimean hemorrhagic fever (CHF) in Bulgaria, *Mater. 15. Nauchn. Sess. Inst. Polio. Virus. Entsefalitov,* 3, 90, 1968; in Russian. (In English, NAMRU3-T857.)

562. **Vasilenko, S. M., Katsarov, G., Kirov, I., Radev, M., and Arnaudov, G.,** Etiological diagnosis of Crimean hemorrhagic fever in Bulgaria, *Tezisy 17. Nauchn. Sess. Inst. Posvyashch. Aktual. Probl. Virus. Profilakt. Virus. Zabolev.,* Moscow, October 1972, 337; in Russian. (In English, NAMRU3-T1049.)

563. **Vasilenko, S. M., Katsarov, G., Levi, V., Minev, G., Kovacheva, O., Genov, I., Arnaudov, G., Pandryov, S., Arnaudov, Kh., and Kutsarova, Yu.,** Certain epidemiological characteristics of Crimean hemorrhagic fever (CHF) in Bulgaria, *Tezisy 17. Nauchn. Sess. Inst. Posvyashch. Aktual. Probl. Virus. Zabolev.* Moscow, October 1972, 338; in Russian. (In English, NAMRU3-T1050.)

564. **Vasilenko, S. M., Katsarov, G., Mikhailov, A., Teokharova, M., Levi, V., Levi, S., Kebedzhiev, G., Kirov, I. D., and Radev, M.,** Crimean hemorrhagic fever (CHF) in Bulgaria, *Tr. Inst. Polio. Virusn. Entsefalitov Akad. Med. Nauk SSSR,* 19, 100, 1971; in Russian. (In English, NAMRU3-T943.)

565. **Vasilenko, S. M., Kirov, I. D., Katsarov, G., Mikhailov, A., Radev, M., Kebedzhiev, G., Levi, V., and Levi, S.,** Studies on the Crimean type haemorrhagic fever in Bulgaria, *Letop. Chig. Epidem. Inst.,* 4, 153, 1970; in Bulgarian.

566. **Vesenjak, J., Calisher, C. H., Brudnjak, Z., and Tovornik, D.,** Report from the Andrija Stampar School of Public Health, Medical Faculty, University of Zagreb, Zagreb, Yugoslavia, *Arthropod-Borne Virus Inf. Exch.,* 28, 89, 1975.

567. **Walker, J. B.,** *Rhipicephalus pulchellus* Gerstäcker 1873: a description of the larva and nymph with notes on the adults and on its biology, *Parasitology,* 45, 95, 1955.

568. **Walker, J. B.,** *Notes on the Common Tick Species of East Africa,* Cooper, McDougall and Robertson, Nairobi, 1960, 23.

569. **Walker, J. B.,** *Notes on the Common Tick Species of East Africa,* 3rd ed., Cooper, McDougall and Robertson, Nairobi, 1970, 23.

570. **Walker, J. B.,** The ixodid ticks of Kenya, in *A review of Present Knowledge of Their Hosts and Distribution,* Commonwealth Institute of Entomology, London, 1974, 220.

571. **Walker, M. L., Rayburn, J. D., Shaw, J. H., Kirby, M. D., and Edwards, S. J.,** Index-Catalogue of Medical and Veterinary Zoology. Parasite-Subject Catalogue: Subject Headings and Treatment, Suppl. 19, Part 6, U.S. Department of Agriculture, Washington, D.C. 1974, 498.

572. **Weilgama, D. J. and Seneviratna, P.,** The Boophilids in Ceylon. Preliminary communication, *Ceylon Vet. J.,* 18, 39, 1970.

573. **Weinbren, M. P., Knight, E. M., Ellice, J. M., and Hewitt, L. E.,** Hitherto unknown strains of virus isolated from human serum, *Rep. E. Afr. Virus. Res. Inst. (1958—1959),* 9, 7, 1959.

574. **Williams, M. C., Tukei, P. M., Lule, M., Mujomba, E., Mukuye, A.,** Virology: identification studies, *Rep. E. Afr. Virus. Res. Inst. (1966),* 16, 24, 1967.

575. **Williams, M. C. and Woodall, J. P.,** Isolation studies on ticks collected in the Rift Valley, Kenya, *Rep. E. Afr. Virus. Res. Inst. (1959—1960),* 10, 34, 1960.

576. **Williams, R. E., Hoogstraal, H., Casals, J., Kaiser, M. N., and Moussa, M. I.,** Isolation of Wano-wrie, Thogoto, and Dhori viruses from *Hyalomma* ticks infesting camels in Egypt, *J. Med. Entomol.,* 10, 143, 1973.

577. **Williams, R. W., Causey, O. R., and Kemp. G. E.,** Ixodid ticks from domestic livestock in Ibadan, Nigeria as carriers of viral agents, *J. Med. Entomol.,* 9, 443, 1972.

578. **Woodall, J. P. and Williams, M. C.,** Two cases of Semunya virus infection, *Rep. E. Afr. Virus Res. Inst. (1960—1961),* 11, 20, 1961.

579. **Woodall, J. P., Williams, M. C., Santos, D. F., and Ellice, J. M.,** Virology: laboratory studies, *Rep. E. Afr. Virus Res. Inst. (1961—1962),* 12, 21, 1962.

580. **Woodall, J. P., Williams, M. C., and Simpson, D. I. H.,** Congo virus: a hitherto undescribed virus occurring in Africa. II. Identification studies, *East Afr. Med. J.,* 44, 93, 1967.

581. **Woodall, J. P., Williams, M. C., Simpson, D. I. H., Ardoin, P., Lule, M., and West, R.,** The Congo group of agents, *Rep. E. Afr. Virus Res. Inst. (1963—1964),* 14, 34, 1965.

582. **Work, T. H.,** Isolation and identification of arthropod-borne viruses, in *Diagnostic Procedures for Viral and Rickettsial Diseases,* 3rd Ed., Lennette, E. H. and Schmidt, N. J., Eds., American Public Health Association, New York, 1964, 312.

583. **Yanovich, T. D.,** Reports of the committee on coordinated study of prophylactic measures against Crimean hemorrhagic fever in Rostov Oblast, *Mater. 3. Oblast. Nauchn. Prakt. Konf.,* Rostov-on-Don, May 1970, 3; in Russian. (In English, NAMRU3-T521.)

584. **Yarovaya, O. P.,** Epidemiology and clinical picture of little studied endemic viral neuroinfections; hemorrhagic fever in Stavropol Region, encephalomeningitis, and lymphadenitis, (Avtoref. Diss. Soisk. Uchen. Step. Kand. Med. Nauk), Sverdlov. Gos. Med. Inst., Minist. Zdravookhr. RSFSR, Stavropol; 1970, in Russian. (In English, NAMRU3-T1181.)

585. **Yarovoy, L. V.,** Hemorrhagic fever endemics in Stavropol Region, *Tr. Stavrop. Obshch. Mikrobiol. Epidem. Infekts. im. Mechnikova (1955—1956),* 1956; in Russian.

586. **Yarovoy, L. V.,** Clinico-epidemiologic characteristics of hemorrhagic fever in Stavropol Region, *Tr. Inst. Polio. Virusn. Entsefalitov Akad. Med. Nauk SSSR,* 7, 255, 1965; in Russian. (In English, NAMRU3-T192.)

587. **Yarovoy, L. V. and Yarovaya, O. P.,** Endemic viral natural focal infections in Stavropol Region, *Sov. Med.,* 3, 80, 1969; in Russian. (In English, NAMRU3-T933.)

588. **Yeoman, G. H. and Walker, J. B.,** *The Ixodid Ticks of Tanzania. A study of the Zoogeography of the Ixodidae of an East African Country,* Commonwealth Institute of Entomology, London, 1967, 215.

589. **Yunker, C. E. and Cory, J.,** Plaque production by arboviruses in Singh's *Aedes albopictus* cells, *Appl. Microbiol.,* 29, 81, 1975.

590. **Zalutskaya, L. I.,** Reports of zoological and parasitological observtions in a hemorrhagic fever focus, *Mater. Konf. Kleshch. Entsefalitov Virus. Gemorragich. Likhoradki,* Omsk, December 1963, (1964) 359; in Russian. (In English, NAMRU3-T861.)

591. **Zarubinsky, V. Ya., Klisenko, G. A., Kuchin, V. V., Timchenko, V. V., and Shanoyan, N. K.,** Application of the indirect hemagglutination inhibition test for serological investigation of Crimean hemorrhagic fever focus in Rostov Oblast, *Sb. Tr. Inst. Virus. imeni D. I. Ivanovsky Akad. Med. Nauk SSSR,* 2, 73, 1975; in Russian. (In English, NAMRU3-T1145.)

592. **Zarubinsky, V. Ya., Kondratenko, V. F., Blagoveshchenskaya, N. M., Zarubina, L. V., and Kuchin, V. V.,** Susceptibility of calves and lambs to Crimean hemorrhagic fever virus, *Tezisy Dokl. 9. Vses. Konf. Prirod. Ochag. Bolez. Chelov. Zhivot.,* Omsk, May 1976, 130; in Russian. (In English, NAMRU3-T1178.)

593. **Zavodova, T. I., Butenko, A. M., Tkachenko, E. A., and Chumakov, M. P.,** Properties of the neutralization test in Crimean hemorrhagic fever, *Tr. Inst. Polio. Virusn. Entsefalitov Akad. Med. Nauk SSSR,* 19, 61, 1971; in Russian (In English, NAMRU3-T926.)

594. **Zavodova, T. I., Chumakov, M. P., Butenko, A. M., Tkachenko, E. A., and Karmysheva, V. Ya.,** Plaque formation in rodent-pathogenic strains of Crimean hemorrhagic fever (CHF) virus, *Mater. 16. Nauchn. Sess. Inst.* Polio. Virusn. Entsefalitov, 2, 132, 1969; in Russian. (In English, NAMRU3-T843.)

595. **Zeitlenok, N. A. and Mart'yanova, L. I.,** Serological investigations on hemorrhagic fever, *Tezisy Dokl. 4. Nauchn. Sess. Inst. Neurol. Akad. Med. Nauk SSSR,* 1949; in Russian.

596. **Zeitlenok, N. A., Vanag, K. A., and Pille, E. R.,** Cases of illness of the Crimean haemorrhagic fever type observed in the Astrakhan Oblast, *Probl. Virol. USSR,* 2, 90, 1957.

597. **Zgurskaya, G. N., Berezin, V. V., and Smirnova, S. E.,** Threshold levels of blood infectiousness for *Hyalomma p. plumbeum* tick during viremia in hares and rabbits caused by CHF virus, *Tezisy Konf. Vop. Med. Virus,* Moscow, October 1975, 291; in Russian. (In English, NAMRU3-T997.)

598. **Zgurskaya, G. N., Berezin, V. V., Smirnova, S. E., and Chumakov, M. P.,** Investigation of the question of Crimean hemorrhagic fever virus transmission and interepidemic survival in the tick *Halomma plumbeum plumbeum* Panzer, *Tr. Inst. Polio. Virusn. Entsefalitov Akad. Med. Nauk SSSR,* 19, 217, 1971; in Russian. (In English, NAMRU3-T911.)

599. **Zgurskaya, G. N. and Chumakov, M. P.,** Titration of antibodies to Crimean hemorrhagic fever virus in a drop from infected tissue culture suspension by the indirect immunofluorescence method, *Vopr. Virusol.,* 22, 606, 1977; in Russian. (In English, NAMRU3-T1289.)

600. **Zgurskaya, G. N., Chumakov, M. P., and Smirnova, S. E,** Titration of anibodies to CHF virus in drops of cell suspensions from infected tissue cultures by the indirect immuno-fluorescence method, *Tezisy Konf. Vop. Med. Virus.,* Moscow, October 1975, 293; in Russian. (In English, NAMRU3-T998.)

601. **Zgurskaya, G. N., Popov, G. V., Berezin, V. V., Smirnova, S. E., and Chumakov, M. P.,** Application of fluorescent antibody method (FAM) in detecting CHF virus in tick vectors, *Tezisy Dokl. Vop. Med. Virus. Inst. Virus. imeni Ivanovsky, D. I. Akad. Med. Nauk SSSR* (19-21 October), 2, 135, 1971; in Russian. (In English, NAMRU3-T509.)

602. **Zgurskaya, G. N., Smirnova, S. E., Berezin, V. V., and Chumakov, M. P.,** Investigation of susceptibility of *Hyalomma p. plumbeum* Panz. ticks to experimental infection with Crimean hemorrhagic fever (CHF) virus, *Tezisy 17. Nauchn. Sess. Inst. Posvyashch. Aktual. Probl. Virus. Profilakt. Virus. Zabolev.,* Moscow, October 1972, 360; in Russian. (In English, NAMRU3-T1068.)

603. **Zgurskaya, G. N., Smirnova, S. E., and Chumakov, M. P.,** Immunofluorescent antibody technique (FAT) application to detect Crimean hemorrhagic fever (CHF) virus in naturally infected ticks, *Tezisy 17. Nauchn. Sess. Inst. Posvyashch. Aktual. Probl. Virus. Profilakt. Virus. Zabolev.,* Moscow, October 1972, 362; in Russian. (In English, NAMRU3-T1069.)

604. **Zhdanov, V. M.,** Construction of a phylogenetic classification of viruses, *Mikrobiologiya,* 22, 206, 1953; in Russian.

605. **Zhdanov, V. M.,** Viruses of transmissive fevers and encephalitides, *Opred. Virus. Chelov. Zhivot,* 1953, 111; in Russian.

606. **Zhdanov, V. M.,** Order IV. Arthropodophiliales ord. nov., *Opred. Virus. Chelov. Zhivot.,* 1953, 273; in Russian.

607. **Zhmaeva, Z. M. and Pchelkina, A. A.,** Ixodoidea ticks and *Rickettsia burneti,* in *Biological Interrelationships of Bloodsucking Arthropods with the Agents of Human Diseases,* Petrishcheva, P. A., Ed., Akad. Med. Nauk SSR, Moscow, 1967, 59; in Russian.

608 **Zhmurova, O. P., Belokon', A. P., Khodykina, Z. S., Konstant, E. G., Leibman A. L., Andreeva, S. K., Klyushkina, E. A., and Domrachev, V. M.,** Liquidation methods of brucellosis, tularemia, malaria, and mosquito-borne and hemorrhagic fever in Crimea Oblast, *Vrach. Delo,* 10, 1964; in Russian.

609. **Zhukova, L. I.,** Test on individual protection of humans against ixodid ticks, *Tezisy Dokl. 3. Vses. Soveshch. Teoret. Priklad. Akarol.,* Tashkent, October 1976, 112; in Russian. (In English, NAMRU3-T1162.)

610. **Zhumatov, Kh. Zh. and Dmitrienko, N. K.,** *Features Specific to Natural Foci of Tick-Borne Encephalitis in Kazakhstan,* Medgiz, Moscow, 1961, 8.

611. **Zimina, Yu. V, Birulya, N. B., Berezin, V. V., Zalutskaya, L. I., Povalishina, T. P., and Stolbov, D. N.,** Materials on zoologico-parasitologic characteristics of Crimean hemorrhagic fever in Astrakhan Oblast, *Tr. Inst. Polio. Virusn. Entsefalitov Akad. Med. Nauk SSSR,* 7, 288, 1965; in Russian. (In English, NAMRU3-T197.)

612. **Zimina, Yu. V. and Ivanova, N. A.,** Importation of certain ixodid ticks to Astrakhan Oblast, *Tezisy Dokl. 3. Vses. Soveshch. Teoret. Priklad. Akarol.,* Tashkent, October 1976, 121; in Russian. (In English, NAMRU3-T1163.)

613. **Zubri, G. L., Savinov, A. P., Smirnova, S. E., and Chumakov, M. P.,** Histological and immunofluorescent investigations of newborne white mice infected with CHF virus, *Tezisy 17. Nauchn. Sess. Inst. Posvyashch. Aktual. Probl. Virus. Profilakt. Virus. Zabolev,* Moscow, October 1972, 346; in Russian. (In English, NAMRU3-T1056.)

RIFT VALLEY FEVER*

C. J. Peters and J. M. Meegan**

NAME AND SYNONYMS

The first detailed description of this disease was based on a sheep epizootic in an area where the great Rift Valley runs through Kenya, and the term Rift Valley fever (RVF) was applied to the disease and to the virus isolated as the causative agent of the epizootic.[1] The synonym "enzootic hepatitis" appears in the early literature but is now used infrequently.

HISTORY

RVF is a viral disease causing arthropod-borne epidemics in domestic animals, during which man is also infected. Sheep epizootics resembling RVF occurred in Kenya during the first two decades of the 20th century, but it was not until 1930 that Daubney, Hudson, and Garnham studied the disease in detail and established the viral etiology of RVF.[1] Initial scientific progress was rapid. Field observations and laboratory studies revealed that: (1) a wide variety of domestic, wild, and laboratory animals were susceptible to RVF virus infection with the characteristic pathological lesion being focal liver necrosis; (2) the virus could be isolated from, and transmitted by, a number of mosquito species; and (3) many African nations had serological evidence of human or animal infection by RVF virus.[2]

The disease caused periodic epizootics, but until 1977 was always geographically limited to sub-Saharan Africa. During many epizootics (and as a result of numerous laboratory infections), human RVF was described as a mild, dengue-like, febrile illness.[3,4] However, during the 1975 epizootic in South Africa, severe clinical disease was reported in a small number of people, and the first fatalities directly ascribable to RVF were documented.[5] In 1977, the disease was reported in a new geographic area, Egypt, and extensive human involvement with numerous fatalities occurred during the epizootic.[6,7]

The Egyptian epizootic re-emphasized the importance of this disease, as well as our lack of detailed understanding of the epidemiology, virology, and pathogenesis of RVF. It also served as a graphic example of the potential of RVF to circulate in a number of differing geographic and climatic settings, since the virus has now spread in a 7000-km north-south range throughout Africa. The reader is referred to two excellent reviews of RVF by Weiss[8] and Easterday.[2] This chapter will briefly review and update our current scientific knowledge of RVF.

ETIOLOGY

Classification

The virus was, until recently, classified as an ungrouped, arthropod-borne virus, with no serological relationship to other viruses.[9] However, accumulating morphological and molecular evidence now indicates that RVF virus is similar to viruses in the family Bunyaviradae.[10] Furthermore, Shope has recently discovered that Rift Valley

* The views of the authors do not purport to reflect the positions of the Department of the Army, the Department of the Navy, or the Department of Defense.

** Dr. Meegan was supported by funds from research project MR 041.09.01-0165, Naval Medical Research and Development Command, National Naval Medical Center, Bethesda, Md.

fever virus crossreacts serologically with the Phlebotomus fever group (Gordil, St. Floris, Punta Toto, Candiru, and perhaps others) by hemagglutination-inhibition tests.[11] This antigenic cross reactivity has been confirmed by indirect fluorescent antibody tests.[12]

Physical and Molecular Characterization

Electron micrographs of virions reveal a spherical viral particle, 90 to 100 nm in diameter, apparently with surface projections similar to other Bunyaviridae viruses.[10,13] The virion has a density of 1.21 in CsCl, and mild detergent treatment frees a nucleocapsid of density 1.29. The nucleocapsid contains a 23,000-dalton molecular weight, nonglycosylated protein as determined by sodium dodecyl sulfate polyacrylamide gel electrophoresis (SDS-PAGE). Two surface glycoproteins have been identified with apparent molecular weights of 65,000 and 70,000 daltons.[14] The virion contains three unique RNA species (designated L, M, and S) with molecular weights by SDS-PAGE of 2.7, 1.7, and 0.6×10^6 daltons.[15] These properties are similar to those shared by the family Bunyaviradae,[16] and by extrapolation, the RNA of RVF virus will probably be found to be of single, negative strandedness, and associated with an RNA polymerase.

The presence of a segmented genome provides a mechanism for high-frequency genetic recombination or reassortment of the segments if a cell is infected with more than one virus. This phenomenon is used to engineer vaccines, and may well participate in the natural evolution of the myxovirus influenza A.[17] Two closely related bunyaviruses, LaCrosse and Snowshoe Hare, have been shown to exchange segments under laboratory circumstances,[18] but the role of reassortment in the evolution of RVF or other bunyaviruses in nature is unknown.

The virus is sensitive to lipid solvents, hemagglutinates sheep erythrocytes, and is inactivated quickly at low pH (≤ 6.8). However, the virus is very resistant to temperatures less than 60°C, and can readily be recovered from serum after several months storage at 4°C or 3 hr at 56°C.[4, 19-22]

RVF virus readily grows in most commonly used cell cultures, except lymphoblastoid cell lines.[12,23,24] Like other bunyaviruses, the virions form by budding from membranes of the endoplasmic reticulum and the Golgi apparatus, and are released by exocytosis and/or cell lysis.[10] Plaques form readily under agar in many cell culture systems, including Vero, LLC-MK$_2$, and BHK-21.[23,24]

Virus strains

Most field virus isolates are regarded as identical. Weinbren, Williams, and Haddow[25] made three isolates of an unusual variant of RVF in the Lunyo forest in Uganda. The Lunyo isolates differ from classical RVF virus strains in being less pathogenic for adult mice by peripheral inoculation, by producing a more encephalitic clinical picture in adult mice, by decreased stability on storage, and by failure to hemagglutinate goose erythrocytes. There may be serological differences as well.[26] Nevertheless, serial mouse liver passage results in the emergence of classical RVF virus.

Recently the prototype isolate from the Egyptian outbreak was compared to 1951 and 1975 South African isolates and a 1944 Ugandan isolate. They were indistinguishable by polyacrylamide gel electrophoresis of virion polypeptides,[14] plaque reduction neutralization tests, or pathogenicity for six laboratory rodents.[12] The Egyptian strain was 100,000-fold more pathogenic for the appropriate laboratory rat.[12] Although this enhanced pathogenicity for rats has been confirmed for other Egyptian isolates, the biological significance of this observation is unclear.

With the exception of the Lunyo variant, recently isolated RVF strains kill adult mice after peripheral or intracranial inoculation by producing extensive hepatic necrosis and are referred to as "pantropic".[27,28] These viruses are also capable of causing encephalitis in the occasional infected mouse surviving acute hepatitis,[12,29,30] or in situations where the liver is protected by therapeutic measures which have low efficiency in the central nervous system, such as passive antibody administration.[12] When pantropic RVF strains are cloned,[12,31] passed in tissue culture,[32] passed intracerebrally in mice,[32-34] or otherwise manipulated,[29,32,35] virus stocks with very different properties may be generated. Some of these strains are truly "neurotropic" and produce encephalitis after peripheral inoculation. Others (which are also referred to as "neurotropic") are attenuated and produce no disease after peripheral inoculation, but retain the ability to cause encephalitis after intracranial injection. Some of these strains have been used as animal vaccines[32,34,36] (*vide infra*) although their stability on further passage is controversial.

DEFINITION

RVF is an acute, infectious disease of man and domestic animals, at this time probably confined to the African continent. The virus is maintained in a poorly understood sylvatic cycle; under appropriate conditions it produces typical arthropod-borne epidemics, particularly in sheep and cattle. Domestic livestock is both a major amplifier of virus transmission and a major impact of the epidemic. Adult animals may die with hepatic necrosis; pregnant animals abort, and, as a rule, neonates die. Man may be infected by arthropods, aerosols, or contact with infected tissues. Human beings usually suffer a self-limited acute febrile disease, but a small proportion may die from hemorrhagic fever, develop severe encephalitis, or be blinded by retinal lesions.

ANIMAL INFECTION

Clinical Manifestations in Domestic Animals

The two initial papers on RVF, the field observations of Daubney and his colleagues in Kenya[1] and the laboratory studies of Findlay at the Wellcome Laboratories,[21] are still unsurpassed for accurate descriptions of the disease and are combined with the other field and laboratory observations in this summary.[37-42] The most susceptible field animals of veterinary interest are the lamb, calf, and kid, with the adults of these species being more resistant to fatal RVF.

In lambs, calves, and kids (less than 7 days old) there is an incubation period of 12 to 18 hr with death in 24 to 48 hr. The animals first appear listless and anorectic; this is followed by rapid onset of vomiting, a staggering gait, and frequently pyrexia, a mucopurulent discharge from the nose, and diarrhea. The adult sheep experiences a distinctly less severe but similar clinical syndrome, including: temperature rise (104 to 106°F) which lasts for 1 to 4 days, rapid pulse, unsteady gait, and sometimes, nasal discharge, erosion of the tongue and skin of the scrotum, and death. Pregnant ewes abort; this may be the only overt clinical sign of disease in these animals. Adult cattle and goats display a disease similar to that of adult sheep.

Field studies and laboratory investigations indicate that within 2 to 6 days after RVF infects a flock of sheep, 90 to 100% of lambs under 7 days of age die, 20 to 60% of older lambs and adult sheep die, and 95 to 100% of the pregnant ewes abort. The statistics are less definitive for cattle, but 10 to 70% of calves and 10 to 20% of adult cattle die, milk production decreases, and 80 to 100% of the pregnant cows abort. Other domestic animal data are limited, but losses could be extensive among goats and probably domestic African buffaloes and camels. Swine and horses do not become ill.

Experimentally infected lambs, sheep, calves, cattle, and goats may have peak serum virus titers as high as 10^{10} MICLD$_{50}$/mℓ and viremias last 1 to 7 days. Viremia is followed by the development of antibodies measurable by the hemagglutination-inhibition (HI), complement fixation (CF), neutralization (N) and fluorescent antibody (FA) tests.[43,44]

Pathology of Domestic Animals

The characteristic pathologic lesion in all species carefully investigated is focal liver necrosis, usually midzonal in distribution. Several workers have studied lambs and sheep in detail; the following description was formulated from their observations.[2,21,37,45,46] In lambs, the liver usually appears yellow or discolored, but is infrequently enlarged. Necrotic foci associated with hemorrhages are scattered beneath the capsule and extend throughout the liver, sometimes resulting in complete loss of normal architecture.

Serial sacrifice experiments[46] showed that minute foci appeared beneath the capsule in the parenchyma 30 to 40 hr postinoculation. These areas enlarged, and just prior to death the liver became irregularly congested, focally or extensively . ...orrhagic and soft. Late in the disease the serosal surfaces, endocardium, and gastrointestinal mucosa develop petechiae and ecchymoses. The spleen showed subcapsular petechiae and the kidneys displayed congestion of the cortical and medullary blood vessels. The alimentary tract was inflamed to varying degrees, and cyanosis was apparent in visible mucous membranes and skin.

Lesions in adult sheep are somewhat less severe, the liver usually being mottled, brown, and frequently enlarged. Degeneration of the liver cells occurs, with characteristic intranuclear eosinophilic inclusions. The lesions, which are usually focal and not panlobular, accumulate polymorphonuclear leukocytes and histiocytes. Pathology in other organs appears similar to that observed in lambs. Lesions in other domestic or laboratory animals are similar to those in lambs and sheep, but vary in severity with the susceptibility of the host.[2,8,21,38]

Pathogenesis in Laboratory Animals

RVF virus can infect a wide variety of animals ranging from the laboratory mouse to the hippopotamus.[47] The disease manifestations vary according to species and age, with the younger animals generally being more susceptible. Some animals, such as the monkey (Indian, South American, and African)and the adult dog and cat, experience a milder, sometimes subclinical infection. Guinea pigs, rabbits, chickens, and pigeons appear somewhat resistant to infection and infrequently show clinical disease.[2,8] Mice and hamsters behave much like lambs or calves; they are readily infected by low doses of virus and die from hepatic necrosis, with very high viremias presumably originating in large part from the liver.[21,27,46,48,49] Colonized gerbils (*Meriones unguiculatus*) and cotton rats do not die from liver disease, but rather develop encephalitis.[12] Different species of wild-caught African rodents may be resistant to viremia, may develop viremia without overt disease, or may die after laboratory inoculation.[50,51]

Inbred rat strains provide an important insight into the genetic basis for host resistance to RVF.[12] Some strains (e.g., Wistar-Furth or Brown Norway) die of massive liver necrosis within 3 to 5 days after subcutaneous inoculation of only 5 plaque-forming units (p.f.u.) whereas others (e.g., Lewis, Buffalo, F344) resist even 5×10^5 p.f.u. Resistance seems to be determined by a single Mendelian dominant gene. Other inbred rats (ACI, MAXX) are intermediate in resistance and develop encephalitis 2 or 3 weeks after inoculation, at a time when high levels of circulating antibody are present. A similar genetic mechanism may determine why human beings develop hemorrhagic fever or encephalitis or why only some adult sheep succumb to fulminant hepatic necrosis.

Diagnosis

In the field, an outbreak of RVF would be suspected if there were increased rates of abortion among sheep, cattle, and goats; an elevated mortality in lambs, calves, and kids, especially in animals under 7 days of age; a milder disease with lower levels of mortality in adult animals; and liver lesions observed at postmortem examination. Other animals, including dogs or cats,[52] might experience disease, abort, or die.[40,41,45] The outbreak would most likely occur during climatic conditions favorable for arthropod multiplication, particularly after wet periods when mosquito population densities have increased. Human disease would also be present, occurring particularly among (but not limited to) those involved with necropsy, handling of infected meat, or laboratory investigation of the disease.

There are a few infections which cause such extensive human and animal disease. The differential diagnosis[40,45] varies geographically, but often includes: bluetongue, Wesselsbron, and Middleburg viruses, ephemeral fever or 3-day sickness of cattle, and enterotoxemia of sheep. Consideration should also be given to: brucellosis, vibriosis, trichomoniasis, Nairobi sheep disease, heartwater, and ovine enzootic abortion. Definitive diagnosis can only be made in the virological laboratory.

If RVF is suspected, unusually extreme precautions must be taken during collection, transport, and testing of specimens (see sections which follow). Virus isolation and identification, demonstration of serologic conversion, and, to a lesser extent, histopathologic examination, must be employed to confirm the diagnosis. Samples for virus isolation should be obtained during the febrile period or at autopsy, and preferably refrigerated or frozen prior to testing. The virus can be isolated from numerous body organs; samples of blood or plasma, abortus, and liver are commonly tested. The most sensitive laboratory system for virus isolation remains i.c. inoculation in 1- to 2-day-old suckling mice; however, adult hamsters and Vero, LLC-MK$_2$, or other cell cultures should also be employed. The i.p. inoculation of adult mice is an important diagnostic test, since many other viruses causing diseases similar to RVF are not lethal for adult mice. With RVF virus, experimental animals die in 1 to 4 days and cytopathic effects appear in cell culture in 3 to 5 days. Virus stocks can be prepared from suckling mouse brains or cell cultures, then identified serologically (cell cultures produce smaller amounts of CF or HI antigens).

The methodology for the CF, HI, FA, agar gel diffusion, and N (mouse or cell culture) tests has been employed to identify suspected RVF virus isolates and to detect serological conversion in serum samples.[26,43,44,53,54] Inoculation of cell culture followed in 18 to 22 hr by the FA test yields the fastest diagnosis.[55] The FA techniques (either direct or indirect) can also be applied to frozen postmortem specimens.[56] Identification of a virus isolate by any of these serological techniques was formerly thought to be diagnostically significant, since no crossreactions with RVF virus had been reported.[9] Recent demonstrations of antigenic relations between RVF and the Phlebotomus fever group by HI[11] and indirect immunofluorescent antibody[12] tests may require revision of these principles. Serological tests to determine a rise in antibodies to RVF virus should be performed on paired sera, one sample taken during the acute phase of illness and another after 10 or more days. In an endemic area, the demonstration of RVF virus antibodies in a single serum sample does not necessarily have diagnostic significance, since antibodies can be detected by the common serological tests for years after RVF virus infection. Histopathological examination of autopsy material or specimens from experimental animals reveal typical pathology of RVF.

The diagnosis of RVF in a previously uninfected area is difficult since the disease is not usually considered in the differential diagnosis, and laboratory methodology is either unavailable or not rigorously employed. During epizootics in the Union of South Africa in 1950 and 1951 and in the Sudan in 1973, diagnosis of the disease was finalized

6 months after the report of initial cases. However, by using the modern diagnostic methods outlined here, and through international collaboration of laboratories, the Egyptian RVF epizootic was confirmed in less than three weeks.

HUMAN INFECTION

Uncomplicated Illness[1,3,4,41,57-59]

After an incubation period estimated to be 2 to 6 days, the disease usually begins abruptly. Shaking chills, malaise, retroorbital pain, headache, abdominal pain, lumbar aches, myalgia, and nausea are common. Fever and prostration usually last 2 to 3 days, but may persist as long as 7 to 10 days with a "saddle-back" fever curve. An uneventful convalescence of 1 to 3 weeks usually follows. Conjunctival and pharyngeal injection are common. Epistaxis is occasionally seen, but petechiae or other hemorrhagic manifestations are absent. Hepatosplenomegaly is not a feature of RVF, but other causes may be common in affected regions. "Joint pains" were described in Ugandan cases, but this may reflect a language problem.[59,60] This form of the disease is virtually never fatal, unless some predisposing or intercurrent medical condition is involved.[61] Limited observations of blood and platelet counts, urinalysis, and serum SGOT levels have all been normal.[3,4,58] Nothing is known of the pathology of these patients. Clinical differential diagnosis from other undifferentiated tropical virus infections is difficult. The diagnosis can be suspected from knowledge of local RVF virus activity, particularly if the patient is involved in livestock slaughter. If RVF virus activity has not been established, presence of livestock disease and/or complicated human cases (particularly ocular lesions) may suggest the diagnosis. Specific virological tests will be necessary to confirm any clinical impression.

In Zimbabwe, virus isolations from sick patients seen at various stages of disease were uncommon and convalescent sera had to be examined for antibody in order to diagnose cases.[54] During epidemic disease in Egypt, viremia was common (>70%) when acutely ill patients were sampled.[6] When six infected field workers were examined serially, viremia lasted 3 to 4 days after onset of illness and HI, CF, and FA antibodies appeared within 8 to 10 days of onset.[58]

Hemorrhagic Fever With Liver Necrosis

This complication was first recognized in South Africa in 1975.[5] It is not clear whether the spectrum of the disease shifted or clinical recognition improved, but in any event there is now ample confirmation from Egypt[6,58,62] and Zimbabwe.[54] The disease usually begins as typical RVF, but petechiae, scleral icterus, and hypotension supervene 2 to 5 days after the acute febrile period. When these symptoms occur, death usually occurs in 5 to 10 days of illness in a deeply jaundiced, anuric patient in shock.[58] Peripheral vascular damage contributes to the severity of the disease, but liver necrosis is extensive and may be a major factor in the fatal outcome.[5,58,62] Zimbabwean patients presented pulmonary symptoms, pharyngitis, and anemia as well.[54] Limited laboratory data have shown hyperbilirubinemia, thrombocytopenia, and prolongation of clotting parameters.[54,58] The differential diagnosis includes the viral hemorrhagic fevers (particularly yellow fever, Ebola, dengue, Marburg, or Lassa), causes of fulminant liver necrosis, and a variety of other medical conditions which may result in jaundice and a bleeding diathesis. When studied, the pathological examination has shown diffuse hepatic necrosis with centrilobular accentuation.[5,54,62]

These patients are often viremic when they present hemorrhagic signs (4 of 7 in the Egyptian epidemic).[6] The liver is not only a major target organ, but also a major source of diagnostic material; virus can be isolated from postmortem tissue or visualized by electron microscopy.[54] Immunodiffusion[54] or possibly fluorescent antibodies can be used directly to detect hepatic viral antigens.

The frequency of fulminant infection must be low, but no data exist to define the risk. Estimates from the Egyptian experience suggest that less than 1% of cases develop this complication.[58] The determinants of this severe form of RVF are not known. If it is indeed a new manifestation, it may represent a shift in viral virulence. If only our perceptions have changed, then it is still necessary to explain why only a small fraction of human beings develop severe disease. Hepatic schistosomiasis may have contributed in Egypt; however, a careful study would be necessary to prove this because of the high prevalence of *Schistosoma mansoni* infection in the involved areas. Certainly, apparently healthy young Egyptian men died from hemorrhagic fever; South African or Zimbabwean cases were not complicated by schistosomiasis. Experimental studies with inbred rat strains suggest that host heredity may play a strong part in determiming the outcome.[12]

Encephalitis[5,6,58,63]

This complication of RVF has also only been recognized recently. Unlike the hemorrhagic fever/liver necrosis syndrome, symptoms usually subside from the acute illness and then central nervous system involvement appears 3 to 12 days after the febrile period. Meningismus, focal motor signs, hallucinations, confusion, stupor, and coma are common manifestations. A recrudescence of fever may occur. Recovery may require several days to several months; residual damage is not uncommon, but fatalities appear infrequent. Lumbar puncture reveals slightly elevated protein, normal sugar, and a modest pleocytosis with lymphocytic predominance. Differential diagnosis centers around other viral or postviral encephalitides.

Specific viral diagnosis depends on demonstration of a rising antibody titer, since virus appears to be cleared from the blood by the time encephalitis develops. Determination of CSF antibodies may also be useful.[63] Virus isolation from organs at autopsy has proved negative.

Ocular Complications[64-68]

Retinal macular lesions were one of the earliest suspected complications of human RVF.[64,65] Blurring or decrease in visual acuity develops rather abruptly from 7 days to up to 3 weeks after the febrile attack. When the patients are seen by the ophthalmologist they usually are asymptomatic, other than their eye complaints and often have severe retinal hemorrhages, exudates, and macular edema to account for the decrease in visual acuity. In many patients, vision returns toward normal in ensuing weeks, but partial loss may persist indefinitely in up to half the severely affected patients.[67] No treatment is known; steroids have not been impressive in their therapeutic effects. The frequency of reported lesions is low, probably less than 1% of all cases, but a careful prospective ophthalmological study has never been performed to detect lesser involvement. Patients with retinal disease do not have an unusual course as far as the other manifestations of RVF are concerned. The pathology in human beings has never been described. Patients are not viremic by the time they are seen and specific diagnosis depends on demonstrating a changing antibody titer to RVF virus.[67] Ocular fluids have never been tested for presence of virus.

Other

We still have much to learn about the uncommon manifestations of RVF. Certainly one would not be surprised to find patients with transverse myelitis or Guillain-Barré syndrome in the wake of acute infection. Hepatic involvement may lead to cirrhosis or trigger autoimmune chronic hepatitis. Since RVF is highly abortogenic in most species tested, human fetal loss or malformation is an undocumented, but real, possibility. A limited study addressing this during the Egyptian epidemic was inconclusive.[68a] Myocarditis is seen in kittens and puppies[52] and pneumonia in ferrets.[3] These have been suggested as complications of human disease[62] but evidence is slight.

In the mouse model, therapy with immune serum, the new antiviral drug ribavirin, or an interferon-inducer has had prophylactic and therapeutic value against hepatic infection, but not against encephalitis.[12] Their potential role in human therapy remains to be defined.

EPIDEMIOLOGY

Occurrence

Since the initial isolation of RVF virus in Kenya in 1930, serological surveys have provided evidence of RVF virus infection in most countries of sub-Saharan Africa. Table 1 depicts the geographical distribution of RVF and reviews the major outbreaks of the disease. The history of RVF in South Africa, Kenya, and Zimbabwe is comparable, and includes epizootics interspersed among enzootic periods where the virus "disappears" except for occasional isolations from mosquitoes. Davies[69] has studied extensively the interepizootic maintenance cycle in Kenya; it appears that the virus circulates in forest or forest-edge areas. Presumably epizootics result either after an environmental change favors spread of virus in nearby flocks and herds, or after people or animals enter the sylvatic area, become infected, and then disseminate the virus to an area with susceptible hosts. However, in Uganda and the Tongaland area of South Africa, RVF does not appear to have a similar epizootic period, but instead circulates in an enzootic pattern with only limited extension to people and animals (Table 1). Attempts to discover a virus reservoir in many countries have yielded negative results. Considering the varying ecological areas of Africa where RVF virus circulates, maintenance of the virus and occurrence of epizootics must depend on the interaction of a wide variety of local hosts, arthropods, and environmental factors.

The extension of the disease to Egypt in 1977 represents an incursion into a climatically rainless zone, which apparently had never previously been seeded with the virus. This epidemic clearly demonstrated the devastating potential of RVF. Eighteen thousand human cases were reported the first year; the actual number may have reached 200,000.[6,7] The Egyptian epidemic was the first in which large-scale human disease was associated with an appreciable number of human fatalities from encephalitis and hemorrhagic fever, perhaps on the order of 1% of the total cases. In 1978, the disease extended its range within Egypt (see Figure 1)[6] and may now pose a threat to other Middle Eastern countries. It is possible that the virus has already spread from mainland Africa to the Sinai.[70]

Transmission

A common feature of many epizootics has been the appearance of the virus after unusual climatic conditions which allowed for increases in arthropod densities. This was noted during the first described epizootic; movement of animals to higher, drier pastures or insect-proof pens stopped the spread of the disease.[1] However, the arthropod-borne nature of the disease was not proven until Smithburn et. al. in 1948 derived six RVF virus isolates from pools of wild-caught mosquitoes representing species in two genera.[76] Entomological studies have concentrated on either virus isolations from field collections, or demonstrating virus transmission with laboratory-bred mosquitoes. Approximately 23 species of mosquitoes have been implicated as possible RVF vectors, including *Aedes tarsalis, Ae. (Stegomyia) de-boeri, Ae. aegypti, Ae. triseriatus, Ae. circumbuleolus, Ae. africanus, Ae. lineatopennis, Ae. dentatus, Ae. caballus,*

Table 1
GEOGRAPHIC DISTRIBUTION OF RIFT VALLEY FEVER

Country	Date	Evidence of RVF	Reference[a]
Kenya	1912	Clinically diagnosed outbreak	8
	1930-1931	Extensive epizootic	1,21
	1936,1937,1947, 1952-1954	Limited outbreaks	71
	1968	Extensive epizootic	69
South Africa	1950-1951	Extensive epizootic	57,73
	1952,1953,1955, 1958,1959	Limited outbreaks	2,72,73
	1969	Extensive epizootic	74
	1956,1967,1971	Clinically diagnosed outbreaks	2,72
	1950-1975	Periodic isolations of virus from animals and mosquitoes	73-75
	1974-1975	Extensive epizootic[b]	5
Rhodesia	1957-1958, 1968,1969	Extensive outbreaks in cattle	54,74
	1970	Extensive outbreak in cattle	74
	1970-1978	Periodic isolations of virus from mosquitoes and animals	54,63,74
	1978	Extensive epizootic[b]	54,63
Uganda	1968	Limited human outbreak (7 cases)	59
	1948-1968	Periodic isolations of virus from mosquitoes and man	25,59,60, 76,76a
Mozambique	1969	Limited outbreak in cattle	74,77
Sudan	1973	Extensive epizootic	78,79
	1976	Clinically diagnosed outbreak	80
Egypt	1977	Extensive epizootic[b]	6,7,58,81
	1978	Extensive epizootic[b]	6,7,58,81
Nigeria	1959	Virus isolation from imported sheep	82
	1970-1972	Antibodies detected in serological survey; isolates from mosquitoes and *Culicoides*	83
Mali	1936	Antibodies detected in human serological survey (formerly part of French Sudan)	84
Gabon	1936	Antibodies detected in human serological survey (formerly part of French Equatorial Africa)	84
Congo	1954	Antibodies detected in subhuman primate serological survey	85
Chad	1969	Antibodies detected in animal serological survey	85
Botswana	1959	Antibodies detected in human sera	86
Angola	1960	Antibodies detected in human sera	87

[a] Outbreaks were frequently reported in internal documents of each country and are not readily accessible. Consequently, whenever possible we have attempted to list more widely available references, which review each outbreak and give additional citations.
[b] Outbreaks during which human fatalities were documented.

Culex theileri, C. neavei, C. pipiens, C. zombaensis, Eretmapodites quinquevittatus, E. chrysogaster, Mansonia africana, and *Anopheles coustani.*[25,37,59,73-76,76a,81,88] In most countries, detailed studies have not been done on the prevalence of each species, population dynamics, feeding preferences, and efficiency as vectors of RVF virus. More extensive entomological investigations in South Africa and Zimbabwe strongly implicate *C. theileri* and *Ae. caballus* as the main RVF virus vectors.[74,75] In Egypt, *C. pi-*

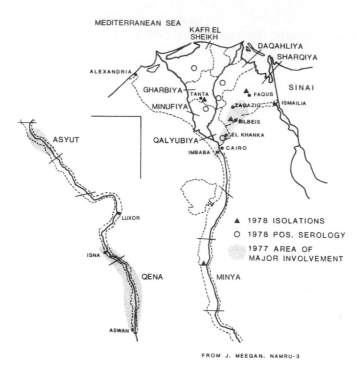

FIGURE 1.   Distribution of Rift Valley fever in Egypt in the 1977 to 1978 outbreaks.

piens is the most prevalent species. RVF virus has been isolated from wild-caught *C. pipiens* and transmitted by a laboratory strain.[81]

Arthropods undoubtedly act as the main vector of the disease among animals. However, in addition to biological transmission of the virus after replication in an arthropod, the unusually high RVF viremias in a number of hosts suggest that any hematophageous arthropod might mechanically transmit the virus. This possibility, and the role of other arthropods, such as *Culicoides*[83] and *Simulium*,[5] is in need of definitive investigation. In some experimental situations, transmission of the disease from sheep to sheep has occurred, but careful documentation of the presence of virus in saliva or excrement is still needed; the role of such contact transmission in the field is probably negligible.[1,12,41]

Observations by a number of South African investigators suggest that the primary means of virus transmission to man is contact with infected animal tissues during slaughter, food preparation, necropsy, or laboratory studies.[4,5,41,54] This viewpoint is supported by studies showing infection of experimental animals through skin abrasions, and by numerous case reports of veterinarians contracting the disease 2 to 4 days after performing a postmortem examination.[1,57] In the Egyptian epizootic, arthropod transmission of the disease to man was thought to have occurred, and it appears that contact with infected meat and, to a lesser extent, aerosols also were means of transmission of the virus to man.[81] Patient-to-patient transmission has not been demonstrated, although virus is present in blood and saliva. In most laboratories that have studied RVF virus, uncomplicated laboratory-acquired infections, probably from aerosol, have been common.

Reservoirs

Several investigations on the natural reservoirs of RVF in East Africa have been unproductive. Rodents had originally been suggested[89] but this was later refuted.[50,51,59] The investigations of Davies in Kenya argue against a role for many wild ruminants and monkeys.[69] In Egypt, the common rodent species apparently do not act as reservoirs and also appear unimportant as amplifying hosts in comparison to domestic animals and man.[6,81] Definitive data are not available on birds, bats, or reptiles, but the limited studies of these animals are not promising.[89a] The possibility of the virus overwintering in mosquitoes by either transovarial transmission or short-term hibernation is under investigation. *Culicoides* isolates in Nigeria may also be significant.[83]

Environment

The infectivity of RVF virus is unusually stable at temperatures below 60°C if the pH is maintained between 6.8 and 8.0.[19,22] This stability increases the likelihood of transmission of the disease through contact with infected tissue. Infection at necropsy or in the laboratory is an obvious concern, but reports from South Africa indicate that transmission might occur during food preparation in the home.[41] It was also speculated that the disposal of carcasses into canals as RVF decimated flocks in Egypt might have allowed further virus transmission, since these canals are used for bathing and sanitation purposes, and also are main breeding sites for mosquito larvae.[81] RVF virus is quite stable in aerosols and this undoubtedly has contributed to the numerous laboratory infections.[90]

Human Host

The human host probably had a greater impact on the natural history of RVF in Egypt than was recognized in previous epidemics. The high density of human beings and animals in the Nile delta and valley areas may well have contributed to the substantial infection rates in man.

Viremia titers as high as $10^{8.6}$ MICLD$_{50}$/mℓ of blood and persistence of viremia for up to 10 to 11 days, make it possible that man may act as an amplifying host during epizootics.[4,6] Since Egypt is a crossroad between Africa and other parts of the world, there is a real possibility that man might play a role in the dessemination of the virus into new areas.[70]

CONTROL

Epizootic Control Measures

Preventive vaccination of animals in endemic areas and in areas adjacent to epizootic foci should be practiced. Control of any outbreak must also include arthropod eradication and restriction of movement of animals (domestic, wild, and pets) and man from the infected area. The unusually wide invertebrate and vertebrate host range of RVF virus makes such restrictions vitally important in prevention of disease spread. Extreme caution must be exercised when disposing of diseased animals, and during collection, transport, and study of possibly contaminated tissue samples. Vaccination should be considered for high risk field and laboratory workers. Only government approved laboratories with high containment biohazard equipment are allowed to study RVF virus in the U.S. and many other nations. Unfortunately, only limited supplies of animal and human vaccine are currently available. Because of our lack of definitive knowledge about the natural cycle and potential of RVF virus, virologic and epidemiologic study of an epidemic is an essential part of control measures.

Regulatory Measures

Within endemic areas, regulatory procedures vary greatly, but generally center around encouragement of the use of animal vaccine and restriction on movement of animals. The regulations in the U.S. are designed to prevent the introduction of RVF, especially since a number of proven arthropod vectors are prevalent in various sections of the country. Regulations governing laboratories performing research on RVF virus are also intended to prevent possible introduction into the animal populations.

Health Education

Because RVF had previously been limited to restricted foci in southern Africa, the disease has received only cursory attention in educational courses. A definite effort is needed to update knowledge about RVF virus among veterinary, medical, research, and public health personnel.

Human Vaccine

A safe and effective formalin-inactivated, human vaccine was developed by Randall and co-workers.[91] This vaccine is still investigational, but has been administered to several hundred laboratory personnel with only occasional mild local reaction; its use has resulted in complete protection from illness. A few persons have experienced asymptomatic rises in antibody titer while working with the virus. There have been no formal field tests, but several thousand doses have been used by at-risk laboratory personnel in endemic/epidemic areas, with no significant adverse effects reported, and apparent protection. Lyophilized vaccine has been stored at $-20°C$ for as long as 10 years with no loss in potency. With an existing effective inactivated vaccine, it seems unlikely that a live attenuated vaccine will be developed for human use.

Veterinary Vaccines

Evaluation of immunity induced by existing animal vaccines has been hampered by the insensitivity of the constant-serum varying-virus mouse N test usually employed. As this test is customarily performed, a log neutralization index (LNI) of 1.7 is required to be statistically confident that antibody exists in the serum sampled assayed. It is clear that both inactivated and attenuated animal vaccines can give significant protection to animals with serum LNI of 1.0 or less.[12,72] Thus actual challenge with virulent RVF was necessary to assess protection. Recently two laboratories[92,101] have measured antibodies induced in sheep by an inactivated RVF vaccine using the sensitive plaque reduction neutralization test, and have found that very low titers (1:40 or greater) protect from viremia and illness.

An inactivated vaccine exists and is used extensively in South Africa.[72] Using 2 mℓ of this formalin-inactivated BHK-21 cell culture supernatant with alum adjuvant administered to sheep protects against illness or viremia when they are challenged with RVF several months later, even though no significant serum LNI can be measured. Cattle develop marginal N antibody responses and presumably would be protected also. This vaccine has been successfully used to interdict the spread of epidemic RVF in South African sheep; the duration of protection, fetal protection, colostral transfer of immunity and the stability of the vaccine are uncertain.

Serial passage i.c. in mice results in attenuated RVF preparations, e.g., the Smithburn neurotropic strain. The Smithburn strain is highly immunogenic[34,36,93] and has been used as an animal vaccine; it is abortogenic and teratogenic[94] and thus is not entirely satisfactory. Further attempts at attenuation apparently led to loss of immunogenicity.[2]

RVF virus propagated repeatedly in tissue culture acquires similar properties to the high mouse-passage virus. These strains are also potential immunogens for sheep and cattle, but are also highly reactogenic in field use.[32,36] Modern technology may well produce a safe effective attenuated vaccine.[17,18,31]

PUBLIC HEALTH IMPORTANCE

Economic Impact and Social Implications

Rift Valley fever epidemics can be associated with tremendous economic losses. In affected sheep, goat, cattle, or camel herds, high attack rates occur. Many adult animals die, and virtually all pregnant animals abort. In the affected areas of Africa this may represent a major blow to the economy and a significant limitation of animal protein available for human consumption. The personal tragedy to the small herdsman who may lose most of his livelihood should not be discounted. Other losses occur from restriction on exportation of animals to unaffected areas and cost of control measures within the country.

In people, the uncomplicated disease results in temporary disability and represents one more tropical fever which may extract its toll from a nutritionally-marginal populace. Although only a small fraction of the total number of patients develops hemorrhagic fever, the large number of total infections may lead to an appreciable number of deaths in the involved areas. These cases cannot be successfully managed medically without modern facilities, if then. Encephalitis has been severe, calling for careful supportive care, and has resulted in appreciable residua in some of the survivors, a further burden for society. Blindness also appears to be an uncommon sequela, but may be permanent and incapacitating. We urgently need adequate population-based data on these complications of human RVF infections, as well as a delineation of less severe complications or other residua of infection which may occur, e.g., cirrhosis from liver involvement, mental impairment from milder encephalitis cases, nonmacular retinal lesions, abortion, or teratogenesis.

Reporting and Surveillance

In previously affected areas the occurrence of abortions, illness, and death among susceptible domestic animals quickly suggests the disease diagnosis. Trained personnel can add weight to the diagnosis from the gross appearance of the liver at autopsy. Confirmation by virus isolation is possible in most cases, since RVF virus is stable even under adverse field conditions. Thus the only prerequisites to definitive diagnosis in known areas of RVF activity are communications, minimum veterinary skills, and the presence of basic viral diagnostic services. Unfortunately, these elements are often unavailable and may be distorted by political or other considerations.

In areas where RVF has never been active, diagnosis may be considerably delayed because of lack of familiarity with the symptoms and pathologic findings. This presumably will lead to spread to a wider area, human cases (particularly among unvaccinated veterinary personnel), and a greater likelihood of establishing endemic foci.

Surveillance in unaffected areas is relatively straightforward in principle. Reporting of characteristic clinical and pathologic findings should lead to immediate virologic confirmation by alert veterinary authorities. Formal surveillance and serologic surveys can then define the involved area. In known regions of RVF activity or contiguous regions, vaccination of livestock theoretically could delay recognition of RVF activity in wild animal populations or even hypothetical human-to-human spread by arthropods. It is worth mentioning in this context that natural infection or infection of vaccinated animals leads to much higher antibody titers (especially in the CF test) than vaccination alone, so that sero-surveillance in the presence of a vaccination campaign may still be feasible. Unfortunately, because of the infectiousness of RVF for laboratory workers, prototype strains cannot be maintained without special precautions, viz., vaccination of laboratory personnel and containment facilities to protect the environment. Inactivated antigens can be prepared for HI or CF tests.

BIBLIOGRAPHY

We have attempted to provide a synthesis of current understanding of RVF as well as indicate uncertainties and emerging research findings. Weiss[8] has provided a classical review of RVF and Easterday[2] later exhaustively catalogued the RVF literature. The classical studies on RVF infection of laboratory animals are summarized in Findlay's article[21]; Mims' articles[19,27,29,49] on the pathogenesis of murine infection have yet to be surpassed.

ADDENDUM

Several developments have occurred since the main body of this review was assembled. Shope's discovery of the serological relatedness of RVF to the Phlebotomus fever group has sparked investigators to compare these viruses in greater detail.[95,96] The HI test is the most broadly reactive measurement; FA also shows extensive crossreactivity within the group. The neutralization test is relatively specific, although low-level reactions between some agents and RVF virus can be readily demonstrated with hyperimmune antisera. The CF test is less sensitive and appears to be specific. When sera are tested by agar gel diffusion with heterologous antigens there are often minor lines, but the patterns are readily distinguishable from the homologous reaction which usually gives two to three heavy lines of identity with a standard antigen. Thus serological surveys conducted with the commonly used HI test would, if positive, require further confirmation. Preliminary results suggest that a positive virus-dilution mouse N test, a high titered plaque-reduction N ($\geqslant$1:320), or CF test ($\geqslant$1:8) would indicate previous RVF; however, further experience with field sera is needed. It is always preferable to conduct simultaneous tests with related agents suspected to be active in the area.

Inclusion of RVF virus in the Phlebotomus fever group may give clues as to its natural cycle. Although the biology of the group is not well understood, transmission by sandflies is common, transovarial infection of sandflies is well-described, and antibody or virus isolation often implicate forest rodents as reservoirs.[9,97,98] Conversely, we should be more alert to the possibility that other members of the group may produce serious or fatal human disease, infect domestic animals, or be infectious by aerosol. Infection in nature may regulate the distribution of RVF; group members might serve as animal vaccines for RVF, either as they exist or after laboratory manipulation to produce attenuated or reassortant strains.

A graphic example of the threat of exportation of RVF was provided by a case recently reported by Mahdi et. al.[99] A Canadian woman visiting Kenya participated in a game safari and subsequently developed a febrile illness consistent with RVF. She remained in Kenya until improving, but then flew to Jeddah, Saudi Arabia, where she developed visual impairment. A clinical diagnosis of RVF was made in Jeddah; upon return to Canada she was found to have high titer antibodies to RVF. She could easily have returned viremic to her rural Canadian home if her schedule had been different. Meegan et al.[70] have also emphasized this possibility in a recent report describing RVF antibodies thought to have been acquired by human beings in the Sinai peninsula.

A workshop on RVF was held in Herzlia, Israel, March 18 to 21, 1980; the proceedings contain more extensive discussions of several topics, including the biochemistry of the virus, the pathogenesis of the disease, the human vaccine, relationship of RVF to the Phlebotomus fever group, and RVF epidemiology in several countries.[100]

REFERENCES

1. **Daubney, R., Hudson, J. R., and Garnham, P. C.,** Enzootic hepatitis or Rift Valley fever. An undescribed virus disease of sheep, cattle and man from East Africa, *J. Pathol. Bacteriol.,* 34, 545, 1931.
2. **Easterday, B. C.,** Rift Valley fever, *Ad. Vet. Sci.,* 10, 65, 1965.
3. **Francis, T. and Magill, T. P.,** Rift Valley fever: a report of 3 cases of laboratory infection and the experimental transmission of the disease to ferrets, *J. Exp. Med.,* 62, 433, 1935.
4. **Smithburn, K. C., Mahaffy, A. F., Haddow, A. J., Kitchen, S. F., and Smith, J. F.,** Rift Valley fever: accidental infections among laboratory workers, *J. Immunol.,* 62, 213, 1949.
5. **Van Velden, D. J. J., Meyer, J. D., Olivier, J., Gear, J. H. S., and McIntosh, B.,** Rift Valley fever affecting humans in South Africa: a clinicopathological study, *S. Afr. Med. J.,* 51, 867, 1977.
6. **Meegan, J. M.,** The Rift Valley fever epizootic in Egypt 1977-1978. 1. Description of the epizootic and virological studies, *Trans. R. Soc. Trop. Med. Hyg.,* 73, 618, 1979.
7. **Meegan, J. M., Hoogstraal, H., and Moussa, M. I.,** An epizootic of Rift Valley fever in Egypt in 1977, *Vet. Rec.,* 105, 124, 1979.
8. **Weiss, K. E.,** Rift Valley fever — a review, *Bull. Epizoot. Dis. Afr.,* 5, 431, 1957.
9. **Berge, T. O., Ed.,** International Catalogue of Arboviruses, Pub no. (CDC) 75-8301, 2nd ed., Public Health Service, U.S. Department of Health, Education and Welfare, Atlanta, 1975.
10. **Murphy, F. A., Harrison, A. K., and Whitfield, S. B.,** Bunyaviridae: morphologic and morphogenetic similarities of Bunyamwera serologic supergroup viruses and several other arthropod-borne viruses, *Intervirology,* 1, 297, 1973.
11. **Shope, R. E.,** personal communication, 1979.
12. **Peters, C. J.,** unpublished data, 1979.
13. **Lecatsas, G. and Weiss, K. E.,** Electron microscopic studies on BHK-21 cells infected with Rift Valley fever virus, *Arch. Gesamte Virusforsch.,* 25, 58, 1968.
14. **Rice, R. M.,** in *Annual Progress Report FY 1978,* Summers, P. W., Ed., U.S. Army Medical Research Institute of Infectious Diseases, Fort Detrick, Frederick, Md., 1979, 309.
15. **Erlick, B., Rice, R., Cash, P., Peters, C. J., and Bishop, D. H. L.,** unpublished data, 1980.
16. **Obijeski, J. F. and Murphy, F. A.,** Bunyaviradae: recent biochemical developments, *J. Gen. Virol.,* 37, 1, 1977.
17. **Tyrrell, D. A. J.,** Using the genetics of influenza virus to make live attenuated vaccines, *Lancet,* 1, 196, 1978.
18. **Bishop, D. H. L.,** Genetic potential of bunyaviruses, *Curr. Top. Microbiol. Immunol.,* 86, 1, 1980.
19. **Mims, C. A. and Mason, P. J.,** Rift Valley fever virus (RVF) in mice. V. The properties of a hemagglutinin present in infective serum, *Br. J. Exp. Pathol.,* 37, 423, 1956.
20. **Craig, D. E., Thomas, W. J., and DeSanctis, A. N.,** Stability of Rift Valley fever virus at 4°C, *Appl. Environ. Microbiol.,* 15, 446, 1967.
21. **Findlay, G. M.,** Rift Valley fever or enzootic hepatitis, *Trans. R. Soc. Trop. Med. Hyg.,* 25, 229, 1932.
22. **Klein, F., Walker, J. S., Mahlandt, B. G., Carter, R. C., Orlando, M. D., Weirether, F. J., and Lincoln, R. E.,** Interacting factors that influence long-term storage of live *Pasteurella tularensis* vaccine and Rift Valley fever virus, *Appl. Environ. Microbiol.,* 17, 427, 1969.
23. **Easterday, B. C. and Murphy, L. C.,** The growth of Rift Valley fever virus in cultures of established lines of cells, *Cornell Vet.,* 53, 3, 1963.
24. **Klein, F., Mahlandt, B. G., Eyler, S. L., and Lincoln, R. E.,** Relationship between plaque assay and the mouse assay for titering Rift Valley fever virus, *Proc. Soc. Exp. Biol. Med.,* 134, 909, 1970.
25. **Weinbren, M. P., Williams, M. C., and Haddow, A. J.,** A variant of Rift Valley fever virus, *S. Afr. Med. J.,* 31, 951, 1957.
26. **Tomori, O. and Oseni, G.,** Discontinuous counter-immunoelectrophoresis in the study of viruses, *Intervirology,* 10, 102, 1978.
27. **Mims, C. A.,** Rift Valley fever in mice. I. General features of the infection, *Br. J. Exp. Pathol.,* 37, 99, 1956.
28. **MacKenzie, R. D. and Findlay, G. M.,** The production of a neurotropic strain of Rift Valley fever virus, *Lancet,* 1, 140, 1936.
29. **Mims, C. A.,** Rift Valley fever in mice. IV. Incomplete virus; its production and properties, *Br. J. Exp. Pathol.,* 37, 129, 1956.
30. **Findlay, G. M. and MacKenzie, R. D.,** Studies on a neurotropic Rift Valley fever virus: "spontaneous" encephalomyelitis in mice, *Br. J. Exp. Pathol.,* 17, 441, 1936.
31. **Koyama, H. and Higashihara, M.,** Selection of avirulent variants of Rift Valley fever virus, *Kitasato Arch. Exp. Med.,* 47, 201, 1974.

32. **Coackley, W.**, Alteration of virulence of Rift Valley fever virus during serial passage in lamb testis cells, *J. Pathol. Bacteriol.*, 89, 123, 1965.

33. **Kitchen, S. F.**, The development of neurotropism in Rift Valley fever virus, *Ann. Trop. Med. Parasitol.*, 44, 132, 1950.

34. **Smithburn, K. C.**, Rift Valley fever: the neurotropic adaptation of virus and experimental use of this modified virus as a vaccine, *Br. J. Exp. Pathol.*, 30, 1, 1949.

35. **Takemori, N., Nakano, M., Hemmi, M., and Kitaoka, M.**, Propagation of Rift Valley fever virus in ascites hepatoma cells of the rat: production of a new variant of the virus, *Virology*, 1, 58, 1955.

36. **Coackley, W., Pini, A., and Gosden, D.**, The immunity induced in cattle and sheep by inoculation of neurotropic or pantropic Rift Valley fever viruses, *Res. Vet. Sci.*, 8, 406, 1967.

37. **Easterday, B. C., Murphy, L. C., and Bennett, D. G.**, Experimental Rift Valley fever in lambs and sheep, *Am. J. Vet. Res.*, 23, 1231, 1962.

38. **Easterday, B. C., Murphy, L. C., and Bennett, D. G.**, Experimental Rift Valley fever in calves, goats, and pigs, *Am. J. Vet. Res.*, 23, 1224, 1962.

39. **Coackley, W., Pini, A., and Gosden, D.**, Experimental infection of cattle with pantropic Rift Valley fever virus, *Res. Vet. Sci.*, 8, 399, 1967.

40. **Kaschula, V. R.**, Rift Valley fever as a veterinary and medical problem, *J. Am. Vet. Med. Assoc.*, 131, 219, 1957.

41. **Gear, J., de Meillon, B., Measroch, V., Harwin, R., and Davis, D. H. S.**, Rift Valley fever in South Africa. 2. The occurrence of human cases in the Orange Free State, the north-western Cape Province, the western and southern Transvaal. B. Field and laboratory investigations, *S. Afr. Med. J.*, 25, 908, 1951.

42. **McIntosh, B. M., Dickinson, D. B., and Dos Santos, I.**, Rift Valley fever. 3. Viremia in cattle and sheep, *J. S. Afr. Vet. Assoc.*, 44, 167, 1973.

43. **Pini, A., Lund, L. J., and Davies, F. G.**, Fluorescent and neutralizing antibody response to infection by Rift Valley fever virus, *J. S. Afr. Vet Assoc.*, 44, 161, 1973.

44. **Binn, L. N., Randall, R., Harrison, V. R., Gibbs, C. J., Jr., and Aulisio, C. G.**, The serological reactions in a case of Rift Valley fever, *Am. J. Trop. Med. Hyg.*, 12, 236, 1963.

45. **Murphy, L. C. and Easterday, B. C.**, Rift Valley fever: a zoonosis, *Annu. Proc. U. S. Livestock Sanit. Assoc.*, 65, 397, 1961.

46. **Easterday, B. C., McGavran, M. H., Rooney, J. R., and Murphy, L. C.**, The pathogenesis of Rift Valley fever in lambs, *Am. J. Vet. Res.*, 23, 470, 1962.

47. **Weinbren, M. P. and Hewitt, L. E.**, Virus neutralization tests on hippopotamus sera, *East African Virus Research Institute Annual Report*, 9, 13, 1958-1959.

48. **Easterday, B. C. and Murphy, L. C.**, Studies on Rift Valley fever in laboratory animals, *Cornell Vet.*, 53, 423, 1963.

49. **Mims, C. A.**, Rift Valley fever in mice. VI. Histological changes in the liver in relation to virus multiplication, *Aust. J. Exp. Biol. Med. Sci.*, 35, 595, 1957.

50. **Swanepoel, R., Blackburn, N. K., Efstration, S., and Condy, J. B.**, Studies on Rift Valley fever in some African murids (*Rodentia: Muridae*), *J. Hyg. Camb.*, 80, 183, 1978.

51. **McIntosh, B. M.**, Susceptibility of some African wild rodents to infection with various arthropod-borne viruses, *Trans. R. Soc, Trop. Med. Hyg.*, 55, 63, 1961.

52. **Mitten, J. Q., Remmele, N. S., Walker, J. S., and Carter, R. C.**, The clinical aspects of Rift Valley fever virus in household pets. III. Pathologic changes in the dog and cat, *J. Infect. Dis.*, 121, 25, 1970.

53. **Casals, J.**, Immunological techniques for animal viruses, *Methods Virol.*, 3, 113, 1967.

54. **Swanepoel, R., Manning, B., and Watt, J. A.**, Fatal Rift Valley fever of man in Rhodesia, *Cent. Afr. J. Med.*, 25, 1, 1979.

55. **Easterday, B. C. and Jaeger, R. F.**, The detection of Rift Valley fever virus by a tissue culture fluorescein-labeled antibody method, *J. Infect. Dis.*, 112, 1, 1963.

56. **Pini, A., Lund, L. J., and Davies, F. G.**, Detection of Rift Valley fever virus by the fluorescent antibody technique in organs of experimentally infected animals, *Res. Vet. Sci.*, 11, 82, 1970.

57. **Mundel, B. and Gear, J.**, Rift Valley fever: I. The occurrence of human cases in Johannesberg, *S. Afr. Med. J.*, 25, 797, 1951.

58. **Laughlin, L. W., Meegan, J. M., Strausbaugh, L. J., Morens, D. M., and Watten, R. H.**, Epidemic Rift Valley Fever in Egypt; Observations of the spectrum of human illness, *Trans. R. Soc. Trop. Med. Hyg.*, 73, 630, 1979.

59. **Henderson, B. E., McCrae, A. W. R., Kirya, B. G., Ssenkubuge, Y., and Sempala, S. D. K.**, Arbovirus epizootics involving man, mosquitoes and vertebrates at Lunyo, Uganda 1968, *Ann. Trop. Med. Parasitol.*, 66, 343, 1972.

60. **Williams, M. H., Simpson, D. I. H., Knight, E. M., Woodall, J. P., Santos, D. F., and Lule, M.**, Virology isolations from man, *E. Afr. Virus Res. Inst. Annu. Rep.*, 13, 12, 1963.

61. **Schwentker, F. F. and Rivers, T. M.**, Rift Valley fever in man. Report of a fatal laboratory infection complicated by thrombophlebitis, *J. Exp. Med.*, 59, 305, 1934.

62. **Abdel-Wahab, K. S. E., El Baz, L. M., El Tayeb, E. M., Omar, H., Ossman, M. A. M., and Yasin, W.**, Rift Valley fever virus infections in Egypt: pathological and virological findings in man, *Trans. R. Soc. Trop. Med. Hyg.*, 72, 392, 1978.

63. **Maar, S. A., Swanepoel, R., and Gelfand, M.**, Rift Valley fever encephalitis. A description of a case, *Cent. Afr. J. Med.*, 25, 8, 1979.

64. **Schrire, L.**, Macular changes in Rift Valley fever, *S. Afr. Med. J.*, 25, 926, 1951.

65. **Freed, I.**, Rift Valley fever in man complicated by retinal changes and loss of vision, *S. Afr. Med. J.*, 25, 930, 1951.

66. **Cohen, C. and Luntz, M. H.**, Rift Valley fever and rickettsial retinitis including fluorescein angiography, *Klin. Monatsbl. Augenheilkd.*, 169, 685, 1976.

67. **Siam, A. L., Meegan, J. M., and Gharbawi, K. F.**, Rift Valley fever ocular manifestation: observations during the 1977 epidemic in the Arab Republic of Egypt, *Br. J. Ophthalmol.*, 64, 366, 1980.

68. **Siam, A. L. and Meegan, J. M.**, Rift Valley fever virus infection causes ocular manifestations, *Trans. R. Soc. Trop. Med. Hyg.*, 74, 540, 1980.

68a. **Abdel-Aziz, A. A., Meegan, J. M., and Laughlin, L. W.**, Rift Valley Fever as a possible cause of human abortions, *Trans. R. Soc. Trop. Med. Hyg.*, 1980, in press.

69. **Davies, F. G.**, Observations on the epidemiology of Rift Valley fever in Kenya, *J. Hyg. Camb.*, 75, 219, 1975.

70. **Meegan, J. M., Niklasson, B., and Bengtsson, E.** Spread of Rift Valley fever virus from continental Africa, *Lancet*, 2, 1184, 1979.

71. **Scott, G. R., Weddell, W., and Reid, D.**, Preliminary finding on the prevalence of Rift Valley fever in Kenya cattle, *Bull. Epizoot. Dis. Afr.*, 4, 17, 1956.

72. **Barnard, B. J. H. and Botha, M. J.**, An inactivated Rift Valley fever vaccine, *J. S. Afr. Vet. Assoc.*, 48, 45, 1977.

73. **Gear, J., de Meillon, B., Le Roux, A. F., Kofsky, R., Rose-Innes, R., Steyn, J. J., Oliff, W. D., and Schulz, K. H.**, Rift Valley fever in South Africa. A study of the 1953 outbreak in the Orange Free State, with special reference to the vectors and possible reservoir hosts, *S. Afr. Med. J.*, 29, 514, 1955.

74. **McIntosh, B. M.**, Rift Valley fever: vector studies in the field, *J. S. Afr. Vet. Assoc.*, 43, 391, 1972.

75. **Steyn, J. J. and Schulz, K. H.**, *Aedes (Ochlerotatus) caballus* Theobald, the South African vector of Rift Valley fever, *S. Afr. Med. J.*, 29, 1114, 1955.

76. **Smithburn, K. C., Haddow, A. J., and Gillett, J. D.**, Rift Valley fever: isolation of the virus from wild mosquitoes, *Br. J. Exp. Pathol.*, 29, 107, 1948.

76a. **Woodall, J. P.**, Summary of virus isolations at the East African Virus Research Institute to the end of 1964, *E. Afr. Virus Res. Inst. Annu. Rep.*, 14, 18, 1963 — 1964.

77. **Valadao, F. G.**, Nota previa sobre a ocorrencia de uma nova, doenca em mocambique — a febre do vale de Rift, *Vet. Mocamb.*, 2, 13, 1969.

78. **Eisa, M., Obeid, H. M. A., and El Sawi, A. S. A.**, Rift Valley fever in the Sudan. I. Results of field investigations of the first epizootic in Kosti District 1973, *Bull. Anim. Health Prod. Afr.*, 25, 343, 1977.

79. **Eisa, M. and Obeid, H. M. A.**, Rift Valley fever in the Sudan. II. Isolation and identification of the virus from a recent epizootic in Kosti District 1973, *Bull. Anim. Health Prod. Afr.*, 25, 349, 1977.

80. **Eisa, M., Kheir El Sid, E. D., Shomein, A. M., and Meegan, J. M.**, An outbreak of Rift Valley fever in the Sudan — 1976, *Trans. R. Soc. Trop. Med. Hyg.*, 74, 417, 1980.

81. **Hoogstraal, H., Meegan, J. M., Kahlil, G. M., and Adham, F.K.**, The Rift Valley fever epizootic in Egypt 1977-1978. 2. Ecological and entomological studies, *Trans. R. Soc. Trop. Med. Hyg.*, 73, 624, 1979.

82. **Ferguson, W.**, Identification of Rift Valley fever in Nigeria, *Bull. Epizoot. Dis. Afr.*, 7, 317, 1959.

83. **Fagbami, A. H., Tomori, O., and Kemp, G. E.**, A survey of Nigerian domestic and wild animals for neutralizing antibody to indigenous Rift Valley fever virus, *Nigerian Vet. J.*, 2, 45, 1973.

84. **Findlay, G. M., Stefanopoulo, G. J., and MacCallum, F. O.**, Pre'sence d'anticorps contra la fie'vre de la Valle'e du Rift dans le sang des Africain, *Bull. Soc. Pathol. Exot.*, 29, 986, 1936.

85. **Pellissier, A. and Rousselot, R.**, Enquete se'rologique sur l'incidence des virus neurotropes chez quelque singes de l'afrique equitoriale francaise, *Bull. Soc. Pathol. Exot.*, 47, 228, 1954.

85a. **Maurice, Y. and Provost, A.**, Sondages serologiques sur les arboviroses animales en Afrique Centrale, *Recl. Elev. Méd. Vet. Pays-Trop.*, 22, 179, 1969.

86. **Kokernot, R. H., Szlamp, E. L., Levitt, J., and McIntosh, B. M.**, Survey for antibodies against arthropod-borne viruses in the sera of indigenous residents of the Caprivi Strip and Bechuanaland Protectorate, *Trans. R. Soc. Trop. Med. Hyg.*, 59, 553, 1965.

87. **Kokernot, R. H., Casaca, V. M. R., Weinbren, M. P., and McIntosh, B. M.**, Survey for antibodies against arthropod-borne viruses in the sera of indigenous residents of Angola, *Trans. R. Soc. Trop. Med. Hyg.*, 59, 563, 1965.

88. **McIntosh, B. M., Jupp, P. G., Anderson, D., and Dickinson, D. B.**, Rift Valley fever. 2. Attempts to transmit virus with seven species of mosquito, *J. S. Afr. Vet. Assoc.*, 44, 57, 1973.

89. **Weinbren, M. P. and Mason, P. J.**, Rift Valley fever in a wild rat (*Arvicanthus abyssinicus*): a possible natural host, *S. Afr. Med. J.*, 31, 427, 1957.

89a. **Davies, F. G. and Addy, P. A. K.**, Rift Valley fever. A survey for antibody to the virus in bird species commonly found in situations considered to be enzootic, *Trans. R. Soc. Trop. Med. Hyg.*, 73, 584, 1979.

90. **Miller, W. S., Demchak, P., Rosenberger, C. R., Dominik, J. W., and Bradshaw, J. L.**, Stability and infectivity of airborne yellow fever and Rift Valley fever viruses, *Am. J. Hyg.*, 77, 114, 1963.

91. **Randall, R., Binn, L. N., and Harrison, V. R.**, Immunization against Rift Valley fever virus. Studies on the immunogenicity of lyophilized formalin-inactivated vaccine, *J. Immunol.*, 93, 293, 1964.

92. **Yedloutschnig, R. J., Dardiri, A. H., Walker, J. S., Peters, C. J., and Eddy, G. A.**, Immune response of steers, goats, and sheep to inactivated Rift Valley Fever vaccine, Proc. 83rd Ann. Meeting U.S. Animal Health Assn., p. 253, 1979.

93. **Weiss, K. E.**, Studies on Rift Valley fever—passive and active immunity in lambs, *Onderstepoort J. Vet. Res.*, 29, 3, 1962.

94. **Wetzer, J. A. W. and Barnard, B. J. H.**, Hydrops Amnii in sheep associated with Wesselbron disease and Rift Valley fever viruses as aetiological agents, *Onderstepoort J. Vet. Res.*, 44, 119, 1977.

95. **Shope, R. E., Peters, C. J., Walker, J. S.**, Serologic relationship between Rift Valley fever virus and viruses of the phlebotomus fever group, *Lancet*, I, 886, 1980.

96. **Shope, R. E., Tesh, R. B., Meegan, J. M., and Peters, C. J.**, personal communication, 1980.

97. **Tesh, R. B., Peralta, P. H., Shope, R. E., Chaniotis, B. M., and Johnson, K. M.**, Antigenic relationships among phlebotomus fever group arboviruses and their implications for the epidemiology of sandfly fever, *Am. J. Trop. Med. Hyg.*, 24, 135, 1975.

98. **Tesh, R. B., Saidi, S., Gajdamovic, S. J., Rodhain, F., Vesenjak-Hirjan, J.**, Serological studies on the epidemiology of sandfly fever in the Old World, *Bull. WHO*, 54, 663, 1976.

99. **Mahdy, M. S., Bansen, E., Joshua, J. M., Parker, J. A., and Stuart, P. F.**, A case report of Rift Valley fever with retinopathy, *Can. Dis. Wkly Rep.*, 5, 189, 1979.

100. **Rift Valley Fever Workshop**, *Contributions to Epidemiology and Biostatistics*, S. Karger, Basel, in press, 1980.

101. **Harrington, D. G., Lupton, H. W., Crabbs, C. L., Peters, C. J., Reynolds, J. A., and Slone, T. W.**, Evaluation of a formalin inactivated Rift Valley Fever vaccine in sheep, *Am. J. Vet. Res.*, 41, 383, 1980.

DENGUE AND DENGUE HEMORRHAGIC FEVER

S. B. Halstead

NAME AND SYNONYMS

There are no synonyms for dengue viruses in the English language. Currently, there is general agreement that there are four antigenically distinct members of the dengue subgroup.[9,37,76,77] These are named dengue types 1 through 4. Dengue viruses cause human syndromes which vary markedly in severity and prognosis. The mild forms are called dengue, dengue fever, and break-bone fever. The severe forms are called dengue hemorrhagic fever (DHF), hemorrhagic dengue, acute infectious thrombocytopenic purpura, dengue shock syndrome, and Philippine, Thai, or Singapore hemorrhagic fever.

HISTORY

The first outbreak of a disease resembling virologically confirmed dengue fever was that described by Benjamin Rush in Philadelphia in 1780.[75] Outbreaks surmised to be of dengue etiology based upon their clinical or epidemiological features were common in North America during the 18th and 19th centuries in inhabitants of the Atlantic coast, the Caribbean islands, and the Mississippi basin.[83] Dengue viruses were almost certainly the cause of the 5- and 7-day fevers which occurred among European colonists in tropical Asia.[11] Similar epidemics occurred among settlers in tropical Australia.[56] During most of the previrological era, dengue viruses were thought to be the cause of a generally benign, self-limited febrile exanthem. Observations which culminated in the recognition of dengue as arthropod-borne were initiated by Graham in Lebanon in 1902.[29] *Aedes aegypti* mosquitoes were identified as vectors by Bancroft.[3] This was confirmed and substantiated by the definitive studies by Cleland, Bradley, and McDonald,[15] Chandler and Rice,[14] Siler et al.,[83] and Simmons et al.[84] Ashburn and Craig, using human volunteers, demonstrated that the etiological agent of dengue was present in the blood of patients and that it passed through a Lilliput diatomaceous earth filter.[2] Siler et al. and Simmons et al. identified an intrinsic incubation period in human beings of 3 to 8 days and an extrinsic incubation period in mosquitoes of 8 to 11 days.[83,84] They also documented post-infection immunity in people and monkeys, and the insusceptibility of dengue infections of most domestic animals. The etiological viruses were almost surely dengue types 1 and 4.[43] With the first isolations of dengue viruses in 1943 and 1944 the modern era of dengue research began.[53,78] In human volunteer studies, two dengue strains were identified as failing to crossprotect, and were named dengue types 1 and 2.[78,79] From 1897 to 1902 in Australia, 1928 in Greece, and 1931 in Taiwan, a clinically severe infection with shock, hemorrhagic manifestation, and death were described during dengue epidemics.[17,46,56,69] This "new" syndrome was described in Manila, Philippines in 1954 and called Philippine hemorrhagic fever because of supposed similarities to epidemic hemorrhagic fever in the Korean peninsula.[71] Philippine hemorrhagic fever was associated with dengue virus in 1956, and is now recognized throughout tropical Asia.[33,47,48,81] Dengue virus type 2, plus two previously unrecognized types, 3 and 4, were recovered from patients during the 1956 Manila outbreak, and all types, 1 through 4 were recovered from patients during an outbreak in Bangkok in 1958.[47,48] Since 1967, the terms dengue hemorrhagic fever and dengue shock syndrome have been in general use.[33]

ETIOLOGY

Classification

By epidemiological criteria, dengue viruses are arthropod-borne (arboviruses) since they are biologically transmitted by various members of the genus *Aedes*.[81,83,84] Using antigenic relationships demonsrated by hemagglutination-inhibition, dengue viruses are placed in the genus *Flavivirus* of the family Togaviridae.[13,81] At present there are 57 members of the flavivirus group, 29 of which are established as human pathogens.[4] Cross comparisons by plaque reduction neutralization tests have shown dengue viruses to be an antigenic subgroup with little relationship to other flaviviruses.[19] Four clearly defined types are identified on the basis of plaque reduction neutralization (N) tests using antisera produced in monkeys or complement-fixation (CF) tests with nonstructural proteins.[37,62,76] From limited data, an antigenic and biologic variant of type 3 has been proposed as a subtype.[77] TH-36 and TH-Sman strains which were initially classified as dengue types 5 and 6,[49,50] are now considered to be closely related or identical to dengue types 2 and 1, respectively.[37,76] Different strains within each dengue serotype show a degree of antigenic heterogeneity.[37,76] The biochemical basis of this heterogeneity and its biological significance are not understood. In addition to their close antigenic interrelationships and their ability to be transmitted by *Aedes spp.* mosquitoes, all 4 types of dengue viruses produce similar clinical syndrome in susceptible human beings.[81,83,84]

Characteristics

Dengue virions are spherical particles, approximately 50 nm in diameter.[60,81] They possess a lipid-containing envelope which carries knob-like projections.[20] The central "core", approximately 25 nm in diameter, is roughly hexagonal in cross section and contains a nucleocapsid of uncertain symmetry.[60,81] The dengue virus genome is ribonuclease sensitive and lacks base pairing; hence it is classified as a linear single stranded RNA.[86] It has a sedimentation coefficient of 45S and a presently accepted molecular weight of approximately 4.2×10^6 daltons.[81] Phenol extracts of dengue infected material are infectious, indicating that the RNA is of the "plus" (messenger) polarity.[81] By analogy with group A togaviruses, one would expect the lipid composition of dengue virions to reflect that of the host cells from which they are derived and to vary accordingly, but no data on this are as yet available. Research on structural proteins has been reviewed by Schlesinger.[81] They may be separated into complete (RHA) and incomplete (SHA) hemagglutinating particles.[87] Polyacrylamide gel electrophoresis of virions degraded with sodium dodecyl sulfate has resulted in the resolution of three proteins, VP-1, VP-2, and VP-3. These are now considered to be VP-3 (mol. wt. ~59,000) — the major envelope glycoprotein; VP-1 (mol. wt. ~8,000), a second envelope protein and VP-2 (mol. wt. ~13,000), the nucleocapsid protein. According to the cryptogram proposed by Gibbs et al., the properties of the dengue viruses are R/1:4.2/7:S/*:V,I/Di.[27]

DEFINITION

Dengue fever is a benign syndrome caused by several arthropod-borne viruses and characterized by biphasic fever, myalgia or arthralgia, rash, leukopenia, and lymphadenopathy. Dengue hemorrhagic fever is a severe, often fatal, febrile disease caused by dengue viruses. It is characterized by abnormalities of hemostatis and in severe cases by a protein-losing shock syndrome (dengue shock syndrome) and is currently thought to have an immunopathological basis.

ANIMAL INFECTION

Clinical

Monkeys are generally susceptible to dengue viruses and a number of species of *Macacus, Cynomolgus, Cercopithicus, Cercocebus,* and *Papio* may be infected by bites of virus-infected mosquitoes or by injection of infectious virus preparations.[81,84] Resulting infections are essentially asymptomatic. Viremias occur from 1 to 7 days after inoculation. Fever has not been unequivocally demonstrated. A mild leukopenia has been reported.[41]

Experimental inoculation of dengue strains of known human pathogenicity into chickens, lizards, newborn or adult guinea pigs, rabbits, hamsters, or cotton rats have not produced clinical disease.[81,84] On the other hand, 1- to 2-day-old mice and hamsters have succumbed to intracerebrally (i.c.) injected virus and high mouse passaged virus has produced deaths in weanling mice inoculated by the i.c. route.[78,79] Individual reports of fatal infections in Japanese ground squirrels inoculated by i.c. or intranasal i.n. route have not been confirmed.[81]

Pathology

Laboratory mice infected by i.c. inoculation of mouse-adapted dengue strains develop neuronal degeneration. Brains and spinal cords show cell infiltration, perivascular cuffing, glial proliferation, and nerve cell degeneration. Small petechial hemorrhages are often present in the meninges, on the surface of the lungs, and hemorrhages of varying degrees are recognized in many organs. Lungs show congestion. Extravasation of erythrocytes is frequently observed into the pulmonary alveolar lumen and into the spleen and lymph nodes with activation of follicles and hyperplasia of lymphoid and reticuloendothelial cells, and swelling and proliferation of vascular endothelial cells.[44]

No pathological findings in dengue infected monkeys have been published. In experimental infections in rhesus monkeys, inoculated by the subcutaneous (s.c.) route, virus was rapidly carried to regional lymph nodes and then transported to lymphatic tissues throughout the body. Early in the viremic period, virus could be recovered only from lymph nodes, but two to three days later there was evidence of dissemination to skin and other leucocyte-rich tissues where it persisted for up to three days after termination of viremia when recoverability ended abruptly.[59] Animals infected with dengue 1, 3, or 4 viruses and subsequently with dengue 2 circulated this latter virus at higher titer than when the same strain was inoculated into susceptible animals.[42] This phenomenon, in vivo immunological enhancement of dengue infection, has formed the basis for the hypothesis of the immunopathogenesis of dengue in human beings.

Diagnosis

The diagnosis of dengue infection in subhuman primates may be important since there is evidence that these animals may be zoonotic hosts.[74] Dengue infected monkeys and gibbons circulate virus in the blood for a period of hours or days and develop hemagglutination-inhibiting (HI), CF, and N antibodies.[38,41,92] Virus recovery techniques are identical to those for human beings. Serological methods for measuring antibody levels in monkey and human serum are similar except that monkey complement must be inactivated at 60° C for 30 min rather than at 56°.[41]

HUMAN INFECTION

Clinical

Dengue Fever

Biphasic fever and rash are the most characteristic features of the dengue fever syndrome. Manifestations vary with age and from patient to patient. In infants and young children, the disease may be undifferentiated or characterized by a 1- to 5-day fever, pharyngeal inflammation, rhinitis, and mild cough.[34] A distinctive range of incubation periods, duration of illness, and clinical findings may characterize disease with different dengue types, although there are insufficient confirmatory studies to document this unequivocally.[43,83,84] In outbreaks, a majority of infected adults have most of the findings summarized below. After an incubation period of 2 to 7 days, there is a sudden onset of fever, rising rapidly to 39.5 to 41.0° C, usually accompanied by frontal or retro-orbital headache. Occasionally, back pain precedes or accompanies the fever. A transient, macular, generalized rash which blanches under pressure may occur during the first 24 to 48 hr of fever. The pulse may be slow in proportion to the degree of fever. Myalgia or bone pain occurs soon after onset of fever and increases in severity. During the second to the sixth day of fever, nausea and vomiting are apt to occur, and during this phase generalized lymphadenopathy, cutaneous hyperaesthesia or hyperalgesia, taste aberrations, and pronounced anorexia may develop.

Coincident with, or 1 to 2 days after, defervescence, a second generalized, morbilliform, maculopapular rash appears, which spares the palms and soles, though in some patients there is edema of the palms and soles. About the time of appearance of this second rash, the body temperature, which has fallen to normal, may become slightly elevated and establish the biphasic temperature curve. The rash disappears in 1 to 5 days, sometimes followed by desquamation of the epithelium.

Epistaxis, petechiae, and purpuric lesions, though uncommon, may occur at any stage of the disease. Swallowed blood from epistaxis may be passed from the rectum or vomited, and may be misinterpreted as bleeding of gastrointestinal origin. GI bleeding, menorrhagia, and bleeding from other organs have been observed in a few patients during large outbreaks.[14] The pathogenesis of the hemorrhage in these cases has not been described, and it is not possible to relate these hemorrhagic phenomena to the hemorrhagic diathesis which accompanies dengue hemorrhagic fever. After the febrile stage, prolonged asthenia, mental depression, bradycardia, and ventricular extrasystoles are common in adults.

Dengue Hemorrhagic Fever

The incubation period of DHF is unknown but is presumed to be that of dengue fever. In children, the progression of the illness is characteristic.[16,67,88] A relatively mild first phase with abrupt onset of fever, malaise, vomiting, headache, anorexia, and cough is followed after 2 to 5 days by rapid deterioration and physical collapse. In this second phase, patients usually manifest cold, clammy extremities, warm trunks, flushed faces, and diaphoresis. They are restless and irritable and complain of mid-epigastric pain. Frequently, there are scattered petechiae on the forehead and extremities, spontaneous ecchymoses may appear, and easy bruising and bleeding at sites of venipuncture are common. There may be circumoral and peripheral cyanosis. Respirations are rapid and often labored. Pulses are weak, rapid and thready, and heart sounds are faint. Pulse pressures are frequently narrow (20 mm Hg or less); the systolic and diastolic pressures may be low or unobtainable. Livers may become palpable two or three finger breadths below the costal margin and are usually firm and nontender. Less than 10% of patients manifest gross ecchymosis or GI bleeding.

After a 24- or 36-hr period of crisis, convalescence is fairly rapid in children who recover. Temperatures may return to normal before or during the stage of shock. Bradycardia and ventricular extrasystoles are common during convalescence. Infrequently, there is residual brain damage apparently due either to prolonged shock or occasionally to intracranial hemorrhage. Death occurs in 10 to 40% of patients, depending greatly on the phase of the illness during which patients reach the hospital and upon the appropriateness and vigor of replacement and supportive therapy.

Pathology and Pathogenesis

The pathogenesis of shock and hemorrhage in human dengue infection is incompletely understood. It is postulated that circulating antibodies may promote cellular infection and thus paradoxically enhance disease severity,[39,45] as demonstrated in cell cultures of human mononuclear phagocytes prepared from dengue immune donors or cultures which are supplemented with non-neutralizing dengue antibodies in which dengue viruses demonstrate enhanced growth.[40,45] Fluorescent antibody (FA) studies on blood leukocytes, and virus isolations from necropsy tissues have suggested that dengue viruses invade leukocytes and lymphatic tissues. It has been proposed on this basis that the number of infected mononuclear phagocytes in individuals with naturally or passively acquired antibody may exceed the number in nonimmune persons.[40] In this context, increased production of viral antigen could contribute to shock, possibly through a second immunopathologic mechanism. Early in the acute stage of secondary dengue infection there is rapid activation of the complement system, presumably caused by complexes of antidengue IgG and viral antigens. During shock, blood levels of Clq, C3, C4, and C5 though C8, and C3 proactivator are depressed and C3 catabolic rates elevated,[7,63] but the kinin system apparently is not involved.[25] Shock may be mediated by histamine released from mast cells by the peptides, C3a and C5a.[7,63] Specific mediator(s) of vascular permeability in dengue hemorrhagic fever have not yet been identified, but a mild degree of disseminated intravascular coagulation, plus liver damage and thrombocytopenia could contribute additively to produce hemorrhage.[7,16,63,67] Capillary damage allows fluid, electrolytes, protein, and, in some instances, red blood cells to leak into intravascular spaces. This internal redistribution of fluid, together with deficits due to fasting, thirsting, and vomiting, results in hemoconcentration, hypovolemia, increased cardiac work, tissue hypoxia, metabolic acidosis, and hyponatremia.[16]

On postmortem examination there are usually no gross or microscopically visible lesions which might account for death except in rare instances in which death may be due to gastrointestinal or intracranial hemorrhages. Minimal to moderate hemorrhages are usually seen in the upper gastrointestinal tract and petechial hemorrhages are frequently observed in the intraventricular septum of the heart, on the pericardium, and on the subserosal surfaces of major viscera organs. Focal hemorrhages are occasionally seen in the lungs, liver, adrenals, and subarachnoid space. The liver is usually enlarged, often with fatty changes. Yellow, watery, at times blood-tinged, effusions are present in serous cavities in about three fourths of patients. Retroperitoneal tissues are markedly edematous. Microscopically, there is perivascular edema in the soft tissues and widespread diapedesis of red blood cells. There may be maturational arrest of megakaryocytes in the bone marrow, and increased numbers are seen in capillaries of the lungs, in renal glomeruli, and in sinusoides of the liver and spleen. Proliferation of lymphocytoid and plasmacytoid cells, lymphocytolysis and lymphophagocytosis occur in the spleen and lymph nodes. In the spleen, Malpighian corpuscle germinal centers are necrotic. There is depletion of lymphocytes in the thymus. In the liver there are varying degrees of fatty metamorphosis, focal midzonal necrosis, and hyperplasia of the Kupffer cells. In the sinusoids are seen non-nucleated cells with vaculoated acidophilic cytoplasm, resembling Councilman bodies. There is a mild, proliferative glomerulonephritis.[8] Biopsies of the skin rash reveal swelling and minimal necrosis of endothelial cells, subcutaneous deposits of fibrinogen, and in a few cases, dengue antigen has been found in extravascular mononuclear cells and on blood vessel walls.[6]

Using cell cultures or suckling mice for virus recovery, dengue virus is almost invariably absent in tissues at the time of death. Rarely isolations have been reported from lymphatic tissues.[68] Tissue suspensions contain large quantities of dengue neutralizing substances.[68]

Diagnosis
Dengue Fever

Clinical diagnosis is based on a high index of suspicion in endemic areas and a knowledge of the geographical distribution and environmental cycle of dengue viruses. Activities of patients during periods preceding the onset of illness may give important clues to the possibilities of infection.

Differential diagnosis includes many viral, respiratory, and influenza-like diseases and the early stages of malaria, scrub typhus, hepatitis, and leptospirosis. Abortive forms of these latter diseases may never evolve beyond a dengue-like stage. Three arboviral diseases are dengue-like with rash: chikungunya and O'nyong-nyong fevers (alphaviruses) and West Nile fever (flavivirus).[4] Three others are dengue-like but without rash: Colorado tick fever, sandfly fever, and the mild form of Rift Valley fever. Because of the variation in clinical findings and the multiplicity of possible causative agents, the descriptive term "dengue-like disease" should be used until a specific etiologic diagnosis is provided by the laboratory.

Dengue Hemorrhagic Fever

In areas endemic for dengue, hemorrhagic fever should be suspected in children with a febrile illness who exhibit shock ahd hemoconcentration with thrombocytopenia. Hypoproteinemia, hemorrhagic manifestations, and hepatic enlargement are frequently accompanying findings.[16,36,38,67] Hemorrhagic manifestations have been described in several viral diseases, including virus hemorrhagic fevers of Argentina, Bolivia, and West Africa (Lassa, Ebola); tick-borne hemorrhagic fevers of India and U.S.S.R., and hemorrhagic fever with renal syndrome which occurs across Northern Eurasia, from Scandinavia to Korea. A number of rickettsial diseases, meningococcemia, and other severe illness caused by a variety of agents may produce similar clinical pictures so diagnosis of DHF should be made only when epidemiological, serological, or virological evidence strongly support dengue etiology.

Laboratory confirmation of DHF diagnosis is based on serological changes between acute and convalescent serum samples, or by isolation of the virus.[88] Blood samples should be obtained during the febrile period, preferably before the 4th day after onset of illness and 2 weeks or more after the first sampling. The acute phase sera or plasma should be frozen, optimally at $-65°$ C or colder, to preserve the specimens for later virus isolation as well as serological testing. Serologic diagnosis is depending on a fourfold or greater increase in antibody titers by HI, CF or N tests, but often similar titers are found in both sera when there has been prior infection with another member of the dengue subgroup and serological findings are difficult to interpret. Sequential infections with dengue and nondengue flaviviruses or vice versa may result in the production of type specific IgM directed to the second infecting virus,[24] and a second antibody which is a group specific IgG, masking the type specific IgM in untreated sera.

A large number of techniques are available for recovery and identification of dengue viruses. Pertinent references can be found in the review by Schlesinger,[81] and recommendations for general use have been made by a World Health Organization (WHO) Expert Committee.[88] Acute phase sera, postmortem tissues, sentinel monkey sera, mosquito suspensions, or other materials thought to contain dengue virus may be inoculated by the i.c. route into suckling mice. Following a suitable period, the mice may be sacrificed and examined for subtle neurological signs or challenged at 14 days with a neurovirulent strain of dengue virus. Suspected materials may be inoculated into any of several cell cultures; primary rhesus kidney, or LLC-MK2, BSC-1, Vero, or other cell lines and examined for plaques under agar or methyl cellulose overlay, or for cytopathic effect or resistance to a challenge cytopathic virus using a fluid overlay.

Intrathoracic inoculation of *Aedes albopictus* or *Ae. aegypti* mosquitoes is a highly sensitive dengue recovery system. Presence of dengue viruses in mosquitoes may be detected by FA or CF tests or by subinoculation of mosquito suspensions into susceptible cell cultures.

Differentiation of a primary- from a secondary-type antibody response may have epidemiologic significance. Criteria for distinguishing these responses have been proposed by a WHO Committee.[88] HI tests using 8 units of antigen measure as a primary response an HI antibody titer generally less than 1:20 in sera obtained on or before the 4th day after onset of illness; or as the presence of antibodies in the acute phase specimen with a four-fold or greater increase in antibody titers between paired sera, with titers in the convalescent sera not exceeding 1:1280. By CF tests, there should be no antibodies demonstrable in acute phase sera collected during the first week of illness and a relatively type-specific CF response in samples collected 3 or more weeks after the onset of illness.

A secondary-type response is (1) one in which HI antibody is detected in acute sera collected before the fifth day after onset followed by four-fold or greater antibody rises in convalescent sera; (2) no HI antibody in acute sera collected prior to the 5th day after onset followed by a rise in antibody titer to at least 1:2560 in convalescent sera; (3) there are HI antibody titers of 1:1280 or greater in paired acute and convalescent sera. CF antibodies are present during the acute phase of illness and may either rise or show high-fixed titers in convalescent samples. When tested against dengue 1 through 4 or other flavivirus antigens, both HI and CF antibodies are broadly reactive.

EPIDEMIOLOGY

Occurrence
Dengue Fever

Dengue outbreaks have been described on every continent except Antarctica.[10,26,51,54,56,80,81,89] There is some evidence to suggest that human dengue may have originated from endemic foci in tropical Asia.[61] The probable spread of vector *Ae. aegypti* mosquitoes by people moving from Africa throughout the world during historical times is postulated to have provided an ecological niche quickly occupied by several human viral pathogens — yellow fever, chikungunya, and dengue viruses. During the 18th and 19th centuries, epidemics or pandemics occurred in newly settled lands largely in the Americas and Australia,[11,56] possibly associated with mosquito habitats provided by domestic water storage in newly developed urban areas. Isolated shipboard or garrison outbreaks often confined among nonindigenous settlers or visitors were reported in Africa, the Indian sub-continent and Southeast Asia.[11,56,83] During World War II, dengue infections were common in combatants of the Pacific war and appeared in staging areas not normally infected; Japan, Hawaii, and Pacific islands.[81] During the past 20 years epidemic dengue fever has centered in the Caribbean and Pacific islands. Dengue type 3 caused human disease in Puerto Rico and other Caribbean islands in 1963 and in Tahiti in 1964 to 1969.[66,85] After a lapse of 6 years, dengue type 2 appeared in the Caribbean basin.[26] In 1977, dengue 1 was introduced, has spread to Mexico, and threatens the southwestern U.S. Extensive dengue type 2 activity occurred throughout Polynesia and Micronesia in 1971 to 1972,[58,85] replaced by dengue type 1 in many of the same populations in 1974 to 1975.[21] Dengue virus types 1 and 2 have been recovered from patients with mild clinical illness in Nigeria in the absence of epidemic disease.[10]

Dengue Hemorrhagic Fever

Outbreaks of dengue-like disease accompanied by cases which clinically resemble

DHF were recorded in Australia over a period of 50 years from 1897, in Greece in 1928, and Taiwan in 1931.[30] Dengue hemorrhagic fever is now endemic in many countries in tropical Asia. It seems probable that the disease was first recognized in Thailand in 1950, in the Philippines in 1953, in Singapore and Malaysia in 1962, in Vietnam in 1963, in India in 1963, in Sri Lanka in 1965, in Indonesia in 1969, and in Burma in 1970.[30,32,52,64,90] DHF has occurred at consistently high endemicity in Thailand and was third among diseases which caused hospitalization or death in children in 1972.[44] Intermittent epidemic activity has been the rule in the Philippines, South Vietnam, Malaysia, and Indonesia, while DHF has apparently disappeared from India and Sri Lanka.[44,57] The present status of DHF in Vietnam, Cambodia, and Laos is unknown.

Reservoir

Numerous species of subhuman primates are readily infected in the laboratory following subcutaneous inoculation of dengue viruses,[81,84] developing viremia levels sufficient to infect mosquitoes.[84,91] Simmons et al. were the first to note that wild-caught *Macaca philippinensis* resisted dengue infection while *Macaca fuscatus* (Japanese macaque) were susceptible.[84] Recent work by Rudnick in Malaysia has revealed a jungle cycle of dengue transmission involving canopy-feeding monkeys and *Ae. niveus,* a vector species which feeds both on monkeys and human beings.[74] Although the existence of a jungle dengue cycle in the Malaysian rain forest has been carefully documented, the geographic range of this subhuman primate zoonotic reservoir of dengue is not known.[74] Because of contiguity of primate populations, it may be possible that jungle dengue is present throughout all of Southeast Asia, possibly extending to southern India and Sri Lanka. Although African and South American monkeys are susceptible to experimental dengue infection by peripheral inoculation, the possibility of jungle dengue in these geographic areas has not been documented nor carefully investigated. From epidemiological studies, it is apparent that urban human dengue and jungle monkey dengue are effectively compartmentalized. Dengue outbreaks are vectored by anthropophilic mosquitoes, and travel along routes of transportation. At present urban dengue vectors and susceptible human beings are so abundant and so wide spread that any possible impact of exchange of dengue viruses between people and monkeys in the jungle is not discernable. If urban dengue may be eliminated in the future, virus from a jungle cycle could become a matter of importance.

Transmission

Ae. aegypti, a daytime biting mosquito, is the principal vector. All four virus types have been recovered from naturally infected *Ae. aegypti.*[32] In most tropical areas *Ae. aegypti* is highly domesticated, breeding in water stored for drinking or bathing, or in any containers collecting fresh water. Dengue viruses have also been recovered from naturally infected *Ae. albopictus,* and outbreaks in the Pacific area have been attributed to *Ae. albopictus* which breeds in bamboo stumps.

Dengue outbreaks in urban areas infested with *Ae. aegypti* may be explosive, involving as many as 70 to 80% of the population.[83] Because *Ae. aegypti* has a limited flight range, spread of epidemics usually follows transportation routes carried by mobile viremic human beings.

Dengue viruses replicate in the gut, brain, and salivary glands of infected mosquitoes without apparent harm to adult mosquitoes.[73] Once infected, mosquitoes remain infectious for their life time; in experimental circumstances as long as 70 days.[84] Since female mosquitoes of *Aedes* spp. take repeated blood meals, long-lived individuals have great potency as vectors. *Aedes* spp. mosquitoes are exquisitely sensitive to intrathoracic inoculation although the threshold of infection by oral feeding is higher.[73] Dengue virus can be transmitted transovarially; larvae do not become infected through contamination of water.[84] *Ae. aegypti* and *Culex quinquefasciatus* can transmit dengue mechanically by interrupted feeding.[84] The contribution of mechanical feeding to the spread of dengue virus during epidemics has never been measured, but because of the "skittishness" of *Ae. aegypti,* and its habit of feeding during the day when its intended victims are awake and often moving, interrupted feeding and thus mechanical transmission may actually be common.

Environment

Ae. aegypti preferentially feed on human beings; hence they are found most abundantly in and around human habitations. Biting activity is greatest above wet bulb readings of 14° C,[22] and increases with higher temperature and humidity.[82] In temperate countries dengue transmission is interrupted during winter months and dengue has not become established endemically at latitudes above 25° N. *Ae. aegypti* mosquitoes prefer small vessels containing clean water for breeding. Breeding sites may be provided by people through cultural customs, as in Thailand where water is stored in and around homes in large earthenware jars.[32] By contrast, *Ae. aegypti* is not abundant in tropical India because small amounts of water are commonly brought from village wells as needed throughout each day.[72] Water in flower vases, household offerings, ant traps, coconut husks, tin cans, and rubber tires may supply breeding sites for *Ae. aegypti.*[56.58] The eggs are resistant to dessication and are deposited inside water containers above the water line.[56] In outdoor containers, the eggs remain dormant until the beginning of monsoonal rains, at which time large hatches emerge and adult populations become large.[31] Indoor mosquito populations are more stable.

Human Host

Infection of human beings is determined both by host immunity patterns and by ecological conditions which vary from country to country and place to place. Where *Ae. aegypti* habitats are largely indoors, attack rates are greatest in persons who spend most of their time in the house, i.e., preschool children and adult women,[66] and dengue mostly attacks the urban poor. Where breeding occurs outdoors in large compounds, dengue may be a disease of the upper classes.[44] During epidemics of DHF in Thailand, foreign residents were largely unaffected because they used piped water and did not store water in jars suitable for mosquito breeding on the premises.[35] Dengue transmission may occur in public buildings and outbreaks among hospital staffs have been reported.[12] There is no information concerning differential attractiveness of people of different ages to *Ae. aegypti.* Severity of dengue, however, is age-related with infections in infants and children generally less severe than those in older children and adults.[14]

CONTROL

Prevention

Dengue type 1 attenuated live virus vaccine of suckling mouse brain origin is efficacious but not available for general use.[93] Prevention of human exposure to biting mosquitoes through the use of insecticides, repellents, protective clothing, and screening of houses is usually the most practical measure. Destruction of *Ae. aegypti* breeding sites is also effective. If water storage is mandatory, use containers with tight-fitting lids or pour a thin layer of oil on the water to prevent egg-laying or hatching. Special larvicides such as Abate® which is available as a 1% sand granule formulation and is effective at a concentration of 1 ppm, may be added safely to drinking water.[28.88] Ultra-low volume (ULV) environmental spraying of malathion or fenetrothion by truck- or airplane-mounted sprayers may rapidly destroy the adult mosquito population.[55.88]

Treatment

Dengue Fever

Treatment is supportive. Bed rest is advised during the febrile period. Anti-pyretics or cold sponging should be used to keep body temperature below 40° C. Analgesics or mild sedation may be required to control pain. Fluid and electrolyte replacement therapy is required when there are deficits due to sweating, fasting, thirsting, vomiting, or diarrhea.

Dengue Hemorrhagic Fever

Management requires immediate evaluation of vital signs and degrees of hemoconcentration, dehydration, and electrolyte inbalance.[16,88] Close monitoring is essential for at least the first 48 hr during which there is greatest danger that shock may occur or recur precipitously coincident with the defervescence of fever. Patients who become cyanotic or develop labored breathing should be given oxygen. Intravenous replacement of fluids and electrolytes is frequently sufficient to sustain patients until spontaneous recovery occurs, but when elevation of the hematocrit value persists after replacement of fluids, plasma or plasma protein preparations should be administered. Care must be taken to avoid overhydration which may contribute to cardiac failure. Transfusion of fresh blood or of platelets suspended in plasma may be required to control bleeding, but should only be given after evaluation of hemoglobin or hematocrit values and never in a patient with hemoconcentration. Salicylates, because of their hemorrhagenic potential, are contraindicated.

Paraldehyde or chloral hydrate sedation may be indicated for children who are markedly agitated. Pressor amines, alpha-adrenergic blocking agents, and aldosterone have been widely utilized but have not reduced mortality below that observed with simple supportive therapy. Heparin may be used with caution in patients with intractable bleeding who show objective evidence of severe disseminated intravascular coagulation. A recent study has demonstrated some decreased mortality in patients treated with corticosteroids,[65] but the more general experience has been that steroids have not shortened the duration of disease nor improved prognosis in children receiving careful supportive therapy.[70]

Regulatory Measures

Dengue is not subject to international quarantine or surveillance regulations. An intensive and effective voluntary reporting system has been devised.

Epidemic Measures

WHO has recommended guidelines for application of mosquito adulticides.[88] Based upon epidemiological and entomological information, the size of the area which requires adult mosquito abatement should be determined. Using technical Malathion® or fenitrothion at 438 mℓ/ha, two adulticidal treatments at 10-day intervals should be made using vehicle-mounted or portable ULV aerosol generators or mist-blowers. It is suggested that moderate-size cities stockpile at least one vehicle-mounted aerosol generator each, five mist-blowers, ten swing foggers and 1000 ℓ of ULV insecticides in order to be prepared to rapidly carry out adulticidal operations over a 20 km² area. Where funds are limited, such equipment and insecticides can be stockpiled regionally for rapid transportation to communities requiring them. Ground applications should be made in areas or neighborhoods where there are concentrations of cases, focusing especially on areas where people congregate during daylight hours such as hospitals and schools. Where outbreaks are widespread or large, ULV sprays may be applied from aircraft. C47 or similar aircraft, small agricultural spray planes, and helicopters have been used to make aerial applications.[55] Because of wind effects the density of spray droplets and effectiveness of coverage of target areas should be carefully monitored.

Upon occurrence of an index case or during the early stages of epidemics before massive rapid action must be taken, 4% Malathion® or other residual insecticides may be sprayed within all houses within a 100-m radius of a residence of a DHF patient.

Eradication

During the early 20th century, *Ae. aegypti* was successfully eradicated from countries and from entire continents using techniques pioneered by the Rockefeller Foundation in its world-wide program to control urban yellow fever.[94] With time, however, the species has successfully re-established itself in much of its former range.[1] An *Ae. aegypti* eradication campaign in the U.S. was abandoned and replaced by a program of disease surveillance and containment of dengue virus should it be reintroduced. Mosquito control or eradication programs require the simultaneous use of two approaches: (1) reduction in breeding sites and application of larvicides, and (2) closely spaced application of adulticides.[88] Source reduction requires the support of the population either by legal sanctions or voluntary actions. Community campaigns should be well organized, supervised, and evaluated. Residential disposal of discarded cans, bottles, tires, and other potential breeding sites not used for storage of drinking or bathing water must be thoroughly carried out. Where water is stored in reservoirs, the sides should be scrubbed to remove eggs when water levels are low. Residential drinking and bathing water storage containers and flower vases should be completely emptied weekly. Water containers which cannot be emptied may be treated with Abate® 1% sand granules at a dosage of 1 ppm (e.g., 10 g sand to 100 ℓ water) at 2- 3-month intervals.[88]

Adulticides should be applied using vehicle-mounted or portable ULV aerosol generators or mist-blowers to apply technical grade Malathion® or fenitrothion at 438 mℓ/ha. Three applications made at one-week intervals can suppress *Ae. aegypti* populations for about 2 months.

Health Education

The object of health education is to make the population aware of the identity of the mosquito vector of DHF, to describe its daytime biting habits and its breeding habits in household water containers, and to motivate people to reduce breeding sources by emptying water from containers on a regular basis. The use of piped water rather than of water storage is encouraged. In some tropical areas, *Ae. aegypti* control has been effectively maintained through the simple expedient of emptying water containers once each week.[94] During the yellow fever campaigns in the Western Hemisphere, strong sanitary laws were adopted in some countries making the presence of mosquitoes on premises a crime punishable by fines or jail sentences.[94] In the modern era, Singapore has successfully adopted these measures. Through enforcement of stiff fines and frequent premises inspections, Singapore has drastically reduced *Ae. aegypti* infestation. Health education through mass media or through schools has been organized in Burma, Thailand, Malaysia, and Indonesia though without spectacular success.[44] Studies in Malaysia following the 1973 epidemic ofDHF indicated a very low level of functional knowledge among the inhabitants of Kuala Lumpur about the vector of DHF, and those persons who were correctly informed, in most instances, took little or no action to protect themselves against mosquito breeding in their homes.[23]

PUBLIC HEALTH ASPECTS

Economic and Social Impact

The economic and social impact of epidemic DHF has not been objectively measured. Throughout much of tropical Asia, DHF is now the most feared epidemic disease, and even small outbreaks cause panic, commanding attention in national and international headlines. In Thailand where between 8,000 and 38,000 DHF patients are hospitalized annually, the financial impact of the disease must be enormous.

A 1972 cost-benefit study of the dengue outbreaks in the Americas estimated a cost for eradication of *Ae. aegypti* of $436 million versus present annual losses in the work force, in tourism and in medical care of patients due to dengue of $450 million.[1]

Reporting

WHO has asked member governments to report cases and deaths from DHF with and without shock by age and sex to the Epidemiological Surveillance Unit, WHO, Geneva, weekly, with copies to the Communicable Disease Adviser in the appropriate regional office — New Delhi for the Southeast Asia region, and Manila for the Western Pacific region. Reports may be submitted in narrative or tabular form and should be signed and dated by the national medical officer responsible for the reporting section.

Surveillance

Surveillance is indicated in all dengue endemic areas as well as in "receptive areas" where *Ae. aegypti* is known to be present. Rapid exchange of technical information is essential. Publication of quarterly Dengue Newsletters is encouraged to facilitate information exchange on morbidity and mortality, epidemiological reports, results of clinical studies, dengue virus isolation by sources and dates, entomological studies, surveys for *Aedes* vectors, control measures planned or accomplished, new developments in insecticides and spray equipment, and other pertinent findings on dengue and DHF. Three newsletters are currently published: Dengue Newsletter for the Americas, editorial office, Department of Health, Education, and Welfare, Center for Disease Control, San Juan Tropical Disease Laboratories, GPO Box 4532, San Juan, Puerto Rico; Dengue Newsletter for the Southeast Asian and Western Pacific Regions, editorial office c/o Project Leader, WHO/VRCRU, P.B. 302, Jakarta, Indonesia; and The South Pacific Commission Dengue Newsletter, editorial office, South Pacific Commission, P. O. Box D5, Noumea Cedex, New Caledonia.

REFERENCES

1. **Anon.**, *The Prevention of Diseases Transmitted by Aedes aegypti* in the Americas — A Cost Benefit Study, Arthur D. Little, Cambridge, Mass., 1972.
2. **Ashburn, P. M. and Craig, C. F.**, Experimental investigations regarding the etiology of dengue fever, *J. Infect. Dis.,* 4, 440, 1907.
3. **Bancroft, T. L.**, On the etiology of dengue fever, *Austral. Med. Gaz.,* 25, 17, 1906.
4. **Berge, T. O., Ed.**, *International Catalogue of Arboviruses,* 2nd ed., Publ. No. (CDC) 75-8301, Public Health Service, U.S. Department of Health, Education and Welfare, Atlanta, 1975.
5. **Bhamarapravati, N., Toochinda, P., and Boonyapaknavik, V.**, Pathology of Thailand hemorrhagic fever: a study of 100 autopsy cases, *Ann. Trop. Med. Parasitol.,* 61, 500, 1967.
6. **Bhamarapravati, N.**, personal communication, 1977.
7. **Bokisch, V. A., Top, F. H., Jr., Russell, P. K., Dixon, F. J., and Muller-Eberhard, H. J.**, The potential pathogenic role of complement in dengue hemorrhagic shock syndrome, *N. Engl. J. Med.,* 289, 996, 1973.
8. **Boonpucknavig, V., Bhamarapravati, N., Boonpucknavig, S., Futrakaul, P., and Tampaichitr, P.**, Glomerular changes in dengue hemorrhagic fever, *Arch. Pathol. Lab. Med.,* 100, 206, 1976.
9. **Boonpucknavig, S., Bhamarapravati, N., Nimmannitya, S., Phalavadhtana, A., and Siripont, A.**, Immunofluorescent staining of the surfaces of lymphocytes in suspension from patients with dengue hemorrhagic fever, *Am. J. Pathol.,* 85, 37, 1976.

10. **Carey, D. E., Causey, O. R., Reedy, S., and Cooke, A. R.,** Dengue viruses from febrile patients in Nigeria, 1964-1968, *Lancet,* 1, 105, 1971.
11. **Carey, S. E.,** Chikungunya and dengue: a case of mistaken identity? *J. Hist. Med.,* 26, 243, 1971.
12. **Carey, D. E., Myers, R. M., Rueben, R., and Rodriques, F. M.,** Studies on dengue in Vellore, South India, *Am. J. Trop. Med. Hyg.,* 15, 580, 1966.
13. **Casals, J. and Brown, L. V.,** Hemagglutination with arthropod-borne viruses, *J. Exp. Med.,* 99, 429, 1954.
14. **Chandler, A. C. and Rice, L.,** Observations on the etiology of dengue fever, *Am. J. Trop. Med.,* 3, 233, 1923.
15. **Cleland, J. B., Bradley, B., and McDonald, W.,** On the transmission of Australian dengue by the mosquito Stegomyia fasciata, *Med. J. Aust.,* 2, 179, 1916.
16. **Cohen, S. N. and Halstead, S. B.,** Shock associated with dengue infection. I. The clinical and physiologic manifestations of dengue hemorrhagic fever in Thailand, 1964, *J. Pediatr.,* 68, 448, 1966.
17. **Copanaris, P.,** L'épidémie de dengue en Grece au cours de l'éte 1928. *Inst. Hyg. Publ.,* 20, 1950, 1928.
18. **Craighead, J. E., Sather, G. E., Hammon, W. McD., and Dammin, G. J.,** Pathology of dengue virus infections in mice, *Arch. Pathol.,* 81, 232, 1966.
19. **DeMadrid, A. T. and Porterfield, J. S.,** The flaviviruses (group B arboviruses): a cross neutralization study, *J. Gen. Virol.,* 23, 91, 1974.
20. **Demsey, A., Steere, R. L., Brandt, W. E., and Veltri, B. J.,** Morphology and development of dengue 2 virus employing the freeze-fracture and thin-section techniques, *J. Ultrastruct. Res.,* 46, 102, 1974.
21. South Pacific Commission, Dengue Newsletter, Vol. 4, Noumea, New Caledonia, 1976.
22. **Derrick, E. H. and Bicks, V. A.,** The limiting temperature for the transmission of dengue, *Australasian Ann. Med.,* 7, 102, 1958.
23. **Dobbins, J. G. and Else, J. G.,** Knowledge, attitudes and practices related to control of dengue hemorrhagic fever in an urban Malay kampung, *Southeast Asian J. Trop. Med. Public Health,* 6, 120, 1975.
24. **Edelman, R. and Pariyonda, A.,** Human immunoglobulin M antibody in the serodiagnosis of Japanese encephalitis virus infections, *Am. J. Epidemiol.,* 98, 29, 1973.
25. **Edelman, R., Nimmannitya, S., Colman, R. W., Talamo, R. C., and Top, R. H., Jr.,** Evaluation of the plasma kinin system in dengue hemorrhagic fever, *J. Lab. Clin. Med.,* 86, 410, 1975.
26. **Ehrenkranz, N. J., Ventura, A. K., Cuadrado, P. R., Pond, W. L., and Porter, J. E.,** Pandemic dengue in Caribbean countries and the Southern United States — past, present and potential problems, *N. Engl. J. Med.,* 285, 1460, 1971.
27. **Gibbs, A. J. and Harrison, B. D.,** Realistic approach to virus classification and nomenclature, *Nature (London),* 218, 927, 1968.
28. **Gould, D. J., Mount, G. A., Scanlon, J. E., Sullivan, M. F., and Winter, P. E.,** Dengue control on an island in the Gulf of Thailand. I. Results of an Aedes aegypti control program, *Am. J. Trop. Med. Hyg.,* 20, 705, 1971.
29. **Graham, H.,** The dengue: a study of its pathology and mode of propagation, *J. Trop. Med.,* 6, 209, 1903.
30. **Halstead, S. B.,** Dengue and Hemorrhagic Fevers in Southeast Asia, *Yale J. Biol. Med.,* 37, 434, 1965.
31. **Halstead, S. B. and Yararat, C.,** Recent epidemics of hemorrhagic fever in Thailand. Observations related to pathogenesis of a "new" dengue disease, *J. Am. Publ. Health. Assoc.,* 55, 1386, 1965.
32. **Halstead, S. B.,** Mosquito-borne hemorrhagic fevers of South and Southeast Asia, *Bull. WHO,* 35, 3, 1966.
33. **Halstead, S. B., Nimmannitya, S., Yamarat, C., and Russell, P. K.,** Hemmorhagic fever in Thailand. Newer knowledge regarding etiology, *Jpn. J. Med. Sci.,* Suppl. 20, 96, 1967.
34. **Halstead, S. B., Nimmannitya, S., and Margiotta, M. R.,** Dengue and chikungunya virus infection in man in Thailand, 1962-1964. Observations on disease in out-patients, *Am. J. Trop. Med. Hyg.,* 18, 972, 1969.
35. **Halstead, S. B., Udomsakdi, S., Singharah, P., and Nisalak, A.,** Dengue and chikungunya virus infection in man in Thailand, 1962-1964. III. Clinical, epidemiological and virological observations on disease in non-indigenous white persons, *Am. J. Trop. Med. Hyg.,* 18, 984, 1969.
36. **Halstead, S. B., Nimmannitya, S., and Cohen, S. N.,** Observations related to pathogenesis of dengue hemorrhagic fever. IV. Relation of disease severity to antibody response and virus recovered, *Yale J. Biol. Med.,* 42, 311, 1970.
37. **Halstead, S. B., Udomsakdi, S., Simasthien, O., Singharah, P., Sukhavachana, P., and Nisalak, A.,** Observations related to pathogenesis of dengue hemorrhagic fever. I. Experience with classification of dengue viruses, *Yale J. Biol. Med.,* 42, 261, 1970.

38. **Halstead, S. B., Casals, J., Shotwell, H., and Palumbo, N.,** Studies on the immunization of monkeys against dengue. I. Protection derived from single and sequential virus infection, *Am. J. Trop. Med. Hyg.,* 22, 365, 1973.

39. **Halstead, S. B., Chow, J., and Marchette, N. J.,** Immunologic enhancement of dengue virus replication, *Nature N. Biol.,* 243, 24, 1973.

40. **Halstead, S. B., Marchette, N. J., and Chow, J. S. S.,** Enhancement of dengue virus replication in immune leukocytes as a mechanism in the immunopathogenesis of dengue shock syndrome, *Adv. Biosci.,* 12, 401, 1973.

41. **Halstead, S. B., Shotwell, H., and Casals, J.,** Studies on the pathogenesis of dengue infection in monkeys. I. Clinical laboratory responses to primary infections, *J. Inf. Dis.,* 128, 7, 1973.

42. **Halstead, S. B., Shotwell, H., and Caslals, J.** Studies on the pathogenesis of dengue infection in monkeys. II. Clinical laboratory responses to heterologous infection, *J. Infect. Dis.,* 128, 15, 1973.

43. **Halstead, S. B.,** Etiologies of the experimental dengue of Siler and Simmons, *Am. J. Trop. Med. Hyg.,* 23, 974, 1974.

44. **Halstead, S. B.,** unpublished observations,

45. **Halstead, S. B. and O'Rourke, E. J.,** Antibody-enhanced dengue virus infection in primate leukocytes, *Nature,* 265, 739, 1977.

46. **Hare, R. E.,** The 1897 epidemic of dengue in North Queensland, *Aust. Med. Gaz.,* 17, 98, 1898.

47. **Hammon, W. McD., Rudnick, A., and Sather, G. E.,** Viruses associated with hemorrhagic fevers of the Philippines and Thailand, *Science,* 131, 1102, 1960.

48. **Hammon, W. McD., Rudnick, A., Sather, G., Rogers, K. D., and Morse, L. J.,** New hemorrhagic fevers of children in the Philippines and Thailand, *Trans. Assoc. Am. Physicians,* 73, 140, 1960.

49. **Hammon, W. McD. and Sather, G. E.,** Problems of typing dengue viruses, *Mil. Med.,* 129, 130, 1964.

50. **Hammon, W. McD. and Sather, G. E.,** Virological findings in the 1960 hemorrhagic fever epidemic (dengue) in Thailand, *Am. J. Trop. Med. Hyg.,* 13, 629, 1964.

51. **Hotta, S., Yamamoto, M., Tokuchi, M., and Sakakibara, S.,** Long persistence of anti-dengue antibodies in serum of native residents of Japanese Main Islands, *Kobe J. Med. Sci.,* 14, 149, 1968.

52. **Kho, L. K., Wulur, H., Himawan, T., and Thaib, S.,** Dengue hemorrhagic fever in Jakarta, *Paediatrica Indones.,* 12, 1, 1972.

53. **Kimura, R. and Hotta, S.,** On the inoculation of dengue virus into mice, *Nippon Igaku,* 3379, 629, 1944.

54. **Kokernot, R. H., Smithburn, K. C., and Weinbren, M. P.,** Neutralizing antibodies to arthropod-borne viruses in human beings and animals in the Union of South Africa, *J. Immunol.,* 77, 313, 1956.

55. **Lofgren, C. S., Ford, H. R., Tonn, R. J., and Jatanasen, S.,** The effectiveness of ultra-low volume applications of malathion at a rate of 6 fluid ounces per acre in controlling Aedes aegypti in a large-scale test at Nakohn Sawan, Thailand, *Bull WHO,* 42, 15, 1970.

56. **Lumley, G. F. and Taylor, F. H.,** Dengue, School of Public Health and Tropical Medicine, Australasian Medical Pub. Glebe, N.S.W., 1943, 74.

57. **Macasaet, F. F., Nakao, J. C., Villamil, P. T., Reala, A. C., and Beran, G. W.,** Epidemiology of arbovirus infections in Negros Oriental. III. Arbovirus infections in man and other vertebrates with emphasis on hemorrhagic fever, *J. Philipp. Med. Assoc.,* 46, 339, 1970.

58. **Maquire, T., Miles, J. A. R., MacNamara, F. N., Wilkinson, F. J., Austin, F. J., and Mataika, J. U.,** Mosquito-borne infections in Fiji, Part V. The 1971-1973 epidemic, *J. Hyg.,* 73, 263, 1974.

59. **Marchette, N. J., Halstead, S. B., Falkler, W. A., Jr., Stenhouse, A., and Nash, D.,** Studies on the pathogenesis of dengue infection in monkeys. III. Sequential distribution of virus in primary and heterologous infections, *J. Inf. Dis.,* 128, 23, 1973.

60. **Matsumura, R., Stollar, V., and Schlesinger, R. W.,** Studies on the nature of dengue viruses. V. Structure and development of dengue virus in Vero cells, *Virology,* 46, 344, 1971.

61. **Mattingly, P. F.,** Symposium on the evolution of arbovirus diseases. II. Ecological aspects of the evolution of mosquito-borne virus diseases, *Trans. R. Soc. Trop. Med. Hyg.,* 54, 97, 1960.

62. **McCloud, T. G., Cardiff, R. D., Brandt, W. E., Chiewslip, D., and Russell, P. K.,** Separation of dengue strains on the basis of a nonstructural antigen, *Am. J. Trop. Med. Hyg.,* 20, 964, 1971.

63. **Memoranda,** Pathogenetic mechanisms in dengue haemorrhagic fever: report of an international collaborative study, *Bull. WHO,* 48, 117, 1973.

64. **Ming, C. K., Thein, S., Thaung, U., Myint, U. T., Swe, T., Halstead, S. B., and Diwan, A. R.,** Clinical and laboratory studies on haemorrhagic fever in Burma, 1970-1972, *Bull. WHO,* 51, 227, 1974.

65. **Ming, M., Tin, U., Aye, M., Shwe, T. N., Swe, T., and Aye, B.,** Hydrocortisone in the management of dengue shock syndrome, *Southeast Asian J. Trop. Med. Public Health,* 6, 573, 1975.

66. **Neff, J. M., Morris, L., Gonzalea-Alcover, R., Coleman, P. H., Lyss, S. B., and Negron, H.,** Dengue fever in a Puerto Rican community, *Am. J. Epidemiol.,* 86, 162, 1967.

67. **Nimmannitya, S., Halstead, S. B., Cohen, S. N., and Margiotta, M. R.,** Dengue and chikungunya virus infections in man in Thailand, 1962-1964. I. Observations on hospitalized patients with hemorrhagic fever, *Am. J. Trop. Med. Hyg.,* 18, 954, 1969.

68. **Nisalak, A., Halstead, S. B., Singharaj, P., Udomsakdi, S., Nye, S. W., and Vinijchaikul, K.,** Observations related to pathogenesis of dengue hemorrhagic fever. III. Virologic studies of fatal disease, *Yale J. Biol. Med.,* 42, 293, 1970.

69. **Nomura, S. and Adashi, K.,** On fatal cases with hemorrhage caused by dengue fever (in Japanese), *Taiwan Igakkai Zasshi,* 30, 1154, 1931.

70. **Ponpanich, B., Bhanchet, P., Phanichyakarn, P., and Valyasevi, A.** Studies on dengue hemorrhagic fever. Clinical study: an evaluation of, steroids as a treatment, *J. Med. Assoc. Thailand,* 55, 6, 1973.

71. **Quitos, F. N., Lim, L. E., Juliano, L., Reyes, A., and Lacason, P.,** Hemorrhagic fever observed among children in the Philippines, *Philipp. J. Pediatr.,* 3, 1, 1954.

72. **Reuben, R.,** A note on the seasonal prevalence of adults of *Aedes aegypti* in Vellore, *Indian J. Med. Res.,* 58, 854, 1970.

73. **Rosen, L. and Gubler, D.,** The use of mosquitoes to detect and propagate dengue viruses, *Am. J. Trop. Med. Hyg.,* 23, 1153, 1974.

74. **Rudnick, A.,** personal communication, 1977.

75. **Rush, B.,** An account of the bilious remitting fever, as it appeared in Philadelphia in the summer and autumn of the year 1780, *Medical Inquiries and Observations,* Philadelphia, 1789, 102.

76. **Russell, P. K. and Nisalak, A.,** Dengue virus identification by the plaque reduction neutralization test, *J. Immunol.,* 99, 291, 1967.

77. **Russell, P. K. and McCown, J. M.,** Comparison of dengue 2 and dengue 3 virus strains by neutralization tests and identification of a subtype of dengue 3, *Am. J. Trop. Med. Hyg.,* 21, 97, 1972.

78. **Sabin, A. B. and Schlesinger, R.W.,** Production of immunity to dengue with virus modified by propagation in mice, *Science,* 101, 640, 1945.

79. **Sabin, A. B.,** The dengue group of viruses and its family relationships, *Bacteriol. Rev.,* 14, 225, 1950.

80. **Sabin, A. B.,** Recent advances in our knowledge of dengue and sandfly fever, *Am. J. Trop. Med. Hyg.,* 4, 198, 1955.

81. **Schlesinger, R. W.,** Dengue viruses, *Virol. Monogr.,* 16, 1, 1977.

82. **Sheppard, P. M., MacDonald, W. W., Tonn, R. J., and Grab, B.,** The dynamics of an adult population of *Aedes aegypti* in relation to dengue haemorrhagic fever in Bangkok, *J. Anim. Ecol.,* 38, 661, 1969.

83. **Siler, J. F., Hall, M. W., and Hitchens, A. P.,** Dengue: its history, epidemiology, mechanisms of transmission, etiology, clinical manifestations, immunity and prevention, *Philipp. J. Sci.,* 29, 1, 1926.

84. **Simmons, J. S., St. John, J. H., and Reynolds, F. H. K.,** Experimental studies of dengue, *Philipp. J. Sci.,* 44, 1, 1931.

85. **Sougrain, J., Moreau, J. A., and Rosen, L.,** L'epidemie de dengue de Tahiti en 1971. Evolution de la tendence hemorrhagique et comparisons avec les epidemie precedentes, *Bull. Soc. Pathol. Exot.,* 66, 381, 1973.

86. **Stollar, V., Stevens, T. M., and Schlesinger, R. W.,** Studies on the nature of dengue viruses. II. Characterization of viral RNA and effects of inhibitors of RNA synthesis, *Virology,* 30, 303, 1966.

87. **Stollar, V.,** Studies on the nature of dengue viruses. IV. The structural proteins of type 2 dengue virus, *Virology,* 39, 426, 1969.

88. Technical Advisory Committee on Dengue Haemorrhagic Fever for the South-East Asian and Western Pacific Regions, *Technical Guides for Diagnosis, Treatment, Surveillance, Prevention, and Control of Dengue Haemorrhagic Fever,* World Health Organization, Geneva, 1975.

89. **Theiler, M., Casals, J., and Moutousses, C.,** Etiology of the 1927-28 epidemic of dengue in Greece, *Proc. Soc. Exp. Biol. Med.,* 103, 244, 1960.

90. Dengue haemorrhagic fever in the South-East Asia and Western Pacific regions, *Weekly Epidimiol. Rec.,* 49, 277, 1974.

91. **Whitehead, R. H., Yuill, T. M., Gould, D. J., and Simasthien, P.,** Experimental infection of *Aedes aegypti* and *Aedes albopictus* with dengue viruses, *Trans. R. Soc. Trop. Med. Hyg.,* 65, 661, 1971.

92. **Whitehead, R. H., Chaicumpa, V., Olson, L. C., and Russell, P. K.,** Sequential dengue virus infections in the white-handed gibbon *Hylobates lar, Am. J. Trop. Med. Hyg.,* 19, 94, 1970.

93. **Wisseman, C. L., Jr., Sweet, B. H., Rosenzweig, E. C., and Eylar, O. R.,** Attenuated living type 1 dengue vaccines, *Am. J. Trop. Med. Hyg.,* 12, 620, 1963.

94. **Stode, G. K., Ed.,** *Yellow Fever,* McGraw-Hill, New York, 1951.

CHIKUNGUNYA FEVER

S. B. Halstead

NAME AND SYNONYMS

Chikungunya (CHIK) fever derives the name from the Swahili word meaning "that which bends up" referring to the characteristic symptom, arthralgia.[67] Chikungunya fever infection in man is dengue-like, and in historical times the terms "knokkel koorts," "abu rokab," "mal de genoux," "dengue," "dyenga", and 3-day fever have been given to epidemics probably caused by chikungunya virus.[9]

HISTORY

The classical account widely cited as being the initial description of epidemic dengue fever but more probably chikungunya fever with its acute onset and joint involvement, is that of David Bylon who was "stads chirurgyn" to the city of Batavia (Jakarta) in the year 1779.[7] Dr. Bylon, who himself contracted the illness, wrote that "it was last May 25, in the afternoon at 5:00 when I noted while talking with two good friends of mine, a growing pain in my right hand, and the joints of the lower arm, which, step by step proceeded upward to the shoulder and then continued onto all my limbs; so much so that at 9:00 that same evening I was already in my bed with a high fever ....."

"It's now been three weeks since I ... was stricken by the illness, and because of that had to stay home for 5 days; but even until today I have continuously pain and stiffness in the joints of both feet, with swelling of both ankles; so much so, that when I get up in the morning, or have sat up for a while and start to move again, I can not do so very well and going up and down stairs is very painful..."

"Natives, Chinese, slaves; no race escaped, as both sexes, children, adults, and old people were all affected equally; not only in this city of Batavia, but also in the surrounding area...."

Remarkably, in 1779 in Cairo and Alexandria another outbreak of disease occurred which bears close resemblance to chikungunya fever.[31] Another interesting pandemic of "dengue" which was probably actually chikungunya fever occurred in the years 1870 to 1873, when it appeared first on the East African Coast, then on the Arabian Coast and in Port Said.[73] From here it was carried by an emigrant steamer to Bombay, Calcutta, and to Java. The 1870 outbreak led to the discovery that the Swahili word for this disease was "ki-dinga pepo."[15] The term "denga" or "dyenga" was used to designate the disease in Africa in an earlier outbreak in 1823.[15] It is assumed that dengue spread with the slave trade to the Caribbean, where in 1827 to 1828 an extensive outbreak occurred in the West Indies.[9] It was in Cuba that the Spanish word dengue was first used.[9] There is epidemiological or serological evidence of pandemics in India in 1824 to 1825, 1871 to 1872, 1923, and 1964 to 1965.[9]

ETIOLOGY

Classification

By epidemiological criteria chikungunya virus is arthropod-borne since it is biologically transmitted by several species of mosquitoes. On the basis of antigenic relationships demonstrated by hemagglutination-inhibition (HI) and complement-fixation (CF) tests, chikungunya is placed in the genus *Alphavirus* of the family Togaviridae.[4,42]

Antisera prepared to chikungunya virus show strong cross reactions by CF and virus-dilution neutralization (N) tests with O'nyong-nyong, Mayaro, and Semliki Forest viruses but little relationship to other group A viruses.[4] Antisera prepared to O'nyong-nyong, Mayaro, and Semliki Forest virus, however, demonstrate only weak cross reactions by HI and no reactions by CF with chikungunya antigen. Cross comparisons by plaque reduction N tests have shown little relationship among alphaviruses.[76] Similar results have been obtained by fluorescent antibody (FA) techniques.[6]

African and Asian strains of chikungunya virus are not antigenically separable using mouse immune sera.[57] Although differences in plaque size and heat stability have been described between these strains, there is a possibility that these may be due to the relatively greater number of mouse passages of the African strains.[57]

Characteristics

Chikungunya virions are spherical, approximately 42 nm in diameter.[30] They possess a lipid-containing envelope with fine projections.[30] The central core approximately 25 to 30 nm in diameter, is roughly hexagonal in cross section and contains a nucleocapsid of uncertain symmetry. Together with other alphaviruses, the genome is a single stranded RNA.[32] It has a sedimentation coefficient of 46 S and a molecular weight of approximately 4.2×10^6 daltons.[32] Phenol extracts of chikungunya virus infected material remain infectious.[32] Virus precursors form in the cytoplasmic matrix and become aligned in the region of cell membranes or apposed to vacuolar membranes.[30] Assembly of virus particles at the cell surfaces occur by a budding process involving incorporation of the core virus precursor into the virion. Host cell membranes are modified during infection and contain viral antigens when incorporated into viral envelopes. The protein hemagglutinin spikes are mounted on phospholipid envelopes.[34] Three major structural proteins have been observed in chikungunya viruses by electrophoresis on polyacrilamide gel.[35,65] Two proteins are associated (VP1, VP2) with the hemagglutinin and the other with the core. Low passage strains recovered in suckling mice characteristically demonstrate autointerference when inoculated at dilutions below 1:100.[69]

DEFINITION

Chikungunya virus is the cause of a benign dengue-like syndrome characterized by abrupt onset of fever, arthralgia, maculopapular rash, and leukopenia.

ANIMAL INFECTION

Clinical

Serological studies indicate that chikungunya virus produces infection in subhuman primates, bats, and possibly wild birds transmitted in nature by a large number of different arthropod vectors. The role of domestic animals as zoonotic reservoirs of CHIK is controversial. CHIK infections in wild species have not been shown to cause sickness or death.

Pathology

Intracerebral inoculation of wild chikungunya virus strains into suckling mice, or of mouse adapted virus into weanling mice produces an acute encephalitis. The virus affects mainly the neuroglial cells, pericytes, neurons, and mononuclear leukocytes.[37] Fresh isolates of Southeast Asian and African strains of CHIK virus produce a hemorrhagic enteritis in suckling mice, hamsters, and white rats following intracerebral inoculation.[25] This syndrome is characterized by loss of erythrocytes through GI mucosa by diapedesis.[82] Hemostasic disorders include thrombocytopenia, prolonged bleeding time, prolonged clotting time, decrease in prothrombin time, and decrease in factor V, VII, and X. The severity of hemorrhage can not be moderated by pretreatment with antibiotics or steroids but animals pretreated with heparin appeared to be somewhat protected against hemorrhage but not against encephalitis and death.[82]

HUMAN INFECTION

Clinical

While chikungunya fever is generally regarded as producing a dengue fever syndrome, careful study demonstrates significant differences between dengue and chikungunya fever. Chikungunya fever characteristically has a more abrupt onset; 65 to 70% of patients seek medical care on the day of onset of fever or during the next day[26,59] in contrast with southeast Asian dengue patients who usually seek medical care considerably later in their illnesses. In one study, the median duration of fever in patients with chikungunya fever was 72 hr whereas the duration of fever in children hospitalized with dengue infections was two days longer.[59]

The similarities and dissimilarities in constitutional symptoms in dengue and chikungunya infections in adults are illustrated in Table 1. A maculopapular rash occurs with greater frequency in chikungunya than in dengue infections. In chikungunya fever a single episode of rash accompanies the crisis of fever, usually on the 2nd and 3rd day after onset of symptoms compared to the biphasic rash common dengue. Arthralgia, not as marked in children as in adults, occurs in a high proportion of chikungunya fever patients but not in dengue patients. Chikungunya infections are frequently accompanied not only by arthralgia, but arthritis, evidenced by redness, swelling, and tenderness of the inflamed joints.[10,18] Myalgia, frequently at the sites of insertion of muscles, is observed in dengue patients in whom it may be confused by patients or physicians as arthralgia. Leukocyte counts in chikungunya fever are normal or low normal, while marked leukopenia is relatively common in dengue. Other distinctive findings in dengue not often reported in chikungunya fever are (1) a change in taste perception, (2) a post-illness bradycardia, and (3) a variety of neurological and psychological symptoms which may extend into the post-illness period.[18,73,74] Isolated instances of neurological and myocardial involvement has been reported during chikungunya infections in adults.[13,54,78]

Petechial rashes are seen in dengue, rarely in chikungunya fever, but in some instances chikungunya virus isolations have been made from persons with severe hemorrhagic manifestations.[70] Those hemorrhagic phenomena are probably very rare.[10,36] Spontaneous hematemesis or melena are more frequently associated with secondary dengue infections.[10,18,26,36,59,74] Prospectively studied, virologically confirmed chikungunya cases have shown neither thrombocytopenia nor severe neutropenia.[36] The author considers it probable that under epidemic conditions, severe hemorrhage may occur in some patients with preexisting hemorrhagic diathesis who are superinfected with chikungunya virus.[55] Chikungunya fever is considered to be an arthropod-borne viral febrile exanthem, and a febrile illness accompanied by minor hemorrhagic manifestations but not a "viral hemorrhagic fever." Accordingly, chikungunya should not be listed as a mosquito-borne hemorrhagic fever. Only with careful study will it be possible to assess the etiological role of chikungunya virus in cases with severe hemorrhage, death, or other findings.

Pathology

The lesions in fatal human chikungunya illnesses have not been extensively studied. Reports in the literature resemble those described in dengue shock syndrome.[78]

Table 1
CLINICAL FEATURES OF SEROLOGICALLY PROVEN CASES OF DENGUE AND CHIKUNGUNYA FEVER IN ADULTS[18]

Clinical manifestation	Dengue (31 cases)		Chikungunya (10 cases)	
	No.	%	No.	%
Fever	31	100	10	100
Chills	31	100	10	100
Headache	31	100	8	80
Malaise	27	87.1	7	70
Anorexia	23	74.2	6	60
Backache	18	58.1	5	50
Myalgia	18	58.1		
Ocular pain	11	35.5		
Nausea/vomiting	9	29.0		
Sore throat	8	25.8		
Cough	7	22.6		
Restlessness	5	16.1		
Arthralgia	4	12.9	9	90
Adenopathy	19	61.3	7	70
Rash	14	45.2	6	60
Arthritis			8	80
Positive tourniquet test	6	19.4	1	10
Conjunctival suffusion	11	35.5		
Pharyngitis	6	19.4	3	30
Splenomegaly	5	16.1		
Wheezes			2	20
Abdominal tenderness	30	96.8		
WBC/mm³				
< 3000	9	29.0		
3000 — 5000	12	38.7		
< 5000			3	30
5000 — 7000	6	19.4	6	60
< 7000	4	12.9		
>10000			1	10

Diagnosis

Diagnosis is usually based on a significant increase in antibody titer following an illness episode. Ordinarily, a serum sample collected within 5 days of the onset of fever will be free of HI, CF, and N antibodies.[10,59] A sample collected 2 weeks or more after onset should have HI and low level N antibodies; CF antibodies develop more slowly.[10,59] In individuals without prior alphavirus infection, the initial antibody response is of the IgM class. As with dengue, IgG antibodies which may fix complement in the presence of viral antigen appear relatively late. Neutralizing antibodies can be measured by the virus dilution method in suckling mice (or in weanling mice using the Ross high mouse passage CHIK strain), or by the serum dilution method in cell cultures by cytopathic effect (cpe) or by plaque assay methods.

Virus isolation may be made by inoculating acute phase serum or other suspect tissues intracerebrally (i.c.) in 1 to 2-day-old mice.[69] On initial passage, deaths may occur within 2 to 5 days after inoculation.[69] Mouse brain seed virus suspensions inoculated into susceptible mice at a 1:5 or 1:10 final concentration, may result in no deaths, delayed deaths, or sporadic deaths due to autointerference.[69]

Chikungunya virus produces cpe in primary hamster kidney cell cultures and in BHK-21, BSC-1, Vero, FL, HeLa. and rhesus kidney cell lines.[17,33,41,79] Virus replicates in *Aedes aegypti, Ae. vittatus, Ae. albopictus, Anopheles stephensi,* and *Culex fatigans* continuous cell lines and in a cell line derived from Drosophila.[4] Plaque assays are described in LLC-MK2, Vero, BHK-21 cell lines and in primary duck and chicken embryo cell cultures. Vero cells and suckling mice are equally sensitive for primary isolation.[79]

EPIDEMIOLOGY

Occurrence

Chikungunya appears to be endemic throughout much of East, Central, South, and West Africa; spread over other parts of the world has apparently come from this area. Subhuman primate populations are involved in epidemics; critical numbers of the susceptible population become infected leading to disappearance of the virus in an area. By a constantly moving epizootic activity, chikungunya virus may cycle in wild primate populations, returning when a sufficient number of susceptibles have developed, in much the same fashion as do respiratory and enteric virus infections in human beings. It seems reasonable to expect that intercurrent and epidemic human infections in Africa are related to wild primate virus cycles. Many putative or identified chikungunya virus vectors feed on people as well as on subhuman primates. As is the case for yellow fever and dengue viruses, chikungunya is capable of being transmitted by *Ae. aegypti.* When a sufficient number of susceptible people and a high enough *Ae. aegypti* population are present in an area, a human-mosquito-human cycle may become established. This cycle is probably responsible for the large or predominantly urban outbreaks of chikungunya which have been studied within the past 20 years. In Africa, chikungunya outbreaks have been reported from Uganda, Tanzania, Zimbabwe, South Africa, Angola, Zaire, Nigeria and Senegal.[5,21,44,53,60,61,67,68,81] This distribution represents the location of virus research laboratories on the continent and allows the reasonable conclusion that chikungunya occurs throughout sub-Saharan Africa.

There is historical evidence that chikungunya has spread from the African endemic focus causing large pandemics throughout both the American and Asian tropics.[9,73] In North America during summer months, outbreaks have extended up the Atlantic coast as far as Philadelphia and along the Asian coast to Hong Kong.[73] Epidemics swept across India in 1824, 1871, 1902, 1923, and 1963 to 1964, reaching Sri Lanka in 1965.[9,51] During the late 1950s and early 1960s chikungunya appears to have established itself endemically in Southeast Asia and was continuously transmitted in urban populations in Thailand, Cambodia, and Vietnam, possibly into the 1970s. Involvement of urban populations in Burma appears to have been intermittent with outbreaks being recorded in 1963 and 1970 to 1973.[52] There is serological evidence of chikungunya infection throughout the Philippines, possibly as early as World War II. Since then, localized outbreaks have occurred in Manila in 1967 and Negros Oriental in 1968.[2,8,39,62] In the 19th century chikungunya epidemics were reported in the Indonesian archipelago.[73] An extensive serologic survey using the plaque reduction test has suggested chikungunya activity during World War II on Kalimantan and Sulawesi islands in Indonesia.[76] However, since 1952, there have been only sporadic documented human cases in Indonesia, Malaysia, and Singapore. Little or no chikungunya infection has occurred on New Guinea, the Solomon Islands, New Hebrides, or West Caroline Islands.[76]

Reservoir

Chikungunya antibodies have been found in vervet monkeys, baboons, chimpanzees, and red tailed monkeys in Zimbabwe, South Africa, and Uganda.[43,46,48] Vervet monkeys and baboons are readily infected, possibly producing clinical illness although this has not been clearly established.[45] Rhesus monkeys may be subclinically infected by intravenous (i.v.) or intramuscular (i.m.) inoculations, developing viremia titers in excess of 10^7 mouse LD_{50}.[64] *Ae. aegypti* have transmitted virus to rhesus monkeys and can readily be infected by biting viremic monkeys.[64] The zoonotic status of chikungunya virus in Asia has not been carefully studied. Chikungunya virus has the ability to produce infection in a broad spectrum of vertebrate species. Newborn mice, hamsters, rats, rabbits, guinea pigs, and kittens can all be infected by subcutaneous inoculation with field strains of chikungunya virus, leading to viremia, sickness, and in most instances, death.[11] Adult rabbits, mice, rats, and chickens inoculated peripherally develop asymptomatic viremias followed by antibody response.[11] Although chikungunya HI or N antibodies have occasionally been reported in sera obtained from domestic animals, experimental attempts to infect cattle, goats, sheep, or horses have failed to produce either viremias or antibody responses.[5,14,45]

Transmission

Chikungunya virus has been recovered from wild-caught *Ae. aegypti* mosquitoes in Tanzania, Nigeria, India, and Thailand; from *Ae. africanus* in Uganda and Bangui, and from *Ae. luteocephalus* in Senegal.[1,16,43,53,56,67,81] Occasional isolates have been made from *Mansonia fuscopenatta* in Uganda and from *Cx. fatigans* in Thailand and Tanzania.[27,43]

Transmission to human beings has been demonstrated with *Ae. furcifer-Ae. taylori* group,[63] while transmission to monkeys or mice has been demonstrated with *Ae. aegypti*, *Ae. albopictus*, *Ae. calceatus*, *Ae. triseriatus*, *Ae. togoi*, *Ae. pseudoscutellaris*, *Ae. polynesiensis*, *Anopheles albinanus*, *Mansonia africana*, *Eretmapodites chrysogaster*, and *Ae. apicoargenteus*.[22,40,47,49,50,63,71,72,75]

Tesh et al. examined *Ae. albopictus* strains collected in 13 geographical locations from Hawaii to Africa. They found considerable variation in susceptibility of these mosquitoes to infection by oral feeding.[77] The 50% oral ID_{50} for *Ae. albopictus* of a wild-caught strain from India was $10^{5.4}$ /mℓ. The virus levels recorded in infected mosquitoes varied between $10^{4.6}$ and $10^{7.4}$ pfu per mosquito.[77] These observations plus a mathematical model of chikungunya virus transmission developed by deMoor and Steffens suggest that major factors in determining endemicity of chikungunya may be arthropod-related.[19] Tesh et al. have suggested that susceptibility to oral infection and amount of virus replicated in mosquitoes may be under genetic control,[77] while deMoor and Steffens have postulated that mosquito longevity is the most important determinant in epidemic transmission of chikungunya.[19]

In studies on chikungunya transmission between *Ae. aegypti* and laboratory mice, Rao et al. have demonstrated mechanical transmission.[66] Viremia in humans may be as high as 10^8 mouse ID_{50} /mℓ.[10] Mosquitoes which interrupt feeding on an infected patient and bite several susceptible people in succession should be able to transmit the virus mechanically. Since the extrinsic incubation period in *Ae. aegypti* is relatively long, a part of explosive nature of chikungunya outbreaks may be explained by mechanical transmission.

Environment

Zoonotic transmission to subhuman primates is surmised to take place in a wide variety of habitats, with transmission occurring in the canopy, or at ground level, or both.[50] The vast geographic area of zoonotic involvement of chikungunya and the multiplicity of potential arthropod vectors suggest a very broad natural ecosystem for chikungunya in Africa.

Although both chikungunya and dengue viruses may be transmitted by *Ae. aegypti* mosquitoes, they are quite different in geographical distribution. Singh and Pavri showed that the infection threshold of chikungunya virus in *Ae. aegypti* is very high, approximately $10^{5.6}$ mouse ID_{50}.[75] By contrast, a female *Ae. aegypti* feeding upon dengue-infected monkeys may become infected from viremia levels too low to be detected by conventional cell culture assays.[23]

Human Host

Almost all recorded chikungunya infections in human beings have paralleled the distribution and abundance of *Ae. aegypti* mosquitoes. Where those mosquitoes are abundant in occupied dwellings, infection rates can be expected to be highest in women and children who are at home during daylight hours. Where they are most abundant in public buildings such as schools and hospitals, outbreaks often show occupational patterns.

CONTROL

Prevention

Several experimental chikungunya vaccines have been produced. Formalin-treated chikungunya virus (Ross strain) vaccine grown in African green monkey kidney cell cultures have elicited satisfactory antibody responses as well as resistance to challenge when administered to monkeys using three divided doses.[28] A vaccine prepared under similar conditions has elicited HI, CF, and N antibody responses in susceptible human volunteers.[29] A comparative study was made on two formalin-inactivated chikungunya vaccines, one prepared of virus propagated in African green monkey kidney monolayers, and the other a concentrated virus harvested from chicken embryo suspension cultures. The latter vaccine was significantly more protective to mice against live homologous virus challenge and stimulated the production of 4 to 5 times more circulating antibodies than the vaccine prepared with virus grown in African green monkey kidney cell cultures.[83] Nakao and Hotta, studying chikungunya vaccines prepared from viruses grown in BHK-21 cells found that UV inactivated preparations were significantly more immunogenic than were formalin treated virus.[58] Tween-ether extracted virus preparations have also been found to be acceptably immunogenic.[20] Despite these laboratory successes, commercial production of chikungunya vaccine has not been attempted. In view of the low mortality associated with chikungunya fever infections, commercial development of a chikungunya vaccine probably will have a low public health priority. Were a vaccine produced in large amounts and stockpiled, it would be useful in combatting epidemics such as have occurred repeatedly in India and which, based upon historic precedents, can be expected again within the next 10 to 20 years.

At present, prevention consists in avoiding exposure by infected mosquitoes. In urban outbreaks in most of the Asian and African tropics where *Ae. aegypti* are the predominant vectors, individual and area control measures are the same as for dengue. When other vectors are involved, particularly if biting is occurring outside of houses, measures designed to combat *Ae. aegypti* may fail and expert entomological advice is needed to design appropriate preventive measures.

Treatment

Treatment is supportive. Bed rest is advised during the febrile period. Anti-pyretics or cold sponging should be used to keep body temperatures below 40° C. Febrile convulsions are frequent in chikungunya infections in children. Salicylates, because of their hemorrhagic potential, are contraindicated. Analgesics or mild sedatives may be required to control pain. Post-illness arthritis may require continued treatment with anti-inflammatory agents and graduate physiotherapy. Children who have lost excessive fluids due to vomiting, fasting, or thirsting, and who cannot take oral fluids, may require intravenous replacement. Individuals with severe hemorrhagic phenomena should be studied for underlying hemostatic disorders.

Regulatory measures

Chikungunya is not a disease subject to international quarantine or surveillance. Reporting of cases to the World Health Organization (WHO) is largely limited to extensive epidemics.

PUBLIC HEALTH ASPECTS

Economic and Social Impact

In India and Burma, epidemic chikungunya fever was widely assumed by the medical and lay community to be an acute hemorrhagic fever. This resulted in much public interest and consternation in both countries. The explosiveness of chikungunya fever outbreaks in susceptible populations, together with inevitable hospitalizations, produce the potential for great social impact by this disease. In the African outbreaks described thus far, chikungunya fever seems to have been regarded as little more than a nuisance. The arthralgia and articular disability which are the aftermath of chikungunya fever in adults can result in prolonged morbidity and the disease may be a significant cause of absenteeism in the work force. In large outbreaks the cost of treatment, whether out-patient or in-patient, must be enormous.

Reporting

There is no requirement to report chikungunya outbreaks to WHO, although reports which are submitted will be published in the *Weekly Epidemiological Record.* Reports of epidemic occurrences, unusual cases, studies on vectors and vertebrate reservoir hosts may be reported informally to the Arthropod-Borne Virus Information Exchange, Editor, Center for Disease Control, Atlanta, Georgia, 30333. Because of the similarity of dengue and chikungunya and the fact that the same vectors are involved, informal reports may also be submitted to Dengue newsletters.

Surveillance

No formal surveillance program has been devised for chikungunya virus transmission. However, the same activities developed for dengue could apply.

REFERENCES

1. **Anderson, C. R., Singh, K. R. P., and Sarkar, J. K.,** Isolation of chikungunya virus from *Aedes aegypti* fed on naturally infected humans in Calcutta, *Curr. Sci.,* 34, 579, 1965.
2. **Basaca-Sevilla, V. and Halstead, S. B.,** Recent virological studies of haemorrhagic fever and other arthropod-borne virus infections in the Philippines, *J. Trop. Med. Hyg.,* 69, 203, 1966.
3. **Bedekar, S. D. and Pavri, K. M.,** Studies with chikungunya virus II. Serological survey of humans and animals in India, *Indian J. Med. Res.,* 57, 1193, 1969.
4. **Berge, T. O., Ed.,** International Catalog of Arboviruses Including Certain Other Viruses of Vertebrates, 2nd ed., Publ. No. (CDC) 75-8301, *Public Health Service, U.S. Department of Health, Education and Welfare,* Atlanta, 1975.
5. **Brès, P., Camicas, J. L., Cornet, M., Robin, Y., and Taufflieb, R.,** Considérations sur l'épidemiologie des arboviroses au Sénégal, *Bull. Soc. Path. Exot.,* 62, 253, 1969.

6. **Buckley, S. M. and Clarke, D. H.**, Differentiation of group A arboviruses chikungunya, Mayaro, and Semliki Forest by the fluorescent antibody technique, *Proc. Soc. Exp. Biol. Med.*, 135, 533, 1970.

7. **Bylon, D., Korte Aatekening, Wegens eene Algemeene Ziekte, Doorgans Genaamd de Knokkel-Koorts**, *Verh. Bataviaasch Genoot. Kunsten Wet.*, 2, 17, 1780.

8. **Campos, L. E., San Juan, A., Cenabre, L. C., and Almagro, E. F.**, Isolation of chikungunya virus in the Philippines, *Acta Med. Philipp.*, 5, 152, 1969.

9. **Carey, D. E.**, Chikungunya and dengue: a case of mistaken identity? *J. Hist. Med. Allied Sci.*, 26, 243, 1971.

10. **Carey, D. E., Myers, R. M., De Ranitz, C. M., Jadhav, M., and Reuben, R.**, The 1964 chikungunya epidemic at Vellore, South India, including observations on concurrent dengue, *Trans. R. Soc. Trop. Med. Hyg.*, 63, 434, 1969.

11. **Chakravarty, S. K. and Sarkar, J. K.**, Susceptibility of new born and adult laboratory animals to chikungunya virus, *Indian J. Med. Res.*, 57, 1157, 1969.

12. **Chastel, C.**, Human infections in Cambodia with chikungunya or a closely allied virus. III. Epidemiology, *Bull. Soc. Path. Exot.*, 57, 65, 1964.

13. **Chatterjee, S. N., Chakravarti, S. K., Mitra, A. C., and Sarkar, J. K.**, Virological investigation of cases with neurological complications during the outbreak of haemorrhagic fever in Calcutta, *J. Indian Med. Assoc.*, 45, 314, 1965.

14. **Chatterjee, S. N., Chakravarty, M. S., Chakravarty, S. K., Ray, S., and Sarkar, J. K.**, Survey of antibodies against chikungunya virus in the sera collected in Calcutta during 1964 and 1965, *Indian J. Med. Res.*, 55, 665, 1967.

15. **Christie, J.**, Remarks on "kidinga Pepo": a peculiar form of exanthematous disease, *Br. Med. J.*, 1, 577, 1872.

16. **Cornet, M. and Chateau, R.**, Quelques donnees biologiques sur *Aedes* (Stegomyia) *luteocephalus* (Newstead) en zone de savane soudanienne dan l'ouest du Senegal, *Cah. O.R.S.T.O.M. Ser. Entomol. Med. Parasitol.*, 12, 97, 1974.

17. **Davis, J. L., Hodge, H. M., and Campbell, W. E., Jr.**, Growth of chikungunya virus in baby hamster kidney cell (BHK-21-clone 13) suspension cultures, *Appl. Microbiol.*, 21, 338, 1971.

18. **Deller, J. J., Jr. and Russell, P. K.**, Fevers of unknown origin in American soldiers in Vietnam, *Ann. Intern. Med.*, 66, 1129, 1967.

19. **deMoor, P. P. and Steffens, F. E.**, A computer-simulated model of an arthropod-borne virus transmission cycle, with special reference to chikungunya virus, *Trans. R. Soc. Trop. Med. Hyg.*, 64, 927, 1970.

20. **Eckels, K. H., Harrison, V. R., and Hetrick, F. M.**, Chikungunya virus vaccine prepared by Tween®-ether extraction, *Appl. Microbiol.*, 19, 321, 1970.

21. **Filipe, A. R. and Pinto, M. R.**, Arbovirus studies in Luanda, Angola: 2. Virological and serological studies during an outbreak of dengue-like disease caused by the chikungunya virus, *Bull. WHO*, 49, 37, 1973.

22. **Gilotra, S. K. and Shah, K. V.**, Laboratory studies on transmission of chikungunya virus by mosquitoes, *Am. J. Epidemiol.*, 86, 379, 1967.

23. **Gubler, D. J.**, personal communication, 1977.

24. **Halstead, S. B.**, unpublished data, 1977.

25. **Halstead, S. B. and Buescher, E. L.**, Hemorrhagic disease in rodents infected with virus associated with Thai hemorrhagic fever, *Science*, 134, 475, 1961.

26. **Halstead, S. B., Nimmannitya, S., and Margiotta, M. R.**, Dengue and chikungunya virus infection in man in Thailand, 1962-64. II. Observations on disease in out-patients, *Am. J. Trop. Med. Hyg.*, 18, 972, 1969.

27. **Halstead, S. B., Scanlon, J. E., Umpaivit, P., and Udomsakdi, S.**, Dengue and chikungunya virus infection in man in Thailand, 1962-1964. IV. Epidemiologic studies in the Bangkok metropolitan area, *Am. J. Trop. Med. Hyg.*, 18, 997, 1969.

28. **Harrison, V. R., Binn, L. N., and Randall, R.**, Comparative immunogenicities of chikungunya vaccines prepared in avian and mammalian tissues, *Am. J. Trop. Med. Hyg.*, 16, 786, 1967.

29. **Harrison, V. R., Eckels, K. H., Bartelloni, P. J., and Hampton, C.**, Production and evaluation of a formalin-killed chikungunya vaccine, *J. Immunol.*, 107, 643, 1971.

30. **Higashi, N., Matsumoto, A., Tabata, K., and Nagatomo, Y.**, Electron microscope study of development of chikungunya virus in green monkey kidney stable (Vero) cells, *Virology*, 33, 55, 1967.

31. **Hirsch, A.**, Dengue, a comparatively new disease: its symptoms-geographical distribution — characteristics of dengue as an epidemic disease of the tropics, *Handbook of Geographical and Historical Pathology*, Vol. 1, 1883, 55.

32. **Igarashi, A., Konosuke, F., and Tuchinda, P.,** Studies on chikungunya virus. III. Infective ribonucleic acid from partially purified virus: its biological assay and some of its basic characteristics, *Biken J.,* 10, 195, 1967.

33. **Igarashi, A. and Tuchinda, P.,** Studies on chikungunya virus. I. Plague titration on an established cell line, *Biken J.,* 10, 37, 1967.

34. **Igarashi, A., Fukuoka, T., Nithiuthai, P., Hsu, L. C., and Fukai, K.,** Structural components of chikungunya virus, *Biken J.,* 13, 93, 1970.

35. **Igarashi, A., Nithiuthai, P., and Rojanasuphot, S.,** Immunological properties of chikungunya virus and its components, *Biken J.,* 13, 229, 1970.

36. **Jadhav, M., Namboodripad, M., Carman, R. H., Carey, D. E., and Myers, R. M.,** Chikungunya disease in infants and children in Vellore: a report on clinical and haematological features of virologically proved cases, *Indian J. Med. Res.,* 53, 764, 1965.

37. **Karmysheva, V. Y. and Borisov, V. M.,** Some problems of comparative cytopathology in virus infection in vitro and in vivo, *Tsitologiya,* 13, 593, 1971.

38. **Macasaet, F. F., Rustia, F. S., Buscato, N. S., Nakao, J. C., and Beran, G. W.,** Epidemiology of arbovirus infections in Negros Oriental. I. Clinical features of an epidemic in Amlan, *J. Philipp. Med. Assoc.,* 45, 207, 1969.

39. **Macasaet, F. F., Villamil P. T., Wexler, S., and Beran, G. W.,** Epidemiology of arbovirus infections in Negros Oriental. II. Serologic findings of the epidemic in Amlan, *J. Phillipp. Med. Assoc.,* 45, 311, 1969.

40. **Mangiafico, J. A.,** Chikungunya virus infection and transmission in five species of mosquito, *Am. J. Trop. Med. Hyg.,* 20, 642, 1971.

41. **Mantani, M., Igarashi, A., Tuchinda, P., and Kato, S.,** Cytoplasmic RNA synthesis and viral antigen in FL cells infected with chikungunya virus, *Biken J.,* 10, 203, 1967.

42. **Mason, P. J. and Haddow, A. J.,** An epidemic of virus disease in Southern Province, Tanganyika Territory, *Trans. R. Soc. Trop. Med. Hyg.,* 51, 238, 1957.

43. **McCrae, A. W. R., Henderson, B. E., Kirya, B. G., and Sempala, S. D. K.,** Chikungunya virus in the Entebbe area of Uganda: Isolations and epidemiology, *Trans. R. Soc. Trop. Med. Hyg.,* 65, 152, 1971.

44. **McIntosh, B. M., Harwin, R. M., Paterson, H. E., and Westwater, M. L.,** An epidemic of chikungunya in South-Eastern Southern Rhodesia, *Cent. Afr. J. Med.,* 9, 351, 1963.

45. **McIntosh, B. M., Paterson, H. E., Donaldson, J. M., and De Sousa, J.,** Chikungunya virus: viral susceptibility and transmission studies with some vertebrates and mosquitoes, *S. Afr. J. Med. Sci.,* 28, 45, 1963.

46. **McIntosh, B. M., Paterson, H. E., McGillivray, G., and De Sousa, J.,** Further studies on the chikungunya outbreak in Southern Rhodesia in 1962. I. Mosquitoes, wild primates and birds in relation to the epidemic, *Ann. Trop. Med. Parasitol.,* 58, 45, 1964.

47. **McIntosh, B. M., Sweetnam, J., McGillivray, G. M., and De Sousa, J.,** Laboratory transmission of chikungunya virus by *Mansonia* (Mansonioides) *africana* (Theobald), *Ann. Trop. Med. Parasitol.,* 59, 390, 1965.

48. **McIntosh, B. M.,** Antibody against chikungunya virus in wild primates in Southern Africa, *S. Afr. J. Med. Sci.,* 35, 65, 1970.

49. **McIntosh, B. M. and Jupp, P. G.,** Attempts to transmit chikungunya virus with six species of mosquito, *J. Med. Entomol.,* 7, 615, 1970.

50. **McIntosh, B. M., Jupp, P. G., and De Souza, J.,** Mosquitoes feeding at two horizontal levels in gallery forest in Natal, South Africa, with reference to possible vectors of chikungunya virus, *J. Entomol. Soc. South. Afr.,* 35, 81, 1972.

51. **Mendis, N. M. P.,** Epidemiology of dengue-like fever in Ceylon, *Ceylon Med. J.,* 12, 67, 1967.

52. **Ming, C. K., Thein, S., Thaung, U. T., Myint, R. S., Swe, T., Halstead, S. B., and Diwan, A. R.,** Clinical laboratory studies on haemorrhagic fever in Burma, 1970-1972, *Bull. WHO,* 51, 227, 1974.

53. **Moore, D. L., Reddy, S., Akinkugbe, F. M., Lee, V. H., David-West, T. S., Causey, O. R., and Carey, D. E.,** An epidemic of chikungunya fever at Ibadan, Nigeria, 1969, *Ann. Trop. Med. Parisitol.,* 68, 59, 1974.

54. **Munasinghe, D. R., Amarasekera, P. J., and Fernando, C. F. O.,** An epidemic of dengue-like fever in Ceylon (chikungunya) — a clinical and haematological study, *Ceylon Med. J.,* 11, 129, 1966.

55. **Munasinghe, D. R. and Rajasuriya, K.,** Haemorrhage in Christmas disease following dengue-like fever, *Ceylon Med. J.,* 11, 39, 1966.

56. **Myers, R. M., Carey, D. E., Reuben, R., Jesudass, E. S., De Ranitz, C., and Jadhav, M.,** The 1964 epidemic of dengue-like fever in South India: isolation of chikungunya virus from human sera and from mosquitoes, *Indian J. Med. Res.,* 53. 694, 1965.

57. **Nakao, E.,** Biological and immunological studies on chikungunya versus: a comparative observation of two strains of African and Asian origins, *Kobe J. Med. Sci.,* 18, 133, 1972.

58. **Nakao, E. and Hotta, S.,** Immunogenicity of purified, inactivated chikungunya virus in monkeys, *Bull. WHO,* 48, 559, 1973.

59. **Nimmannitya, S., Halstead, S. B., Cohen, S. N., and Margiotta, M. R.,** Dengue and chikungunya virus infection in man in Thailand, 1962-64. I. Observations on hospitalized patients with hemorrhagic fever, *Am. J. Trop. Med. Hyg.,* 18, 954, 1969.

60. **Osterrieth, P. and Blanes-Ridaura, G.,** Studies on chikungunya virus in the Congo. I. Isolation of the virus in Upper Uele Region, *Ann. Soc. Belge Med. Trop.,* 40, 199, 1960.

61. **Osterrieth, P.,** Deleplanque-Liegeois, P., and Renoirte, R., Studies on chikungunya virus in the Congo. II. Serological survey, *Ann. Soc. Belge Med. Trop.,* 40, 205, 1960.

62. **Paguia, L. A.,** A report on the clinical manifestations, laboratory examinations and viral studies of a newly observed viral infection in the Philippines, *J. Philipp. Med. Assoc.,* 44, 532, 1968.

63. **Paterson, H. E. and McIntosh, B. M.,** Further studies on the chikungunya outbreak in Southern Rhodesia in 1962. II. Transmission experiments with the *Aedes furcifer-taylori* group of mosquitoes and with a member of the Anopheles gambiae complex, *Ann. Trop. Med. Parasitol.,* 58, 52, 1964.

64. **Paul, S. D. and Singh, K. R. P.,** Experimental infection of *Macaca radiata* with chikungunya virus and transmission of virus by mosquitoes, *Indian J. Med. Res.,* 56, 802, 1968.

65. **Pedersen, C. E., Jr., Marker, S. C., and Eddy, G. A.,** Comparative electrophoretic studies on the structural proteins of selected group A arboviruses, *Virology,* 60, 312, 1974.

66. **Rao, T. R., Devi, P. S., and Singh, K. R. P.,** Experimental studies on the mechanical transmission of chikungunya virus by *Aedes aegypti, Mosq. News,* 28, 406, 1968.

67. **Robinson, M. C.,** An epidemic of virus disease in Southern Province, Tanganyika Territory, in 1952-53. I. Clinical features, *Trans. R. Soc. Trop. Med. Hyg.,* 49, 28, 1955.

68. **Rodger, L. M.,** An outbreak of suspected chikungunya fever in northern Rhodesia, *S. Afr. Med. J.,* 35, 126, 1961.

69. **Ross, R. W.,** The Newala epidemic. III. The virus: isolation, pathogenic properties and relationship to the epidemic, *J. Hyg.,* 54, 177, 1956.

70. **Sarkar, J. K., Chatterjee, S. N., Chakravarti, S. K., and Mitra, A. C.,** Chikungunya virus infection with haemorrhagic manifestations, *Indian J. Med. Res.,* 53, 921, 165.

71. **Sempala, S. D. K. and Kirya, B. G.,** Laboratory transmission of chikungunya virus by *Aedes* (Stegomyia) *apicoargenteus* Theobald, *Am. J. Trop. Med. Hyg.,* 22, 263, 1973.

72. **Shah, K. V., Gilotra, S. K., Gibbs, C. J., Jr., and Rozenboom, L. E.,** Laboratory studies of transmission of chikungunya virus by mosquitoes, *Indian, J. Med. Res.,* 52, 703, 1964.

73. **Siler, J. F., Hall, M. W., and Hitchens, A. P.,** Dengue: its history, epidemiology, mechanisms of transmission, etiology, clinical manifestations, immunity, and prevention, *Philip. J. Sci.,* 29, 1, 1926.

74. **Simmons, J. S., St. John, J. H., and Reynolds, R. H. K.,** Experimental studies of dengue, *Philipp. J. Sci.,* 44, 1, 1931.

75. **Singh, K. R. P. and Pavri, K. M.,** Experimental studies with chikungunya virus in *Aedes aegypti* and *Aedes albopictus, Acta Virol.,* 11, 517, 1967.

76. **Tesh, R. B., Gadjusek, D. C., Carruto, R. M., Cross, J. H., and Rosen, L.,** The distribution and prevalence of group A arbovirus neutralizing antibodies among human populations in Southeast Asia and the Pacific Islands, *Am. J. Trop. Med. Hyg.,* 24, 664, 1975.

77. **Tesh, R. B., Gubler, D. J., and Rosen, L.,** Variation among geographic strains of *Aedes albopictus* in susceptibility to infection with chikungunya virus, *Am. J. Trop. Med. Hyg.,* 25, 326, 1976.

78. **Thiruvengadam, K. V., Kalyanasundaram, V., and Rajgopal, J.,** Clinical and pathological studies on chikungunya fever in Madras City, *Indian J. Med. Res.,* 53, 720, 1965.

79. **Umrigar, M. D. and Kadam, S. S.,** Comparative sensitivity of suckling mice and Vero cells for primary isolation of chikungunya virus, *Indian J. Med. Res.,* 62, 1893, 1974.

80. **Vu-Qui, D., Nguyen-Thi, K. T., and Ly, Q. B.,** Antibodies to chikungunya virus in Vietnamese children in Saigon, *Bull. Soc. Path. Exot.,* 60, 353, 1967.

81. **Weinbren, M. P., Haddow, A. J., and Williams, M. C.,** The occurrence of chikungunya virus in Uganda, *Trans. R. Soc. Trop. Med. Hyg.,* 52, 253, 1958.

82. **Weiss, H. J., Halstead, S. B., and Russ, S. B.,** Hemorrhagic disease in rodents caused by chikungunya virus. I. Studies of hemostasis, *Proc. Soc. Exp. Biol. Med.,* 119, 427, 1965.

83. **White, A., Berman, S., and Lowenthal, J. P.,** Comparative immunogenicities of chikungunya vaccines propagated in monkey kidney monolayers and chick embryo suspension cultures, *Appl. Microbiol.,* 23, 951, 1972.

JAPANESE ENCEPHALITIS

T. W. Lim and G. W. Beran

NAME AND SYNONYMS

Japanese encephalitis (JBE) has also been called Japanese B encephalitis, Russian autumnal encephalitis, and summer encephalitis.

HISTORY

Japanese encephalitis virus was initially isolated from brain tissue collected at necropsy of a 19-year-old man who died of encephalitis in a hospital in Tokyo, Japan in 1935. Clinical records of Japanese encephalitis identify the disease in Japan in the late 1800s. A severe epidemic was recorded in Japan in 1924 and several workers demonstrated that filtered extracts of brain tissues remained infectious to rabbits. In 1934, Hayashi transmitted the disease to monkeys by intracerebral inoculation and the following year the viral etiology of the disease was proven in virological and serological studies in mice. The seasonal occurrence of the disease with the active season of culicine mosquitoes suggested a vector relationship, and in 1938, Mitamura et al. reported the isolation of JBE virus from *Culex tritaeniorhyncus* mosquitoes. In other temperate and subtropical adjoining areas, the clinical disease was probably recognized as early as 1932 in Korea and epidemics were reported in 1935 and 1939. The virus was isolated and identified in 1946. Years during which over 3000 human cases were diagnosed have been 1949, 1958, 1966. In Taiwan, 1958 and 1961 were epidemic years with 1800 and 704 reported cases, respectively, and a case fatality rate above 28% each year. Epidemics recur in maritime Siberia, U.S.S.R., in China, in Taiwan,[14] in the Ryukyus, and have been reported in Guam.[16]

In tropical Southeast and South Asia, Japanese encephalitis is endemic in animal reservoirs, and serological evidence of widespread human infections has been reported from many countries, but clinical encephalitis has been recognized only sporadically or in small outbreaks.[38] In Malaysia, a serological survey showed a 10% prevalence of neutralizing antibodies in 1 to 2-year-old children of rubber estate workers, but reached 90% in 14-year-old and older persons. Among forest-dwelling aboriginal adults, the rate was 22%, reflecting a much lower environmental exposure rate.[2] Japanese encephalitis virus has most frequently been isolated from *Culex* spp. of a wide variety of species which feed on birds, wild and domestic animals, and people.

ETIOLOGY

Classification

JBE is classified in the genus *Flavivirus* (group B arboviruses) of the family Togaviridae.[50] The "B" designation of the earlier term Japanese B encephalitis referred not to the group B identification of the virus but served to separate the clinical syndrome from Von Economos type A encephalitis.

Characterization

The virions are spherical, lipoprotein-enveloped particles about 20 nm in diameter by electron microscopic measurement. The genomes are single stranded RNA of molecular weight 3×10^6 daltons. The virus produces hemagglutinin peptides in projections on the envelope in infected suckling mouse brains active against chick or goose erythrocytes.[36] The virus is sensitive to ether, trypsin,[47] sodium deoxycholate, and urea. The virus is transmitted by mosquitoes to a variety of amplifying hosts in nature, principally swine, herons, egrets, and perhaps other animals and birds, and tangentially to human beings and horses. The virus undergoes intrinsic incubation periods in the vertebrate hosts and extrinsic incubation in the mosquito vectors.

DEFINITION

Japanese encephalitis is an inapparent to acute arboviral infection characterized in human patients by fever, headache, prostration, stiff neck, and central nervous system signs including encephalitis. In animals and birds infection is common and usually inapparent. Horses may develop encephalitis, and gestating swine may give birth, frequently prematurely, to infected and often dead pigs. A variety of mosquitoes of *Culex, Anopheles,* and perhaps *Aedes* and *Armigeres* spp. serve as vectors. In temperate and subtropical areas of East Asia, the human disease occurs in human beings in epidemics which are often clinically severe, whereas in tropical areas of Southeast and South Asia, it is commonly clinically recognized in sporadic cases and small outbreaks.

ANIMAL INFECTION

Clinical

A number of vertebrate hosts act as amplifiers of the virus. In Japan and neighboring areas, swine, herons, egrets, and perhaps other birds provide an annual susceptible population for rapid build-up of the virus through mosquito transmission.[42] Infection in gestating swine may be transmitted to their fetuses in utero, causing stillbirths or farrowing of weak pigs which may succumb during the first week in up to 42% of infections.[5,42,43] Except for gestating swine, infections in these animals are subclinical but with high titered viremias and very widespread occurrence, with serological surveys at the end of mosquito seasons often showing 100% seropositive rates. Infections in horses are often equally prevalent, and while usually inapparent, may be characterized by acute, even fatal encephalitis. Virus is commonly isolated only at necropsy from horses and they are not considered important amplifying hosts. Many serological surveys in other domestic and wild animals and birds have shown susceptibility to infection, but virological studies have indicated that only a few species are involved in the cycles of transmission. Cattle, sheep, and goats have shown antibody prevalence rates of 9 to 100% in different surveys, dogs 17% in one survey, bats 2 to 12.5% in two surveys, and domestic chickens 0 to 20% with most findings indicating such infections are rare.[9,11,19,20,25,30,32,34] Among these, viremia has been found only in swine. The black crowned night heron, the little egret, and the plumed egret are considered to be important in transmission cycles, showing both high levels of viremia and high prevalence of antibody titers. Among other birds, antibody prevalence rates of 7 to 27% have been recorded in house swallows. Indian kingfishers and other birds but viremias have not been detected[21,22] Frogs and snakes have been suggested as overwintering hosts on the basis of both field and laboratory studies. Viremias have been detected in frogs in nature and variably in laboratory-inoculated frogs, but antibody production has not been demonstrated.[6,7,8,27] Virus has been detected in snakes in nature and hemagglutination inhibiting (HI) antibodies, neutralizing antibodies, and increased levels of gamma globulin have been reported in snakes in nature or following laboratory inoculations.[24,26] Experimental infections with viremia have also been produced in toads.

In the tropical areas of Southeast and South Asia, serological surveys in Malaysia have shown that infection is prevalent in cattle, swine, and dogs, with neutralizing antibodies in approximately 80%, and in dogs and cats with approximately 50% seropositive, but less common in goats or house rats.[3] Clinical disease has not been reported in association with infections in any of these animals. Antibody titers have occasionally been detected in wild swine, feral rodents, wild cats, monitor lizards, and snakes, and in one survey were reported in 4% of emerald doves, tree sparrows, white headed munias, and house swifts.

Experimentally, suckling and adult mice inoculated by the intracerebral (i.c.) route develop fatal encephalitis; following intraperitoneal (i.p.) inoculation, fatal encephalitis is produced in suckling mice but only with some strains in adult mice. Rhesus and cynomolgous monkeys and adult hamsters develop fatal encephalitis following i.c. injection but only asymptomatic viremia following inoculation by peripheral routes. Guinea pigs and rabbits inoculated i.c. or by peripheral routes, and bats, chickens and herons inoculated by peripheral routes develop only asymptomatic viremia. Bats may retain persistent infections through hibernation, followed by recurrence of viremia.

Diagnosis

Viral isolation from blood samples of viremic animals, from tissues of stillborn pigs,[31] or from brains of horses or neonatal pigs which die of suspected Japanese encephalitis provide definitive diagnosis. Isolation and identification may be performed in suckling mice, in a variety of cell cultures or in embryonating hens' eggs. In Vero and LLC-MK$_2$ cell lines, the virus is replicated but produces little cytopathic effect (CPE); and in primary cell cultures of chick embryo and monkey or other kidney tissues, the virus is replicated with minimal or no cpe. Embryonic death is produced in embryonating hens' eggs inoculated by yolk sac or other routes. Serodiagnosis of infection is based on antibody titer rises between paired acute and convalescent serum samples. HI and neutralizing antibodies appear within a week after onset while complement fixing (CF) antibodies appear only after several weeks. Plaque reduction neutralization tests have been found to be most specific in differentiating infections with JBE from other flaviviruses. In retrospective serological surveys, neutralizing and HI antibody titers can be depended upon to persist for years following infection whereas CF antibodies have seldom been detectable for 5 years.

HUMAN INFECTION

Clinical

Human infections vary from clinically inapparent to acute fatal encephalitic disease. The incubation period varies widely, usually between 7 and 10 days, but may be 4 to 14 days. The onset of clinical disease is usually abrupt with fever, headache, and signs of meningeal irritation. Marked and increasing sensorial disturbances usually appear in the first 48 hr with convulsions common in children. Manifestations of upper motor neuron and extrapyramidal tract involvement are frequent. Fever usually peaks at 4 to 5 days, then gradually subsides. Patients who succumb usually progress into fatal coma within 7 to 10 days. Prognosis varies with the age of patients varying from 20% or below in children to nearly 50% in patients above 50 years of age. In persons 5 to 40 years of age, sequelae remain in 30 to 40% of convalescent patients but in children under 4 years of age, the occurrence is much higher. Sequelae may be motor, neural, psychological, or combinations of all three.[12,49]

Pathology

During the first week of illness, moderate to appreciable leucocytosis appears, gradually subsiding to normal levels. Cerbrospinal fluid (CSF) shows mononuclear pleocytosis to 100 to 500/mm^3 in almost all patients, moderate protein elevation in many patients, and normal to slight elevation of glucose levels. At necropsy, edema and congestion of the brain and meninges are usually present. Histologically, neuronal degeneration and necrosis with neuronophagia and associated cellular infiltration of perivascular and damaged areas of the cerebral cortex, cerebellum, and spinal cord are frequently seen, as is extensive destruction of Purkinje cells in the cerebellum.[51]

A hypersensitive destruction of selected neurons by antigen-antibody complexes rather than primary viral destruction has been proposed.[40] This would be in accord with the excessive case fatality rate in older patients in the temperate areas where it is probable that most such cases did not represent primary infections but occurred in persons whose early acquired antibody levels had fallen below protective levels.

Diagnosis

Clinical diagnosis is considered to be fairly accurate only in large epidemics. Virus isolation from patients who succumb to suspected infection may be made from brain tissue in suckling mice, cell cultures, or embryonated hens' eggs, or specific antigens may be demonstrated in brain tissues by fluorescent antibody (FA) techniques. Virus isolations may usually be made from patients who succumb in the first week of illness but are almost never possible after the tenth day. In patients who die during the second week of illness, the FA test on sections containing nerve cells is very useful. Virus isolations from CSF have been rare. For serological diagnosis, acute serum samples should be collected between the first and fifth day of illness and convalescent samples between 2 and 6 weeks after onset. In patients with acute disease manifestations, an acute serum sample should be collected as early as possible to be followed by a post-mortem sample in the event death intervenes. HI tests on paired serum samples are at least 80% definitive in areas where vaccination has not been used and other flavivirus infections are not present. Neutralization tests, especially by plaque reduction techniques, and CF tests are most definitive in areas as the tropics where many flavivirus infections may occur.[4] Recent studies have indicated that the CF antibodies are found in the IgG fraction which appears in primary infections about 10 days after onset. The 2-mercaptoethanol (2-ME) test to distinguish IgM antibodies which develop early in primary infections from IgG antibodies is promising to be of value. In secondary infections with encephalitic manifestations IgG antibodies may appear very early, making further study of this procedure essential.

EPIDEMIOLOGY

Occurrence

Japanese encephalitis occurs in epidemics in people in maritime areas of the western Pacific region from eastern Siberia southward to Taiwan. In the subtropical area, the epidemic period is usually July-August, spreading northward and occurring in the temperate area usually in August-September. In the tropical area sporadic human cases appear throughout the year but incidence usually rises at the peak of the monsoon season.[18] Overwintering of the virus in the temperate area has not been elucidated. Lee, in Korea, has proposed that the virus is carried through the winters in snakes or other hibernating animals. As these animals come out of hibernation in spring, viremias recur, infecting *Culex pipiens* and *Aedes vexans* in spring, which transmit the virus to other snakes and to swine, horses, birds, and possibly other animals. Rapid transmission cycles then develop involving susceptible swine and wild birds by *Cx. tritaeniorhynchus* mosquitoes. During the summer period these mosquitoes, plus *Cx. pipiens* and *Ae. vexans,* may tangentially expose people, setting off summer epidemics. The autumn transmission cycle carries the virus back into snakes in which it overwinters.[25] In warmer climates, the transmission of the virus to human beings appears to be related to population levels of the vector mosquitoes.

Transmission

Cx. tritaeniorhynchus, a rice paddy breeding mosquito has been shown to be the most important vector of JBE virus in Japan and neighboring countries and to a lesser extent in tropical Asia.[15,33] In addition to rice paddies, *Cx. tritaeniorhynchus* mosquitoes breed in drains, ditches, ground pools, and fish ponds.[17] Peak populations occur at times when rice fields are flooded. This mosquito preferentially feeds on swine and birds and between 10:00 P.M. and 2:00 A.M. on hosts which are outdoors. Thus people are less frequently exposed to this mosquito than outdoor animals and enter transmission cycles only when mosquito populations become large.[33,39] *Cx. gelidus* appears to be the major vector farther south.[13,35] The populations of this mosquito are relatively constant throughout the year. It feeds predominantly on swine but does also bite people. *Cx. pipiens* and *Cx. annulus* which are widely distributed in East Asia;[28] *Ae. curtipes, Anopheles* spp., and *Mansonia* spp. mosquitoes in Sarawak, East Malaysia;[44] and *An. barbirostris, An. hyrcanus,* and mosquitoes of the *Cx. vishnui* complex in South Asia have all been found infected in nature.[10] Viral transmission has been demonstrated in laboratory studies with a variety of *Culex, Aedes,* and *Armigeres* spp. mosquitoes but transovarial transmission could not be demonstrated in these vectors.

Human Host

In temperate East Asia, cycles of viral transmission recur each year in swine, birds, and possibly other animals, but susceptible human populations build up by lack of transmission from the amplifying hosts or by loss of protective antibody levels with increasing age. Spill-over of virus into populations of susceptible people make possible the appearance of epidemics. In tropical East Asia, seroconversions appear about 5 to 6% per year, ensuring that large susceptible human populations do not build up on any widespread basis.[45] The role of antibody titers acquired from infection by other flaviviruses in affecting the status of resistance of people in the tropics to Japanese encephalitis has not been assessed. There is strong evidence, however, that frequent re-exposures to JBE virus by infected mosquitoes act as a periodic antigenic booster to maintain immunity levels in the human population.[29]

CONTROL

Prevention and Therapy

There is no specific therapeutic regimen for Japanese encephalitis. Treatment of patients is based on palliative and supportive measures. Comprehensive care is most important as the clinical disease can be very severe, convalescence may be protracted and prolonged hospitalization is frequently necessary. As in the control of other arboviral infections, vector control is important if it is feasible. Control of the ubiquitous *Cx. tritaeniorhynchus* mosquito has been difficult because it breeds in economically essential rice paddies as well as in a variety of other fresh-water habitats. Insecticides which can be used in rice paddies as Dursban,® Sumithion,® and Fenthione,® and the older Paris green may give simultaneous control of mosquitoes and insect pests of rice.[1,41] Integration of agricultural and public health use of insecticides is pertinent in areas where this can be affectively achieved.

Vaccination of people in high risk areas has long been desired for prevention of Japanese encephalitis in Japan, Korea, and Taiwan. A formalin-inactivated mouse brain vaccine using the Nakayama strain of JBE virus was developed for immunization of children in Japan in 1954. Attempts to improve its antigenicity led to concentration of the virus and use of Freund's adjuvant, but allergic encephalomyelitic reactions were caused in some guinea pigs. Although allergic encephalitis had not been reported in children vaccinated with the earlier crude extract vaccine, field trials of the adjuvant vaccine were not undertaken.[40] Recent vaccine studies have focused on cell culture cultivated virus. A primary hamster kidney cell culture vaccine produced with an attenuated strain inactivated with formalin has given satisfactory serological response in 92% of 41 adult volunteers given three doses each, but field trials have not yet been conducted. A hamster embryonic kidney diploid cell line vaccine has elicited good serological response in volunteer children but has not yet been tried in the field. A highly purified vaccine concentrated by ultra-centrifugation is currently in a field trial in nearly 40,000 first grade school children 6 and 7 years of age in Cholla Pukdo Province in Korea, using two injections of 1 mℓ., each at intervals of 2 weeks. Another group of 40,000 children in the same province has been selected as a control population. An elaborate case-control study is in progress with a program of serological and virological monitoring. Over 80% of the vaccinated population showed a positive serological response.[40] Experimental formalin-inactivated vaccines have been effective in preventing stillbirths in swine in Japanese and Korean studies.[37,46,48] In tropical Asia, no control or regulatory measures and no vaccine trials have been considered applicable at this time.

PUBLIC HEALTH ASPECTS

Losses up to 50% of litters of swine farrowed during active transmission periods in Japan and Korea have had a serious impact on agriculture in these countries. Immigrants or travellers from non-endemic areas into endemic tropical countries may place themselves at risk, and personal protective measures against mosquito exposure are recommended.

REFERENCES

1. **Ahn, S. K., Lee, H. I., and Park, D. W.,** On the susceptibility of several insecticides against the larvae of *Culex tritaeniorhynchus summorosus, Report of National Institute of Health* (Korea), 5, 156, 1968.
2. Institute for Medical Research, *Annual Report,* Kuala Lumpur, 80, 1953.
3. Institute for Medical Research, *Annual Report,* Kuala Lumpur, 58, 1955.
4. **Buescher, E. L., Scherer, W. F., Rosenberg, M. Z., Gresser, I., Hardy, J. L., and Bullock, H. R.,** Ecologic studies of Japanese encephalitis virus in Japan. II. Mosquito infection, *Am. J. Trop. Med. Hyg.,* 8, 651, 1959.
5. **Burns, K. F.,** Congenital Japanese B encephalitis infection of swine, *Proc. Soc. Exp. Biol. Med.,* 75, 621, 1950.
6. **Chang, I. C.,** Studies of Japanese B encephalitis in cold-blooded animals. 1. Experimental infection of frog, *Rana rugosa,* Schlegel with Japanese B encephalitis virus, *J. Korean Pediatr. Assoc.,* 3 (2), 27, 1960.
7. **Chang, I. C.,** Studies of Japanese B encephalitis in cold-blooded animals. 3. Epidemiological significance and persisting period of Japanese B encephalitis virus in frog, *J. Korean Pediatr. Assoc.,* 4 (1), 37, 1961.
8. **Chang, I. C.,** Studies on Japanese B encephalitis in cold-blooded animals. 3. Isolation of Japanese B encephalitis virus from naturally infected frogs, Rana nigramaculata, Hallowell collected in Chollapuk — To, *J. Korean Pediatr. Assoc.,* 4 (1), 42, 1961.
9. **Chung, Y. C., Moon, J. B., Kang, B. J., Kwon, H. J., and Choi, H. I.,** Serologic studies of Japanese encephalitis in domestic animals, *Korean J. Vet. Res.,* 11 (2), 163, 1971.
10. **Clarke, D. H. and Casals, J.** Japanese encephalitis virus, in *Viral and Rickettsial Infections of Man,* Horsefall, F. L. and Tamm, I., Eds., J. B. Lippincott Co., Philadelphia, 1965, 625.
11. **Deuel, R. E., Bawell, M. B., Matumono, M., and Sabin, A. B.,** Status and significance of inapparent infection with virus of Japanese B encephalitis in Korea and Okinawa in 1946, *Am. J. Hyg.,* 51, 13, 1950.

12. **Dickerson, R. B., Newton, J. R., and Hansen, J. E.,** Diagnosis and immediate prognosis of Japanese B encephalitis, *Am. J. Med.,* 12, 277, 1952.

13. **Gould, D. J., Barnett, H. C., and Suyemoto, W.,** Transmission of Japanese encephalitis virus by *Culex gelidus* Theobald, *Trans. R. Soc. Trop. Med. Hyg.,* 56, 429, 435, 1962.

14. **Green, J. J., Wang, S. P., Yen, C. H., and Hung, S. C.,** The epidemiology of Japanese encephalitis virus in Taiwan in 1961, *Am. J. Trop. Med. Hyg.,* 12, 668, 1963.

15. **Gressler, I., Hardy, J. L., Hu, S. M. K., and Scherer, W. F.,** Factors influencing transmission of Japanese B encephalitis virus by a colonized strain of *Culex tritaeniorhynchus* Giles, from infected pigs and chicks to susceptible pigs and birds, *Am. J. Trop. Med. Hyg.,* 7, 365, 1958.

16. **Hammon, W. M., Tigertt, W. D., and Sather, G. E.,** Epidemiologic studies of concurrent virgin epidemics of Japanese B encephalitis and of mumps on Guam, 1947-1948, with subsequent observations including dengue, through 1957, *Am. J. Trop. Med. Hyg.,* 7, 441, 1958.

17. **Heathcoate, O. H. V.,** Japanese encephalitis in Sarawak: studies on juvenile mosquito populations, *Trans. R. Soc. Trop. Med. Hyg.,* 64, 483, 1970.

18. **Hill, M. N., Varma, M. G. R., Mahadevan, S., and Meers, P. D.,** Arbovirus infections in Sarawak: observations on mosquitoes in the premonsoon period, September to December, 1966, *J. Med. Entomol.,* 6, 398, 1969.

19. **Hullinghorst, R. L., Burns, K. H., Choi, Y. T., and Whatley, L. R.,** Japanese B encephalitis in Korea the epidemic of 1949, *JAMA,* 145 (7), 460, 1951.

20. **Kim, C. S.,** Problems on overwintering of Japanese encephalitis virus. I. Serologic survey of Japanese encephalitis virus infection in bats and birds, *Rep. Ewha Womans Univ. Korean Res. Inst. For Better Living,* (Korea), 4, 159, 1970.

21. **Kim, I. H. and Chang, I. C.,** Serologic survey of Japanese encephalitis virus infection in wild birds in Korea, *Korean J. Int. Med.,* 9 (3), 37, 1966.

22. **Kim, K. H., Paik, S. B., Choi, H., Kim, J. H., Pack, H. J., Paik, Y. H., Oh, H. S., Chung, H. C., and Yang, S. J.,** Epidemiological study of Japanese encephalitis virus in south Korea. Report 1, serological survey of Japanese encephalitis virus in Korea, *J. Korean Soc. Microbiol.,* 2 (1), 49, 1961.

23. **LaMotte, L. C.,** Japanese B encephalitis in bats during simulated hibernation, *Am. J. Hyg.,* 67, 101, 1958.

24. **Lee, H. W.,** Multiplication and antibody formation of Japanese encephalitis virus in snakes. II. Proliferation of the virus, *Seoul J. Med.* (Korea), 9 (3), 1, 1968.

25. **Lee, H. W.,** Study on overwintering mechanisms of Japanese encephalitis virus in Korea, *J. Korean Med. Assoc.,* 14 (11), 65, 1971.

26. **Lee, H. W. and Kee, R. S.,** Multiplication and antibody formation of Japanese encephalitis virus in snakes. I. Antibody responses to the virus and serum, *J. Korean Soc. Microbiol.,* 3 (1), 43, 1968.

27. **Lee, H. W., Lee, K. C., Paik, N. E., Lee, J. S., and Kim, Y. S.,** Experiments to demonstrate multiplication of Japanese encephalitis virus and antibodies in frogs, *N. Med. J. (Korea),* 13 (11), 41, 1970.

28. **Lee, H. W., Min, B. W., and Lee, Y. W.,** Japanese encephalitis virus isolation from mosquitoes of Korea, *J. Korean Med. Assoc.,* 12 (4), 69, 1969.

29. **Lee, H. W. and Scherer, W. F.,** The anamnistic antibody response to Japanese encephalitis virus in monkeys and its implications concerning naturally acquired immunity in man, *J. Immunol.,* 85, 151, 1961.

30. **Lee, K. M., Lee, H. W., Park, C. Y., Pyun, K. K., Park, D., Kim, C. S., and Chung, Y. C.,** Serologic studies of Japanese encephalitis in domestic animals and chickens, *Seoul J. Med.* (Korea), 3 (2), 5, 1962.

31. **Lee, N. S., Moon, J. B., and Kim, Y. H.,** Studies on Japanese B encephalitis I. Isolation of Japanese B encephalitis virus from a pig fetus of stillbirth, *Rep. Nat. Inst. Vet. Res.* (Korea), 3, 1-16, 1955.

32. **Lee, N. S., Moon, J. B., and Kim, Y. H.,** Studies on Japanese B encephalitis. III. Distribution of complement fixation antibody among pigs and cattle, *Rep. Nat. Inst. Vet. Res.* (Korea), 3, 27, 1955.

33. **Lee, S. W., Ree, H. I., Hong, H. K., Park, D. W., Lee, K. W., and Ahn, S. K.,** Studies on the Behavior and Possible Control Measures of the Confirmed Vector of Japanese Encephalitis in Korea, National Malaria Eradication Service, Ministry of Health and Social Affairs, Korea, July, 1968.

34. **Lee, S. Y.,** Inapparent infection on Japanese B encephalitis among horses and several species of Mammalia in Korea, *Bull. Nat. Inst. Prevention Infect. Dis.* (Korea), 2 (1), 83, 1953.

35. **Macdonald, W. W., et al.,** Arbovirus infections in Sarawak: further observations on the mosquito, *J. Med. Entomol.,* 4, 146, 1967.

36. **Mitsunobu A.,** Study on the basic morphology of Japanese encephalitis virus: the isolation of purified haemagglutinin and the detection of core membrane, *Trop. Med.,* 18 (1), 11, 1976.

37. **Nakamura, H.,** Use of vaccine in pigs. C. Field trials of Japanese encephalitis vaccine for prevention of viral stillbirth among sows, in *Immunization for Japanese Encephalitis,* Hammon, W. M., Kitaoka, M., and Downs, W. G., Eds., Williams & Wilkins Co., Baltimore, 1971, 305.

38. **Pond, W. L., Russ, S. B., Lancaster, W. E., Audy, J. R., and Smadel, J. E.,** Japanese Encephalitis in Malaya. II. Distribution of neutralizing antibody in man and domestic animals, *Am. J. Hyg.,* 59, 17, 1954.

39. **Ree, H. I., Chen, Y. K., and Chow, C. Y.,** Methods of sampling population of the Japanese encephalitis vector mosquitoes in Korea (a preliminary report), *Korean J. Parasitol.,* 7 (1), 25, 1969.

40. World Health Organization, Rep. 2nd Reg. Semin. Virus Diseases: Mosquito-borne Virus Diseases (Arboviruses), 1969, WHO, Manila, 4.

41. World Health Organization, Rep. 2nd Reg. Semin. Virus Diseases: Mosquito-borne Virus Disease (Arboviruses), 1969, WHO, Manila, 10.

42. **Scherer, W. F., Buescher, E. L., and McClure, H. E.,** Ecologic studies of Japanese encephalitis virus in Japan. V. Avian factors, *Am. J. Trop. Med. Hyg.,* 8, 689, 1959.

43. **Shimizu, T., Kawakami, Y., Fukuhara, S., and Matumoto, M.,** Experimental stillbirth in pregnant swine infected with Japanese encephalitis virus, *Jpn. J. Exp. Med.,* 24, 363, 1954.

44. **Simpson, D. I. H., et al.,** Arbovirus infections in Sarawak: virus isolations from mosquitoes, *Ann. Trop. Med. Parasitol.,* 64, 137, 1970.

45. **Smith, C. E. G., et al.,** Arbovirus infections in Sarawak: human serological studies, *Trans. R. Soc. Trop. Med. Hyg.,* 68, 96, 1974.

46. **Takahashi, K., Matsuo, R., Kuma, M., Baba, S., Noguchi, H., Inoue, Y. K., Sasaki, N., and Kodama, K.,** Use of vaccine in pigs. Effect of immunization of swine upon the ecological cycle of Japanese encephalitis virus, in *Immunization for Japanese Encephalitis,* Hammon, W. M., Kitaoka, M., and Downs, W. G., Eds., Williams & Wilkins Co., Baltimore, 1971, 292.

47. **Takehara, M. and Hotta, S.,** Effect of enzymes on partially purified Japanese B encephalitis and related arbor viruses, *Science,* 134, 1878, 1961.

48. **Watanabe, M.,** Use of vaccine in pigs. B. Formalized vaccine, antibodies and swine fetus resistance to Japanese encephalitis virus infections, in *Immunization for Japanese Encephalitis,* Hammon, W. M., Kitaoka, M., and Downs, W. G., Eds., Williams & Wilkins Co., Baltimore, 1971, 304.

49. **Weaver, O. M., Haymaker, W., Pieper, S., and Kurland, R.,** Sequelae of the arthropod-borne encephalitides. V. Japanese encephalitis, *Neurology,* 8, 887, 1958.

50. **Wildy, P.,** Classification and nomenclature of viruses, first report of the ICTV, *Monogr. Virol.,* 5, 53, 1971, 1971, 53.

51. **Zimmerman, H. M.,** The pathology of Japanese B encephalitis, *Am. J. Pathol.,* 22, 965, 1946.

ARBOVIRUSES OF SOUTHEAST ASIA

N. J. Marchette

There are 24 arthropod-borne viruses known to occur in Southeast Asia in addition to chikungunya, Japanese encephalitis, and the four dengue viruses. Most have not been adequately studied, and in some cases, the only published account is in the International Catalogue of Arboviruses.[1]

BEBARU VIRUS

Bebaru virus is in the genus *Alphavirus,* formerly called the group A arboviruses, in the family Togaviridae. It is considered to be a subtype of Getah virus. Infant mice are susceptible to infection by the intracerebral route; adult mice are not. Infection of rabbits and guinea pigs results in the production of antibody but no disease. No human disease is known.

Bebaru virus has been isolated only from large pools of *Culex (Lophoceratomyia)* spp. and *Aedes butleri* complex mosquitoes collected in mangrove swamp forest in West Malaysia. Nothing is known of its distribution or natural transmission cycle, but the occurrence of neutralizing antibodies in residents of various localities in Malaysia suggests that it may exist in habitats other than coastal mangrove swamps.

GETAH VIRUS

Getah virus is in the genus *Alphavirus,* and is considered the prototype of a closely related subgroup of viruses consisting of Bebaru (described above), Sagiyama virus in Japan, and Ross River virus in Australia. Infant mice and chick embryos are susceptible to infection and lesions are produced on the chorioallantoic membrane. Adult mice and rabbits do not develop disease, but neutralizing antibodies are produced in rabbits. Wild monkeys (*Macaca* spp. and *Presbytis* spp.) in West Malaysia have getah antibody,[2] but experimental infection of *M. fascicularis* did not produce disease. Antibodies occur in domestic animals, principally buffaloes, cows, and pigs in West Malaysia. Viremia in sheep and clinical disease in calves is reported after experimental infection.[3]

Antibodies to getah virus without human disease are widespread throughout Malaysia[4] and has been reported in Australia.[5] Getah virus was once thought to be a cause of epidemic polyarthralgia and rash in Australia, but Ross River virus, another *Alphavirus,* is now known to be the etiologic agent.[6,7] No similar disease has been reported in Southeast Asia where Ross River virus does not occur.

Getah virus is distributed widely and infects a variety of mosquitoes. The first isolations were made from *Culex gelidus* and *Cx. tritaeniorhynchus*[1,4] in West Malaysia. It was subsequently reported from *Cx. tritaeniorhynchus* in Cambodia,[8] *Cx. bitaeniorhynchus* and *Anopheles amictus* in Australia,[9] *Aedes vexans* and pigs in Japan.[1] A closely related *Alphavirus,* Sagiyama virus, also infects *Ae. vexans* in Japan.[1] The natural transmission cycle is not known, but the mosquitoes it infects mainly feed on domestic mammals and fowl suggesting their involvement in a transmission cycle. There may also be a jungle cycle involving wild vertebrates.

SINDBIS VIRUS

Another *Alphavirus,* Sindbis is most closely related antigenically to western encephalitis virus of North America. Reports that Sindbis virus, unlike other togaviruses, contains a double-stranded RNA genome[1] are incorrect. The genome consists of a single strand of RNA.[10] Infant mice are susceptible to intracerebral and intraperitoneal infection, with paralysis and death occurring in 2 to 4 days. Adult mice can be infected by adapted strains.[11] The virus grows in embryonated eggs after yolk sac inoculation. African green monkeys (*Cerocopithecus aethiops*) and rhesus monkeys (*Macaca mulatta*) can be infected by the bite of infected mosquitoes. A variety of wild and domestic birds can be infected by inoculation, with subsequent circulation of virus and antibody development. Viremia, illness, and death were produced in young chickens and viremia without overt disease in adult fowl.[12] Wild birds and domestic fowl are naturally infected.

Sporadic cases of disease in man have occurred in Uganda, South Africa, and Australia.[13-15] Serological conversion without apparent disease occurred in a study population in West Malaysia; and an earlier case with fever, headache, general body ache, and erythematous rash was reported on the basis of HI serological conversion to Sindbis virus. However, the patient's acute serum had high titer Sindbis HI antibody and there was no conversion of neutralizing antibody.[16] This seems to have been an *Alphavirus* infection, but was probably not Sindbis. A serologically confirmed case of infection in a young girl in Australia was characterized by fever, malaise, and vesicular rash mostly on the face and extremities.[14] The disease was relatively mild and the child recovered completely in a few days.

A reported case in South Africa was more severe, lasting several weeks with fever, vesicular rash, vomiting, and swelling of fingers and feet.[13] In general, however, the illness lasts 4 to 8 days with lassitude, headache, sore throat, lymphadenopathy, muscle and tendon pain, joint pain, and a maculopapular rash, often with vesicles between fingers and toes.[17] Occasionally there may be a slight jaundice.[18]

Sindbis virus is widely distributed in Africa, India, Southeast Asia, and Australia, and has been reported from Czechoslovakia[19] and the U.S.S.R.[1] *Culex sinensis, Cx. vishnui, Cx. pseudovishnui, Cx. tritaeniorhynchus,* and *Cx. bitaeniorhynchus* are naturally infected in the Philippines, West Malaysia, and Sarawak.[2,16,20,21] A high proportion of domestic fowl contains Sindbis antibody suggesting a natural bird-mosquito cycle in this region.[2] Wild birds and *Culex* mosquitoes probably constitute the natural cycle, with man and other mammals peripherally involved. Experimental transmission has been accomplished with *Cx. univittatus* in South Africa and it is assumed that most or all the four *Culex* species in which the virus occurs in Southeast Asia actively transmit it. These mosquitoes are rural, farmland, and paddy field mosquitoes, breeding in fresh or stagnant water. They bite at night, feeding readily on domestic animals and fowl with activity peaks just after dark and again before dawn. Approximately 10% of more than 4000 West Malaysian human serum samples tested had neutralizing antibody to Sindbis virus.[4]

BAKAU VIRUS

Bakau is one of two viruses in the Bakau group of *Bunyvirus*-like arboviruses. It produces fatal infection in infant and adult mice in 4 to 5 days. Nothing is known of natural infections in animals or man. It is associated with *Culex* mosquitoes in nippah palm-mangrove and fresh water swamps in West Malaysia[1] and *Argas abdussalami* ticks in Pakistan.[22] Long-tailed macaques (*M. fascicularis*), slow loris (*Nyctacebus coucang*), and silvered leaf monkeys (*Presbytis cristatus*) in mangrove forests in West Malaysia have neutralizing antibodies, and a strain of Bakau virus was isolated from the blood of a wild *M. fascicularis*. Antibodies also occur in bats, rodents, wild birds, and domestic fowl.[23]

Human disease is not known, but antibodies are prevalent in persons living near mangrove swamps. In one case, a patient with pyrexia of unknown origin developed a diagnostic rise in antibody titer to Bakau virus during the illness.[23]

The principal vector appears to be *Culex (Eumelanomyia) malayensis* and the vertebrate hosts are a wide variety of animals, but the natural cycles are not completely known.

KETAPANG VIRUS

Also in the Bakau group, kepatang virus is antigenically distinct from Bakau virus. Infant and adult mice are susceptible to infection, with an average survival time of 3 days. Rabbits produce neutralizing antibody upon inoculation with the virus, but there are no signs of illness. No human disease is known, but neutralizing antibodies are prevalent in West Malaysia.

Ketapang virus is known only from West Malaysia where a single isolation from a pool of *Culex (Lophoceratomyia)* spp. mosquitoes has been reported.[1] Nothing is known of its natural cycle.

BATAI VIRUS

Its synonyms are Calovo Virus (Czechoslovakia) and Olyka (U.S.S.R.).

Batai virus is one of approximately 86 members of the genus *Bunyavirus* in the Bunyamwera supergroup of Togaviridae. It is closely related to several Bunyamwera sub-group viruses in Africa. It produces death in 3 to 5 days in infant and adult mice when inoculated intracerebrally. Rabbits produce neutralizing antibodies without signs of illness. No natural human or animal disease is known.

Batai virus has been isolated only from *Culex gelidus* and *Aedes vexans* mosquitoes in West Malaysia and Thailand, respectively, but several species of *Anopheles* are naturally infected in India[25] and Eurasia.[26,27] There is an unconfirmed report of the isolation of a Batai-like virus from a pool of *Aedes nocturnus* mosquitoes in Cambodia. In Thailand antibodies is prevalent in wild birds, rodents, and bats. Domestic ungulates have a high prevalence of antibodies in India.[28] Antibodies in man in West Malaysia and India occur at a much lower rate. The natural cycles of infection are not known, but domestic animals in Southeast Asia are probably involved as they are in India, since they are the preferred hosts of *C. gelidus* mosquitoes.

KAENG KHOI VIRUS

Kaeng Khoi virus is the second member of the *Bunyavirus* genus in Southeast Asia. It produces fatal infection in infant and adult mice. Nothing is known of natural infections in animals or man.

This is a bat virus, having been recovered from the brains and salivary glands of numerous cave bats, *Tadarida plicata* and *Taphozous theobaldi* and from sentinel mice and rats placed in bat caves. Guano miners have a high prevalence of antibodies to Kaeng Khoi virus. The vector is not known, and the virus may not even be transmitted by arthropods. No human disease is known.[1]

PATHUM THANI VIRUS

Pathum Thani virus is a member of the Dera Ghazi Khan group of unclassified arboviruses. Infant mice inoculated intracerebrally or intraperitoneally die in 7 to 11 days. Adult mice, hamsters, rabbits, and guinea pigs produce antibodies but no signs of illness. Natural infection in animals or humans is not known.[1]

Pathum Thani virus has been isolated only from the soft-bodied bird tick *Argas robertsi* in Thailand and Sri Lanka.[29]

KAO SHUAN VIRUS

Kao Shuan virus is a third member of the Dera Ghazi Khan group in Asia and the second in Southeast Asia. It is very similar to Pathum Thani virus and has been recovered only from *Argas robertsi* ticks in Taiwan, Java,[29] and the Northern Territories in Australia.[30] The natural vertebrate hosts are not known, but are assumed to be one or more of the various species of birds on which *A. robertsi* feeds.

Another Asian member of this group, Dera Ghazi Khan virus, infects camel ticks, *Hyalomma dromedarii* in West Pakistan.[31] Nothing is known of vertebrate hosts or natural cycles of infection.

KUNJIN VIRUS

Kunjin virus is in the *Flavivirus* genus in the Togaviridae. With the exception of dengue and Japanese encephalitis viruses (covered in separate chapters), Kunjin is the only flavivirus in Southeast Asia known to be pathogenic for man. It is most closely related to West Nile virus.[32] It produces fatal illness in infant and adult mice and chick embryos. Pocks are produced on the chorioallantoic membrane of chick embryos. Clinical disease occurs in calves.[33]

Naturally occurring disease in man due to Kunjin virus is not known, but there have been two documented laboratory infections.[34] In both cases there was low grade fever of short duration. In one, nausea, anorexia, and tremor were the only symptoms recorded. The other began as a rubella-like illness with lymphadenopathy and maculopapular rash, which became extensively papular with small vesicles on parts of the trunk. This patient did not feel ill, and her temperature never exceeded 98.8°C.

First isolated from *Culex annulirostris* mosquitoes in Australia, Kunjin virus is known only from Sarawak in Southeast Asia. It was isolated from pools of *Cx. pseudovishnui* mosquitoes in a rural farming area.[35] Nothing is known of its host range or natural cycles of infection, but presumably domestic animals or fowl are involved, as they are with Tembusu and JBE viruses.

TEMBUSU VIRUS

Another *Flavivirus,* Tembusu is antigenically distinct and does not crossreact by neutralization test with other flaviviruses. Fatal infection in 4 to 8 days is produced in infant and adult mice, but no disease occurs in guinea pigs or rabbits. Pocks are produced on the chorioallantoic membrane (CAM) of 10 day chick embryos. Chickens are readily infected and circulate virus, but do not become ill.[36] No human disease has been reported.

Tembusu is reported to occur only in West Malaysia, Sarawak, and Thailand where *Cx. tritaeniorhynchus, Cx. vishnui,* and *Cx. pseudovishnui* are the major vectors with *Cx. gelidus* and *Cx. sitiens* playing a minor role.[36,37] The results of prospective studies in Malaysia showed that sentinel chickens become infected during almost every month of the year, whereas in the same area Sindbis virus is active only in the summer months. No antibodies were found in wild birds. The natural cycles of infection are not known, but a chicken-mosquito-virus cycle is quite evident.

WESSELSBRON VIRUS

Wesselsbron virus is a *Flavivirus* forming a closely related complex with Uganda S,

Banzi, and yellow fever viruses.[38] It causes fatal infection in infant and adult mice in 6 to 12 days; a febrile response in cattle, horses, pigs, and monkeys (*Cercopithecus aethiops*); abortion in ewes and fatal infection in lambs. Human disease reported from South Africa is characterized by fever, headache, myalgia, arthralgia, and rash.[39]

Wesselsbron virus is mainly associated with *Aedes* spp. mosquitoes and sheep in Africa although it has been isolated occasionally from species of *Culex* and *Anopheles*.

In Thailand *An. mediolineatis* and *An. lineatopennis* are naturally infected.[40] Both *Aedes aegypti* and *Culex quinquifasciatus* are efficient experimental vectors,[41] suggesting the potential for a human-mosquito cycle. However, no human or animal disease associated with Wesselsbron virus has been reported in Thailand. The natural cycles of infection are not known, but neutralizing antibodies were found in wild rodents and children residing in the area where the infected mosquitoes were captured.

ZIKA VIRUS

Zika virus is a flavivirus, closely related antigenically to Spondweni virus in Africa and is ecologically related to dengue, Uganda S., and yellow fever viruses.[38] Infant and adult mice become paralyzed and die after i.c. or i.p. inoculation. Monkeys are readily infected, becoming viremic and producing antibodies but no clinical signs of illness. The original isolation was made from the blood of a sentinel monkey in Uganda.[42]

Only one human case, a laboratory infection, has been reported, although the virus was also recovered from the blood of a febrile mosquito catcher in Senegal.[41] The laboratory infection was a short, mild febrile illness with headache.

Aedes mosquitoes, primarily *Ae. africanus* in Africa, are naturally infected. In West Malaysia the only reported isolation was from *Ae. aegypti* collected in a small town in the west central part of the country.[43] Neutralizing antibodies were found in wild monkeys in Malaysia and has been reported in human beings throughout Southeast Asia.[44-46] However, since dengue viruses are endemic in the same area and induce cross-reacting antibody, interpretation of Zika antibody survey data must be made with some reservations.

LANGAT VIRUS

Langat virus is a tick-borne *Flavivirus* in the Russian spring summer encephalitis (RSSE) subgroup. Paralysis and death result from inoculation of infant and adult mice. Viremia occurs in monkeys, and antibody is produced, but no illness. No natural disease is known in man, but experimental infection of patients with malignant tumors produced fever and encephalitis.[47] Laboratory strains have been administered to man as experimental vaccines against Kyasanur Forest Disease and RSSE.[48-50]

Langat virus has been isolated from *Ixodes granulatus* ticks only in Ulu Langat Forest Reserve in West Malaysia where the wild rat hosts of the ticks also possess neutralizing antibodies.[51] All attempts to isolate the virus from Malaysian ticks collected outside the Ulu Langat Reserve have failed.[2] Recently, however, the virus was isolated from *Haemaphysalis papuana* ticks in Thailand.[52] The natural cycle appears to involve only forest rats and ticks. No natural human infections are known.

JUGRA VIRUS, CAREY ISLAND VIRUS, BATU CAVE VIRUS, AND PHNOM-PENH BAT VIRUS

These flaviviruses are all associated with bats in Malaysia or Cambodia. None of them has been associated with natural human or animal disease.[1]

Jugra virus causes death in infant and adult mice. It has been isolated from *Aedes (Cancraedes)* spp. and *Uranotaenia* spp. mosquitoes and from the blood of a bat, *Cynopterus brachyotis* in mangrove swamp forests, suggesting a natural mosquito-bat cycle.

Carey Island virus causes death of infant mice but no disease in adult mice. It has been isolated only from the salivary glands of bats (*C. brachyotis* and *Macroglossis lagochilus*) collected in the same mangrove swamp forest as Jugra virus. No vector and no natural human animal disease is known.

Batu Cave virus causes death in infant mice in 5 days. It has been isolated only from salivary glands of bats (*Eonycteris spelaea* and *C. brachyotis*) whose natural habitat includes limestone caves and houses. No vector and no human or animal disease are known.

Phnom-Penh bat virus causes paralysis and death of infant and adult mice and death of young guinea pigs, but no disease in white rats. It has been isolated only from salivary glands and brown fat of frugivorus bats (*C. brachyotis*) collected in attics of houses in Cambodia. No vector or natural animal or human disease is known.

LANJAN VIRUS

Lanjan virus is a member of the Kaisodi group of tick-borne viruses,[53] which also contains Kaisodi virus in India and Silverwater virus in North America. They are characterized as *Bunyavirus*-like,[1] but are not yet officially included in the *Bunyavirus* genus. Paralysis and death are caused by intracerebral inoculation of Lanjan virus into infant and adult mice. No illness is produced in rabbits, guinea pigs, hamsters, or monkeys. There is no known human disease.

Lanjan virus naturally infects *Dermacentor* spp. and *Haemaphysalis* spp. ticks in West Malaysian forests.[54] A few species of wild rodents have antibody, but nothing is known of the natural cycles of infection. No antibody surveys of human populations have been conducted.

SELETAR VIRUS

Seletar virus belongs to the Kemerovo group of tick-borne viruses in the genus *Orbivirus* in the family Reoviridae. Unlike members of the Togaviridae, these viruses have a double stranded RNA genome. They are of medium size (60 to 80 nm) with cubic symmetry and, unlike most arboviruses, are ether resistant. The genus includes bluetongue virus, African horse sickness virus, and Colorado tick fever virus, all of which produce significant disease in animals or man. Seletar virus is most closely related to Wad Medani virus in North Africa, India, Pakistan, and Jamaica. It produces illness and death only in infant mice as far as known.

Seletar virus has been recovered only from the one-host cattle tick *Boophilus microplus* in Singapore and West Malaysia.[55] Neutralizing antibody occurs in cattle, carabao, and pigs. Since *B. microplus* is a one-host tick, spending its entire life span on a single host, transovarial transmission would seem to be necessary for preservation of the virus. There is no information available on possible natural cycles involving wild vertebrates and other tick species. No human involvement is known.

PUCHONG VIRUS

Puchong virus belongs to the Malakal serogroup of arboviruses. It causes illness and death of infant and adult mice after intracerebral inoculation. Nothing is known of natural infection or disease in animals or man.

A single strain of Puchong virus was isolated from *Mansonia uniformis* mosquitoes collected from a carabao shed in West Malaysia.[1] Malakal virus, the other member of the serogroup, was also recovered from *M. uniformis* in the Sudan. There is no information on natural cycles of infection.

INGWAVUMA VIRUS

Ingwavuma virus (synonym: Balagodu virus) is one of 16 viruses comprising the Simbu subgroup in the genus *Bunyavirus*. It causes death in infant and adult mice and guinea pigs after intracerebral inoculation. Nothing is known about disease in animals or man.

Ingwavuma virus infects *Culex vishnui* mosquitoes and domestic animals and fowl in Thailand.[56] Pigs are considered to be the natural vertebrate hosts in Thailand, but numerous isolations of the virus have been made from wild birds in Africa and India, suggesting a bird-mosquito natural cycle. No antibodies were detected in a large sample of residents of Thai villages in the natural focus. This is in contrast to the relatively high prevalence of antibodies in human sera in India.[57] Natural cycles of infection are yet to be elucidated, but probably involve domestic animals and birds. Man may be an accidental host.

UMBRE VIRUS

Umbre virus belongs to the *Bunyavirus*-like Turlock subgroup of arboviruses, which includes two other viruses, one from Africa (Mopoko virus) and one from North and South America (Turlock virus). Paralysis and death occur in infant mice and sickness and death in adult mice inoculated intracerebrally. Naturally infected chickens become viremic but exhibit no visible signs of illness. There are no reports of human disease.

Umbre virus naturally infects *Culex* mosquitoes (principally *Cx. vishnui* and *Cx. pseudovishnui*) in India and West Malaysia. In one study, sentinel chickens were infected in almost every month of the year.[36] Wild birds in Malaysia have antibodies and the virus was isolated from the blood of a bird in India, suggesting that natural cycles of infection may include wild birds as well as domestic fowl. No human disease is recognized, but neutralizing antibodies are prevalent in man in Malaysia and several persons acquired antibodies during the previously cited study.[36]

KETERAH VIRUS

Keterah virus, an ungrouped arbovirus, was initially isolated from *Argas pusillus* ticks and *Scotophilus kuhlii castaneus* (= *S. temmenckii*) house bats in West Malaysia.[1] Subsequently, L'vov et al. reported the isolation of Issyk-Kul-virus from bats and *Argas vespertilionis* ticks in Kirgiz S.S.R.[58] Keterah and Issyk-Kul are closely related, if not identical, to each other and to two strains isolated from bats in Japan.[59,60]

Keterah virus causes illness and death in infant and adult mice after intracerebral inoculation. It produces viremia in bats, but no apparent illness. Human disease has not been reported, but Miura[60] found antibodies to the Japan strain of Keterah virus in patients with diabetes mellitus, suggesting that natural infection may occur.

TANJONG RABOK VIRUS

Tanjong Rabok virus is ungrouped and unrelated to any other arboviruses with which it has been tested. It was isolated from the blood of a pig-tailed macaque (*Macaca nemestrina*) in West Malaysia, and antibodies were demonstrated in other monkeys, flying squirrels, bats, and human beings. It causes illness and death in infant and adult mice after intracerebral inoculation and viremia, but no apparent illness in cynomalogous monkeys.

This virus is known only from West Malaysia where it exists in swamp forest canopy-dwelling mammals (monkeys, flying squirrels, and bats). It is presumed to be an arbovirus, but no vector has been discovered. Two possible cases of human illness, one with hemorrhagic manifestations, have been attributed to infection with Tanjong Rabok virus but the etiological relationship has not been confirmed.

NYAMANINI VIRUS

Nyamanini virus is an ungrouped virus of *Argas arboreus* and *A. persicas* ticks and birds in Africa. It has also been isolated from *A. robertsi* in Sri Lanka and Thailand.[61] Nothing is known of its life cycle in Southeast Asia.

OTHER VIRUSES

There are unconfirmed reports of isolations of eastern encephalitis virus (*Alphavirus*) from *Culex pipiens* mosquitoes in Thailand[1] and from the brain of an infected monkey in the Philippines.[62] However, it is doubtful that eastern encephalitis virus occurs naturally in this part of the world. Human infection has not been reported.

Several other viruses, mostly alphaviruses and flaviviruses indigenous to Africa, have been reported in East and West Malaysia on the basis of serological surveys by early investigators.[42,45] It is now thought that the antibodies in the human donors were against related viruses now known to be endemic or enzootic in the region and were crossreacting with the antigens used. Thus antibodies reacting with Semliki Forest virus (*Alphavirus*) were probably crossreacting chikungunya, Getah, or Bebaru antibodies. The antibodies to Ntya, Uganda S, West Nile, Murray Valley encephalitis, Ilheus, St. Louis encephalitis, and RSSE (all flaviviruses) were probably reacting with the other flaviviruses such as dengue, Japanese encephalitis, and Tembusu which are widespread throughout the entire region. It is especially unlikely that Ilheus and St. Louis encephalitis viruses occur in Southeast Asia since they are enzootic in the Western Hemisphere.

REFERENCES

1. **Berge, T. O., Ed.,** *International Catalogue of Arboviruses Including Certain Other Viruses of Vertebrates,* 2nd ed., Publ. No. (CDC) 75-8301, Public Health Service, U.S. Department of Health, Education and Welfare, Atlanta, 1975.
2. **Marchette, N. J., Rudnick, A., Garcia, R., and MacVean, D. W.,** Alphaviruses in Peninsular Malaysia. I. Virus isolation and animal serology, *Southeast Asian J. Trop. Med. Public Health,* 9, 317, 1978.
3. **Spradbrow, P. B.,** Arbovirus infections of domestic animals in Australia, *Aust. Vet. J.,* 48, 181, 1972.
4. **Marchette, N. J., Garcia, R., Rudnick, A., and Dukellis, E.,** 1980. Group A arboviruses in West Malaysia. II. Serological evidence of human infection, *Southeast Asian J. Trop. Med. Public Health,* 11, 14, 1980.
5. **Doherty, R. L.,** Arboviruses of Australia, *Aust. Vet. J.,* 48, 172, 1972.
6. **Shope, R. E. and Anderson, S. G.,** The virus etiology of epidemic exanthem and polyarthritis, *Med. J. Aust.,* 1, 156, 1960.

7. **Doherty, R. L., Gorman, B. M., Whitehead, R. H., and Carley, J. G.**, Studies of epidemic polyar-thritis: the significance of three group A arboviruses isolated from mosquitoes in Queensland, *Aust. Ann. Med.*, 13, 322, 1964.
8. **Chastel, C. and Rageau, J.**, Isolement d'arbovirus au Cambodge a partir de mostiques naturellement infectes, *Med. Trop. Marseilles*, 26, 391, 1966.
9. **Doherty, R. L., Carley, J. G., Mackerras, M. J., and Marks, E. N.**, Studies of arthropod-borne virus infections in Queensland. III. Isolation and characterization of virus strains from wild-caught mosquitoes in North Queensland, *Aust. J. Exp. Biol. Med. Sci.*, 41, 17, 1963.
10. **Arif, B. M. and Falkner, P.**, Genome of Sindbis virus, *J. Virol.*, 9, 102, 1972.
11. **Weinbren, M. P., Kokernot, R. H., and Smithburn, K. C.**, Strains of Sindbis-like virus isolated from culicine mosquitoes in the Union of South Africa, *S. Afr. Med. J.*, 30, 631, 1956.
12. **Whitehead, R. H.**, Experimental infection of vertebrates with Ross River and Sindbis viruses, two group A arboviruses isolated in Australia, *Aust. J. Exp. Biol. Med. Sci.*, 41, 11, 1969.
13. **Malherbe, H., Strickland-Cholmley, M., and Jackson, A. L.**, Sindbis virus infection in man: report of a case with recovery of virus from skin lesions, *S. Afr. Med. J.*, 37, 547, 1963.
14. **Doherty, R. L., Bodey, A. S., and Carew, J. S.**, Sindbis virus infection in Australia, *Med. J. Aust.*, 2, 1016, 1969.
15. **Doherty, R. L.**, Surveys of Hemagglutination inhibition antibody to arboviruses in aborigines and other population groups in northern Australia, *Trans. R. Soc. Trop. Med. Hyg.*, 67, 197, 1973.
16. **Lim, T. W., Burhainuddin, M., and Abbas, A.**, A case of Sindbis virus infection in Kuala Lumpur, *Med. J. Malaysia*, 27, 147, 1972.
17. **Gear, J. H. S., MacIntosh, B. M., Spence, I. M., Donaldson, J. M., Dickenson, D. B., McGillivray, G. M., and Gauntlett, J. T.**, Human infection with Sindbis and West Nile viruses, *Rep. S. Afr. Inst. Med. Res.*, 1963, 211.
18. **Knight, E. M., Woodall, J. P., Williams, M. C., and Ellice, J. M.**, Sindbis infection in man, *Rep. E. Afr. Virus Res. Inst.*, 13, 17, 1962.
19. **Ernek, E., Kozuch, O., Nosek, J., and Labudu, M.**, Evidence for circulation of Sindbis and other arboviruses by using sentinel animals in Western Slovakia, *Intervirology*, 2, 186, 1973.
20. **Rudnick, A., Hammon, W. McD., and Sather, G. E.**, A strain of Sindbis virus isolated from *Culex bitaeniorhynchus* mosquitoes in the Philippines, *Am. J. Trop. Med. Hyg.*, 11, 546, 1962.
21. **Simpson, D. H., Smith, C. E. G., Bowen, E. T. W., Platt, G. S., Way, H., McMahon, D., Bright, W. F., Hill, M. N., Mahadevan, S., Macdonald, W. W.**, Arbovirus infections in Sarawak: virus isolations from mosquitoes, *Ann. Trop. Med. Parasitol.*, 64, 137, 1970.
22. Subcommittee on Information Exchange, American Committee on Arthropod-borne Viruses Cata-logue of arthropod-borne viruses of the world, *Am. J. Trop. Med. Hyg.*, 19, 1082, 1970.
23. **MacVean, D.**, The Natural History of Bakau Virus in West Malaysia, Ph.D. thesis, University of California, Berkeley, 1976.
24. **Hunt, A. R. and Calisher, C. H.**, Relationships of Bunyamwera group viruses by neutralization, *Am. J. Trop. Med. Hyg.*, 28, 740, 1979.
25. **Singh, K. R. P. and Pavri, K. M.**, Isolation of Chittoor virus from mosquitoes and demonstration of serological conversions in sera of domestic animals at Manjri, Poona, India, *Indian J. Med. Res.*, 54, 220, 1966.
26. **Gaidamovich, S. Y., Obuklova, V. R., Vinograd, A. H., Klisenko, G. A., and Melnikoog, E. E.**, Olyka, an arbovirus of the Bunyamwera group in the USSR, *Acta Virol.*, 17, 444, 1973.
27. **Bardos, V. and Cupkova, E.**, The Calovo virus—the second virus isolated from mosquitoes in Czechoslovakia, *J. Hyg. Epidemiol. Microbiol. Immunol.*, 6, 18, 1962.
28. **Pavri, K. M. and Sheikh, B. M.**, Distribution of antibodies reacting with Chitoor virus in humans and domestic ungulates in India, *Indian J. Med. Res.*, 54, 225, 1966.
29. **Hoogstraal, H., Kaiser, M. N., and McClure, H. E.**, The subgenus *Persicargas* (Ixodoidea:Argasidae:*Argas*) 20. *A. (P.) robertsi* parasitizing nesting wading birds and domestic chickens in the Australian and Oriental regions, viral infections and host migration, *J. Med. Ento-mol.*, 11, 513, 1974.
30. **Doherty, R. L., Carley, J. G., Filippich, C., and Kag, B. H.**, Isolation of virus strains related to Kao Shuan virus from *Argas robertsi* in Northern Territory, *Search (Australia)* 7, 484, 1976.
31. **Begum, F., Wisseman, C. L., and Casals, J.**, Tick-borne viruses of West Pakistan. III. Dera Ghazi Khan, A new agent isolated from *Hyaloma drommedarii* ticks in the D.G. Khan district of West Pakistan, *Am. J. Epidemiol.*, 92, 195, 1970.
32. **Westaway, E. G.**, The neutralization of arboviruses. II. Neutralization in heterologous virus-serum mixtures with four group B arboviruses, *Virology*, 26, 528, 1965.
33. **Spradbrow, P. B. and Clark, L.**, Experimental infection of calves with a group B arbovirus (Kunjin virus), *Aust. Vet. J.*, 42, 65, 1966.
34. **Allan, B. C., Doherty, R. L., and Whitehead, R. H.**, Laboratory infections with arboviruses includ-ing reports of two infections with Kunjin virus, *Med. J. Aust.*, 2, 844, 1966.

35. **Bowen, E. T. W., Simpson, D. I. H., Platt, G. S., Way, H. J., Smith, C. E. G., Ching, C. Y., and Casals, J.,** Arbovirus infections in Sarawak; the isolation of Kunjin virus from mosquitoes of the *Culex pseudo-vishnui* group, *Ann. Trop. Med. Parasitol.,* 64, 263, 1970.

36. **Wallace, H. G., Rudnick, A., and Rajagopal, V.,** Activity of tembusu and Umbre viruses in a Malaysian community: mosquito studies, *Mosq. News,* 37, 35, 1977.

37. **Platt, G. S., Way, H. J., Bowen, E. T. W., Simpson, D. I. H., and Hill, M. N.,** Arbovirus infections in Sarawak, October 1968-February 1970. Tembusu and Sindbus virus isolations from mosquitoes, *Ann. Trop. Med. Parasitol.,* 69, 65, 1975.

38. **Theiler, M. and Downs, W. G.,** *The arthropod-borne viruses of vertebrates,* Yale University Press, New Haven, 1973, 177.

39. **Smithburn, K. C., Kokernot, R. H., Weinbren, M. P., and De Meillon, B.,** Studies on arthropod-borne viruses of Tongaland. IX. Isolation of Wesselsborn virus from a naturally infected human being and from *Aedes (Banksinella) circumluteolus* Theo., *S. Afr. J. Med. Sci.,* 22, 113, 1957.

40. **Simasathien, P. and Olson, L. C.,** Factors influencing the vector potential of *Aedes aegypti* and *Culex quinquefasciatus* for Wesselsbron virus, *J. Med. Entomol.,* 10, 587, 1973.

41. **Simpson, D. I. H.,** Zika virus infection in man, *Trans. R. Soc. Trop. Med. Hyg.,* 58, 335, 1964.

42. **Dick, W. W. A., Kitchen, S. F., and Haddow, A. J.,** Zika virus. I. Isolations and serological specificity, *Trans. R. Soc. Trop. Med. Hyg.,* 46, 509, 1952.

43. **Marchette, N. J., Garcia, R., and Rudnick, A.,** Isolation of Zika virus from *Aedes aegypti* mosquitoes in Malaysia, *Am. J. Trop. Med. Hyg.,* 18, 411, 1966.

44. **Smithburn, K. C.,** Neutralizing antibodies against arthropod-borne viruses in the sera of long-term residents of Malaya and Borneo, *Am. J. Hyg.,* 59, 157, 1954.

45. **Pond, W. L.,** Arthropod-borne virus antibodies in sera from residents of South-East Asia, *Trans. R. Soc. Trop. Med. Hyg.,* 57, 364, 1963.

46. **Hammon, W. McD., Schrack, W. D., Jr., and Sather, G. E.,** Serological survey for arthropod-borne virus infections in the Philippines, *Am. J. Trop. Med. Hyg.,* 7, 323, 1958.

47. **Webb, H. E., Wetherley-Mein, G., Smith, C. E. G., and McMahon, D.,** Leukemia and neoplastic processes treated with Langat and KFD viruses; a clinical and laboratory study of 28 patients, *Br. Med. J.,* 1, 258, 1966.

48. **Il'enko, V. I., Smorodintsev, A. A., Prozorova, I. N., and Platonov, V. G.,** Experience in the study of a live vaccine made from TP-21 strain of Malayan Langat virus, *Bull. WHO,* 39, 425, 1968.

49. **Price, W. H., Thine, I. S., Teasdall, R. D., and O'Leary, W.,** Vaccination of human volunteers against Russian spring-summer (RSS) virus complex with attenuated Langat E5 virus, *Bull. WHO,* 42, 89, 1970.

50. **Smith, C. E. G.,** Langat virus and vaccination against infections by the tick-borne complex of group B arboviruses, *Jpn. J. Med. Sci. Biol.,* 20 (Suppl.), 130, 1966.

51. **Smith, C. E. G.,** A virus resembling RSSE virus from an ixodid tick in Malaya, *Nature (London),* 178, 581, 1956.

52. **Bancroft, W. H.,** Scott, R. M., Snitbalm, R., Weaver, R. E., Jr., and Gould, D. S., Isolation of Langat virus from *Haemaphysalis papuana* Thorell in Thailand, *Am. J. Trop. Med. Hyg.,* 25, 500, 1976.

53. **Pavri, K. M. and Casals, J.,** Kaisodi virus, a new agent isolated from *Haemaphysalis spinigera* in Mysore State, South India. II. Characterization and identification, *Am. J. Trop. Med. Hyg.,* 15, 961, 1966.

54. **Tan, K. S. K., Smith, C. E. G., McMahon, D. A., and Bowen, E. T. W.,** Lanjan virus, a new agent isolated from *Dermacentor auratus* in Malaya, *Nature (London),* 214, 1154, 1967.

55. **Rudnick, A., Marchette, N. J., and Garcia, R.,** Seletar, A new Wad Medani-related arbovirus from Malaysia and Singapore, *First Southeast Asian Reg. Sem. Trop. Med., Bangkok* (Abstr.), 40, 1967.

56. **Top, F. H., Jr., Kraivapan, C., Grossman, R. A., Rozmiarek, H., Edelman, R., and Gould, D. J.,** Ingwavuma virus in Thailand. Infection of domestic pigs, *Am. J. Trop. Med. Hyg.,* 23, 251, 1974.

57. **Pavri, K., Sheikh, B. H., Singh, K. R. P., Rajogopalan, P. K., and Casals, J.,** Balagodu virus, a new arbovirus isolated from *Ardeola grayii* (Sykes) in Mysore State, South India, *Ind. J. Med. Res.,* 57, 785, 1969.

58. **L'vov, D. K., Karas, F. R., Timofeev, E. M., Tsyrkin, Yu M., Vargina, S. G., Veselovskaya, O. V., Opisova, N. Z., Grebenyuk, Yu I., and Gromashevski, V. C.,** Issyk-Kul virus, a new arbovirus isolated from bats and *Argas (Casios) vespertilionis* (Latr, 1802) in the Kirghiz S.S.R. Brief Report, *Arch. Gesamte Virusforsch.,* 42, 207, 1973.

59. **Miura, T.,** Virus isolations from Japanese bats, *Med. Biol. Tokyo,* 91, 291, 1975.

60. **Miura, T.,** Serological characteristics of Japan bat viruses and the relation of the viruses to man, *Med. Biol., Tokyo,* 92, 135, 1976.

61. **Hoogstraal, H.,** Viruses and ticks, in *Viruses and Invertebrates,* Gibbs, A., Ed., North-Holland Pub. Co., Amsterdam, 1973, 349.

62. **Mace, D. L., Ott, R. I., and Cortez, F. S.,** Evidence of the presence of the equine encephalomyelitis virus in Philippine animals, U.S. Army, *Dept. Army Med. Bull.,* 9, 504, 1949.

ARBOVIRAL ZOONOSES IN AUSTRALASIA

MURRAY VALLEY ENCEPHALITIS

R.L. Doherty

NAME AND SYNONYMS

The disease has been known as the "mysterious disease"[12] (1917), "Australian X disease"[16] (1918 to 1951), and "Murray Valley encephalitis"[28] (MVE) (1951 to the present). The name "Australian encephalitis" has been proposed recently.[40]

HISTORY

Epidemics of encephalitis in southern Australia in 1917, 1918, 1922, 1925, 1951, 1956, 1971, and 1974 are generally accepted to have been due to MVE,[5,22,24] although specific laboratory diagnostic tests did not become available until 1951. During the earliest recorded epidemics in 1917 and 1918, an infectious agent was recovered in the laboratory by inoculation of monkeys,[13,16] but the strains could not be maintained. From 1925 to 1950 the etiology remained unclear, although suggestions were made that the disease was a southern extension of Japanese encephalitis[41] or a variant of louping ill.[42] The MVE virus was isolated in 1951[28] and shown to be related but recognizably distinct from Japanese encephalitis (JBE) virus.[43] Serological tests were developed which allowed confirmation of clinical diagnoses and demonstrated widespread subclinical infections in human beings and animals, especially water birds.[2] No evidence was found of viral activity in southern Australia outside epidemic years,[3] and extensive investigations were made for possible mechanisms of endemic survival.[8,19,39] *Culex annulirostris* mosquitoes were proposed on epidemiological grounds in 1951[44] to be vectors of MVE virus; this was proven by laboratory isolation of the virus in 1960.[20] The presence of the disease in New Guinea was discovered in 1956.[29]

ETIOLOGY

Classification

MVE virus is classified in the genus *Flavivirus* (group B arbovirus) of the family Togaviridae. It is antigenically closely related to JBE, St. Louis encephalitis, West Nile, and several other flaviviruses[43] which form a definable antigenic complex within the group.[18] Strains from human patients and mosquitoes isolated from 1951 to 1974 are all antigenically very similar.[10,35]

Characteristics

MVE virus has a single-stranded RNA genome[1] and a lipid-containing envelope[7] characteristic of flaviviruses. The genome codes for three virion and seven non-virion proteins, together representing 400×10^3 daltons of polypeptide synthesis, close to the maximum coding content of its RNA.[47] Sucrose-acetone extracts of virus-infected mouse brain yield high titering hemagglutinin which provides a sensitive and broadly reactive test for antibodies to many flaviviruses. The virus multiplies in mouse brain, embryonated chicken eggs, and various cell cultures which can be used for virus isolation and/or neutralization tests.[31]

DEFINITION

Murray Valley encephalitis is an acute and commonly severe disease intermittently epidemic in the Murray-Darling basin and occasionally other areas of Australia, and occurring in sporadic cases in northern Australia or New Guinea. It is caused by a specific flavivirus, currently believed to survive in cycles involving various species of water birds and the mosquito *Cx. annulirostris*.

ANIMAL INFECTION

Serological surveys suggest that subclinical infection of birds and mammals is widespread during epidemics in southern Australia[2,4,33] and in the endemic areas of northern Australia and New Guinea.[21,26,32,48] Species infected include horses,[21] cattle,[21] swine,[32] buffaloes,[26] dingoes,[26] foxes,[2] opossums,[2] dogs,[2] domestic fowls,[4,21] and many species of wild birds.[4,48] No evidence has been presented that the animal infections are associated with disease, with the single exception of recent and still equivocal associations with encephalitis in horses.[33]

HUMAN INFECTION

Clinical

The human disease is characterized by sudden onset of headache, anorexia, vomiting, drowsiness, malaise, irritability, mental confusion, and meningism. The clinical disease progresses with continued fever, cerebrospinal fluid pleocytosis, and polymorphonuclear leucocytosis, and in some cases hyperactive reflexes, rigidity of limbs with purposeless movements, convulsions, coma, and death.[11,14,46] Paresis of either the upper or lower motor neuron type may be associated with difficulty in swallowing or breathing. Death or recovery usually occur within 2 weeks, but some patients show serious neurological or psychiatric sequelae. Case fatality rates were as high as 60% in early epidemics but have fallen to 20% in the most recent epidemic, probably due to modern intensive care and assisted respiration. This decline in fatality rate has been accompanied by an increase in the rate of survivors with serious neurological defects. Subclinical infections are perhaps 500 times more common than overt encephalitis in human beings; when clinical disease occurs it is in the form of encephalitis and no evidence has been found that MVE virus causes minor febrile illness or aseptic meningitis.[2,11,24]

Pathology

Lesions are restricted to tissues of the central nervous system (CNS) and include lymphocytic infiltration of the meninges, perivascular cuffing especially in the cortex, and neuronal degeneration and neuronophagia in the cerebrum and spinal cord, especially involving Purkinje and anterior horn cells.[13,16,42,45] These changes do not distinguish MVE from other arboviral encephalitides.

Diagnosis

Clinical (rapid onset of severe central nervous system disease) and epidemiological (geographical, seasonal, and age distribution) features may be strongly suggestive of the disease, but the differential diagnosis from other forms of encephalitis or encephalopathy may be difficult in any individual case. Specific diagnosis depends on virus isolation or serological confirmation of MVE infection. The virus has been isolated repeatedly from brain or spinal cord taken at necropsy, but not from cerebrospinal fluid or blood. The most sensitive laboratory method for virus isolation has been inoculation of the chorioallantoic membranes of embryonated eggs with CNS tissues.[28,35] Most patients develop both hemagglutination-inhibition (HI) and complement-fixing (CF) antibodies and both tests should be used in parallel for serological diagnosis.[24] Hi tests are broadly crossreactive and neutralization (N) tests may be needed to distinguish MVE from infection with related viruses such as Kunjin. The early appearance of HI antibody in the IgM serum fraction is of diagnostic value.[49]

EPIDEMIOLOGY

Occurrence

MVE epidemics have been recorded on eight occasions between 1917 and 1974 in southern Australia, mostly limited to the Murray-Darling River basin.[5] Epidemics outside this area have been recorded in north Queensland (1917, 1918, 1925), southeast Queensland (1922), central Australia, and east central and western Queensland (1974).[5,24] Sporadic cases and small epidemics have occurred in northwestern Australia[17,46a] and New Guinea[27,29] and serological surveys have suggested that MVE is more widespread in northern Australia[21,26] and New Guinea[6] than clinical recognition has indicated.

Reservoir

The virus is believed to survive in cycles involving water birds and mosquitoes in northern Australia and New Guinea. It has been proposed that the virus disappears from southern Australia following epidemic periods and is reintroduced from the north when bird-mosquito cycles build up in years of high rainfall in western Queensland and the Northern Territory.[5,30] There is only partial evidence for this mechanism; the virus has only been isolated once from a bird[37] and virus activity has been difficult to detect in northern Australia except during the rainy season of January-April.[23] Recently evidence that the virus may persist in an alternate host in southern Australia has been obtained in feral swine in southeast Australia outside known epidemic periods.[32]

Transmission

The mosquito *Cx. annulirostris* has been incriminated as the major vector of MVE by field isolations of virus in epidemic[25,37] and enzootic[20,36,50] areas, by its high populations during epidemics,[44] and by its high sensitivity to experimental infection.[34] Other mosquitoes such as *Aedes normanensis* may play a secondary role in virus transmission.[20]

Environment

Summer and autumn epidemics of MVE in southern Australia have been associated with abnormally high rainfall during the preceding spring in northern Australia rather than in the areas of the epidemics. Several rainfall patterns have been proposed as means of predicting high virus cycles in nature and risk of ensuing epidemics.[3,38]

Human Host

Early epidemics showed highest incidence in children,[5] but more recently a second peak in old age has been recognized.[24] A high subclinical infection rate has been repeatedly documented.

CONTROL

Prevention and Treatment

No attempts have been made to develop vaccines for MVE. Prevention depends on interruption of mosquito-man transmission through health education and control of *Cx. annulirostris* vector mosquitoes.

No specific therapy is available for MVE. Comatose patients require controlled respiration and careful management of fluid balance, nutrition, and bladder function. Prolonged periods of rehabilitation may be required.

Regulatory and Epidemic Measures and Eradication

The control of MVE, usually an epidemic disease which occurs on widely separated occasions over large areas, presents many problems. The vector mosquito *Cx. annulirostris* breeds widely each summer in eastern Australia in shallow pools, in both urban and rural areas, making area eradication manifestly impossible. A basic program of mosquito control by application of larvicides such as Abate ® to recognized breeding areas is carried out near major towns and tourist centers in the Murray-Darling Basin each year.[9] It is proposed to supplement this by more extensive use of larvicides and by use of adulticides such as Malathion® in and near centers of population in years when climatic patterns, serological evidence of MVE virus activity or occurrence of cases indicate a period of risk.

Health Education

Appropriate personal protective measures can greatly reduce exposure to MVE. The vector mosquito, *Cx. annulirostris* is most active outdoors before dawn and after dusk. Sensible use of screens, mosquito nets, protective clothing, and household insecticides, combined with avoidance of outdoor activities during high risk periods, can afford a considerable degree of protection during periods of known epidemic activity.

PUBLIC HEALTH ASPECTS

Economic and Social Impact

The most recent epidemic of MVE caused much community concern in the Murray Valley region, an economic impact estimated at several million dollars. In particular, the tourist trade and recruitment of labor for agricultural work in the area were seriously disrupted.

Reporting

The disease is notifiable to the Health departments of all mainland Australian states, as 'Murray Valley encephalitis" in Victoria or as "virus encephalitis" or "acute infective encephalitis" in other states.

Surveillance

Several Australian states have in recent years supplemented the reporting of human cases by serological surveillance of sentinel chickens.[15,25] This program was of very limited predictive value in the 1974 epidemic and detected no evidence of MVE virus activity in the Murray-Darling basin in 1975 and 1976.

REFERENCES

1. **Ada, G. L., Anderson, S. G., and Abbot, A.,** Purification of Murray Valley encephalitis virus, *J. Gen. Microbiol.,* 24, 177, 1961.
2. **Anderson, S. G., Donnelley, M., Stevenson, W. J., Caldwell, N. J., and Eagle, M.,** Murray Valley encephalitis: surveys of human and animal sera, *Med. J. Aust.,* 1, 110, 1952.

3. **Anderson, S. G. and Eagle, M.,** Murray Valley encephalitis: the contrasting epidemiological picture in 1951 and 1952, *Med. J. Aust.,* 1, 478, 1953.

4. **Anderson, S. G.,** Murray Valley encephalitis: a survey of avian sera, 1951-1952, *Med. J. Aust.,* 1, 573, 1953.

5. **Anderson, S. G.,** Murray Valley encephalitis and Australian X disease, *J. Hyg.,* 52, 447, 1954.

6. **Anderson, S. G., Price, A. V. G., Nanadai-Koia, and Slater, K.,** Murray Valley encephalitis in Papua and New Guinea. II. Serological survey, 1956-1957, *Med. J. Aust.,* 2, 410, 1960.

7. **Anderson, S. G. and Ada, G. L.,** The action of phospholipase A and lipid solvents on Murray Valley encephalitis virus, *J. Gen. Microbiol.,* 25, 451, 1961.

8. **Anderson, S. G., Price, A. V. G., and Williams, M. C.,** Antibody to Murray Valley encephalitis and louping-ill viruses in Australia and Papua-New Guinea, *Med. J. Aust.,* 1, 444, 1961.

9. **Anonymous.** Commonwealth, States pool resources to control encephalitis, *Health, Canberra,* 26, 18, 1976.

10. **Barrett, E. J.,** Intratypic antigenic variation among strains of the group B arboviruses Murray Valley encephalitis and Kunjin, *Am. J. Epidemiol.,* 93, 212, 1971.

11. **Bennett, N. McK.,** Murray Valley encephalitis, 1974: clinical features, *Med. J. Aust.,* 2, 446, 1976.

12. **Breinl, A.,** The mysterious disease, *Med. J. Aust.,* 1, 454, 1917.

13. **Breinl, A.,** Clinical pathological and experimental observations on the 'mysterious disease', a clinically aberrant form of acute poliomyelitis, *Med. J. Aust.,* 1, 209 and 229, 1918.

14. **Burnell, G. H.,** The Broken Hill epidemic, *Med. J. Aust.,* 2, 157, 1917.

15. **Campbell, J. and Hore, D. E.,** Isolation of Murray Valley encephalitis virus from sentinel chickens, *Aust. Vet. J.,* 51, 1, 1975.

16. **Cleland, J. B., Campbell, A. W., and Bradley, B.,** *Rep. Dir. Gen. Public Health, N.S.W.,* 8, 150, 1918.

17. **Cook, I., Allan, B. C., Horsfall, W. R., and Flanagan, J. E.,** A fatal case of Murray Valley encephalitis, *Med. J. Aust.,* 1, 1110, 1970.

18. **de Madrid, A. T. and Porterfield, J. S.,** The flaviviruses (group B arboviruses): a cross-neutralization study, *J. Gen. Virol.,* 23, 91, 1974.

19. **Doherty, R. L., Carley, J. G., and Lee, P. E.,** Studies of arthropod-borne virus infections in Queensland. I. A serological survey of Aboriginal missions bordering the Gulf of Carpentaria, *Aust. J. Exp. Biol. Med. Sci.,* 37, 365, 1959.

20. **Doherty, R. L., Carley, J. G., Mackerras, M. J., Trevethan, P., and Marks, E. N.,** Studies of arthropod-borne viruses in Queensland. III. Isolation and characterization of virus strains from wild-caught mosquitoes in north Queensland, *Aust. J. Exp. Biol. Med. Sci.,* 41, 17, 1963.

21. **Doherty, R. L., Carley, J. G., and Gorman, B. M.,** Studies of arthropod-borne virus infections in Queensland. IV. Further serological investigations of antibodies to group B arboviruses in man and animals, *Aust. J. Exp. Biol. Med. Sci.,* 42, 149, 1964.

22. **Doherty, R. L., Carley, J. G., Cremer, M. R., Rendle-Short, J., Hopkins, J., Caro, A. S., and Stephens, W. B.,** Murray Valley encephalitis in eastern Australia, 1971. *Med. J. Aust.,* 2, 1170, 1972.

23. **Doherty, R. L.,** Arthropod-borne viruses in Australia and their relation to infection and disease, *Progr. Med. Virol.,* 17, 136, 1974.

24. **Doherty, R. L., Carley, J. G., Filippich, C., White, J., and Gust, I. D.,** Murray Valley encephalitis in Australia, 1974: antibody response in cases and community, *Aust. N.Z. J. Med.,* 6, 446, 1976.

25. **Doherty, R. L., Carley, J. G., Kay, B. H., Filippich, C., and Marks, E. N.,** Murray Valley encephalitis virus infection in mosquitoes and domestic fowls in Queensland, 1974, *Aust. J. Exp. Biol. Med. Sci.,* 54, 237, 1976.

26. **Doherty, R. L., Filippich, C., Carley, J. G., and Hancock, J. Y.,** Antibody to togaviruses in the Northern Territory and adjoining areas of Australia, *Aust. J. Exp. Biol. Med. Sci.,* 55, 131, 1977.

27 **Essed, W. C. A. H. and van Tongeren, H. A. E.,** Arthropod-borne virus infections in Western New Guinea. I. Report of a case of Murray Valley encephalitis in a Papuan woman, *Trop. Geogr. Med.,* 17, 52, 1965.

28. **French, E. L.,** Murray Valley encephalitis: isolation and characterization of the aetiological agent, *Med. J. Aust.,* 1, 100, 1952.

29. **French, E. L., Anderson, S. G., Price, A. V. G., and Rhodes, F. A.,** Murray Valley encephalitis in New Guinea. I. Isolation of Murray Valley encephalitis virus from the brain of a fatal case of encephalitis occurring in a Papuan native, *Am. J. Trop. Med. Hyg.,* 6, 827, 1957.

30. **French, E. L.,** A review of arthropod-borne virus infections affecting man and animals in Australia, *Aust. J. Exp. Biol. Med. Sci.,* 51, 131, 1973.

31. **French, E. L.,** Murray Valley encephalitis, in *International Catalogue of Arboviruses,* 2nd ed., Pub. No. (CDC) 75-8301, Berge, T. O., Ed., Public Health Service, U.S. Department of Health, Education and Welfare, Atlanta, 1975.

32. **Gard, G. P., Giles, J. R., Dwyer-Gray, R. J., and Woodroofe, G. M.,** Serological evidence of inter-epidemic infection of feral pigs in New South Wales with Murray Valley encephalitis virus, *Aust. J. Exp. Biol. Med. Sci.,* 54, 297, 1976.

33. **Gard, G. P., Marshall, I. D., Walker, K. H., Acland, H. M., and De Saram, W.,** Association of Australian arboviruses with nervous disease in horses, *Aust. Vet. J.,* 53, 61, 1977.

34. **Kay, B. H., Carley, J. G., and Filippich, C.,** The multiplication of Australian and New Guinean arboviruses in *Culex annulirostris* Skuse and *Aedes vigilax* (Skuse) (Diptera: Culicidae), *J. Med. Entomol.,* 12, 279, 1975.

35. **Lehman, N. I., Gust, I. D., and Doherty, R.,** Isolation of Murray Valley encephalitis virus from the brains of three patients with encephalitis, *Med. J. Aust.,* 2, 450, 1976.

36. **Liehne, C. G., Leivers, S., Stanley, N. F., Alpers, M. P., Paul, S., Liehne, P. F. S., and Chan, K. H.,** Ord River arboviruses — isolations from mosquitoes, *Aust. J. Exp. Biol. Med. Sci.,* 54, 499, 1976.

37. **Marshall, I. D. and Woodroofe, G. M.** Epidemiology of arboviruses, *Rep. John Curtin Sch. Med. Res., Aust. Nat. Univ.,* 1975, 92.

38. **Miles, J. A. R. and Howes, D. W.,** Observations on virus encephalitis in South Australia, *Med. J. Aust.,* 1, 7, 1953.

39. **Miles, J. A. R. and Dane, D. M. S.,** Further observations relating to Murray Valley encephalitis in the Northern Territory of Australia, *Med. J. Aust.,* 1, 389, 1956.

40. **National Health and Medical Research Council, Canberra,** Report of the Seventy-eighth Session, 1974, 8.

41. **Olitsky, P. K. and Casals, J.,** Viral encephalitides, in *Viral and Rickettsial Infections of Man,* Rivers, T. M., Ed., J. B. Lippincott, Philadelphia, 1948, 233.

42. **Perdrau, J. R.,** The Australian epidemics of encephalomyelitis (X-disease), *J. Pathol. Bacteriol.,* 42, 59, 1936.

43. **Pond, W. L., Russ, S. B., Rogers, N. G., and Smadel, J. E.,** Murray Valley encephalitis virus: its serological relationship to the Japanese-West Nile-St. Louis encephalitis group of viruses, *J. Immunol.,* 75, 78, 1955.

44. **Reeves, W. C., French, E. L., Marks, E. N., and Kent, N. E.,** Murray Valley encephalitis: a survey of suspected mosquito vectors, *Am. J. Trop. Med. Hyg.,* 3, 147, 1954.

45. **Robertson, E. G.,** Murray Valley encephalitis: pathological aspects, *Med. J. Aust.,* 1, 107, 1952.

46. **Robertson, E. G. and McLorinan, H.,** Murray Valley encephalitis: clinical aspects, *Med. J. Aust.,* 1, 103, 1952.

46a. **Stanley, N. F.,** Problems related to the epidemiology of Murray Valley encephalitis and Kunjun viruses created by development in north-west Australia, in *Arbovirus Research in Australia, Proc. 2nd Symp. 17—19 July, 1979,* St George, T. D. and French, E. L., Eds., Commonwealth Scientific and Industrial Research Organisation and Queensland Institute of Medical Research, Brisbane, 1979, 41.

47. **Westaway, E. G.,** The proteins of Muray Valley encephalitis virus, *J. Gen. Virol.,* 27, 293, 1975.

48. **Whitehead, R. H., Doherty, R. L., Domrow, R., Standfast, H. A., and Wetters, E. J.,** Studies of the epidemiology of arthropod-borne virus infections at Mitchell River Mission, Cape York Peninsula, north Queensland. III. Virus studies of wild birds, 1964-1967, *Trans. R. Soc. Trop. Med. Hyg.,* 62, 439, 1968.

49. **Wiemers, M. A. and Stallman, N. D.,** Immunoglobulin M in Murray Valley encephalitis, *Pathology,* 7, 187, 1975.

50. **Woodroofe, G. M. and Marshall, I. D.,** Arboviruses from the Sepik District of New Guinea, *Rep. John Curtin Sch. Med. Res., Aust. Nat. Univ.,* 1971, 90.

EPIDEMIC POLYARTHRITIS

R. L. Doherty

NAME AND SYNONYMS

The name epidemic polyarthritis[13] has been accepted as preferable to several other names which continue to have local use in Australia, including epidemic exanthem,[1] Murray Valley rash,[32] and Robinvale disease. Ross River fever, named for the etiological Ross River virus has some currency in medical circles but has not reached the literature.

HISTORY

A syndrome of polyarthralgia and rash was first recognized in small epidemics in residents of N.S.W., Australia in 1927.[14,23] It was seen again in Army groups in northern Australia during World War II.[13,19,28] Large epidemics occurred in residents of the Murray Valley of Victoria[1] and South Australia,[15,32] and in southwest Western Australia[29] in 1956. Serological evidence for an alphavirus (group A arbovirus) as the etiological agent was obtained during these epidemics.[27] The Ross River virus was isolated in 1963[5] and was quickly associated as the alphavirus causing epidemic polyarthritis.[6] Serological studies have shown that the disease occurs in sporadic cases and small outbreaks in eastern Australia each summer and autumn.[9] As medical practitioners become more aware of this disease they are recognizing it as a frequent and important cause of illness.

ETIOLOGY

A single strain of Ross River virus has been isolated from the blood of a febrile child in Australia; it has never been recovered from an epidemic polyarthritis patient there, although isolations have been reported from Fiji.[1a] The evidence that it causes epidemic polyarthritis comes mainly from serological findings, which, over 17 years have strongly supported a causal relationship.

CLASSIFICATION AND CHARACTERISTICS

Ross River virus is an alphavirus antigenically related to the Malaysian Getah and Bebaru viruses[12] of the Semliki Forest virus subgroup. Prior to the discovery of Ross River virus,[4] Getah and Bebaru viruses were used in diagnostic serological tests for epidemic polyarthritis. The prototype strain has not been fully characterized biochemically, but it has three virion polypeptides similar in molecular weight to those of other alphaviruses.[30] The virus replicates in infant mice, affecting especially muscle and brown fat,[21,22] and in various cell cultures.[18] Mouse blood or carcasses may be used to prepare high titering antigens for hemagglutination-inhibition (HI) or complement-fixation (CF) tests.[12] There is some evidence of biological and antigenic diversity among strains of Ross River virus, as recently isolated strains from a focus of infection in coastal New South Wales[2] have shown lower virulence for mice and differences in antigenic composition detectable by kinetic HI tests as compared to the prototype strain.[33]

DEFINITION

Epidemic polyarthritis is a benign human disease characterized by polyarthralgia and rash, caused by a specific alphavirus and occurring in sporadic cases or epidemics in Australia each summer and autumn. The natural history of its causative agent is not fully understood but is believed to depend on summer and autumn cycles of infection between mammals and mosquitoes, and on an unknown mechanism of survival over winter.

ANIMAL INFECTION

Serological surveys have indicated widespread infection by Ross River virus among wild and domestic mammals in Australia.[7,10,25] Specific antibodies have been demonstrated in cattle, sheep, horses, pigs, kangaroos, wallabies, and other marsupials, dogs, and rodents. Among these, the virus has been isolated from wallabies.[10] Antibodies are rarely detected in birds and titers are unconvincingly low, although several virus strains have been isolated from wild birds.[31] It seems unlikely that birds play any important part in the natural history of Ross River virus infections. No evidence has been presented that the virus causes disease in any hosts except human beings, with the exception of a serological association which has been reported with encephalitis and polyarthritis in horses; this requires further study.[17]

HUMAN INFECTION

Clinical

Epidemic polyarthritis in human patients usually occurs as a mild illness with low grade fever, sore throat, pain and swelling of joints, especially small joints of the hands and feet, and in some patients a maculopapular, rarely vesicular, rash involving the trunk and limbs.[1,6,9,19] In some epidemics a significant number of patients develop rash without polyarthralgia.[32] Additional clinical features include lymphadenopathy, paresthesia, and tenderness of palms and soles, enanthem and rarely petechiae. Most patients recover completely within 2 weeks; a minority have persistent or relapsing joint swellings for up to a year after onset,[9] but there is no evidence that any patients go on to chronic joint disease. Virus isolation[11] and serological tests[4] suggest that Ross River virus may also cause brief febrile episodes without joint pain or rash.

Pathology

Because of the benign nature of the disease, no histopathological studies have been carried out. Fluid aspirated from affected joints has been shown to contain monocytes and macrophages rather than neutrophils, and it has been suggested that macrophages may play an important part in the pathogenesis of the clinical disease.[3]

Diagnosis

During identified epidemics, clinical diagnoses of individual cases present no problems but sporadic cases may simulate other, perhaps more serious diseases such as rheumatic fever or early rheumatoid arthritis and be misdiagnosed by practitioners not familiar with the disease. Patients showing fevers above 39° C or with arthritis limited to a single large joint have rarely been serologically confirmed as infected by Ross River virus. Standard clinical laboratory tests are of limited help, but increased erythrocyte sedimentation rates have frequently been found in epidemic polyarthritis patients.[4]

Specific diagnosis of human infections depends on serological tests; both HI and CF tests are of value. HI antibodies appear within a few days of onset and may allow early diagnosis; however, many patients have high HI titers in the first serum collected, and significant rises in titers may be confirmed only by CF tests.[9] HI titers often persist in IgM fractions for considerable periods after infection.[24]

EPIDEMIOLOGY

Occurrence

Epidemic polyarthritis is recognized in eastern Australia each year from December to June, especially January to May. Most cases are reported in Queensland,[9] especially in the outer suburbs of Brisbane, the Townsville and Rockhampton areas, and such southwestern towns as Charleville and Dirranbandi.[8] An increasing number of cases is being reported in New South Wales and northern Victoria, and it seems likely that cases occur there each year also. Epidemics have been described in the Murray Valley area of South Australia,[15,26,32] but there is as yet no evidence that the disease is endemic there. Sporadic cases continue to occur in southwest Western Australia.[20]

Antibody surveys indicate widespread infection with Ross River virus in New Guinea,[30a,30b] where clinical cases of epidemic polyarthritis were described during and after World War II.[27] Epidemics of polyarthritis confirmed by serological test and virus isolation occurred in 1979 in Fiji (April to June) and American Samoa (August to October).[1a,1b,1c]

Reservoir, Transmission, and Environment

Serological evidence of Ross River virus infection has been obtained in several mammals,[7] and the virus has been isolated from *Aedes vigilax*,[5,16] *Culex annulirostris*,[10,16] and other mosquitoes. It has been postulated that the virus is transmitted in nature in animal-mosquito cycles, with exposure of human beings by mosquito bites. Animal reservoirs have not been delineated and may differ from place to place. It has been suggested that the New Holland mouse (*Pseudomys novaehollandiae*) may be the major reservoir host on the central coast of New South Wales,[16] but this rodent has a very limited geographical range and could not play any epidemiological role in most of Australia. The persistence of antigenically and biologically distinguishable strains of Ross River virus over several years in this same focus[16,33] has suggested that the virus has survived continually in southern Australia but no mechanism for this survival during non-mosquito transmission seasons has yet been proposed. Epidemics have commonly followed periods of excess rainfall and consequent mosquito plagues.

Human Host

Several clinical, virological, and epidemiological features of the disease have suggested that the immune response to infection rather than virus infection itself may be the basic mechanism of pathogenesis.[9] Ross River virus has not been isolated from patients seen early in their illness. HI antibodies, at least at low levels, may be detected in most patients within a few days of the recognized onset of disease. The incidence of clinical disease is higher in adolescents and young adults than in children, and in women rather than men.

CONTROL

No specific vaccines or chemotherapy are available. Prevention is directed toward mosquito control in and near centers of population during epidemics, and toward health education on simple protective measures against mosquito exposures. So far no active public health measures have been taken against this disease in Australia.

PUBLIC HEALTH ASPECTS

Epidemic polyarthritis has been viewed as a minor disease in Australia. Community concern during epidemics has responded quickly to diagnosis and reassurance, an attitude which is becoming less justifiable with the recognition of increasing numbers of cases over a wide area in recent years. It is now the most common human arboviral disease in Australia and public demand for preventive measures can be anticipated. Epidemic polyarthritis is not a notifiable disease in any Australian state and surveillance is a function of the four public health laboratories which offer diagnostic tests.

ADDENDUM[20a,30b]

During the 15-month period between April 1979 to June 1980 the significance of Ross River Virus as a cause of epidemic disease in man has increased sharply. For the first time, epidemics have occurred outside Australia and, in almost completely non-immune populations, these have been on a much larger scale than any reported from Australia.

The first began in Fiji in late April 1979 and for the first 10 days, cases were only reported in the Nadi area, close to the main international airport. The disease then spread to all the larger islands, but the smaller islands of the Lomaiviti and Lau groups were spared.

Clinically, the disease did not differ from that seen in Australia, and in young children the infection was usually subclinical. In one village in the Nadi area, where nearly all the population were bled late in the epidemic, over 90% had developed antibodies. The ratio of clinical to inapparent infections was between 1:3 to 1:10 — a much higher proportion of clinical cases than is seen in Australia. It has been estimated that there were 30,000 to 40,000 clinical cases in the Fiji epidemic.

Early in the epidemic Dr. Mataika in Suva made two isolations from the blood of typical adult cases seen during the first 24 hr of illness. As Doherty reports, such isolations have never been obtained in Australia.

In August 1979 the infection spread to Samoa and in American Samoa there was an epidemic of an intensity comparable to that in Fiji. In February 1980 a sharp epidemic occurred in Raratonga in the Cook Islands and early in May, spread occurred to Tonga. It is also reported that there is infection on some Melanesian Islands. In Fiji, cases are still occurring 15 months after the onset of the epidemic and it is likely that the disease is now enzootic in domestic animals and possibly also in wild rodents.

REFERENCES

1. **Anderson, S. G. and French, E. L.,** An epidemic exanthem associated with polyarthritis in the Murray Valley, 1956, *Med. J. Aust.,* 2, 113, 1957.
1a. Australia: Department of Health, Environmental Health Branch, Viral Infections — Fiji, *Communicable Dis. Intelligence Bull.,* 79(12), 3, 1979.
1b. Australia: Department of Health, Environmental Health Branch, Ross River viral infections imported from Fiji, *Communicable Dis. Intelligence Bull.,* 79(15),2, 1979.
2. **Clarke, J. A., Marshall, I. D., and Gard, G.,** Annually recurrent epidemic polyarthritis and Ross River virus activity in a coastal area of New South Wales. I. Occurrence of the disease, *Am. J. Trop. Med. Hyg.,* 22, 543, 1973.
3. **Clarris, B. J., Doherty, R. L., Fraser, J. R. E., French, E. L., and Muirden, K. D.,** Epidemic polyarthritis: a cytological, virological and immunochemical study, *Aust. N.Z. J. Med.,* 5, 450, 1975.
4. **Doherty, R. L., Anderson, S. G., Aaron, K., Farnworth, J. K., Knyvett, A. F., and Nimmo, D.,** Clinical manifestations of infection with group A arthropod-borne viruses in Queensland, *Med. J. Aust.,* 1, 276, 1961.

5. **Doherty, R. L., Whitehead, R. H., Gorman, B. M., and O'Gower, A. K.,** The isolation of a third group A arbovirus in Australia, with preliminary observations on its relationship to epidemic polyarthritis, *Aust. J. Sci.,* 26, 183, 1963.

6. **Doherty, R. L., Gorman, B. M., Whitehead, R. H., and Carley, J. G.,** Studies of epidemic polyarthritis: the significance of three group A arboviruses isolated from mosquitoes in Queensland, *Australas. Ann. Med.,* 13, 322, 1964.

7. **Doherty, R. L., Gorman, B. M., Whitehead, R. H., and Carley, J. G.,** Studies of arthropod-borne virus infections in Queensland V. Survey of antibodies to group A arboviruses in man and animals, *Aust. J. Exp. Biol. Med. Sci.,* 44, 365, 1966.

8. **Doherty, R. L., Wetters, E. J., Gorman, B. M., and Whitehead, R. H.,** Arbovirus infection in western Queensland: serological studies, 1963-1969, *Trans. R. Soc. Trop. Med. Hyg.,* 64, 740, 1970.

9. **Doherty, R. L., Barrett, E. J., Gorman, B. M., and Whitehead, R. H.,** Epidemic polyarthritis in eastern Australia, 1959-1970, *Med. J. Aust.,* 1, 5, 1971.

10. **Doherty, R. L., Standfast, H. A., Domrow, R., Wetters, E. J., Whitehead, R. H., and Carley, J. G.,** Studies of the epidemiology of arthropod-borne virus infections at Mitchell River Mission, Cape York Peninsula, north Queensland. IV. Arbovirus infections of mosquitoes and mammals, 1967-1969, *Trans. R. Soc. Trop. Med. Hyg.,* 65, 504, 1971.

11. **Doherty, R. L., Carley, J. G., and Best, J. C.,** Isolation of Ross River virus from man, *Med. J. Aust.,* 1, 1083, 1972.

12. **Doherty, R. L.,** Ross River virus, in *International Catalogue of Arboviruses Including Certain Other Viruses of Vertebrates, 2nd ed., Publ. No. (CDC) 75-8301,* Berge, T. O., Ed., Public Health Service, U.S. Department of Health, Education and Welfare, Atlanta, 1975.

13. **Dowling, P. G.,** Epidemic polyarthritis, *Med. J. Aust.,* 1, 245, 1946.

14. **Edwards, A. M.,** An unusual epidemic, *Med. J. Aust.,* 1, 664, 1928.

15. **Fuller, C. O. and Warner, P.,** Some epidemiological and laboratory observations on an epidemic rash and polyarthritis occurring in the upper Murray region of South Australia, *Med. J. Aust.,* 2, 117, 1957.

16. **Gard, G., Marshall, I. D., and Woodroofe, G. M.,** Annually recurrent epidemic polyarthritis and Ross River virus activity in a coastal area of New South Wales. II. Mosquitoes, viruses and wildlife, *Am. J. Trop. Med. Hyg.,* 22, 551, 1973.

17. **Gard, G. P., Marshall, I. D., Walker, K. H., Acland, H. M., and De Saram, W.,** Association of Australian arboviruses with nervous disease in horses, *Aust. Vet. J.,* 53, 61, 1977.

18. **Gorman, B. M., Leer, J. R., Filippich, C., Goss, P. D., and Doherty, R. L.,** Plaquing and neutralization of arboviruses in the PS-EK line of cells, *Aust. J. Med. Technol.,* 6, 65, 1975.

19. **Halliday, J. H. and Horan, J. P.,** An epidemic of polyarthritis in the Northern Territory, *Med. J. Aust.,* 2, 293, 1943.

20. **Mackay-Scollay, E. M.,** personal communication, 1976.

20a. **Miles, J. A. R.,** Ross River Fever comes to Fiji, *Fiji Med. J.,* 7(8), 216, 1979.

21. **Mims, C. A., Murphy, F. A., Taylor, W. P., and Marshall, I. D.,** Pathogenesis of Ross River virus infection in mice. I. Ependymal infection, cortical thinning, and hydrocephalus, *J. Infect. Dis.,* 127, 121, 1973.

22. **Murphy, F. A., Taylor, W. P., Mims, C. A., and Marshall, I. D.,** Pathogenesis of Ross River virus infection in mice. II. Muscle, heart and brown fat lesions, *J. Infect. Dis.,* 127, 129, 1973.

23. **Nimmo, J. R.,** An unusual epidemic, *Med. J. Aust.,* 1, 549, 1928.

24. Health and Medical Services of the State of Queensland, Annual Report, 1975—1976, 100.

25. **Sanderson, C. J.,** A serologic survey of Queensland cattle for evidence of arbovirus infection, *Am. J. Trop. Med. Hyg.,* 18, 433, 1969.

26. **Seglenieks, Z. and Moore, B. W.,** Epidemic polyarthritis in South Australia: report of an outbreak in 1971, *Med. J. Aust.,* 2, 552, 1974.

27. **Shope, R. E. and Anderson, S. G.,** The virus aetiology of epidemic exanthem and polyarthritis, *Med. J. Aust.,* 1, 156, 1960.

28. **Sibree, E. W.,** Acute polyarthritis in Queensland, *Med. J. Aust.,* 2, 565, 1944.

29. **Snow, D. J. R.,** in Rep. Commissioner Public Health, West. Aust., for 1956, 1958, 63.

30. **Symons, M. H.,** Biochemistry of Ross River virus, *Rep. Qd. Inst. Med. Res.,* 31, 26, 1976.

30a. **Tesh, R. B., Gajdusek, D. C., Garruto, R. M., Cross, J. H., and Rose, L.,** The distribution and prevalence of Group A Arbovirus neutralizing antibodies among human populations in southeast Asia and the Pacific Islands, *Am. J. Trop. Med. Hyg.,* 24, 664, 1975.

30b. **Thomson, K. B., Austin, F. J., Maguire, T., and Miles, J. A. R.,** Epidemic polyarthritis in Fiji and New Zealand, *N. Z. Med. J.,* 90, 30, 1979.

30c. **Van Tongeren, H. A. E. and van Kammen, A.,** Arthropod-borne virus infections in western New Guinea (Irian Jaya), a serological retrospection, *Trop. Geog. Med.,* 30, 428, 1978.

31. **Whitehead, R. H., Doherty, R. L., Domrow, R., Standfast, H. A., and Wetters, E. J.,** Studies of the epidemiology of arthropod-borne virus infections at Mitchell River Mission, Cape York Peninsula, north Queensland. III. Virus studies of wild birds, 1964-1967, *Trans. R. Soc. Trop. Med. Hyg.,* 62, 439, 1968.
32. **Wilson, J. G.,** The Murray Valley rash, *Med. J. Aust.,* 2, 120. 1957.
33. **Woodroofe, G., Marshall, I. D., and Taylor, W. P.,** Antigenically distinct strains of Ross River virus from north Queensland and coastal New South Wales, *Aust. J. Exp. Biol. Med. Sci.,* 55, 79, 1977.

OTHER ARBOVIRAL INFECTIONS

R. L. Doherty

Over 40 arboviruses have been isolated in Australia and New Guinea,[18] and at least 8 produce specific antibodies in man.[14] Only two, however, Sindbis and Kunjin, have been incriminated as agents of disease additional to MVE and Ross River virus, discussed above. Dengue fever was epidemic on many occasions in the 19th and early 20th centuries,[7] most recently in 1953 to 1955,[5] and antibodies to dengue viruses are prevalent in persons of older age groups in Queensland.[10] There is no evidence of dengue transmission in Australia in recent years and the disease will not be discussed further in this section. Two arbovirus diseases of cattle important in Australia, bovine ephemeral fever[8] and Akabane disease,[11] are not known to infect people.

SINDBIS FEVER

Two patients with fever and rash, a child at Mildura in 1967[1] and a young woman at Brisbane in 1970,[9] showed rising antibody titers to Sindbis virus and not to several other possible agents. Surveys showed a low prevalence of antibodies to Sindbis virus in residents of this Australian community,[2] and the virus was seen as an uncommon cause of human disease. It has been isolated from the mosquito *Culex annulirostris* from a wide area of northern Australia[16,19] and New Guinea,[7] and rarely from other mosquitoes.[16,18] Surveys indicate frequent infection of wild and domestic birds, and less commonly of mammals, especially dogs and cattle.[2,16]

Australian strains of Sindbis virus have been shown to have minor antigenic differences from Asian and African strains.[3] The related virus Whataroa is present in New Zealand.[6]

KUNJIN VIRUS INFECTION

Kunjin virus, a flavivirus of the same antigenic subgroup as Murray Valley encephalitis virus,[15] but most closely related to West Nile virus,[4] has been isolated from the mosquito *Culex annulirostris* at several centers in northern and eastern Australia, and on single occasions from *Aedes tremulus* and *Cx. fatigans*.[14,16,18,19] Antibodies to it have been found in wild and domestic birds, cattle, and people.[16] Evidence that Kunjin virus causes mild febrile human illness comes from laboratory infections,[17] from one patient with rising antibody titers in Murray Valley of Victoria in 1974,[13] and from several cases in northwestern Australia.[17a]

Both Sindbis and Kunjin viruses appear to survive in nature in bird-*Cx. annulirostris* cycles similar to those described for Murray Valley encephalitis virus. Prevention, if ever indicated, could be based on mosquito control and health education as described for MVE.

REFERENCES

1. **Allan, B. C., Doherty, R. L., and Whitehead, R. H.,** Laboratory infections with arboviruses including reports of two infections with Kunjin virus, *Med. J. Aust.,* 2, 844, 1966.
2. **Casals, J.,** Antigenic variants in arthropod-borne viruses, *Abst. Proc. 10th Pacif. Sci. Congr.,* 1961, 458.
3. **Della-Porta, A. J., Murray, M. D., and Cybinski, D. H.,** Congenital bovine epizootic arthrogryposis and hydranencephaly in Australia. Distribution of antibodies to Akabane virus in Australian cattle after the 1974 epizootic, *Aust. Vet. J.,* 52, 496, 1976.
4. **Doherty, R. L. and Carley, J. G.,** Studies of arthropod-borne virus infections in Queensland. II. Serological investigations of antibodies to dengue and Murray Valley encephalitis in eastern Queensland, *Aust. J. Exp. Biol. Med. Sci.,* 38, 427, 1960.
5. **Doherty, R. L., Gorman, B. M., Whitehead, R. H., and Carley, J. G.,** Studies of arthropod-borne virus infections in Queensland. V. Survey of antibodies to group A arboviruses in man and other animals, *Aust. J. Exp. Biol. Med. Sci.,* 44, 365, 1966.
6. **Doherty, R. L., Bodey, A. S., and Carew, J. S.,** Sindbis virus infection in Australia, *Med. J. Aust.,* 2, 1016, 1969.
7. **Doherty, R. L.,** Arboviruses of Australia, *Aust. Vet. J.,* 48, 172, 1972.
8. **Doherty, R. L.,** Arthropod-borne viruses in Australia, 1973-1976, *Aust. J. Exp. Biol. Med. Sci.,* 55, 103, 1977.
9. **Doherty, R. L.,** Surveys of haemagglutination-inhibiting antibody to arboviruses in Aborigines and other population groups in northern Australia, *Trans. R. Soc. Trop. Med. Hyg.,* 67, 197, 1973.
10. **Doherty, R. L.,** Arthropod-borne viruses in Australia and their relation t nfection and disease, *Progr. Med. Virol.,* 17, 136, 1974.
11. **Doherty, R. L.,** Kunjin virus, in *International Catalogue of Arboviruses Including Certain Other Viruses of Vertebrates,* 2nd ed., Pub. No. (CDC) 75-8301, Berge, T.O., Ed., Public Health Service, Department of Health, Education and Welfare, 1975.
12. **Doherty, R. L., Carley, J. G., Filippich, C., White, J., and Gust, I. D.,** Murray Valley encephalitis in Australia, 1974: antibody response in cases and community, *Aust. N.Z. J. Med.,* 6, 446, 1976.
13. **Liehne, C. G., Leivers, S., Stanley, N. F., Alpers, M. P., Paul, S., Liehne, P. F. S., and Chan, K. H.,** Ord River arboviruses — isolations from mosquitoes, *Aust. J. Exp. Biol. Med. Sci.,* 54, 499, 1976.
14. **Lumley, G. F. and Taylor, F. H.,** Dengue, *Serv. Pub., Sch. Public Health Trop. Med.,* No. 3, University of Sydney, 1943.
15. **Mackerras, I. M. and Mackerras, M. J.,** Experimental studies of ephemeral fever in Australia, Bull. Commonw. Sci. Ind. R. Organ. No. 136, Melbourne, 1940.
16. **Miles, J. A. R.,** The ecology of Whataroa virus, an alphavirus in south Westland, New Zealand, *J. Hyg. Camb.* 71, 701, 1973.
17. **Rowan, L. C.,** An epidemic of dengue-like fever, North Queensland, 1954: clinical features with a review of the literature, *Med. J. Aust.,* 1, 651, 1956.
17a. **Stanley, N. F.,** Problems related to the epidemiology of Murray Valley encephalitis and Kunjin viruses created by development in north-west Australia, in *Arbovirus Research in Australia, Proc. 2nd Symp., 17—19 July, 1979,* St George, T. D. and French, E. L., Eds., Commonwealth Scientific and Industrial Research Organization and Queensland Institute of Medical Research, Brisbane, 1979, 41.
18. **Westaway, E. G.,** The neutralization of arboviruses. II. Neutralization in heterologous virus-serum mixtures with four group B arboviruses, *Virology,* 26, 528, 1965.
19. **Woodroofe, G. M. and Marshall, I. D.** Arboviruses from the Sepik District of New Guinea, Ann. Rep. John Curtin Sch. Med. Res. Aust. Nat. Univ., 1971, 90.

Index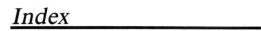

INDEX

A

B

C

D

G

H

J

K

Q

S